Clinical Paediatric Dietetics

Also from Blackwell Publishing

Manual of Dietetic Practice
Third Edition
Edited by Briony Thomas
0-632-03003-8

Counselling Skills for Dietitians
Judy Gable
0-632-04261-3

Journal of Human Nutrition and Dietetics
ISSN 0952-3871

Clinical Paediatric Dietetics
Second Edition

Edited by

Vanessa Shaw

and

Margaret Lawson

Blackwell
Science

© 1994, 2001 by
Blackwell Science Ltd
Editorial Offices:
Osney Mead, Oxford OX2 0EL
25 John Street, London WC1N 2BS
23 Ainslie Place, Edinburgh EH3 6AJ
350 Main Street, Malden
 MA 02148 5018, USA
54 University Street, Carlton
 Victoria 3053, Australia
10, rue Casimir Delavigne
 75006 Paris, France

Other Editorial Offices:

Blackwell Wissenschafts-Verlag GmbH
Kurfürstendamm 57
10707 Berlin, Germany

Blackwell Science KK
MG Kodenmacho Building
7–10 Kodenmacho Nihombashi
Chuo-ku, Tokyo 104, Japan

Iowa State University Press
A Blackwell Science Company
2121 S. State Avenue
Ames, Iowa 50014-8300, USA

First edition published 1994
Reprinted 1995
Second edition published 2001
Reprinted 2002

Set in 10 on 11 pt Ehrhardt MT
by Best-set Typesetters Ltd., Hong Kong
Printed and bound in Great Britain by Antony Rowe Ltd, Chippenham

The Blackwell Science logo is a
trade mark of Blackwell Science Ltd,
registered at the United Kingdom
Trade Marks Registry

DISTRIBUTORS

Marston Book Services Ltd
PO Box 269
Abingdon
Oxon OX14 4YN
(*Orders*: Tel: 01235 465500
       Fax: 01235 465555)

USA and Canada
Iowa State University Press
A Blackwell Science Company
2121 S. State Avenue
Ames, Iowa 50014-8300
(*Orders*: Tel: 800-862-6657
       Fax: 515-292-3348
       Web www.isupress.com
       email: orders@isupress.com)

Australia
Blackwell Science Pty Ltd
54 University Street
Carlton, Victoria 3053
(*Orders*: Tel: 03 9347 0300
       Fax: 03 9347 5001)

A catalogue record for this title
is available from the British Library

ISBN 0-632-05241-4

Library of Congress
Cataloging-in-Publication Data

Clinical paediatric dietetics / edited by Vanessa Shaw and Margaret
 Lawson. – 2nd ed.
   p.; cm.
   Includes bibliographical references and index.
   ISBN 0-632-05241-4 (hb)
   1. Diet therapy for children. I. Shaw, Vanessa. II. Lawson,
 Margaret, MSc.
   [DNLM: 1. Diet Therapy – Child. WS 366 C6405 2001]
 RJ53.D53 C58 2001
 615.8'54'083 – dc21   00-052960

For further information on
Blackwell Science, visit our website:
www.blackwell-science.com

Contents

Contributors

June Brown
Former Senior Dietitian
  Chelsea and Westminster Hospital, London SW10
  9NH

Jayne Butler
Senior Paediatric Dietitian
  St Mary's Hospital, Praed Street, London W2
  1NY

Christine Carter
Specialist Dietitian
  Great Ormond Street Hospital for Children NHS
  Trust, London WC1N 3JH

Janet Coleman
Chief Paediatric Renal Dietitian
  City Hospital, Hucknall Road, Nottingham NG5
  1PB

Mary Deane
Senior Dietitian
  Royal Hospital for Sick Children, Sciennes Road,
  Edinburgh EH9 1LF

Marjorie Dixon
Specialist Dietitian
  Great Ormond Street Hospital for Children NHS
  Trust, London WC1N 3JH

Janice Glynn
Senior Dietitian
  Royal Liverpool Children's NHS Trust, Eaton
  Road, Liverpool L2 2AP

Lesley Haynes
Specialist Dietitian
  Institute of Child Health, 30 Guilford Street,
  London WC1N 1EH

Dona Hileti-Telfer
Senior Dietitian
  Great Ormond Street Hospital for Children NHS
  Trust, London WC1N 3JH

Dearbhla Hunt
Senior Dietitian
  The Children's Hospital, Temple Street, Dublin,
  Eire

Stephanie France (née Jackson)
Senior Paediatric Dietitian
  Kings College Hospital, Denmark Hill, London
  SE5 9RS

Karen Jeffereys
Chief Dietitian
  Services for People with Learning Disabilities, P O
  Box 107, Southsea, Hants PO4 8NG

Tracey Johnson
Senior Dietitian
  The Birmingham Children's Hospital NHS Trust,
  Steelhouse Lane, Birmingham B4 6NH

Alison Johnston
Senior Dietitian
  Royal Hospital for Sick Children, Yorkhill,
  Glasgow G3 8SJ

Caroline King
Chief Paediatric Dietitian
  Queen Charlotte's Hospital, Goldhawk Road,
  London W6 0XG

Margaret Lawson
Nestle Senior Research Fellow
  Institute of Child Health, 30 Guilford Street,
  London WC1N 1EH

Helen McCarthy
Senior Dietitian
  Manchester Children's Hospitals, Charlestown Road, Blackley, Manchester M9 7AA

Anita MacDonald
Head of Dietetic Services
  The Birmingham Children's Hospital NHS Trust, Steelhouse Lane, Birmingham B4 6NH

Sarah Macdonald
Specialist Dietitian
  Great Ormond Street Hospital for Children NHS Trust, London WC1N 3JH

Dasha Nicholls
Clinical Lecturer in Neurosciences and Mental Health
  Institute of Child Health, 30 Guilford Street, London WC1N 1EH

Marion Noble
Former Specialist Dietitian
  Great Ormond Street Hospital for Children NHS Trust, London WC1N 3JH

Patricia Rutherford
Chief Dietitian
  Royal Liverpool Children's NHS Trust, Eaton Road, Liverpool L2 2AP

Vanessa Shaw
Chief Dietitian
  Great Ormond Street Hospital for Children NHS Trust, London WC1N 3JH

Zofia Smith
Senior Dietitian
  St Mary's Hospital, Greenhill Road, Leeds LS12 3QU

Evelyn Ward
Senior Paediatric Dietitian
  St James University Hospital NHS Trust, Beckett Street, Leeds LS9 7TF

Ruth Watling
Chief Dietitian
  Royal Liverpool Children's NHS Trust, Eaton Road, Liverpool L2 2AP

Fiona White
Chief Dietitian
  Manchester Children's Hospitals, Hospital Road, Manchester M27 4HA

Sue Wolfe
Chief Paediatric Dietitian
  St James University Hospital NHS Trust, Beckett Street, Leeds LS9 7TF

Foreword

The first edition of *Clinical Paediatric Dietetics* was published in 1994, contributions being made by many senior dietitians. It is now a great pleasure to write a Foreword to this second edition to which no fewer than 28 experienced colleagues have contributed. Over the years the role of dietetics in the treatment of sick infants and children has become both increasingly important and in many instances far more complex. The Paediatric Group of the British Dietetic Association is to be congratulated for the way it has moved dietetics forwards, with great benefit to their young patients.

As before, the chapters cover a wide variety of subjects ranging from the principles of paediatric dietetics to the treatment of diabetes mellitus, allergic disorders, inherited metabolic disorders, burns and eating disorders to name but a few. As previously, the needs of sick children from ethnic minorities have been included. The practical aspects of dietary management are given a high profile, excellent tables and clear diagrams provide essential information and each chapter has a suitable list of references. All the chapters are full of commonsense and the volume provides lists of commercial products and the addresses of manufacturers.

Once again, Vanessa Shaw and Margaret Lawson have undertaken a huge task; they have contributed chapters themselves and undertaken the editing. Obtaining high standard material from so many colleagues is certainly not easy, and I congratulate Vanessa and Margaret most warmly. This multi-author book will, I am sure, go through numerous editions as the years pass and each edition will help so many sick infants and children. Looking back to 1965 when the first edition of *Diets for Sick Children* appeared, one is conscious of the huge developments which have taken place in dietetics and the ever increasing importance of the dietitians.

Dame Barbara Clayton DBE, MD, PhD, HonDSc, FRCP, FRCPE, HonFRCPI, HonFRCPCH, FMedSci, HonFIBiol, FRCPath

Honorary Research Professor in Metabolism, University of Southampton
Honorary President, British Dietetic Association

Preface

The aim of this manual is to provide a very practical approach to the nutritional management of a wide range of paediatric nutritional disorders that may benefit from nutritional support or be ameliorated or resolved by dietary manipulation. The text will be of particular relevance to professional dietitians, dietetic students and their tutors, paediatricians, paediatric nurses and members of the community health team involved with children requiring therapeutic diets. The growing importance of nutritional support in many paediatric conditions is recognised and reflected in new text for this edition.

The authors are largely drawn from experienced paediatric dietitians around the United Kingdom, with additional contributions from other specialist dietitians and a psychiatrist. The text does not attempt to discuss normal nutrition in healthy children (though references for this topic are addressed), but concentrates on the nutritional requirements of sick infants and children in a clinical setting. Normal dietary constituents are used alongside special dietetic products to provide a prescription that will control progression and symptoms of disease whilst maintaining the growth potential of the child.

There has been an expansion of the range of disorders and treatments described: additional information has been included on nutritional assessment, inborn errors of metabolism, food allergy and intolerance, immunodeficiency syndromes and gastroenterology. Arranged under headings of disorders of organ systems rather than type of diet, and with much information presented in tabular form, the manual is easy to use. Dietary restrictions due either to customs, religious beliefs or environmental conditions which may affect the nutritional adequacy of the diet of the growing child are also discussed.

Appendices list the many and varied special products described in the text, together with details of their manufacturers. The appendices are not exhaustive, but include the products most commonly used in the UK. The information has been updated for this edition and the most recent data has been used in the preparation of the manual, but no guarantee can be given of the validity or availability at the time of going to press.

Vanessa Shaw
Margaret Lawson
January 2001

Acknowledgements

We would like to thank a number of the contributors to the first edition, who were unable to contribute to this second edition, but whose work has formed the basis for the following chapters:

Chapter 2, Provision of Nutrition in a Hospital Setting: Christine Clothier, Former Chief Dietitian, Royal Liverpool Children's NHS Trust

Chapter 3, Enteral Feeding: Debra Woodward, Former Senior Dietitian, The Children's Hospital, Birmingham

Chapter 4, Parenteral Nutrition: Alison Macleod, Former Senior Dietitian, Royal Liverpool Children's Hospital NHS Trust

Chapter 6, The Gastrointestinal Tract: Sheena Laing, Chief Dietitian, Royal Hospital for Sick Children, Edinburgh

Chapter 8, The Liver and Pancreas: Jane Ely, Former Senior Paediatric Dietitian, King's College Hospital, London

Chapter 14, Ketogenic Diet for Epilepsy: Jane Eaton, Former Chief Community Dietitian, Dorset Health Care NHS Trust

Chapter 18, Lipid Disorders: Anne Maclean, Former Senior Paediatric Dietitian, St George's Hospital, London

Chapter 22, Eating Disorders: Bernadette Wren, Former Principal Clinical Psychologist, and Bryan Lask, Former Consultant Psychiatrist, Great Ormond Street Hospital for Children NHS Trust

Chapter 25, Burns: Judith Martin, Former Chief Dietitian, Whittington Hospital, London.

SECTION 1

Introduction

CHAPTER 1

Principles of Paediatric Dietetics

This manual provides a practical approach to the dietary management of a range of paediatric disorders. The therapies describe dietetic manipulations and the nutritional requirements of the infant and child in a clinical setting. It does not attempt to address the nutrition of the healthy child in any detail (see Further Reading at end of this chapter), but illustrates how normal dietary constituents are used alongside special dietetic products to allow the continued growth of the child whilst controlling the progression and symptoms of disease. Dietary restrictions, due either to custom, religious beliefs or environmental conditions are also discussed.

DIETARY PRINCIPLES

The following principles are relevant to the treatment of all infants and children and provide the basis for many of the therapies described later in the text.

Assessment of nutritional status

Assessment and monitoring of nutritional status should be included in any dietary regimen, audit procedure or research project where a modified diet plays a role. There are a number of methods of assessing specific aspects of nutritional status, but no one measurement will give an overall picture of status for all nutrients. There are a number of assessment techniques, some of which should be used routinely in all centres whilst others are still in a developmental stage or suitable only for research. Figure 1.1 outlines the techniques that can be used for nutritional assessment.

Nutritional intake

For children over the age of two years food intake is assessed in the same way as for adults: using a recall diet history taken from the usual carers (or from the child if appropriate), a quantitative food diary over a number of days, a weighed food intake over a number of days or a food frequency questionnaire. The assessment of milk intake for breast-fed infants is difficult and only very general estimations can be made. Infants can be test-weighed before and after a breast-feed and the amount of milk consumed can be calculated. This requires the use of very accurate scales (± 1–$2\,g$) and should be done for all feeds over a 24 hour period as the volume consumed varies throughout the day. Test-weighing should be avoided if at all possible as it is disturbing for the infant, engenders anxiety in the mother and is likely to compromise breast-feeding. Studies have shown that the volume of breast milk consumed is approximately 770 ml at 5 weeks and 870 ml at 11 weeks [1]. In general an intake of 850 ml is assumed for all infants who are fully breast-fed and over the age of 6 weeks. Estimation of food intake is particularly difficult in infants who are taking solids, as it is not possible to assess accurately the amount of food wasted through spitting, drooling etc.

Conversion of food intake into nutrient values for young children may involve the use of manufacturers' data if the child is taking proprietary infant foods and/or infant formula. The composition of breast milk varies and food table values may be inaccurate by up to 20% because of individual variation. Assessment of the adequacy of an individual calculated nutrient intake for sick and for healthy infants and children is discussed in the section on dietary reference values later in this chapter.

Anthropometry

Measurement of weight and height or length is critical as the basis for calculating dietary requirements as

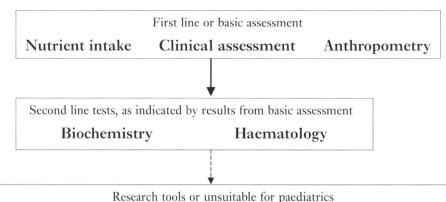

Fig. 1.1 Nutritional assessement methods

well as monitoring the effects of dietary intervention. Other anthropometric measurements are summarised in Table 1.1. Measurement of weight is an easy and routine procedure using an electronic digital scale or a beam balance. Ideally infants should be weighed nude and children wearing just a clean nappy or pants, but if this is not possible it is important to record whether the infant is weighed wearing a clean nappy, and the amount and type of clothing worn by older children. For weighing infants up to 10 kg, scales should be accurate to 10 g; for children up to 20 kg, accuracy should be +/− 20 g and over 20 kg it should be +/− 50–200 g. A higher degree of accuracy is required for the assessment of sick children than for routine measurements in the community. Frequent weight monitoring is important for the sick infant or child and hospitalised infants should be weighed each day or every second day; children over the age of two in hospital should be weighed at least weekly. Healthy infants should be weighed every 2 weeks until the age of 6 months, every month between the ages of 6 months and 24 months and every 2–3 months after the age of 2 years.

Height or length measurement requires a sta-diometer or length-board. Details of suitable equipment, which may be fixed or portable, are available from the Child Growth Foundation (see end of chapter). Measurement of length using a tape measure is too inaccurate to be of use for longitudinal monitoring of growth, although an approximate length may be useful as a single measure (e.g. for cal-culating body mass index). Under the age of about 2 years supine length is measured; standing height is usually measured over this age or whenever the child can stand straight and unsupported. When the method of measurement changes there is likely to be a difference, and measurements should be made by both methods on one occasion when switching from supine length to standing height. Measurement of length is difficult and requires careful positioning of the infant, ensuring that the back, legs and head are straight, the heels are against the footboard, the shoulders are touching the baseboard and the crown of the head is touching the headboard. Two people are required to measure length – one to hold the child in position and one to record the measurement. Posi-tioning of the child is also important when measur-ing standing height and care should be taken to ensure that the back and legs are straight, the heels, buttocks, shoulder blades and back of head are touching the measurement board and that the child is looking straight ahead.

A body mass index (BMI) measurement can be calculated from the weight and height measurements (BMI = weight(kg)/height(m)^2) and provides an indi-cation of fatness or thinness. In adults body fatness is largely unrelated to age and high BMI measurements are related to health risks. In children the amount and distribution of body fat is dependent on age, and does not appear to be related to health. Age-related centile charts for BMI have been developed [2] and indicate how heavy the child is relevant to his height and age.

Table 1.1 Anthropometric measurements

Comments	Measurement	Derived indices
Easy to do Useful <2 years Affected by medical condition	Head circumference	
Easy to do Useful on a day-to-day basis Does not differentiate between lean tissue and fat deposition	Weight	weight for height height for age Body Mass Index Standard Deviation Score
Difficult to do accurately Needs >1 person Best indicator of overall nutritional well-being	Height	
Easy to do Useful <5 years Does not differentiate between muscle and fat	Mid-arm circumference (MAC/MUAC)	arm muscle area arm fat area lean body mass (requires five site measures)
Difficult to do Requires training and practice Triceps most commonly used	Skinfold thickness (SFT)	
Easy to do No standards for children May be useful in defining obesity	Waist-hip ratio	

In some cases it is difficult to obtain length or height measurements, for example in very sick or preterm infants and in older children with scoliosis. A number of proxy measurements can be used which are useful to monitor whether longitudinal growth is progressing in an individual, but there are no recognised centile charts as yet and indices such as body mass index cannot be calculated. In adults arm span is approximately equivalent to height, but body proportions depend upon age and this measurement is not generally useful. Measurements of lower leg length or knee-heel length have been used and are a useful proxy for growth. For infants and small children a kneemometer has been developed which displays knee-heel length digitally [3]. For older children knee-heel length is measured with the child in a supine position (if possible) with the knee bent at a 90° angle using a caliper with a blade at either end. One blade is fitted under the heel of the foot and the other onto the knee, immediately behind the patella, using the outside surface of the leg. Total leg length is rarely measured outside specialist growth clinics

and is calculated as the difference between measured sitting height and standing height. A number of other measures have been used in children with cerebral palsy as a proxy for height, but numbers are too small for reference standards to be established [4].

Head circumference is a useful measurement in children under the age of two years, particularly where it is difficult to obtain an accurate length measurement. After this age head growth slows and is a less useful indicator of somatic growth. A number of genetic and acquired conditions will affect head growth – for example, neurodevelopmental delay – and measurement of head circumference will not be a useful indicator of nutritional status in these conditions. Head circumference is measured using a narrow, flexible, non-stretch tape. Details of a suitable disposable paper tape are available from the Child Growth Foundation. Measurement should be made just above the eyes to include the maximum circumference of the head, with the child supported in an upright position and looking straight ahead.

The measurement of weight and length or height form the basis of anthropometric assessment. However these measurements on their own do not indicate whether weight increments are lean + fat tissue or whether weight gained is merely fat. Supplementary measurements which can be used include mid upper arm circumference (MUAC or MAC). This is a useful measurement in children under the age of 5 years, as MAC increases fairly rapidly up until this age. Age-related standards exist for children over the age of one year [5]. Increases in MAC are more likely to comprise muscle and less likely to be affected by oedema than body weight. In order to fully differentiate between lean and fat, measurement of triceps skinfold thickness (TSF or SFT) is necessary. This can be an unpleasant procedure for young children, who are afraid of the skinfold caliper and may not remain still for long enough for accurate measurements to be taken. The equipment and technique are identical to those in adults and the measurement is subject to the same observer error. Skinfold thickness is not used as a routine anthropometric measure but provides valuable data in research studies. Reference data for children over the age of one year is available [5]. Arm muscle and arm fat area can be calculated and compared to reference data [5]. A calculation of arm fat and muscle area is shown in Table 1.2.

The measurement of the waist:hip ratio in children has not proved to be a useful predictor of obesity

Table 1.2 Arm fat and arm muscle area

$$\text{Arm muscle area } (\text{mm}^2) = \frac{(\text{MAC} - (\pi \times \text{TSF}))^2}{4 \times \pi}$$

$$\text{Arm fat area } (\text{mm}^2) = \frac{\text{TSF} \times \text{MAC}}{2} - \frac{\pi \times (\text{TSF})^2}{4}$$

where MAC = mid arm circumference in mm^2
      TSF = triceps skinfold thickness in mm

For a boy aged 6 years:

MAC = 180 mm	(50th centile* for age)
TSF = 16 mm	(95th centile* for age)

Arm muscle area = 1340 mm^2	(<5th centile* for age)
Arm fat area = 1238 mm^2	(90–95th centile* for age)

Although all measurements are within the normal range for age, this boy is severely depleted in muscle and may be depleted in all lean tissue.

* Reference standards taken from Gibson [5].

in pre-pubertal children [6], and reference data does not exist at present for European children.

Evaluation of anthropometric measurements

Measurements should be regularly plotted on the relevant centile chart. All children in the UK are issued with a growth centile chart as part of the personal child health record held by parents and completed by health care professionals whenever the child is weighed or measured. UK centile charts are available for weight, length/height, head circumference and BMI. There are a number of problems associated with accurate plotting on charts which can lead to inaccuracies in monitoring. The decimal age may need to be calculated using the decimal age calendar on the centile charts, rather than guessing the exact age. In a clinic or a centre where a number of people are involved in plotting measurements, agreement should be reached over whether values which fall between centiles should be rounded up or rounded down. Variations in procedures can result in relatively large errors, particularly in infants, and deviations from centiles can be missed. When assessing height it is important to take parental height into consideration, and the genetic height potential for the child can be approximately estimated using the mid-parental height centile which is included in the weight monitoring chart for use in children with slow weight gain.

For definitions of obesity and failure to thrive see the relevant chapters (pp. 371 and 423).

It is difficult to assess progress or decide upon targets where a measurement falls outside the centile lines – either <0.4 centile or >99.6 centile line. Amended weight charts showing up to −5 standard deviations for monitoring children with slow weight gain are available – details from the Child Growth Foundation. 'Thrive lines' have also been developed to aid interpretation of infants and children with slow weight gain. These are in the form of an acetate overlay for the standard weight centile charts and indicate when failure to progress along a centile line is a cause for concern [7]. The acetates are available from the Child Growth Foundation.

There are a number of methods of overcoming problems in plotting onto charts, which involve converting the weight and height into a finite proportion of a reference or standard measurement. Calculation of the standard deviation score (SDS) or Z score for length/height, weight and BMI gives a numerical score indicating how far away from the 50th centile for age the child's measurements falls. A child on the 0.4 centile will have a SDS of −3SD. A child on the 99.6 centile will have a SDS of +3SD. Because of the distribution of the data, calculation of SDS by hand is extremely difficult. A computer software program is available from the Child Growth Foundation that will calculate SDS scores from height, weight and age data. However this method does not take into account the degree of stunting which often accompanies severe failure to thrive. The calculation of height for age, height age and weight for height are useful when assessing nutritional status initially or when monitoring progress in children who are short for their chronological age. Table 1.3 shows examples of calculations for these measurements. Calculation of height age is necessary when determining nutrient requirements for children who are much smaller (or larger) than their chronological age (see section on Dietary Reference Values later in this chapter). A number of methods of classification of malnutrition have been used in developing countries. The Waterlow classification [8] may be of use when assessing children in the UK with severe failure to thrive. An adaptation of the classification is shown in Table 1.4.

Clinical assessment

Clinical assessment of the child involves a medical history and a physical examination. The medical

Table 1.3 Height for age, height age and weight for height

Example – Six year old girl with cerebral palsy referred with severe feeding problems.

Visit 1	Decimal age = 6.2 years Height = 93 cm (<0.4 centile) Weight = 10 kg (<0.4 centile)
	Height for age – 50th centile for height for a girl aged 6.2 years = 117 cm
	Height for age $= \dfrac{93}{117} = 79.5\%$ height for age
	Height age = age at which 93 cm falls on 50th centile = 2.7 years
	Weight for height – 50th centile for weight for 2.7 years = 14 kg
	Weight for height $= \dfrac{10}{14} = 71\%$ weight for height
Visit 2	(after intervention) Decimal age = 6.8 years Height = 95.5 cm (<0.4 centile) Weight = 12 kg (<0.4 centile)
	Height for age $= \dfrac{95.5}{121} = 79\%$ height for age
	Height age = 3.1 years
	Weight for height $= \dfrac{12}{14.5} = 82.7\%$ weight for height

Improvement in both height and weight has been achieved

Table 1.4 Classification of malnutrition (adapted from Waterlow [8])

Acute malnutrition (wasting)	Chronic malnutrition (stunting +/– wasting)
Weight for height 80–90% standard – grade 1 70–80% standard – grade 2 <70% standard – grade 3	Height for age 90–95% standard – grade 1 85–90% standard – grade 2 <80% standard – grade 3

history will identify medical, social or environmental factors that may be risk factors for the development of nutritional problems. Such factors may include parental knowledge and money available for food purchase, underlying disease, weight changes, food allergies and medications. Clinical signs of poor nutrition, revealed in the physical examination, only appear at a late stage in the development of a deficiency disease and absence of clinical signs should not be taken as indicating that a deficiency is not present. Typical physical signs associated with poor nutrition which have been described in children in western countries are summarised in Table 1.5. Physical signs represent very general changes and may not be due to nutrient deficiencies alone. Other indications such as poor weight gain and/or low dietary intake are needed in order to reinforce suspicions, and a blood test should be carried out to confirm the diagnosis.

Food and nutrient intake, anthropometric measurements and clinical examination and history form the basis of routine nutritional assessment. None of them are diagnostic tests and can only predict which nutrients may be deficient and which children need further investigation. If a nutrient deficiency (or excess) is suspected as a result of the first-line assessment tools, then confirmation using other objective measures should be sought.

Biochemistry and haematology

Methods of confirming suspicion of a nutritional problem include analysis of levels of nutrients or

Table 1.5 Physical signs of nutritional problems

Assessment	Clinical sign	Possible nutrient(s)
Hair	Thin, sparse Colour change – 'flag sign' Easily plucked	Protein and energy, zinc, copper
Skin	Dry, flaky	Essential fatty acids B vitamins
	Rough, 'sandpaper' texture	Vitamin A
	Petechiae, bruising	Vitamin C
Eyes	Pale conjunctiva	Iron
	Xerosis	Vitamin A
	Keratomalacia	
Lips	Angular stomatitis Cheilosis	B vitamins
Tongue	Colour changes	B vitamins
Teeth	Mottling of enamel	Fluorosis (excess fluoride)
Gums	Spongy, bleed easily	Vitamin C
Face	Thyroid enlargement	Iodine
Nails	Spoon shape, koilonychia	Iron, zinc, copper
Subcutaneous Tissue	Oedema	Protein, sodium Over-hydration
	Depleted subcutaneous fat	Energy
Muscles	Wasting	Protein, energy, zinc
Bones	Craniotabes Parietal and frontal bossing Epiphyseal enlargement Beading of ribs	Vitamin D

nutrient-dependent metabolites in body fluids or tissues, or measuring functional impairment of a nutrient-dependent metabolic process.

The most commonly used tissue for investigation is the blood. Either whole blood, plasma, serum or blood cells can be used, depending on the test. Tests may be static – for example, levels of zinc in plasma – or may be functional – for example the measurement of the activity of glutathione peroxidase, a selenium-dependent enzyme, as a measure of selenium status. Although an objective measurement is obtained from a blood test there are a number of factors that can affect the validity of such biochemical or haematological investigations. Age-specific normal ranges need to be established for the individual centre unless the laboratory participates in a regional or national quality control scheme. Recent food intake and time of sampling can affect levels and it may be necessary to take a fasting blood sample for some nutrients. Physiological processes such as infection, disease or drugs may alter normal levels. Contamination from exogenous materials such as equipment or endogenous sources such as sweat or interstitial fluid is important for nutrients such as trace elements, and care must be taken to choose the correct sampling procedure. For a fuller review of the subject see Clayton and Round [9]. A summary of some biochemical and haematological measurements is given in Table 1.6.

Urine is often used for adult investigations, but many tests require the collection of a 24 hour urine sample, and this is difficult in babies and children. The usefulness of a single urine sample for nutritional tests is limited, and needs to be compared with a standard metabolite, usually creatinine. However creatinine excretion itself is age dependent and this needs to be taken into consideration. Hair and nails have been used to assess trace element and heavy metal status in populations, but a number of environmental and physiological factors affect levels and these tissues are not routinely used in the UK. Tissues that store certain nutrients, such as the liver and bone, would be useful materials to investigate but sampling is too invasive for routine clinical use.

Other tests

A number of other tests that are indicative of nutritional status may provide useful information but are not available routinely. Measurement of body composition using isotope dilution or imaging techniques is particularly useful for the clinical dietitian as most methods of assessment do not indicate whether growth consists of normal ratios of fat and protein or whether excess amounts of adipose tissues are being accumulated. Body composition measurements are described by Ruxton *et al.* [10]. Tests which are not routinely carried out but which may be useful research tools are summarised in Table 1.7.

Expected growth in childhood

Normal birthweight for infants in the United Kingdom varies between 3.3 and 3.5 kg for both sexes. There is some weight loss during the first 5–7 days of life whilst feeding on full volumes of milk is

Table 1.6 Biochemical and haematological tests

Nutrient	Test	Normal values in children	Comments
Biochemical tests			
Protein	Total plasma protein	55–80 g/l	Low levels reflect long-term not acute depletion
	Albumin	30–45 g/l	
Protein	Caeruloplasmin	0.18–0.46 g/l	Low levels indicate acute protein depletion, but are acute-phase proteins which increase during infection
	Retinol binding protein (RBP)	2.6–7.6 g/l	
Thiamin	Erythrocyte transketolase activity coefficient (ETK)	1–1.15	High activity coefficient (>1.15) indicates thiamin deficiency
Vit B_{12}	Plasma B_{12} value	263–1336 pmol/l	Low levels indicate deficiency
Riboflavin	Erythrocyte glutathione reductase activity coefficient (EGRAC)	1.0–1.3	High activity coefficient (>1.3) indicates deficiency
Vit C	Plasma ascorbate level	8.8–124 µmol/l	Low levels indicate deficiency
Vit A	Plasma retinol level	0.54–1.56 µmol/l	Low level indicates deficiency
Vit D	Plasma 25–hydroxy cholecalciferol level	30–110 nmol/l	Low level indicates deficiency
Vit E	Plasma tocopherol level	α tocopherol 10.9–28.1 µmol/l	Low levels indicate deficiency
Copper	Plasma level	70–140 µmol/l	Low levels indicate deficiency
Selenium	Plasma level	0.76–1.07 µmol/l	Low levels indicate deficiency
	Glutathione peroxidase activity (GSHPx)	>1.77 µmol/l	Low levels indicate deficiency
Zinc	Plasma level	10–18 µmol/l	Low levels indicate deficiency
Haematology tests			
Folic acid	Plasma folate	7–48 nmol/l	Low levels indicate deficiency
	Red-cell folate	429–1749 nmol/l	Low levels indicate deficiency
Haemoglobin	Whole blood	104–140 g/l	Levels <110 g/l indicate iron deficiency
Red cell distribution width (RDW)	Whole blood	<16%	High values indicate iron deficiency
Mean corpuscular volume (MCV)	Whole blood	70–86 fl	Small volume (microcytosis) indicates iron deficiency. Large volume (macrocytosis) indicates folate or B_{12} deficiency
Mean cell haemoglobin (MCH)	Whole blood	22.7–29.6 pg	Low values indicate iron deficiency
Percentage hypochromic cells	Whole blood	<2.5%	High values (>2.5%) indicate iron deficiency
Zinc protoporphyrin (ZPP)	Red cell	32–102 µmol/mol haem	High levels indicate iron deficiency
Ferritin	Plasma level	5–70 µg/l	Low levels indicate depletion of iron stores. Ferritin is an acute phase protein and increases during infection

Table 1.7 Other tests

Measurement	Method
Body composition	Total body potassium using ^{40}K
	Total body water using water labelled with stable isotopes (^2H_2O, $H_2^{18}O$, $^2H_2^{18}O$)
	Ultrasound
	Bioelectrical impedance
	Computerised tomography
	Dual X-ray absorptiometry (DEXA)
Functional tests	Muscle strength using dynamometer to assess protein energy malnutrition
	Taste acuity to assess zinc status
	Dark adaptation test to assess vitamin A adequacy
	These tests require the co-operation of the subject and none have been used extensively in children
Immunological tests	Leucocyte function, delayed cutaneous hypersensitivity reaction
	These tests are affected by infection and are age-dependent
	There is no reference data for children and immunological tests are not normally used as a measure of nutritional status in paediatrics

established; birthweight is normally regained by the tenth to fourteenth day. Thereafter, average weight gain is as follows:

- 200 g per week for the first 3 months
- 150 g per week for the second 3 months
- 100 g per week for the third 3 months
- 50–75 g per week for the fourth 3 months.

Increase in length during the first year of life: 25 cm.

During the second year, the toddler following the 50th centile for growth velocity gains approximately 2.5 kg in weight and a further 12 cm in length. Average growth continues at a rate of approximately 2 kg per year and 10 cm, steadily declining to 6 cm, per year until the growth spurt at puberty.

Dietary Reference Values

The 1991 Department of Health Report on Dietary Reference Values [11] provides information and figures for requirements for a comprehensive range of nutrients and energy. The requirements are termed dietary reference values (DRV) and are for normal, healthy populations. It is important to remember that these are recommendations for groups, not for individuals; however they can be used as a basis for estimating suitable intakes for the individual, using the Reference Nutrient Intake. This level of intake should satisfy the requirements of 97.5% of healthy individuals in a population group. A summary of these DRVs for energy, protein, sodium, potassium, vitamin C, calcium and iron is given in Table 1.8. The DRVs for other nutrients may be found in the full report.

When estimating requirements for the individual sick child it is important to calculate energy and nutrient intakes based on actual body weight, and not expected body weight. The latter will lead to a proposed intake that is inappropriately high for the child who has an abnormally low body weight. In some instances it may be more appropriate to consider the child's height age rather than chronological age when comparing intakes with the DRVs as this is a more realistic measure of the child's body size and hence, nutrient requirement. An estimation of requirements for sick children is given in Table 1.9.

Fluid requirements in the newborn

Breast feeding is the most appropriate method of feeding the normal infant and may be suitable for sick infants with a variety of clinical conditions. Demand breast feeding will automatically ensure that the healthy infant gets the right volume of milk and, hence, nutrients. If the infant is too ill or too immature to suckle, the mother may express her breast milk; expressed breast milk (EBM) may be modified to suit the sick infant's requirements. If EBM is unavailable or inappropriate to feed in certain circumstances, infant formula milks must be used (Table 1.10). After the age of 6 months a follow-on formula can be used (Table 1.11). Organic infant formulas are also available.

Infants over 2.5 kg birthweight

Fluid offered per 24 hours: 150–200 ml/kg. On the first day, if bottle fed, approximately one seventh of the total volume should be offered, divided into eight feeds and fed every 2–3 hours. The volume offered should be gradually increased over the following days to give full requirements by the seventh day of life, or

Table 1.8 Selected dietary reference values

Age	Weight	Fluid	Energy (EAR)				RNI								
							Protein		Sodium		Potassium		Vitamin C	Calcium	Iron
	kg	ml/kg	kJ/day	kJ/kg/day	kcal/day	kcal/kg/day	g/day	g/kg/day	mmol/day	mmol/kg/day	mmol/day	mmol/kg/day	mg/day	mmol/day	µmol/day
Males															
0–3 months	5.1	150	2280	480–420	545	115–100	12.5	2.1	9	1.5	20	3.4	25	13.1	30
4–6	7.2	130	2890	400	690	95	12.7	1.6	12	1.6	22	2.8	25	13.1	80
7–9	8.9	120	3440	400	825	95	13.7	1.5	14	1.6	18	2.0	25	13.1	140
10–12	9.6	110	3850	400	920	95	14.9	1.5	15	1.5	18	1.8	25	13.1	140
1–3 years	12.9	95	5150	400	1230	95	14.5	1.1	22	1.7	20	1.6	30	8.8	120
4–6	19.0	85	7160	380	1715	90	19.7	1.1	30	1.9	28	1.6	30	11.3	110
7–10	—	75	8240	—	1970	—	28.3	—	50	—	50	—	30	13.8	160
11–14	—	55	9270	—	2220	—	42.1	—	70	—	80	—	30	25.0	200
15–18	—	50	11510	—	2755	—	55.2	—	70	—	90	—	40	25.0	200
Females															
0–3 months	4.8	150	2160	480–420	515	115–100	12.5	2.1	9	1.5	20	3.4	25	13.1	30
4–6	6.8	130	2690	400	645	95	12.7	1.6	12	1.6	22	2.8	25	13.1	80
7–9	8.1	120	3200	400	765	95	13.7	1.5	14	1.6	18	2.0	25	13.1	140
10–12	9.1	110	3610	400	865	95	14.9	1.5	15	1.5	18	1.8	25	13.1	140
1–3 years	12.3	95	4860	400	1165	95	14.5	1.1	22	1.7	20	1.6	30	8.8	120
4–6	17.2	85	6460	380	1545	90	19.7	1.1	30	1.7	28	1.6	30	11.3	110
7–10	—	75	7280	—	1740	—	28.3	—	50	—	50	—	30	13.8	160
11–14	—	55	7920	—	1845	—	42.1	—	70	—	70	—	35	20.0	260
15–18	—	50	8830	—	2110	—	45.4	—	70	—	70	—	40	20.0	260

EAR Estimated average requirement
RNI Reference nutrient intake

Table 1.9 General guide to oral requirements in sick children

	Intants 0–1 year (based on actual weight, not expected weight)		Children
Energy	High: 130–150 kcals/kg/day (545–630 kJ/kg/day) Very high: 150–220 kcals/kg/day (630–920 kJ/kg/day)	**Energy**	High: 120% EAR for age Very high: 150% EAR for age
Protein	High: 3–4.5 g/kg/day Very high: 6 g/kg/day 0–6 months, increasing to maximum of 10 g/kg/day up to 1 year	**Protein**	High: 2 g/kg/day, actual body weight. It should be recognised that children may easily eat more than this
Sodium	High: 3.0 mmol/kg/day Very high: 4.5 mmol/kg/day a concentration >7.7 mmolNa⁺/100 ml of infant formula will have an emetic effect		For severely underweight children, initially an energy and protein intake based on weight, not age, is used
Potassium	High: 3.0 mmol/kg/day Very high: 4.5 mmol/kg/day		

Table 1.10 Infant milk formulas

Whey based	Casein based	Manufacturer
Aptamil First*	Aptamil Extra* Milumil	Milupa Ltd Milupa Ltd
Cow & Gate Premium	Cow & Gate Plus	Cow & Gate Nutricia Ltd
Farley's First Milk*	Farley's Second Milk*	H J Heinz Co Ltd
SMA Gold*	SMA White	SMA Nutrition

* Contain long chain polyunsaturated fatty acids

Table 1.11 Follow-on milks

	Manufacturer
Farley's Follow-on Milk	HJ Heinz Co Ltd
Forward	Milupa Ltd
Progress	SMA Nutrition
Step-up	Cow & Gate Nutricia Ltd

sooner if the infant is feeding well. Breast fed infants will regulate their own intake of milk.

For infants under 2.5 kg, see page 55.

Fluid requirements in the first few weeks

The normal infant will tolerate four hourly feeds, six times daily once a body weight of more than 3.5 kg is reached. By the age of 3–6 weeks (body weight approximately 4 kg) the infant may drop a night feed. A fluid intake of 150 ml/kg should be maintained. Infants should not normally be given more than 1200 ml of feed per 24 hours as this may induce vomiting and, in the long term, will lead to an inappropriately high energy intake. Sick infants may need smaller, more frequent feeds than the normal child and, according to the clinical condition, may have increased or decreased fluid requirements.

Once solids are introduced at 4–6 months of age the infant's appetite for milk will lessen. At 6 months, fluid requirements decrease to 120 ml/kg. At 1 year, the child's thirst will determine how much fluid is taken. Fluid requirements throughout childhood (if all fluid comes from feed and there is no significant contribution to fluid intake from foods) are given in Table 1.8.

Supplementing feeds for infants failing to thrive on normal strength feeds or who are fluid restricted

Supplements may be added to EBM, infant formula milks and special therapeutic formulas to achieve the necessary increase in energy and protein required by some infants. Care needs to be taken not to present an osmotic load of more than 500 mOsm/kg H_2O to the normal functioning gut, otherwise an osmotic diarrhoea will result. If the infant has malabsorption, an upper limit of 400 mOsm/kg H$_2$O may be necessary.

Concentrating infant formulas

Normally infant formula powders, whether whey and casein based formulas or specialised dietetic products, should be diluted according to the manufacturers' instructions as this provides the correct balance of energy, protein and nutrients when fed at the appropriate volume. However, there are occasions when to achieve a feed that is more dense in energy, protein and nutrients it is necessary to concentrate a formula. Most normal baby milks in the UK are made up at a dilution of 13%. By making the baby milk up at a dilution of 15% (15 g powder per 100 ml water), more nutrition can be given in a given volume of feed, e.g. energy content may be increased from 65 kcal (272 kJ) per 100 ml to 75 kcal (314 kJ) per 100 ml and protein content from 1.5 g/100 ml to 1.7 g/100 ml. Similarly special therapeutic feeds that are usually made up at a dilution of for example 15% may be concentrated to a 17% dilution. Carbohydrate and fat sources may be added to the concentrated feed if necessary. This concentrating of feeds should only be performed as a therapeutic procedure and is not usual practice. Table 1.12 shows an example of a 15% feed. The protein : energy ratio of the feed should be kept within the range 7.5%–12% for infants (i.e. 7.5%–12% energy from protein) and 5–15% in older children. In order for accelerated or 'catch-up' growth to occur it is necessary to provide about 9% energy from protein.

If infants are to be discharged home on a concentrated feed the recipe may be translated into scoop measures for ease of use. This will mean that more scoops of milk powder will be added to a given volume of water than recommended by the manufacturer. As this is contrary to normal practice the reasons for this deviation should be carefully explained to the parents and communicated to primary health care staff. There are two nutrient-dense ready-to-feed formulas available for hospital use and in the community, Infatrini and SMA High Energy (Table 1.12). They are nutritionally complete formulas containing more energy, protein and nutrients than standard infant formulas. They are suitable for use from birth and are designed for infants who have increased nutritional requirements or who are fluid restricted. They obviate the need for carers to make up normal infant formulas at concentrations other than the usual 1 scoop of powder to 30 ml water.

Low birthweight formulas are specifically designed for use in the premature infant (page 56). They may be a convenient way to provide an increased energy and protein intake in an infant who is fluid restricted, though the other nutrients provided by

Table 1.12 Examples of energy and nutrient-dense formulas for infants who are failing to thrive or who are fluid restricted

	per 100 ml								
	Energy kcal	kJ	Protein g	CHO g	Fat g	Na mmol	K mmol	Osmolality mOsm/ kg H$_2$O	Energy: protein ratio
13% SMA Gold	67	280	1.5	7.2	3.6	0.7	1.8	294	9.0
15% SMA Gold	79	329	1.8	8.4	4.2	0.8	2.1	347	9.0
Low Birthweight SMA	82	343	2.0	8.6	4.4	1.5	2.2	284	9.8
EBM + 3% SMA Gold	84	353	1.7	8.9	4.9	0.7	1.8	—	8.1
SMA High Energy	91	382	2.0	9.8	4.9	1.0	2.3	415	8.9
Infatrini	100	420	2.6	10.4	5.4	1.0	2.6	325	10.4
15% SMA Gold +Maxijul to 12% CHO +Calogen to 5% fat	100	420	1.8	12.0	5.0	0.9	2.1	—	7.2

Other ready-to-feed low birthweight/preterm formulas are: Nutriprem, Osterprem, Prematil.

Table 1.13 Energy supplements
a) Glucose polymers

Per 100 g	Ingredients	Energy* kcal	kJ	Na mmol	K mmol	PO₄ mmol
Caloreen (Nestle Clinical)	Hydrolysed corn starch	400	1674	<1.8	0.3	—
Super Soluble Maxijul (SHS International)	Hydrolysed corn starch	380	1615	<0.86	0.12	0.16
Polycal (Nutricia Clinical)	Hydrolysed corn starch	380	1615	2.2	1.3	2.3–4.2
Polycose (Abbott Laboratories Ltd)	Hydrolysed corn starch	380	1596	4.8	0.26	0.39
Vitajoule (Vitaflo Ltd)	Hydrolysed corn starch	385	1610	<1.9	<0.2	—

* As quoted by manufacturers

b) Fat emulsions

Per 100 g	Ingredients	Energy kcal	kJ	Na mmol	K mmol
Calogen (SHS)	Arachis oil	450	1850	0.9	0.5
Liquigen (SHS)	MCT oil	416	1740	1.7	0.7

c) Combined fat and carbohydrate supplements

Per 100 g	Ingredients	Energy kcal	kJ	Na mmol	K mmol
Duocal (SHS)	Cornstarch, maize oil, coconut oil	470	1988	<0.2	<0.1
MCT Duocal (SHS)	Cornstarch, coconut oil, sunflower oil	486	2042	1.3	0.09

these formulas may not be appropriate for the term infant. Nutrient intake should be assessed for the individual.

Energy and protein modules

There may be therapeutic circumstances when energy and/or protein supplements need to be added to normal infant formulas or special formulas without necessarily the need to increase the concentration of the base feed. Sometimes a ready to feed formula does not meet the needs of the individual child. Energy and protein modules and their use are described.

Carbohydrate

Carbohydrate provides 4 kcal/g (16 kJ/g). It is preferable to add carbohydrate to a feed in the form of glucose polymer, rather than using mono- or disaccharides, because they exert a lesser osmotic effect on the gut. Hence, a larger amount can be used per given volume of feed (Table 1.13). Glucose polymers should be added in 1% increments each 24 hours, i.e. 1 g per 100 ml feed per 24 hours. This will allow the point at which the infant becomes intolerant (i.e. has loose stools) to the concentration of the extra carbohydrate to be identified. Tolerance depends on the age of the infant and the maturity and absorptive capacity of the gut. As a guideline the following percentage concentrations of carbohydrate (g total carbohydrate per 100 ml feed) will be tolerated if glucose polymer is used:

- 10–12% carbohydrate concentration in infants under 6 months (i.e. 7 g from formula, 3–5 g added)
- 12–15% in infants aged 6 months to 1 year
- 15–20% in toddlers aged 1–2 years
- 20–30% in older children.

If glucose or fructose needs to be added to a feed where there is an intolerance of glucose polymer, an upper limit of tolerance may be reached at a total carbohydrate concentration of 7–8% in infants and young children.

Fat

Fat provides 9 kcal/g (37 kJ/g). Long chain fat emulsions are favoured over medium chain fat emulsions because they have a lower osmotic effect on the gut and provide a source of essential fatty acids. Medium chain fats are incorporated where there is malabsorption of long chain fat (Table 1.13).

Fat emulsions should be added to feeds in 1% increments each 24 hours, so providing an increase of 0.5 g fat per 100 ml per 24 hours. Infants will tolerate a total fat concentration of 5–6% (i.e. 5–6 g fat per 100 ml feed) if the gut is functioning normally. Children over 1 year of age will tolerate more fat, though concentrations above 7% may induce a feeling of nausea and cause vomiting. Medium chain fat will not be tolerated at such high concentrations, and may be the cause of abdominal cramps and osmotic diarrhoea if not introduced slowly to the feed.

There are combined carbohydrate and fat supplements using both long and medium chain

Table 1.14 Schedule for the addition of energy supplements to infant formulas

Day	Energy source added	Additional CHO/fat per 100 ml Feed	Energy Added per 100 ml (kcal)	(kJ)
1	1% Glucose Polymer	1 g CHO	4	17
2	2% Glucose Polymer	2 g CHO	8	33
3	3% Glucose Polymer	3 g CHO	12	50
4	3% Glucose Polymer +1% Fat Emulsion	3 g CHO 0.5 g Fat	16.5	69
5	3% Glucose Polymer +2% Fat Emulsion	3 g CHO 1 g Fat	21	88
6	4% Glucose Polymer +2% Fat Emulsion	4 g CHO 1 g Fat	25	105
7	5% Glucose Polymer +2% Fat Emulsion	5 g CHO 1 g Fat	29	121
8	5% Glucose Polymer +3% Fat Emulsion	5 g CHO 1.5 g Fat	33.5	140

fats (Table 1.13). Again these must be introduced to feeds in 1% increments to determine the child's tolerance of the product. A schedule for the addition of energy supplements to infant formulas is given in Table 1.14.

Protein

Protein may be added to feeds in the form of whole protein, peptides or amino acids (Table 1.15). Protein supplementation is rarely required without an accompanying increase in energy consumption.

Protein supplements are added to feeds to provide a specific amount of protein per kg actual body weight of the child. It is rarely necessary to give intakes of greater than 6 g protein/kg; if intakes do approach this value, blood urea levels should be monitored twice weekly to avoid the danger of uraemia developing. Supplements should be added in small increments as they can very quickly and inappropriately increase the child's intake of protein. The osmotic effect of whole protein products will be less than that of peptides, and peptides less than the effect of amino acids.

Vitamin and mineral requirements

Vitamin and mineral requirements for populations of normal children are provided by the DRVs. In disease states, requirements for certain vitamins and miner- als will be different and are fully described in the dietary management of each clinical condition. The prescribable vitamin and mineral supplements that are most often used in paediatric practice are given in Tables 1.16, 1.17 and 1.18.

Table 1.15 Protein supplements

Per 100 g	Energy kcal	kJ	Protein g	CHO g	Fat g	Na mmol	K mmol
Maxipro HBV whey protein (SHS)	394	1667	80	<5	6.0	5.6	12.0
Casilan 90 whole protein (Heinz)	367	1556	88.5	0.2	1.3	1.1	3.1
Vitapro whole protein (Vitaflo Ltd)	378	1558	75	9.0	6.0	10.0	18.0
ProMod whole protein (Abbott)	392	1658	75	7.5	6.9	7.83	13.95
Protifar whole protein (Nutricia Clinical)	370	1554	88.5	<1	<2	<1.7	<2.3
Peptide Module 767 peptides from hydrolysed meat and soya (SHS)	346	1469	86.4	—	—	—	—
Complete Amino Acid Mix Code 124 l-amino acids (SHS)	328	1374	82	—	—	—	—

Table 1.16 Vitamin supplements

Daily dose		Mother's & Children's Drops 5 drops recommended for all infants from 6 months of age[+]	Abidec 0.3 ml < 1 yr 0.6 ml > 1 yr*	Dalivit 0.6 ml	Ketovites 5 ml liquid + 3 tablets
Thiamin (B$_1$)	mg		1	1	3.0
Riboflavin (B$_2$)	mg		0.4	0.4	3.0
Pyridoxine (B$_6$)	mg		0.5	0.5	1.0
Nicotinamide	mg		5	5	9.9
Pantothenate	mg				3.5
Ascorbic acid (C)	mg	20	50	50	49.8
Alpha-tocopherol (E)	mg				15.0
Inositol	mg				150
Biotin	mg				0.5
Folic acid	mg				0.8
Acetomenaphthone (K)	mg				1.5
Vitamin A	μg	200	1200	1500	750
Vitamin D	μg	7.5	10	10	10
Choline chloride	mg				150
Cyanocobalamin (B$_{12}$)	μg		.		12.5

* Values relate to 0.6 ml dose
+ Unless taking >500 ml infant formula or follow an milk

Table 1.17 Mineral supplements

Daily dose		1.5 g/kg/day up to full dose of 8 g/day*	
		Aminogran Mineral Mixture	Metabolic Mineral Mixture
Sodium	mmol	14	14
Potassium	mmol	17	17
Chloride	mmol	—	4
Calcium	mmol	16	16
Phosphorus	mmol	15	15
Magnesium	mmol	3	3.2
Iron	mg	5	5
Zinc	mg	4	4
Iodine		trace	trace
Manganese	mg	0.4	0.4
Copper	mg	1	1
Molybdenum		trace	trace
Cobalt		trace	—
Aluminium		trace	trace

* Values relate to 8 g dose

Prescribability of products for paediatric use

The majority of specialised formulas, supplements and special dietary foods are prescribable for specific conditions. The Advisory Committee on Borderline Substances of the Department of Health recommends suitable products and defines the conditions for which they can be used. Prescriptions from the general practitioner (FP10) should be marked 'ACBS' to indicate that the prescription complies with recommendations. A list of prescribable items appears in the *Monthly Index of Medical Specialities* (*MIMS*) and in the *British National Formulary* (*BNF*) under the Borderline Substances Appendix. Children under the age of 16 years in the UK are exempt from prescription charges.

Table 1.18 Vitamin and mineral supplements

Daily dose		Paediatric Seravit (powder) Unflavoured (SHS) 17 g powder	Forceval Junior Capsules (Unigreg) 2 caps	Daily dose		Paediatric Seravit (powder) Unflavoured (SHS) 17 g powder	Forceval Junior Capsules (Unigreg) 2 caps
Sodium	mmol	<0.09	—	Riboflavin	mg	0.75	2.0
Potassium	mmol	trace	—	Pyridoxine	mg	0.58	2.0
Chloride	mmol	1.12	—	Nicotinamide	mg	5.95	15.0
Calcium	mmol	10.9	—	Pantothenic acid	mg	2.89	4.0
Phosphorus	mmol	9.4	—	Inositol	mg	119	—
Magnesium	mmol	2.5	0.08	Choline	mg	59.5	—
Iron	mg	11.7	10.0	Vitamin D_3	µg	9.44	10.0
Zinc	mg	7.8	10.0	Vitamin B_{12}	µg	1.46	4.0
Iodine	mg	0.06	0.15	Folic acid	mg	0.05	0.2
Manganese	mg	0.78	2.5	Biotin	mg	0.04	0.1
Copper	mg	0.78	2.0	Vitamin K	mg	0.03	0.05
Molybdenum	mg	0.06	0.1	Carbohydrate		glucose polymer 75 g/100 g	
Selenium	mg	0.02	0.05				
Chromium	mg	0.02	0.1				
Vitamin A	µg	710	750	Osmolality		216 mOsm/kg H_2O at 10% dilution	
Vitamin E	mg	4.9	10.0				
Vitamin C	mg	68	50				
Thiamin	mg	0.54	3.0				

REFERENCES

1 Lucas A, Ewing G, Roberts SB, Coward WA How much energy does the breast-fed infant consume and expend? *Brit Med J*, 1987, **295** 75–7.

2 Cole TJ, Freeeman JV, Preece MA Body mass index curves for the UK, 1990. *Arch Dis Childh*, 1995, **73** 25–9.

3 Michaelson KF Short-term measurements of linear growth in early life: infant kneemometry. *Acta Paed*, 1997, **86** 551–3.

4 Stevenson RD Use of segmental measures to estimate stature in children with cerebral palsy. *Arch Pediatr Adoles Med*, 1995, **149** 658–62.

5 Gibson RS *Principles of Nutritional Assessment*. Appendix A, pp. 649–62. New York: Oxford University Press, 1990.

6 Sangi H, Mueller WH Which measure of body fat distribution is best for epidemiological research among adolescents. *Am J Epidemiol*, 1991, **133** 870–73.

7 Cole TJ Conditional reference charts to assess weight gain in British infants. *Arch Dis Childh*, 1995, **73** 8–16.

8 Waterlow JC Some aspects of protein calorie malnutrition. *Brit Med J*, 1972, **3** 556–69.

9 Clayton BE, Round JM (eds) *Chemical Pathology and the Sick Child*. Oxford: Blackwell Science, 1994.

10 Ruxton CH, Reilly JJ, Kirk TR Body composition of healthy 7- and 8-year-old children and a comparison with the 'reference child'. *Int J Obesity*, 1999, **23** 1276–81.

11 Department of Health. Report on Health and Social Subjects No 41. *Dietary Reference Values for Food Energy and Nutrients for the United Kingdom*. London: The Stationery Office.

FURTHER READING

Gibson RS *Principles of Nutritional Assessment*. Oxford: Oxford University Press, 1986.

Talbot J (ed.) *Infant Feeding in the First Year*. London: Profile Productions Ltd, 1989.

Thompson JM *Nutritional Requirements of Infants and Young Children*. Oxford: Blackwell Science, 1998.

Wardley BL, Puntis JWL, Taitz LS *Handbook of Child Nutrition*, 2nd edn. Oxford: Oxford University Press, 1997.

USEFUL ADDRESS

Child Growth Foundation
2 Mayfield Avenue, Chiswick, London W4 1PW. Tel. 020 8994 7625/8995 0257, email cgflondon@aol.com

CHAPTER 2

Provision of Nutrition in a Hospital Setting

Studies of children in hospital indicate a significant incidence of both acute and chronic malnutrition [1, 2, 3]. Provision of an adequate nutritional intake is an important part of the care of all hospitalised children whether previously malnourished or not.

To meet the nutritional needs of the range of paediatric patients a variety of services are required including:

- Ready-to-feed (RTF) infant milks
- Adapted infant milks and specialised infant formulas
- Enteral feeds
- Hospital food including special diets.

Close co-operation between dietitians, caterers, medical and nursing staff and the child's carers is also an essential part of nutrient provision in hospital.

INFANT AND ENTERAL FEEDS

Infant milks

Many infants admitted to hospital will simply require an adequate volume of infant milk. To minimise hygiene concerns and ensure uniform composition this is best provided in a ready-to-feed (RTF) form. A selection of whey and casein based milks should be available to meet the personal preference of the family. If RTF milks are not available the guidance for preparation of adapted or specialised formula apply.

Adapted infant milks and specialised formulas

To prepare adapted infant milks, e.g. thickened, energy supplemented or specialised infant formulas, a designated feed-making area is required.

Children receiving such feeds are likely to be those at greatest nutritional risk, therefore feeds must be made accurately to ensure the prescribed nutritional content is achieved.

Hygiene standards in feed preparations are of paramount importance as feeds are generally for infants or for older children who are immunologically compromised as a result of illness.

Enteral feeds

The range and presentation of paediatric enteral feeds continues to expand, increasing the possibility that feeds in a ready-to-hang presentation could be available at ward level. In situations where enteral feeds require adaptation, e.g. energy supplementation or decanting into enteral feeding bottles, again these processes should be carried out in a designated feed-making area.

Designated feed-making area

In large hospitals preparing in excess of 15–20 feeds daily a feed-making unit will be required, normally consisting of three separate areas for storage, preparation and cleaning. In smaller hospitals a designated feed-making room or a specific area of the ward kitchen should be available.

Any feed-making operation must comply with the requirements of the Food Safety Act 1990 [4]. The manager of such an operation has a legal obligation to ensure that it operates to acceptable standards of hygiene. To establish and monitor such standards a hazard analysis and critical control point (HACCP) system is recommended [5]. Such a system will ensure that all aspects of feed production are subjected to rigorous assessment for potential hazards and risks, and that adequate control points are incorporated into the process.

Structural design of feed-making areas

A designated feed-making area should be an independent unit or room whose access is restricted to authorised personnel. Designed to prevent the entrance and harbouring of vermin and pests and constructed to be easily cleaned, it must be operated to the highest standards of hygiene.

It is desirable to separate the unit into three areas:

A storage area, situated adjacent to the feed preparation area, where bulk goods are delivered, unpacked and stored. It should be large enough to accommodate adequate storage racks which are constructed and sited to permit segregation of commodities, stock rotation and effective cleaning. Items must be stored on racks or shelves, not directly on the floor. The temperature should be maintained between 10°C and 15°C and should be monitored daily. Entry to this area is restricted to unit and delivery staff.

A feed preparation area where very clean conditions prevail and access is only allowed to feed preparation staff who are suitably clothed (see later); entry should be via an anteroom containing a wash-hand basin and storage facilities for outer protective clothing. Bulk storage of items (e.g. large cardboard cartons) is not recommended. There should be sufficient space to allow clean equipment and small quantities of ingredients to be stored, preferably on wheel-mounted stainless steel solid shelving, leaving worktops clear. During the preparation of feeds all other activities in the area should cease and the doors should be closed and secured against all staff (including dietitians) who are not involved in the manufacturing process. If it is necessary for staff to leave the preparation area they must, on re-entry, wash their hands again, according to the correct hand washing procedure.

A wash up area. A unit re-using feeding bottles will require a designated space, adjoining the feed preparation area, with a separate access for the delivery of dirty bottles. A unit using disposable bottles does not require such a wash-up room if a dishwasher is in operation for preparation equipment. Access to this area should be restricted to cleaning and delivery staff.

Storage of cleaning materials should be separated from ingredients and equipment and requires a designated clean, dry room or cupboard.

A cloakroom with a separate changing room for feed unit staff should be conveniently sited but segregated from the feed-making area. The cloakroom should have a foot operated flush toilet and a wash-hand basin with foot or elbow operated taps; the changing room should contain secure lockers for storage of personal belongings and outdoor clothes and clean storage for protective clothing.

Recommendations for construction of feed units are as follows [6]:

Plant

Walls, floors and ceilings: hardwearing, impervious, free from cracks and open joints. Smooth surfaces to permit ease of cleaning and coved junctions between floors, walls and ceilings to prevent collection of dust and dirt. Light coloured sheen finish to reflect light and increase illumination.

Doors in the production area: self-closing with glass observation panel.

Windows: sealed to prevent opening.

Lighting level: to allow staff to work cleanly and safely without eye strain, and to expose dirt and dust. Light fixtures flush with wall or ceiling.

Ventilation in the production area: mechanical means; air supply filtered with temperature (and preferably humidity) control to give optimum working environment and control bacterial and dust contamination. Steam-producing equipment such as sterilisers, dishwashers and pasteurisers should be fitted with a canopy and exhaust fan system to draw off steam and fumes.

Wash-hand basins: one hand basin provided in each of the storage, wash-up and preparation areas. Hot and cold water with foot or elbow operated taps. Adjacent soap dispenser and either single use disposable towels or a hot air hand dryer.

Water supply: of potable quality from a rising main. Softened water supply to equipment is preferable, but water softened by ion exchange should not be used in feeds.

Hot water: provided from a fixed device such as a gas or electric water boiler to dispense water above 80°C.

Large equipment

- Large equipment such as shelving, tables and refrigerators should be castor mounted with wheel brakes to allow easy access for cleaning. Smooth impervious surfaces free from sharp internal corners, which may act as dirt traps, which can be easily cleaned and disinfected (e.g. stainless steel) are recommended.

- One or more refrigerators which operate at a temperature between 1–4°C is a necessity; the temperature should be monitored and recorded twice daily.

- A blast chiller to allow rapid cooling of all feeds to below 5°C.

- A deep freeze which operates at −18°C will be necessary if feeds of expressed breast milk are to be stored for more than a few hours. Both the refrigerator and freezer should be self-defrosting and have shelves which are easy to clean. An alarm which is activated if the door is left open accidentally or the internal temperature rises is also useful.

- Pasteurisation equipment which is suitable for the range of procedures carried out (see later) and which includes a method of monitoring and recording pasteurisation cycles is desirable.

- Thermal sterilisation or disinfection equipment is desirable in a small unit and essential in a large centralised unit. This can be a washer adapted for bottle and equipment washing, with a rinse cycle which holds a temperature of 85°C for 2 minutes. This ensures a surface temperature of 80°C for 1 minute, which is an effective disinfectant. A drying cycle is useful. For units with a very small workload, a domestic steam steriliser is adequate for non-reusable bottles [7].

- A feed delivery trolley.

Small equipment

- Mixing and measuring equipment including jugs, measures, cutlery, sieves and whisks should be made from plastic or stainless steel. They must be easily washed and cleaned.

- Electric whisks or liquidisers create large froth volumes in feeds, making accurate measurement difficult. They are also difficult to clean and if used, the bowl and blades should be suitable for use in a washing machine, autoclave or chemical disinfectant.

- Weighing equipment should be easy to clean, easy to use and of the appropriate accuracy for the task. It may be battery or electrically operated.

- Feeding bottles are available in glass, polycarbonate or plastic polythene in 100–150 ml and 200–250 ml sizes. Glass is a hazardous material prone to cracking and chipping; polycarbonate shrinks if autoclaved at temperatures greater than 119°C and bottles become scratched or crazed after some time in use. Reusable bottles require washing, sanitising by heat or chemical means; sealing discs or caps need to undergo a similar treatment and are likely to become lost or misshapen with continuous use. Disposable sterile polythene bottles (although apparently more expensive) reduce the workload in the unit as the responsibility for providing clean bottles is transferred to the manufacturer.

Staffing levels and staff procedures

Feed provision is usually required 365 days a year and staffing levels should take this fact and the workload into consideration. Part-time employment of some staff may be particularly appropriate. In large units the dietitian may be managerially responsible for staff and feed preparation. In small areas attached to a ward the supervision and management may be the responsibility of the nursing staff with the dietitian acting in an advisory capacity. As identified in the Food Safety Act [4] all food handlers should hold a Basic Food Hygiene Certificate. No other specific qualifications are required for feed preparation staff, provided that adequate instruction and supervision is provided; in situations such as small units where this is difficult it is an advantage for staff to be trained nurses or nursery nurses.

Training should cover personal hygiene, prevention of bacterial and foreign matter contamination, preparation procedures, cleaning procedures and documentation requirements. All staff should be provided with an agreed job description covering these issues. If staff numbers warrant, then a supervisor should be appointed. Regular meetings between the manager, supervisor, microbiologist and infection control officer will enhance communication and help ensure that standards are maintained.

Suitable protective uniforms and a satisfactory laundry service are required. A disposable plastic apron should be worn during feed preparation and a disposable head covering should completely cover the hair. Shoes should be flat-heeled and cover the foot; jewellery (with the exception of a wedding ring and stud type earrings) is not allowed.

Appointment of staff should be subject to a satisfactory medical examination; bacteriological screening of faecal specimens should take place prior to appointment, after a gastrointestinal upset and on return from a hot climate.

Feed preparation

A policy for documentation of raw materials should be implemented and goods received checked to ensure they meet the required standard and specification. Goods for storage should be marked and dated to aid identification and stock rotation. All raw materials should be dated when the packaging is opened and any surplus discarded after the recommended time or after 1 month.

Details of each feed to be prepared should be in a clearly written or printed form. All ingredients should be weighed or measured accurately. Once decanted into the appropriate bottles all feeds should be labelled. The label should include details of the patient's name, ward, hospital number, feed ingredients and date of preparation. It should also be labelled to refrigerate and discard after 24 hours.

Feed ingredients

Only unopened tins and packets of milk powder or feed ingredients should be allowed into the preparation area. Bulk goods (e.g. glucose polymer) should be decanted into a disinfected container prior to entry. Ultra treated (UHT) cow's milk is recommended as it does not need to be refrigerated until opened. If pasteurised milk is used, its storage conditions and shelf life need to be carefully controlled; pasteurised cow's milk that has not been used should be discarded at the end of each working day.

Expressed breast milk (EBM) should be handled carefully and a procedure adopted for its use on the wards and milk room. Recommendations for the handling and storage of human milk are found in publications from the Department of Health and the Royal College of Paediatricians and Child Health [8a].

Pasteurisation

The type of feeds prepared in the milk room will readily support the growth of harmful microorganisms, particularly if stored at temperatures above 5°C. Pasteurisation can limit the potential microbiological contamination but may be less effective against all potential pathogens, e.g. *Bacillus* sp. [9].

A pasteuriser built to the specifications of the unit should be equipped with a computer printout to show the temperature and process time for each batch of feeds.

There are two methods of pasteurisation:

- *Holder method for breast milk only:* the temperature is raised to 62.5°C for 30 minutes, followed by rapid cooling to less than 10°C
- *Flash method for milk formulas, modular feeds and supplements:* the temperature is raised to 67.5°C for 4 minutes followed by rapid cooling to less than 10°C.

After pasteurisation feed should be stored in a suitable refrigerator (see above) until delivery.

Blast chilling

One of the most important steps in limiting microbial growth in prepared feeds is to rapidly cool to below 5°C.

Delivery

Feed delivery to wards should be compatible with food safety requirements of being refrigerated to 4°C or less without avoidable delay. If the preparation unit is some distance from wards this requires a refrigerated trolley. Feeds should be checked and placed in a designated refrigerator at ward level; this refrigerator should be reserved for milk feeds and should not contain items of food. The temperature of ward refrigerators should be between 1–4°C and should be checked twice daily.

Cleaning procedures

Sterilisation (the destruction of all microorganisms and their spores) is not attainable in a special feeds unit. Sanitation or disinfection of small equipment can be achieved by autoclaving, by a dishwasher or by chemical means.

Autoclaving, although effective, has a number of disadvantages: equipment first has to be washed, dried, packed and sealed; this is costly and time consuming. In addition water condensation forms and remains in feeding bottles, where it can induce bacterial activity.

Thermal disinfection in a dishwasher requires less time and the inclusion of a drying cycle will ensure that all equipment is dry and ready for storage. To achieve thermal disinfection the water in the dishwasher should reach a minimum temperature of 85°C for 2 minutes (see the section on Large equipment earlier in this chapter).

Chemical disinfection (e.g. hypochlorite) reduces levels of harmful bacteria to acceptable levels and is also satisfactory for small (non-metallic) equipment provided recommendations are followed, although heat sanitisation is the preferred method. Disinfection will only be effective if:

- The equipment is adequately cleaned; residual organic matter inactivates the chlorine content of the disinfectant
- The disinfectant is freshly and correctly prepared with all air bubbles removed to ensure the solution reaches each surface of the equipment
- The equipment remains in the disinfectant for the recommended length of time.

After disinfection the equipment should be rinsed free of contaminated hypochlorite with clean water. Feed equipment should be covered with sterile paper or drape and used within 24 hours of disinfection. Equipment which is stored for longer than this should be re-disinfected before use.

Walls of a special feed unit should be washed every 6 months, floors cleaned daily and all cleaning procedures documented. Separate, clearly indentified cleaning equipment should be used for the 'clean' and 'dirty' areas of the unit.

Microbiological surveillance

To ensure satisfactory standards of working practice a microbiological surveillance policy should be implemented and monitored. The following samples should be sent for microbiological analysis once each month: each type of feed (both freshly prepared and after storage); water from boiler, tap and pasteuriser; a swab from work surfaces, sinks, shelving, mixing equipment and feeding bottles. An air sample should be taken if *Staphylococcus aureus* is identified.

Procedures and documentation

To comply with legislative requirements, standards for all procedures within the feed preparation area should be set, implemented, monitored and recorded. To increase staff awareness and to aid training a 'Procedure Manual' should be drawn up which should be available to all staff. It should contain staff job descriptions, guidelines for personal hygiene and prevention of cross-infection, procedures for ordering supplies, feed preparation, instructions for pasteurisation, cleaning and disinfection, procedures for microbiological surveillance and accident procedures. Information about equipment maintenance and emergency telephone numbers in case of breakdown should also be displayed.

Currently there are no accepted published standards for the preparation of enteral feeds for the paediatric age range. Operational practices should be based on standards identified for food products [4, 5, 10].

NORMAL DIET IN A HOSPITAL SETTING

Food in hospital should be seen as an integral part of treatment [11]. Many children admitted to hospital are already malnourished or have chronic diseases which impair their nutritional state [1, 2, 3].

A hospital menu should, over a period of days, provide the minimum nutritional requirements [12]. Whilst a nutritionally sound diet incorporating appropriate nutrition education messages may be desirable, it is vital to encourage children to eat something when they are in unfamiliar surroundings with feelings of anxiety and depression. It is most important, therefore, that familiar foods are included on the menu and that healthy eating guidelines are applied with caution. Where there are paediatric wards in a general hospital a separate children's menu should be available and food items such as full-fat milk provided for the paediatric wards. Patient choice of food is generally recommended [13] and where practically possible choice should also be offered to paediatric patients. Caterers should also be aware of the wide age range encountered in a paediatric setting and provide an appropriate selection of food choices and portion sizes (Table 2.1). At ward level food should be attractively presented with crockery and utensils appropriate to the age range.

If possible children should be encouraged to eat together and they should be adequately supervised. Accurate charting of food and fluid intake in combination with mealtime supervision greatly assists the detection of patients at risk from a poor food intake [14]. Where such a problem does occur, it may be simply solved by increased supervision at mealtimes, use of favourite foods, inclusion of regular snacks and the availability of nutritious supplements such as milk-based drinks.

It is important that all hospital patients are provided with food which is acceptable to them. Choices should be available for vegetarians, vegans and those whose eating habits are based on religious and cultural beliefs.

MODIFIED DIET IN A HOSPITAL SETTING

The major role of the dietitian is to liaise with the medical and nursing staff and to advise on the appropriate therapeutic regimen. The advice and education given to children requiring modified diets and to their carers is the responsibility of the dietitian. In addi-

Table 2.1 Portion sizes for different age groups

	1 year	2–3 years	3–5 years	10 years
Meal pattern	3 small meals and 3 snacks plus milk	3 meals and 2–3 snacks or milky drinks	3 meals and 1–2 snacks or milky drinks	3 meals and 1–2 snacks or milky drinks
Meat, fish etc.	½–1 tablespoon (20–30 g) minced/finely chopped, with gravy/sauce; ½–1 hard cooked egg	1½ tablespoons (20–30 g) chopped; 1 fish finger; 1 sausage; 1 egg	2–3 tablespoons (40–80 g); 1–2 fish fingers/sausages	90–120 g meat; 3–4 fish fingers/sausages
Cheese	20 g grated	25–30 g cubed or grated	30–40 g	50–60 g
Potato	1 tablespoon (30 g) mashed	1–2 tablespoons (30–60 g); 6 smallish chips	2–3 tablespoons (60–80 g); 8–10 chips	4–6 tablespoons (100–180 g); 100–150 g chips
Vegetables	1 tablespoon (30 g) soft or mashed	1–2 tablespoons (30–60 g) or small chopped salad	2–3 tablespoons (60–80 g)	3–4 tablespoons (100–120 g)
Fruit	½–1 piece (40–80 g)	1 piece (80–100 g)	1 piece (100 g)	1 piece (100 g)
Dessert (e.g. custard/yoghurt)	2 tablespoons (60 g)	2–3 tablespoons (60–80 g)	4 tablespoons (120 g); 1 carton yoghurt (150 g)	6 tablespoons (180 g)
Bread	½–1 slice (20–30 g)	1 large slice (40 g)	1–2 large slices (40–80 g)	2–4 large slices (80–160 g)
Breakfast cereal	1 tablespoon (15 g); ½ Weetabix	1–1½ tablespoons (15–20 g); 1 Weetabix	2–3 tablespoons (20–30 g); 1 Weetabix	3–4 tablespoons (30–40 g); 2 Weetabix
Drinks	¾ teacup (100 ml)	1 teacup (150 ml)	1 teacup (150 ml)	1 mug (200 ml)
Milk	500 ml whole milk/day	350 ml whole or semiskimmed/day	350 ml whole or semiskimmed/day	350 ml whole, semiskimmed or skimmed/day

tion to this the dietitian assists in the provision of modified diets within the hospital. Usually this is in a supervisory and advisory capacity to diet cooks employed by the caterer, but rarely dietitians may also be managerially responsible for the diet kitchen. In the majority of cases design and maintenance of the diet preparation area, staff management, supply of provisions and responsibility for hygiene will rest with the catering manager. If these are the responsibility of the dietitian the same principles apply as previously described for feed-making areas [4].

Staff involved in the preparation of modified diets must be aware of the need for accuracy, appropriate portion size for age, consistency of nutrient content and variety. For those on a modified diet the food provided in hospital is taken as an example and must therefore be correct. It is advisable that staff employed to prepare modified diets should have as a minimum qualification City and Guilds 706/2 and have attended a diet cookery course. In-service training of diet cooks should be undertaken by the dietitian particularly to ensure that staff are kept up-to-date with changes to dietary treatment.

The dietitian should specify to the caterer standards of quality and suitability of provisions for use in the diet preparation area. Stocks of specific dietary products such as gluten-free and low protein products should be available and those working in the area should be familiar with the use of these products.

Appropriate equipment for preparation of small quantities of food must be available for the diet cooks. Specifically a sturdy industrial liquidiser, small pots and pans and accurate scales are all essential items. Freezer space is also required, as it is useful to keep frozen portions of rarely used items, e.g. vegetable casserole for low protein diets, low protein bread.

A suitable plating system for diets must be used. Where a bulk catering system is operated, individual foil containers, clearly labelled, are suitable for diet meals. If a plated system is in use the diet meals should be clearly labelled.

The dietitian should always provide the diet cooks with clear written and verbal instructions for each individual diet being prepared. The written information should include the patient's name, age and ward, the diet required and specific instructions regarding the composition of the diet.

Within the diet preparation area there should be a diet manual. This should include instructions regarding commonly requested modified diets and appropriate recipes. It is also useful to include details of any patients on unusual diets if they are likely to be admitted. This manual should be regularly updated.

To ensure consistency and accuracy, the provision of modified diets should be monitored regularly. The following should all be considered: the quality, freshness and suitability of the provisions; the storage methods; the preparation of raw ingredients; and the presentation to the patient. Regular monitoring should ensure a high quality product. Additionally, where the dietitian is responsible for the management of the diet preparation area, then the legal obligations of the Food Safety Act 1990 [4] should be fulfilled.

IMMUNOSUPPRESSION AND 'CLEAN' MEAL PROVISION

Children with a number of conditions (including acute megaloblastic leukaemia, stage IV neuroblastoma, relapsed acute lymphoblastic leukaemia and immunodeficiency syndromes) requiring a bone marrow transplant or autograft, and children undergoing heart-lung transplantation, receive drug therapy which causes severe immunosuppression and neutropenia. They require protective isolation in the immediate post-transplant period and, since they are highly susceptible to food-borne pathogens, must be protected from gastrointestinal infection [15]. In immunosuppressed patients even normally non-pathogenic organisms may cause problems. Particular attention should be paid to personal hygiene in the food handler, and to food purchase, storage and preparation.

There is limited evidence on the use and effectiveness of 'clean' diets. Practice is variable and in general there has been a move away from stringent sterile diets [16]. Three levels of 'clean' diet are generally recognised: sterile diet, clean diet and common-sense food hygiene guidelines.

Sterile meals

In some units food production may be a sterile or near-sterile method incorporating the use of gamma-irradiated and canned foods prepared in a filtered laminar airflow system. Such a system requires specialised facilities and equipment and is labour-intensive and costly. Irradiation adversely affects food flavour and texture and consequently patient acceptability of food [17].

'Clean' meals

A practical and acceptable alternative is the use of a reduced bacterial diet or 'very clean food regimen'. Such regimens avoid the use of raw foods, reheated dishes and foods known to contain high levels of pathogenic and non-pathogenic bacteria, such as soft cheese, chicken and pâté. Details of foods allowed and forbidden are given in Table 2.2.

Practice between centres can vary, for example some allow all meat and poultry providing it is well cooked and served immediately. Other centres follow common sense food hygiene guidelines and avoid high risk foods only (Table 2.3).

Table 2.2 Foods for a 'clean' diet

Food	Allowed	Not allowed	Food	Allowed	Not allowed
Water	Sterile water Boiled tap water	Mineral water Unboiled water		Meat paste in individual jars	Take away meals (e.g. hamburgers) Salami Liver pâté, liver sausage
Drinks	Fruit juice and soft drinks – individual cartons or cans Ice cubes and ice lollies – made with sterile water High energy packaged drinks (e.g. Polycal Liquid) Tea, coffee, cocoa etc. – individual sachets	Squashes unless repacked and pasteurised	Fish	Freshly-cooked fresh or frozen fish Tinned fish Fish fingers, fish paste	Shellfish
			Eggs	Hard boiled egg Fried egg	Raw egg, soft-cooked egg
Milk and dairy products	Milk – UHT, pasteurised, condensed or sterilised in individual portions Cheeses – individually vacuum wrapped portions; cheese spread portions; processed cheese Yoghurt – pasteurised Butter/margarine – individual portions Cream – UHT or sterilised Ice cream – individually wrapped portions	Unpasteurised milk Soft cheeses Unwrapped hard cheese Blue cheeses Unpasteurised or 'live' yoghurt Fresh cream	Vegetables	Fresh leafy vegetables – well washed and cooked Root vegetables, washed, peeled and cooked Jacket potato; oven chips Beans and lentils – well cooked or tinned Tomato and cucumber – raw, peeled Tinned and frozen vegetables	Salad vegetables which cannot be peeled (e.g. lettuce, radish) Raw root vegetables
			Fruit	Fresh fruit that can be peeled Tinned fruit	Unpeeled fruit Dried fruit
Cereals	Breakfast cereals – individual packets Bread from newly opened loaf Biscuits and cakes – individual portions Rice – well cooked Pasta – tinned or dried	Cereals with added milk powder; sugar coated cereals Unwrapped bread Cream cakes Slow-cooked rice (e.g. rice pudding) Fresh pasta	Snacks and Soups	Crisps, sweets etc. – individual packets Tinned soups, packet soups – made with boiled water	Unwrapped sweets
			Miscellaneous	Cooking oils Puddings, pies, custards – freshly made Jelly – made with sterile/ boiled water Salt, salad cream, sauces – individual portions Pepper – gamma irradiated	Instant puddings made with cold water Herbs and spices
Meat and poultry	Pork, lamb, beef, veal – fresh or frozen, well cooked Tinned meats; chicken, sausages, ham, corned beef	Chicken, turkey – fresh or frozen Sausages Pies (unless home made)			

Table 2.3 High risk foods

Mineral water
Raw eggs and cooked egg dishes
Soft and blue veined cheeses
Pâté
Live and bio yoghurts
Take-away foods
Reheated chilled meals
Ready-to-eat poultry
Shellfish
Soft whip ice cream
Nuts and dried fruit

Purchasing

(1) Many chilled and frozen foods contain unacceptably high levels of organisms for the immunosuppressed patient. Before allowing them to be included a sample of the product should be tested. Canned and sterilised products are generally suitable.
(2) The 'Best Before' date should be checked on manufactured foods.
(3) Individual portions of foods (e.g. jams, butter/margarine, breakfast cereals, juices, sugar) should be purchased where these are available.
(4) Foods should be purchased as fresh as possible and cooked shortly after purchase.

Storage

(1) Check temperatures of refrigerators and freezers regularly.
(2) Ideally food for 'clean' meals should be stored in a separate refrigerator; where this is not practical, the top shelf should be used.
(3) Transfer food that is to be eaten cold to the refrigerator as quickly as possible; cover or wrap all foods stored in the refrigerator. Leftover food should be disposed of quickly; leftovers and reheated foods should not be used.

Preparation

(1) Wash hands thoroughly with soap and water and dry with a hand dryer or a clean paper towel before handling food.
(2) In the hospital setting the food handler should wear a fresh plastic apron over the usual kitchen dress.

(3) Use clean utensils, containers and chopping boards which have been through a dishwasher.
(4) In a hospital kitchen, work surfaces should be wiped with a suitable disinfectant solution before 'clean' meals are prepared. This precaution should be unnecessary at home.
(5) Do not use wooden utensils (e.g. chopping boards).
(6) A fresh packet or tin should be used for each meal to avoid re-opening containers. Large packets (e.g. a loaf of bread, a pint of milk etc.) can be divided into convenient size portions and individually wrapped at the beginning of each day.
(7) Before opening packages such as tins the top should be wiped with a clean cloth or paper towel.
(8) Tin openers should be washed daily, preferably in a dishwasher.
(9) Cooking methods employed should ensure a minimum core temperature of 70°C, and this temperature should be maintained until the food is eaten.
(10) There should be minimum delay between food being cooked and consumed.

Acceptable bacterial levels should be determined in consultation with the microbiologist and haematologist/immunologist. There are a few guidelines to assist with this [18]. Additionally guidelines on the bacteriology of enteral feeds may be a useful starting point [10].

The 'very clean food regimen' should be fully explained to the patient and carers prior to transplant as it should be commenced as soon as the patient is able to take anything orally. Prior discussion also allows time to obtain supplies of favourite or unusual foods and to liaise with the catering department regarding provision of supplies.

At discharge neutrophil counts may still be below normal so care to avoid food-borne infection is required. Food hygiene advice and avoidance of high risk foods (Table 2.3) are required.

REFERENCES

1 Moy RJD, Smallman S, Booth IW Malnutrition in a UK children's hospital. *J Hum Nutr Diet*, 1990, 3 93–100.
2 Merritt RJ, Suskind RM Nutritional survey of the hospitalised paediatric patient. *Am J Clin Nutr*, 1979, 32 1320–25.

3 Hendrickse WK, Reilly JJ, Weaver LT Malnutrition in a children's hospital. *Clin Nutr*, 1997, **16** 13–18.

4 *The Food Safety Act*. London: The Stationery Office, 1990.

5 *Assured Safety Catering: A Management System for Hazard Analysis*. London: The Stationery Office, 1993.

6 Sprenger RA *Hygiene for Management*. Doncaster: Highfield Publications, 1991.

7 Health Technical Memorandum 2030: Washer-disinfectors, NHS Estates. London: The Stationery Office, 1995.

8 Department of Health and Social Security Report on Health and Social Subjects No 22. *The Collection and Storage of Human Milk*. London: The Stationery Office, 1981.

8a *Guidelines for the Establishment and Operation of Human Milk Banks in the UK*. 2e London: Royal College of Paediatrics and Child Health, 1999.

9 Anderton A, pers. comm., 1998.

10 BDA *Microbiological Control in Enteral Feeding – a guidance document*. Birmingham: British Dietetic Association, 1986.

11 *Hospital Food as Treatment*. A report by a working party of the British Association for Parenteral and Enteral Nutrition, Maidenhead, Berks, 1999.

12 Department of Health Report on Health and Social Subjects No. 41. *Dietary Reference Values for Food. Energy and Nutrition for the United Kingdom*. London: The Stationery Office, 1991.

13 *Nutrition Guidelines for Hospital Catering*. London: Department of Health, 1995.

14 Todd EA *et al.* What do patients eat in hospital? *Hum Nutr: Appl Nutr*, 1984, **38A** 294–7.

15 Dezenhall A *et al.* Food and nutrition services in bone marrow transplant centres. *J Am Diet Assoc*, 1987, **87** 1351–3.

16 Pattinson AJ Review of current practice in 'clean' diets in the UK. *J Hum Nutr Diet*, 1993, **6** 3–11.

17 Aker SN, Cheney CU The use of sterile and low microbial diets in ultra isolation environments. *J Parent Ent Nutr*, 1983, **7** 390.

18 Pizzo PA, Purvis DS, Waters C Microbiological evaluation of food items. *J Am Diet Assoc*, 1982, **81** 272.

SECTION 2

Enteral and Parenteral Nutrition

CHAPTER 3

Enteral Feeding

Enteral nutrition is the method of supplying nutrients to the gastrointestinal tract. It is the term often used to describe nasogastric, gastrostomy and jejunostomy feeding although it can also include food and drink taken orally.

Enteral feeding is the preferred method of providing nutritional support to children who have a functioning gastrointestinal tract, with parenteral nutrition reserved for children with severely compromised gut function. It is safer and easier to administer than parenteral nutrition both in hospital and at home and can be adapted to meet the individual requirements of infants and children of all ages.

Some children require total nutrition via a nasogastric, gastrostomy or jejunostomy tube, whereas others require nutritional support to supplement their poor oral intake or to meet their increased nutritional requirements. Enteral feeding may be short term but for many children it can be a long term or even life-long method of feeding. As a result of these diverse indications for enteral feeding, regimens need to be adaptable to ensure each child receives the vital nutrients they require for normal growth and development.

Tube feeding children requires the expert knowledge of a paediatric dietitian who, along with a specialist nursing team, has the knowledge to use feeds and feeding equipment appropriate for the individual requirements and clinical condition of the patient. Indications for enteral feeding are given in Table 3.1.

CHOICE OF FEEDS

The choice of feed is dependent on a number of factors:

- Age
- Gut function
- Dietary restrictions and specific nutrient requirements
- Route of administration
- Prescribability and cost.

Infants under 12 months

Mother's expressed breast milk (EBM) may be given to her own baby or pasteurised donor breast milk may be available. The principal benefits of using breast milk are the presence of immunoglobulins, antimicrobial factors and lipase activity. In addition, there is a psychological benefit to the mother if she is able to contribute to the care of her sick child by providing breast milk. These benefits may be outweighed by the possible poorer energy density of EBM, particularly if the fore milk is used which is lower in fat than the hind milk. If the infant fails to gain weight on breast milk alone it can be supplemented either with infant formula, a commercial human milk fortifier or glucose polymer and fat emulsion (p. 13, 14, 61). Pasteurisation of a mother's EBM remains a controversial issue. Pasteurisation will destroy a percentage of the antimicrobial, hormonal and enzymic factors within the milk [1] but may protect against bacterial contamination. Currently there are no national guidelines and individual hospitals and units have developed their own local protocols. The cleanliness of the collection technique can be assessed by microbial analysis and a decision then made as to whether the milk can be used raw or whether it needs to be pasteurised.

Normal infant formulas are suitable for enteral feeding from birth to 12 months of age. They provide an energy density of approximately 65 kcal (272 kJ)/100 ml and meet European Community Regulations [2]. Follow-on formulas may also be used after 6 months of age if their higher protein and iron

Table 3.1 Indications for enteral feeding

Indication	Example
Inability to suck or swallow	Neurological handicap and degenerative disorders
	Severe developmental delay
	Trauma
	Ventilated child
Anorexia associated with chronic illness	Cystic fibrosis
	Inflammatory bowel disease
	Liver disease
	Chronic renal failure
	Congenital heart disease
	Inherited metabolic disease
Increased requirements	Cystic fibrosis
	Congenital heart disease
	Malabsorption syndromes (e.g. short gut syndrome, liver disease)
Congenital anomalies	Tracheo-oesophageal fistula
	Oesophageal atresia
	Orofacial malformations
Primary Disease Management	Crohn's disease
	Severe gastro-oesophageal reflux
	Short bowel syndrome
	Glycogen storage disease
	Very long chain fatty acid disorders

content is thought to be more beneficial to the child. Most infants requiring enteral feeding will have increased nutritional requirements. Concentrating infant formulas and adding glucose polymer powders and fat emulsions has traditionally been practised to increase the energy and nutrient content (p. 13). Nutrient dense infant formulas such as Infatrini (Nutricia) and SMA High Energy (SMA Nutrition) are now commercially available and have been shown to promote better growth [3].

Normal infant formulas are based on cows milk protein and lactose. Infants with impaired gut function who do not tolerate whole protein formulas frequently benefit from the use of hydrolysed protein or amino acid based feeds (p. 74, 75). Such feeds are hypoallergenic and are free of cow's milk and lactose. Many of these formulas also have a proportion of the fat content as medium chain triglycerides (MCT) which can be beneficial in children with fat malabsorption (e.g. liver disease, short gut syndrome).

If a commercial formula is unable to meet the specific requirements of an infant it is possible to formulate the feed from separate ingredients. These modular feeds allow a choice of protein, fat and carbohydrate and give the flexibility to meet the needs of individual patients. However they are expensive and time consuming to prepare and there is a greater risk of bacterial contamination and mistakes during preparation. It will also take several days to establish a child on a full strength modular feed (p. 84). Consequently, modular feeds should only be used if a ready-made feed is unsuitable and should ideally be prepared in a dedicated special feed preparation area.

Children 1–6 years (8–20 kg)

Special paediatric enteral feeds are available for the 1–6 year old age group who weigh between 8–20 kg. These feeds are also suitable for older children who are more than 6 years of age but fall within the weight range. The composition of paediatric enteral feeds ensures an appropriate intake of vitamins and minerals and is based on guidelines published in 1988 [4].

Table 3.2 The nutritional composition of paediatric enteral feeds

	Nutrini* (Nutricia)	Nutrini Extra (Nutricia)	Paediasure** (Ross Laboratories)	Frebini (Fresenius)
Energy (kcal/kJ)	100/420	150/630	101/422	100/420
Protein (g)	2.75	3.4	2.8	2.5
Fat (g)	4.5	6.8	5.0	4.0
Carbohydrate (g)	12.2	18.8	11.2	13.5
Vitamin A (μg)	45	67.5	45	40
Vitamin D (μg)	1.0	1.5	1.0	0.75
Vitamin C (mg)	4.0	6.0	5.0	4.5
Thiamin (mg)	0.06	0.1	0.15	0.2
Riboflavin (mg)	0.09	0.13	0.2	0.2
Niacin (mg)	1.07	1.6	1.2	0.9
Pantothenate (mg)	0.33	0.5	0.3	0.4
Vitamin B_6 (mg)	0.09	0.13	0.1	0.09
Folic acid (μg)	10	15	15	10
Biotin (μg)	4.2	6.25	5.0	6.0
Vitamin B_{12} (μg)	0.17	0.2	0.2	0.2
Vitamin E (mg)	0.6	0.9	1.0	0.6
Vitamin K (μg)	1.3	2.0	3.5	1.3
Sodium (mmol)	2.3	3.5	2.6	2.6
Potassium (mmol)	2.6	4.0	2.8	2.6
Phosphorus (mg)	39	58	53	50
Calcium (mg)	50	75	55	60
Iron (mg)	0.73	1.1	1.0	0.9
Magnesium (mg)	11	16	16	15
Zinc (mg)	0.73	1.1	1.0	0.9
Copper (μg)	87	130	100	100
Chromium (μg)	3.0	4.5	2.5	2.7
Manganese (mg)	0.13	0.2	0.1	0.15
Iodine (μg)	8.7	13	10	10
Selenium (μg)	2.5	3.8	2.5	2.0
Molybdenum (μg)	3.5	5.3	3.5	2.6
Choline (mg)	10	15	15	15
Osmolality (mOsm/kg)	245	370	286	250

* Nutrini Fibre has the same composition as Nutrini with the addition of 0.75 g fibre/100 ml

** Paediasure with Fibre has the same composition as Paediasure with the addition of 0.52 g fibre/100 ml

Paediatric feeds are based on cow's milk protein but are lactose-free and are available at 1 kcal (4 kJ)/ml and 1.5 kcal (6 kJ)/ml concentrations. Children who are troubled by constipation may benefit from an enteral feed supplemented with fibre. The composition of paediatric enteral feeds is outlined in Table 3.2.

Hydrolysed protein feeds are available for older children (e.g. Pepdite 2+). It is also sometimes necessary, as with infants, to use a modular feed (pp. 76, 84).

Children over 6 years (>20 kg)

The requirements of children over 6 years of age who are greater than 20 kg body weight are met using standard adult feeds. These are available in 1 kcal (4 kJ)/ml and 1.5 kcal (6 kJ)/ml concentrations. Adult peptide-based and elemental feeds can be used for children with impaired gut function and it is also necessary in special circumstances to employ the flexibility of a modular feed (pp. 76, 84).

Table 3.3 Choice of feeds for enteral feeding

	Normal gut function	Impaired gut function
Infants	Breast milk or normal infant formulas +/− energy/protein supplements or nutrient-dense infant formula (e.g. Infatrini, SMA High Energy)	Hydrolysed protein formula +/− energy supplements (e.g. Pregestimil, Pepti-Junior, Nutramigen) or modular feed
1–6 years (8–20 kg)	Standard paediatric enteral feed e.g. Nutrini, Paediasure, Frebini, Nutrini Extra	Hydrolysed protein formula +/− energy supplements (e.g. Pepdite 1+, MCT Pepdite 2+) or modular feed
6 years + (>20 kg)	Standard adult enteral feed e.g. Nutrison Standard, Osmolite, Ensure, Nutrison Energy Plus, Fortisip, Ensure Plus	Hydrolysed protein feeds +/− energy supplements (e.g. Pepdite 1+, Nutrison-Pepti) or modular feed

Some adult feeds have a protein content of 6 g/100 ml or more. Care should be taken when using such feeds for children even if they weigh in excess of 20 kg as they may provide an excessively high amount of protein.

The choice of feeds suitable for children is given in Table 3.3.

FEED THICKENERS

Feed thickeners can be a useful dietary intervention for children with gastro-oesophageal reflux. In addition to anti-reflux medication, feed thickeners can help to reduce vomiting. Feed thickeners can also be added to enteral feeds that would otherwise separate out when left to stand (e.g. Comminuted Chicken feed).

There is a wide range of commercially produced feed thickeners (p. 91). Most are suitable for thickening enteral feeds but it is worth remembering that some continue to thicken over time and may therefore be unsuitable for feeds delivered by continuous infusion. Thickened feeds may also be difficult to give as a bolus via a fine bore nasogastric tube, and syringe feeding may be necessary. Another point to consider is the energy contribution of some of the thickening agents. The thickeners based on modified starch given at a concentration of 3 g/100 ml may result in an increased energy content of more than 10%.

ROUTES OF ADMINISTRATION

Nasogastric feeding

Nasogastric is the most common route for enteral feeding and, unless prolonged enteral nutrition is anticipated, it would usually be the route of choice [5]. Passing a nasogastric tube can be distressing for both parents and children and careful preparation is beneficial [6]. Frank discussions and a clear explanation of the procedure can help older children, and play therapy with the use of dolls and picture books has been shown to alleviate anxieties in the younger age group. Older children, particularly teenagers, are naturally sensitive about their body image and they may be reluctant to start nasogastric feeding. Some children successfully pass their own nasogastric tube at night and remove their tube in the daytime which can be a successful way of administering supplementary feeds without the embarrassment of a permanent nasogastric tube.

It is essential to ensure that the nasogastric tube is situated in the stomach before feeding is commenced. The easiest and most common method is to aspirate a small quantity of gastric juice, which will turn litmus paper red. If the litmus test is unsuccessful the tube should be withdrawn and repassed as it is possible that the tube could have been sited or dislodged into the bronchus.

Long term nasogastric feeding in some children can cause inflammation and irritation to the skin

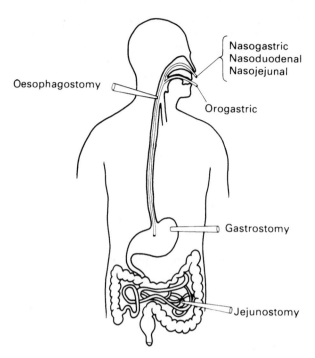

Fig. 3.1 Routes of enteral feeding

where the nasogastric tube is secured to the face. Use of Duoderm or Granuflex placed onto the skin can improve this. Another common problem, particularly with fine bore tubes, is tube blockage. Regular flushing of tubes can help to prevent this problem and the use of carbonated liquids can clear and prevent the build-up of feed within the lumen of the tube.

Gastrostomy feeding

Gastrostomy is a widely used route of feeding when longer term enteral nutrition is indicated [7]. Gastrostomy feeding is generally well accepted with children as it is more comfortable, obviates the need for frequent tube changes and is cosmetically more acceptable. Indications are not solely for long-term feeding; in certain situations gastrostomy feeding is the feeding route of choice. This includes children with congenital abnormalities such as tracheo-oesophageal fistula and oesophageal atresia and children with oesophageal injuries, e.g. following the ingestion of caustic chemicals. Contraindications include children with severe gastro-oesophageal

reflux, which can be worsened with the introduction of a gastrostomy tube [8].

The most popular technique for placing a gastrostomy tube is the percutaneous endoscopic gastrostomy (PEG) method [9]. A general anaesthetic is not usually required for its insertion making it a quicker technique with fewer complications than a surgically placed gastrostomy tube. After about 3 months, once the tract is formed, a child can be fitted with a gastrostomy button that sits almost flush against the skin. This is far more discreet than the tubing associated with a conventional gastrostomy catheter and is a popular choice, particularly with teenagers.

Gastrostomy tubes and buttons require less frequent changes than nasogastric tubes. A device secured by a deflatable balloon is easier to change than one secured by an internal bumper bar or disc. If a tube is inadvertently removed it should be replaced within 6–8 hours or the tract will start to close.

The main complication of gastrostomy feeding is leakage from around the gastrostomy site. This can cause severe inflammation and skin irritation and patients and parents should be taught about skin care.

Feeding into the jejunum

Indications for feeding into the jejunum include:

- Congenital gastrointestinal anomalies
- Gastric dysmotility
- Severe vomiting resulting in failure to thrive
- Children at risk of aspiration.

When children are fed directly into the jejunum, feed enters the intestine distal to the site of release of pancreatic enzymes and bile. Whole protein feeds can be used but malabsorption can occur due to inadequate digestion, so the use of hydrolysed feeds is recommended. Feeds delivered into the jejunum should always be given by continuous infusion. The stomach acts as a reservoir for food in the normally fed child, regulating the amount of food that is delivered into the small intestine. Feed given as a bolus into the small intestine can cause abdominal pain, diarrhoea and dumping syndrome resulting from rebound hypoglycaemia.

Placement of a naso-jejunal tube is difficult and maintaining the position of the tube causes numerous problems. The position of the tube can be checked using pH paper. The tube can spontaneously resite into the stomach or can be inadvertently pulled back, and weighted tubes do not seem to be of much value in preventing this occurring [10]. For longer term feeding a jejunostomy tube or a gastro-jejunal tube is usually a more successful route for nutritional support.

Complications can include bacterial overgrowth, malabsorption, bowel perforation and tube blockage. Like nasogastric and gastrostomy tubes, jejunostomy tubes need regular flushing to maintain patency but in contrast it is recommended that sterile water is always used.

The advantages and disadvantages of the routes of feed administration are given in Table 3.4.

Orogastric feeding

This route is principally used for feeding neonates where nasal access is not feasible or where breathing would be compromised. The tube is passed via the mouth into the stomach. If all feeds are given via the orogastric tube it can be taped in place, but if the infant is taking some breast or bottle feeds the tube can be passed as required and removed between feeds.

Gastrostomy coupled with oesophagostomy

Following surgery in infants born with tracheo-oesophageal fistulas it is not always possible to join the upper and lower ends of the oesophagus in continuity. When the baby has grown, surgical reconnection will be considered at a later date. Until this time the child receives nutrition via a gastrostomy tube but is encouraged to feed orally to learn normal feeding skills. The food that is taken orally is collected at a cervical oesophagostomy site (p. 97).

CONTINUOUS VERSUS BOLUS FEEDING

Enteral feeds can be given continuously via an enteral feeding pump, or as boluses, or a combination of both. A regimen should be chosen to meet the individual requirements of the child and in most cases it can be tailored to the most practical method of feeding to cause minimum disruption to the child's lifestyle and that of their family. Certain situations will dictate a preferred feeding regimen, but a flexible approach to feeding should be taken wherever possible. This enables the child to maintain their usual day-to-day activities and for the family to experience minimal disruption to their lifestyle and routines. Flexibility is especially important in

Table 3.4 Advantages and disadvantages of various routes of feed administration

Nasogastric feeds	Gastrostomy feeds	Jejunostomy feeds
Advantages	*Advantages*	*Advantages*
• No surgical procedure required	• Percutaneous gastrostomy tubes can be inserted without a general anaesthetic	• No possibility of aspiration
• Procedure can be easily taught		• No nightly insertion of tube
• Non-invasive	• No nightly insertion of tube	
Disadvantages	*Disadvantages*	*Disadvantages*
• Nausea	• Nausea	• Nausea
• Dislodgement of the tubes with coughing	• Vomiting associated with coughing and reflux	• Tube blockage
• Vomiting associated with coughing and reflux	• Feeling full	• Placed under general anaesthesia
• Feeling full	• Local infection	• Increase risk of nutrient malabsorption
• Difficulty in inserting nasogastric tube	• Leakage around the tube causing granuloma formation	• Leakage around the tube causing granuloma formation
• Irritation to the nose and throat	• Possibility of aspiration	• Local infection
• Possibility of aspiration	• Tube blockage	• Tube dislodgement

By kind permission of A. MacDonald

children with a need for long-term tube feeding who, as time passes, will need a feed that is appropriate to their age and changing nutritional requirements and a regimen that is adaptable as they grow and develop.

Continuous feeding

Generally children will tolerate a slow, continuous infusion of feed better than bolus feeds and this method is frequently chosen when enteral feeding is first started. Potentially there are fewer problems with intolerance when small feed volumes are infused continuously and there is a smaller time commitment for ward staff and for parents and carers at home. Mobility is affected but is minimised by the use of portable feeding pumps, particularly for children who are on continuous feeding for longer than 12 hours. These portable pumps can be carried by older children as backpacks and for infants can be carried by carers or attached to a pram. Children under 6 years are often too small to carry a heavy backpack, yet cannot be kept still for long periods of continuous feeding. In these children the extra hours of feeding can sometimes be achieved during daytime sleeps and when they are occupied with quieter tasks or watching television and videos.

There are situations where continuous feeding is essential. As discussed above, feeds given through a feeding jejunostomy should always be delivered by continuous infusion. Severe gastro-oesophageal reflux can be managed with a slow continuous infusion of feed as an adjunct to anti-reflux medication and positioning. Infants and children with malabsorption will benefit from a continuous infusion of feed. This will slow transit time and may improve symptoms of diarrhoea, steatorrhoea and abdominal cramps and help to promote weight gain. In children with protracted diarrhoea and short bowel syndrome, continuous enteral feeding with a specialised formula often forms the basis of medical management, and continuous tube feeding with an elemental feed is a well established treatment option for children with Crohn's disease to induce remission of disease. Infants and children with glycogen storage disease type I require a constant supply of dietary glucose to maintain their blood glucose levels within normal limits. Continuous overnight nasogastric feeding is used to provide glucose overnight until children are established on cornstarch therapy at 2–3 years of age.

Intermittent bolus feeding

Bolus tube feeding is successfully used in many children requiring enteral feeding both in hospital and at home. Giving boluses three to four hourly throughout the day via the nasogastric or gastrostomy tube mimics a physiologically normal feeding pattern and can be adapted to fit in with family mealtimes. It is more time consuming than continuous feeding but is the preferred method for many families with children requiring long-term feeding as it gives them greater freedom and mobility.

There are situations where bolus feeding is recommended. Neonates requiring small volumes may need to be given their feed by hourly bolus as the length of tubing between the reservoir and child creates a 'dead space' holding feed. This can be particularly relevant in infants fed EBM as some fat can be lost by adherence to the sides of the burette and tubing [11]. Children who have had a surgical anti-reflux procedure are unable to vomit. Large volumes of feed from a continuous infusion can accumulate in the stomach and remain undetected in children who have gastric stasis or poor gastrointestinal motility. This can lead to gastric rupture. Bolus feeding with a gravity feeding pack will prevent over-filling of the stomach as tubes are routinely aspirated before each feed and further feed will be prevented from entering the stomach from the feeding chamber if the stomach is already full. Children who frequently try to remove their nasogastric tube risk aspiration if the end of the tube is dislodged into the airways. They will benefit from bolus feeding as they can be constantly supervised during the feed. Children with an oesophagostomy who are sham fed should preferably receive bolus feeds to coincide with their oral feeds. Finally, the continuous delivery of enteral feeds may interfere with the absorption of medication. Bolus feeding will provide periods of rest when medication can be given to allow optimal absorption.

A schedule of feeding regimens is given in Table 3.5.

ENTERAL FEEDING EQUIPMENT

Nasogastric feeding tubes

There is a wide range of paediatric feeding tubes available. The tubes are of varying lengths and gauges to meet the requirements of children of all ages. All

Table 3.5 Choosing a suitable feeding regimen

Regimen	Example
Bolus top-up feeding	*Congenital heart disease* Bottle feeds are not completed due to breathlessness and remaining feed is topped up via the nasogastric tube
Exclusive bolus feeding	*Long-term feeding for children with a neurological handicap* Daytime bolus feeding can allow flexibility and mobility and provide a regimen that can fit in with the family mealtimes *Post-fundoplication* Bolus feeding is the method of choice for children following a surgical anti-reflux procedure *Sham feeding* Children who are sham fed should receive a bolus feed to coincide with oral feeds
Combination of bolus and continuous feeding	*Chronic illness* Children with anorexia associated with chronic illness may receive a large proportion of their nutrition via a nasogastric or gastrostomy tube. Daytime boluses allow for a normal meal pattern and overnight feeding with a feeding pump reduces the time commitment at night for parents and ward staff.
Overnight feeding only	*Supplementary nutrition* Children who require enteral feeding to supplement their poor oral intake or to meet their increased nutritional requirements are usually fed overnight only. This allows the children to maintain a normal daytime eating pattern whilst still providing the nutritional support they require.
Continuous feeding only	*Primary disease management* Gastro-oesophageal reflux Malabsorption syndromes (e.g. short gut) Crohn's disease Glycogen storage disease

tubes should conform to British Standards BS 6314 with a male luer connection to avoid connection with intravenous lines and should be radio-opaque to help confirm position. For children, an ideal tube should be of a small gauge with a large internal diameter to make the tube more comfortable and cosmetically acceptable. All tubes will have a syringe adaptor to use for flushing, aspiration or administration of drugs. Some tubes may also have separate side ports.

Polyvinylchloride (PVC) tubes are used for short term enteral feeding. They require changing every week as the tubes stiffen over time and may cause tissue damage. These tubes are less likely to be displaced than a polyurethane tube so can also be used for children who are prone to vomiting (e.g. children with gastro-oesophageal reflux or children receiving chemotherapy).

Fine bore polyurethane or silicone tubes are de-signed for longer term nasogastric feeding and are very much softer and more comfortable than PVC tubes. Each tube comes with a guidewire or stylet to give the tube rigidity when passed. Tubes can remain in situ for 4–6 weeks but can also be used for overnight feeding and removed during the daytime if storage and cleaning instructions are carefully adhered to. When passing polyurethane tubes there is a high risk of continuous tracheal intubation in children who have an impaired swallow or who are ventilated. In these children PVC tubes may be preferable despite the need for longer term feeding.

Gastrostomy devices

Gastrostomy devices evolved considerably in the 1990s with an increasing amount of equipment entering the specialised paediatric market. Gastrostomy tubes, whether inserted by an open procedure or a percutaneous endoscopic method, are manufactured from pliable, biocompatible silicone. PEG tubes are held in place by a cross bar or bumper preventing inadvertent removal and require repeat endoscopy for change of tube or replacement with a gastrostomy button once the tract has formed. Surgically placed gastrostomy tubes are secured by an inflated balloon which allows easy replacement of the tube. They also have a skin level retention disc preventing migration of the tube. Foley catheters may be used as gastrostomy tubes but they require strapping securely in place, as they have no retention disc and may easily migrate into the duodenum. Children requiring long term gastrostomy feeding will usually elect to have a gastrostomy button once a tract has been established. These devices are secured within the stomach by an inflated balloon facilitating removal and replacement.

Enteral feeding pumps

Choice of feeding pumps will depend on the requirements of individual hospitals and individual children but there are a number of features that are either essential or desirable:

- Occlusion and low battery alarms
- Easy to operate
- Durable
- Tamper proof
- Easy to clean
- Low noise
- Small and lightweight if designed to be portable
- Long battery life if designed to be portable
- Accurate flow rate setting (5–10%)
- Small flow rate increments (1 ml preferable)
- Option of bolus feeding
- Good servicing backup

Reservoirs

There are many different reservoirs on the market. Generally children require smaller reservoirs than adults do, especially when using a portable system. Whatever choice is made, the reservoir and giving set should be changed every 24 hours and discarded. Any

practice of sterilisation and re-use potentially leads to infection and is not recommended.

Studies have shown that feed contamination is common [12, 13] so feed should always be decanted in a clean environment. Some standard feeds can be used directly from a pre-filled container connected directly to the giving set. The majority of infants and children requiring feeds will need the feed to be decanted into a reservoir. Infants requiring small volumes of feed may have their feed decanted into a burette, which has a small capacity and is principally for hospital use. Larger volumes of feeds are delivered from either a rigid plastic container or a feeding bag, which are both available in a range of sizes. These are ideal for paediatrics where the use of modified formulas and modular feeds is common.

Home enteral feeding

When a decision is made to commence enteral feeding at home it is important that the parents undergo a training programme that will teach them to look after all aspects of feeding and equipment safely. Correct procedures and adherence to safety are paramount and all parents and carers will require help and supervision to become familiar with the techniques involved prior to hospital discharge. Whilst it is essential that the child receives adequate nutrition the enteral feeding regimen should be planned to fit in as much as possible with the family's lifestyle [14]. The social and emotional aspects of tube feeding are often overlooked [15]. Pictorial teaching aids may be used to help non-English speaking families and those unable to read and follow written guidelines [16]. It is essential to identify and liaise with community staff who will be sharing care when a child is discharged; they will have a key role in supporting the child and family.

Home enteral feeding companies can supply both feeds and feeding equipment directly to the homes. With more companies providing a home delivery service the market has become competitive and hospital and community trusts are benefiting from improved deals. The companies may insist on the use of their own brand of pumps and feeds so it is important to ensure the child gets a suitable infusion pump and the feed that has been prescribed. Enteral feeds are prescribed by the general practitioner; however, the costs for disposable equipment are generally funded by hospital departments or purchasing authorities. BAPEN (the British Association for Parenteral and Enteral Nutrition) continues to lobby government for enteral feeding to be managed as a total package by making equipment, as well as feeds, prescribable items.

FEED ADMINISTRATION AND TOLERANCE

The way in which a feed is administered ultimately depends on the clinical condition of the individual child and there are no set rules for starting enteral feeds. Neonates may need to be started on just 1 ml/hr infusion rates whereas older children may tolerate rates of 100 ml/hr. In most cases feeds can be started at full strength with the volume being gradually increased in stages either at an increased infusion rate or as a larger bolus.

Gastrointestinal symptoms are the most common complications of enteral feeding but with the wide choice of feeds, administration techniques and enteral feeding devices it should be possible to minimise gastrointestinal symptoms.

Some causes of feed intolerance and their resolution are given in Table 3.6.

Table 3.6 Feed intolerance

Symptom	Cause	Solution
Diarrhoea	Unsuitable choice of feed in children with impaired gut function	Change to hydrolysed formula or modular feed
	Fast infusion rate	Slow infusion rate and increase as tolerated to provide required nutrition
	Intolerance of bolus feeds	Frequent, smaller feeds or change to continuous infusion
	High feed osmolarity	Build up strength of feeds and deliver by continuous infusion
	Contamination of feed	Use sterile commercially produced feeds wherever possible and prepare other feeds in clean environments
	Drugs (e.g. antibiotics, laxatives)	Consider drugs as a cause of diarrhoea before feed is stopped or reduced
Nausea and vomiting	Fast infusion rate	Slowly increase rate of feed infusion
	Slow gastric emptying	Correct positioning and drugs
	Psychological factors	Address behavioural feeding issues
	Constipation	Maintain regular bowel motions with adequate fluid intakes and laxatives
	Medicines given at the same time as feeds	Allow time between giving medicines and giving feeds or stop continuous feed for a short time when medicines are given
Regurgitation and aspiration	Gastro-oesophageal reflux	Correct positioning, anti-reflux drugs, feed thickener, fundoplication
	Dislodged tubes	Secure tube adequately and test position of tube regularly
	Fast infusion rate	Slow infusion rate
	Intolerance of bolus feeds	Smaller, more frequent feeds or continuous infusion

MONITORING CHILDREN ON ENTERAL FEEDS

Children who are commenced on enteral feeding require monitoring. At the initiation of enteral feeding, goals will be set with respect to an improvement in nutritional status or control of symptoms, and regular follow-up is required to monitor both short-term and longer-term progress. Anthropometry, blood monitoring and control of symptoms all have a role to play in monitoring progress. As children gain weight and get older their requirements change and follow-up is essential to ensure they continue to receive adequate nutrition. Although enteral feeds are formulated to be nutritionally complete it is wise to check nutritional status with blood tests particularly if tube feeding is the sole source of nutrition (p. 9). Routine checks of albumin, electrolytes and haemoglobin are useful as well as assessment of micronutrient status. Blood tests can also be helpful in assessing response to nutritional therapy, e.g. monitoring of inflammatory markers as well as assessment of symptoms can measure the success of feeding in children with active Crohn's disease. Both hospital and community staff have a role to play in monitoring a child's progress and helping the family cope with tube feeding at home. The needs of a young infant are quite different from those of a toddler or teenager and the individual needs of each child should be considered at different stages of their development.

Regular follow-up can also be important for the family as well as the child. Home enteral feeding has a big impact on family life, resulting in both psychological and practical problems which should be addressed regularly [15, 17].

Another important aspect of follow-up is the encouragement to maintain oral feeding skills. Children who miss out on early experiences of taste and texture are much more likely to develop feeding problems. Offering a small amount of food gives children the chance to use the lips and tongue and develop their oromotor skills whilst experiencing a range of tastes. This is particularly important around the time of weaning from 4–6 months when children are often more willing to accept different food [18].

REFERENCES

1 Balmer SE *et al.* *Guidelines for the collection, storage and handling of mother's breast milk to be fed to her own baby on a neonatal unit.* London: British Association of Perinatal Medicine, 1997.

2 *Infant Formula and Follow-on Regulations.* Statutory Instrument No. 77. London: The Stationery Office, 1995.

3 Clarke SE *et al.* Impaired growth and nitrogen deficiency in infants receiving an energy supplemented standard infant formula. *Proceedings of the Royal College of Paediatrics and Child Health Annual Spring Meeting 1998.* Abstract G132, 2–75.

4 Russell C *et al. Paediatric Enteral Feeding Solutions and Systems.* A Report by the joint working party of the Paediatric Group and Parenteral and Enteral Nutrition Group of the British Dietetic Association. Birmingham: BDA, 1988.

5 Puntis JWL *et al.* Home enteral nutrition in paediatric practice. *Brit J Hosp Med,* 1991, **45** 104–107.

6 Holden CE *et al.* Psychological preparation and support of children undergoing enteral nutrition: an evaluation. *Brit J Nurs,* 1997, **6** 376–85.

7 Taylor E *et al.* Supplementary feeding using a gastrostomy button. *Paed Nurs,* 1990, 16–19 Dec.

8 Khattak IU *et al.* Percutaneous endoscopic gastrostomy in paediatric practice: complications and outcome. *J Paediatr Surg,* 1998 Jan, **33** 67–72.

9 Caulfield MP Percutaneous endoscopic gastrostomy placement in children. *Gastrointest Endosc Clin NAm.* 1994, **4** 179–93.

10 Rees RGP *et al.* Spontaneous transpyloric passage and performance of fine bore polyurethane feeding tubes. A controlled clinical trial. *J Parent Ent Nutr,* 1998, **12** 469–72.

11 Brook OG *et al.* Loss of energy during continuous infusions of breast milk. *Arch Dis Childh,* 1978, **53** 344–5.

12 Patchell CJ Bacterial contamination of enteral feeds. *Arch Dis Childh,* 1994, **170** 327–30.

13 Anderton A *et al.* Problems with the re-use of enteral feeding system. A study of design of enteral feeding sets. *J Hum Nutr Diet,* 1991, **4** 25–32.

14 Sidey A *et al.* Enteral Feeding in Community Setting. *Paediatr Nurs,* 1995, **7** 21–4.

15 Holden CE *Enteral and parenteral nutrition: Feeding at home impact on family life and the implications for home care.* MSc, Wolverhampton University, 1994.

16 Sexton E *et al.* A pictorial assisted teaching tool for families. *Paediatr Nurs,* June 1996, 8 24–6.

17 Holden CE *et al.* Nasogastric feeding at home: acceptability and safety. *Arch Dis Childh,* 1991, **66** 148–51.

18 Feeding Liaison Team 1998: *Parents Positive Action for Feeding.* The Birmingham Childrens Hospital NHS Trust.

SUPPORT GROUP

Patients on Intravenous and Nasogastric Nutrition Therapy (PINNT) is a support group for patients receiving parenteral or enteral nutrition with a sub-group HALF PINNT for children. The group promotes public awareness and encourages contact between patients receiving similar treatment. As well as providing general support the group provides assistance with claiming benefits and can provide members with portable equipment for holidays.

PINNT
P O Box 3126, Christchurch, Dorset BH23 2XS

CHAPTER 4

Parenteral Nutrition

Intravenous feeding was one of the major medical developments of the twentieth century. Parenteral nutrition (PN) is now an established therapy, to which many patients of all ages owe their lives. It has transformed the outcome for many conditions including feeding the preterm infant and for post-surgical short gut neonates [1].

As with many life-saving procedures PN is not without its risks and is associated with fatal complications. PN should, therefore, not be used casually but in a disciplined and organised manner in carefully selected patients [2, 3].

INDICATIONS FOR PARENTERAL NUTRITION

General guidelines

It is widely accepted that enteral feeding should be used wherever possible. If the gut works, use it [3, 4]. Parenteral nutrition is a hazardous and expensive form of nutritional support and should only be used if the enteral route has failed, or is expected to fail. Even during PN it is important to maintain some degree of enteral nutrition whenever possible, as the complete absence of luminal nutrients has been associated with atrophic changes in the gut mucosa [3, 5]. Nutritionally insignificant volumes of enteral nutrition have been found to have a trophic effect on the gut and have been linked to enhanced gut motility, decreased incidence of PN induced cholestasis and bacterial translocation [6, 7].

There is little clinical or nutritional justification for parenteral nutrition for less than 5 days. Many centres gradually build up the concentration of the solutions over 3–4 days, hence achieving maximum concentration and nutritional adequacy at day 4. The risks outweigh any minor nutritional gains in very short courses of PN [8].

Parenteral feeding is not an emergency procedure; electrolyte imbalances should be corrected before PN commences.

Common indications for children

The indications for the use of PN for children listed here have not been determined by controlled clinical trials but are representative of clinical experience in many centres in the UK [2]. PN may be indicated under the following circumstances to supplement or replace enteral feeding:

Limited tolerance of enteral feeding
- Low birthweight/premature infants
- Surgical gastrointestinal abnormalities, e.g. gastroschisis/intestinal atresia
- Short bowel syndrome
- Necrotising enterocolitis
- Protracted diarrhoea
- Malabsorption syndromes
- Inflammatory bowel disease
- Chemotherapy/bone marrow transplants

Patients requiring additional nutrition support
- Trauma/burns
- Chronic renal failure
- Liver disease
- Malignant disease

NUTRITION SUPPORT TEAMS

Parenteral feeding requires considerable clinical, pharmaceutical and nursing skills, and the use of special laboratory facilities for the biochemical monitoring of small blood samples. Children who require PN should be cared for by staff who are experienced in the prescription, production and care of PN and its equipment. This is often facilitated by a multidisciplinary nutrition team, and many centres now follow this principle [3, 9]. The team usually plans regimens and provides training in the care, prescription and monitoring of patients on PN. The nutrition support team is usually monitored by a nutrition steering committee which produces protocols and procedures and organises audit and reviews of the PN service [10, 11].

Core members of the multidisciplinary nutrition team vary from centre to centre. Good interdisciplinary communication is paramount if patient care is to be of the highest standard. Core members are usually:

- Consultants – overseeing the patient care
- Surgical registrar – who inserts feeding lines
- Medical registrar – advising with regard to prescription of PN and other aspects of care
- Senior pharmacist – production of solutions, stability
- Intravenous therapy nurse – advising and care of lines etc.
- Biochemist – advising on monitoring and interpretation of blood biochemistry
- Dietitian – (see section on role of the dietitian below).

Nutrition teams usually review the child's progress at least weekly, with reviews by some individual members daily. In centres where nutrition teams have been established, reported benefits include a reduction in mechanical line problems, reduced sepsis, fewer metabolic complications, shorter courses of PN (due to faster transition to appropriate enteral formulas) and savings on the cost of providing PN [12].

ROLE OF THE DIETITIAN

Patient selection

As paediatric dietitians have a great expertise in nutritional assessment, provision and monitoring of enteral feeds in hospital, they are ideally suited to advise on patient selection for PN. The dietitian will usually be aware if the enteral route has been adequately trialed before considering PN and can advise on the most appropriate enteral feed to use while on PN or during the weaning period.

Baseline nutritional assessment

The dietitian may assess and record the nutritional status of the child, review the feeding history and advise on the degree of malnutrition, and any possible micronutrient inadequacies. For many children who have had long-term poor nutrition it may be necessary to advise the team to consider evaluating micronutrient status before PN commences, as chronic under nutrition may lead to vitamin and mineral deficiences. The dietitian may also perform regular anthropometry as part of the assessment and monitoring processes.

Estimating energy and protein requirements

The dietitian is often the most competent member of the team at estimation of energy and protein requirements and may advise on individual goals for energy and protein intakes. In many centres, dietitians are involved in the production of protocols and procedures to advise on the aims for energy and protein content of PN for each age/weight range in children.

Monitoring

The dietitian may monitor actual intake on PN (from PN and enteral feeds) versus prescription. This is often not the same; flow rates are altered for drugs, time off for investigations, play etc. resulting in missed nutrition. Once highlighted this can be solved by ensuring flow rates allow for these missed hours. The dietitian may assess if enteral feeding is being considered regularly or used appropriately. As with patients on enteral feeds, the dietitian will monitor growth and progress while on PN.

Weaning from PN to enteral nutrition

Ideally some degree of enteral nutrition will be maintained during the period on PN via the most appropriate route and type of feed. The strength and speed of delivery will be gradually increased in line with tolerance and maintained growth parameters.

If fluid restriction is not a major issue, once enteral feeds/diet are providing at least 25% of the total requirements a corresponding reduction could be made to the PN solution. Once 50% of requirements are met by enteral feeds/diet the PN could be decreased to 50%, with a further decrease to 25% once 75% of requirements are met by the enteral route. When more than 75% of requirements are achieved by enteral nutrition the PN could be stopped in most cases [13].

If fluid restriction is a complicating factor the PN will usually need to be decreased by each millilitre that the enteral nutrition is increased (although a greater fluid volume is usually tolerated via the enteral route than parenteral route). Care and attention to actual intake should be employed in these cases to ensure maximum nutrition is achieved, as enteral feeds are often less concentrated than PN. This is especially important in infancy or for malnourished children.

GENERAL PRINCIPLES FOR PN FOR CHILDREN

There are important differences between children and adults which should be taken into account when prescribing PN.

PN for children needs to provide sufficient nutrients to allow normal growth and body composition [3]. The daily requirement for fluid, protein, fat, carbohydrate and electrolytes varies considerably according to age, weight and growth rate. The requirements may also be increased or decreased during periods of nutritional stress as a result of the clinical condition, e.g. in malabsorption or catabolic states [14].

Children have lower nutritional stores than adults and have widely varying abilities to withstand starvation. A low birthweight neonate may only survive 4–7 days without nutrition whereas a one year old child may survive one month [15]. This has important implications for the individual child and must be a major consideration in deciding when to start PN.

Infants are a vulnerable group of patients. The brain grows rapidly during the first year of life and is sensitive during this time to periods of malnutrition and metabolic insult. Special care should be taken to avoid malnutrition and biochemical abnormalities at this time (e.g. hypernatraemia or hyperaminoacidaemia) [14, 16].

PN induced cholestasis is common among paediatric patients, especially neonates on long-term PN. Cholestasis is often reversible after PN stops. Some infants are at risk of irreversible liver failure associated with cholestasis; these infants have usually had intestinal surgery and sepsis. Strategies to avoid/minimise cholestasis include [7, 17]:

- Giving small amounts of enteral feeds each day (even if <10% total energy)
- Cycling PN
- Decreasing a high protein load
- Reducing trace element solutions temporarily
- Giving long term antibiotics to avoid sepsis.

Essential amino acid requirements differ for children. Histidine is an essential acid in infancy in addition to the eight required by older children and adults. Tyrosine, cysteine and taurine are usually included in amino acid solutions used in infancy as they cannot be synthesised in adequate amounts by the young infant; proline and alanine may also be semi-essential [18]. Some amino acid solutions produced for adult use have high levels of some amino acids (e.g. phenylalanine) which may be detrimental to the developing brain [14]. Products have been developed to provide optimal nutritional support for the paediatric patient, especially infants, e.g. Primene and Vaminolact. These products are associated with fewer metabolic complications than the products designed for adult use [19].

Infants have immature organ systems to excrete high sodium loads, and need a high volume of fluid in order to excrete sufficiently. Dehydration can occur, as can metabolic acidosis. Care should always be taken to ensure that adequate fluid requirements are met.

It is important, especially in long-term PN, to ensure oral feeding is maintained. Whenever possible tastes, textures of food and/or use of dummies etc. should be employed to stimulate oral function, especially in infancy. The advice of a speech therapist is invaluable.

Children need to maintain mobility while on PN. Portable IV pumps and PN regimens which allow time off the infusion may be necessary to make longer term PN tolerable and allow for play and development of the child. Once PN is well established the time required for delivery of the infusion should be decreased with an increase in flow rates to allow for this. Many children progress gradually to increase the number of hours off PN each day, the hours on

PN decreasing by 2 hours per day until maximum tolerance is achieved at approximately 12 hours per day for most children. This should not be attempted until the child is stable for at least a week.

There is an increasing number of children who require very long-term PN. These children or their families are taught how to administer PN and care for their catheters to allow the child to be discharged home on PN. Home PN needs a considerable commitment on behalf of the family and medical team to ensure safety and success [3, 20]. This takes many weeks to plan and carry out and for safety's sake should not be undertaken lightly; however it can work well, if supported, for many children whose only option in the past was long-term hospitalisation.

NUTRIENT REQUIREMENTS AND SOLUTIONS

There is no comprehensive guide to the nutritional requirements of infants and children receiving PN. There are very few clinical trials on requirements for children on PN. Nutrient intakes vary at different centres and tend to be based on clinical experience [3, 8, 18, 21].

Fluid

Basic daily fluid requirements and other factors affecting fluid needs are described in detail elsewhere [22]. Age, size, fluid balance, the environment and clinical conditions are all factors affecting fluid requirements. Cardiac impairment, renal disease and respiratory insufficiency are examples of conditions which may limit available fluid volumes, whereas high fluid losses due to diarrhoea, high output fistula and fever may all increase fluid needs.

When considering PN, the available fluid allowance should be considered initially. (*Note* – some of the fluid allowance may be used by medication.) The available fluid volume for PN may influence the choice of nutrient solutions and the route of delivery. If concentrated PN solutions are needed to provide adequate nutrition (due to fluid restrictions), then the peripheral route may be contraindicated as there is a risk that concentrated solutions will cause thrombophlebitis. Children who are severely fluid restricted will only receive adequate nutrition if the concentrated PN is delivered via a central venous catheter.

Normal fluid requirements [3]

Infants up to 10 kg
0–12 months   150–110 ml/kg/day

Volume may be increased by 10 ml/kg/day until the required energy intake is achieved (according to fluid tolerance). Additional fluid may be needed if radiant heaters/phototherapy is used.

Children over 10 kg
1–6 years   100–80 ml/kg/day
6–12 years   80–75 ml/kg/day
12–18 years   75–50 ml/kg/day

Energy

Many well infants and children will achieve their expected growth rate if the energy intakes in Table 4.1 are provided. In illness these requirements may vary depending on the severity of the condition. An appropriate gain in weight for the age, sex, size of the individual child whilst considering the clinical condition is likely to indicate that the prescription is adequate. All children on PN should therefore be weighed and measured regularly and these measurements recorded and plotted on growth charts to ensure appropriate growth is maintained.

Table 4.1 Estimated average requirements (EAR) for energy and protein

Age	Mean weight (a) kg	Energy intake (b) kcal/kg/day	Protein intake (c) g/kg/day	Nitrogen intake (d) g/kg/day
0–3 months	5.0	115	2.9	0.46
4–12 months	8.3	95	2.4	0.38
1–3 years	12.1	95	2.4	0.38
4–6 years	18.0	85	2.1	0.34
7–10 years	26.7	66	1.7	0.26
11–14 years	40.0	47	1.2	0.19
15–18 years	60.0	41	1.0	0.16

(a) Adapted from Annex 1 (Table A.2, Dietary Reference Values, 1991)
(b) Derived from [23] (WHO)
(c) Based on 10% energy intake from protein
(d) Nitrogen intake $(g) = \dfrac{\text{protein intake (g)}}{6.25}$

In the past energy requirements were often over-estimated, especially in burns and trauma, resulting in overfeeding from PN. Recent research suggests that actual energy requirements for many children are less than originally thought and maximum increases of 10–15% above normal requirements are seen in trauma/burns, and not 50% as previously estimated [24]. Whatever estimate of energy requirement is used for an individual child it is essential to monitor closely to ensure appropriate growth achieved without adverse biochemical consequences.

Energy sources

Carbohydrate

Glucose and fat should be used as non-protein energy sources, although the use of intravenous fat has been associated with certain complications:

- Altered immune function
- Fat overload syndrome
- Free radical production.

The use of glucose alone is not recommended [3, 25]. It can cause hyperglycaemia, fatty liver, excessive carbon dioxide production and essential fatty acid deficiency [26]. The use of fats can help prevent thrombophlebitis when PN is given peripherally [27]. In addition the use of a glucose lipid regimen has been shown to reduce whole body protein turnover and produce higher net protein synthesis rates when compared to glucose alone. Approximately 250 kcal (1045 kJ) should be given per gram of nitrogen to allow for nitrogen use [28].

Dextrose (D-glucose) is the most commonly used source of non-protein energy in PN. Solutions which contain 5%, 10% and 50% glucose are mixed to provide the desired concentration. The energy content and approximate osmolality of various glucose concentrations are shown in Table 4.2. Glucose is an essential fuel for infants and is the most important substrate for brain cell metabolism. A continuous supply is essential for normal neurological function.

Dextrose solutions have a high osmolality; most centres use 10% dextrose on the first day of PN. The concentration of dextrose may increase in a stepwise manner as required. Peripheral infusions do not

Table 4.2 Intravenous carbohydrate solutions

Solution	Energy kcal/l	Osmolality mOsm/kg H_2O
5% Dextrose	200	277
10% Dextrose	400	555
20% Dextrose	800	1110
50% Dextrose	2000	2775

usually contain more than 10–12% dextrose due to the increased risk of thrombophlebitis with such a hypertonic solution [29]. A gradual increase in dextrose concentration allows time for an increase in the rate of endogenous insulin production which reduces the risk of glycosuria and osmotic diuresis [30].

The amount of glucose that can be directly oxidised to meet a child's energy need is limited. Reports have suggested that infusion rates should not exceed 7 mg/kg/minute initially [20] but can be increased to 12–14 mg/kg/minute after 5–7 days feeding [8]. Total glucose intake should not exceed 18 g/kg/day (often lower than this before hyperglycaemia occurs) [26]. Hyperglycaemia can easily occur in certain clinical situations at much lower doses, for example, very low birthweight neonates, sepsis, or stress/trauma (often due to insulin resistance – glucose doses may need to be reduced) [26]. Higher infusion rates result in the conversion of carbohydrate to fatty acids. This process consumes up to 15% of the available glucose energy [31].

Fat/lipid

Intravenous fat preparations provide a concentrated source of energy in an isotonic solution. If the fluid intake is not restricted, the use of a lipid emulsion via a peripheral vein will help to provide sufficient energy for growth, avoiding the complications associated with central venous access, and it may prolong the life of peripheral lines in infants [21].

When the fluid volume is limited, maximum energy intake can only be achieved via a central venous catheter by using dextrose : fat mixtures. Lipid emulsions normally contribute 30% of non-protein energy as fat [3].

A range of lipid based products are available in the UK, containing soybean oil, glycerol and phospholipids in 10%, 20% and 30% emulsions. Fat emulsions currently used are either based on long chain

triglycerides or long chain and medium chain triglycerides mixed together. The latter were thought to
have a more rapid clearance from the blood.

The most commonly used fat intakes are
0.5–4 g/kg/day, with serum lipid levels monitored
to ensure adequate clearance and hence utilisation. Clearance of lipids from the plasma is limited by
the rate of activity of lipoprotein lipase. Hyperlipidaemia will result if the enzyme is saturated by excessive doses of fat or by rapid infusion [25, 32]. Maximum fat tolerance is usually achieved by gradually
increasing the volume of the lipid emulsion by
1 g/kg/day over 4 days and by maintaining a steady
rate of infusion, giving 4 hours off the infusion per
24 hours to allow all administered fat to clear the circulation before the next infusion begins. Serum lipids
should be monitored as the volume of fat increases
and should always be taken 4 hours after the infusion
is completed. Peak levels of triglyceride and free
fatty acids normally occur towards the end of the
infusion, returning to fasting levels 2–4 hours later.
Once they are stable, weekly monitoring is likely to be
sufficient.

In malnourished children, it is good practice to
assess baseline serum lipids prior to starting PN.
Children who have failed to thrive frequently have
raised triglyceride levels which return to normal
when sufficient energy is provided. A reduced dose of
fat (0.5–2 g/kg/day) may be indicated for children
with hyperbilirubinaemia, sepsis, impaired immune
function, blood coagulopathies, chronic liver failure,
and very low birthweight infants [33].

As essential fatty acid (EFA) deficiency occurs
more readily in children than in adults, care
should be taken to ensure sufficient fat is provided
to avoid this. Biochemical evidence of deficiency
has been reported after receiving fat-free PN for
only 2 days, yet EFA deficiency can be avoided by
giving only 2–4% total energy as lipid [34]. For
example:

2–5 ml/kg/d   Intralipid   20%   will   provide
   0.5 g fat/kg/d and 5% total energy for an infant
2.4% total energy from n-6 linoleic acid (reference
   nutrient intake 1%)
0.4% total energy from n-3 linolenic acid (reference
   nutrient intake 0.2%)

Therefore, even when fat tolerance is impaired, essential fatty acid deficiency can be avoided in most children. A 20% fat emulsion is most commonly used for
infants and children since it contains half the amount
of phospholipids per gram of fat compared to a 10%
solution. Phospholipids are known to inhibit the
activity of lipoprotein lipase.

Note   In older children some medication may be
given in fat emulsions, for example the sedative
Propofol. Consideration should be made of the fat
content of this.

Carnitine

Carnitine is an amino acid which is needed in the beta
oxidation of long chain fatty acids. It transports them
across the mitochondrial membrane in the form of
carnitine esters. Carnitine can usually be synthesised
from lysine and methionine and under normal circumstances carnitine is not needed by children;
however some groups will need carnitine supplementation of the PN due to impaired ability to synthesise
or to increased losses [35, 36]:

- Premature infants of less than 34 weeks (supple-
  mentation improves growth and nitrogen balance)
- Children with end stage liver disease
- Children on dialysis.

Protein

Crystaline L amino acid solutions are used as the
nitrogen source for PN. The amino acid composition
of the products for adult and older children use is
based on high biological value protein. The products
designed for use in infants, at the time of writing, are
Vaminolact, which is based on breast milk, and
Primene (Clintec Nutrition Ltd) which is based on
cord blood. These solutions contain taurine, essential
for retinal development and bile acid metabolism and
may lead to less biochemical abnormalities [19]. The
ideal amino acid profile for PN solutions for infants
and children is still unclear. A solution which contains
insufficient quantities of essential amino acids will
inhibit protein synthesis and may limit growth [14].
A solution which contains excessive amounts of an
amino acid may result in hyperaminoacidaemia and
metabolic complications which can cause coma and
brain damage. Plasma aminograms should be checked
if insufficient or excess amino acids are administered.
Estimates of protein requirements are often based on
the dietary reference values or based on 10% of the
total energy intake (see Table 4.1).

MICRONUTRIENTS

The requirements for intravenous micronutrients in infants and children remain unclear [37]. Electrolyte requirements vary with age, clinical condition and blood biochemistry. Individual electrolyte solutions are usually added to the PN in response to each individual child's blood biochemistry. Requirements for calcium, phosphorus, magnesium, iron, copper, zinc, sodium and potassium are high during growth periods and especially great during the first year of life or during catch-up growth.

Note Intravenous iron supplementation is controversial due to the risk of adverse side effects [37]. Excess iron may enhance the risk of Gram-negative septicaemia and lead to iron overload syndrome. Iron also has powerful oxidative properties and may increase demand for antioxidants. Iron preparations are rarely added to the intravenous solution due to poor solubility and risk of anaphylaxis; additional iron is usually given by top-up blood transfusions when required, if oral supplementation fails.

The guidelines currently in use appear to maintain blood levels within acceptable ranges for children and infants [3, 38]. A summary is given in Table 4.3.

Intravenous vitamin intake is usually recommended to be higher than enteral intakes. This is to allow for losses of the vitamins by adsorption onto the PN bag and giving set or biodegradation due to light exposure, drastically reducing the child's intake. Vitamin A is most affected by these problems [39].

Trace elements

Trace element (TE) deficiencies have been described in neonates receiving TE-free PN, therefore supplements are essential in long-term PN. Requirements for PN vary according to clinical condition. For example, high fluid losses result in greater losses of magnesium and zinc, whereas obstructive jaundice reduces the loss of copper and manganese (normally excreted in bile). Serum levels of TE should be measured before the child starts PN and 1–3 monthly thereafter (if initially stable) [40]. Trace element mixtures are usually avoided in the first week of life to avoid toxic accumulation; many centres only add TE if the child is fed parenterally for longer than 2 weeks [3, 40].

Table 4.3 Guidelines for micronutrient requirements per day in term infants and children

Micronutrient		Recommended Intake	
Sodium	(mmol/kg/day)	1–5	
Potassium	(mmol/kg/day)	1–5	
Chloride	(mmol/kg/day)	1–5	
A	(µg)	500–800	
D	(µg)	4.0–20	
E	(mg)	2.8–15	
K	(µg)	80.0–200	
C	(mg)	20–40	
B_1	(mg)	0.35–3.0	
B_2	(mg)	0.4–3.0	
B_6	(mg)	0.1–2.0	
Niacin	(mg)	5–20	
B_{12}	(µg)	0.3–100	
Biotin	(µg)	35–300	
Pantothenate	(mg)	2.0	
Folate	(µg)	100–200	
Iron		*	
Copper	µg/kg/day	20 {300}	
Selenium	µg/kg/day	2.0 {30}	
Chromium	µg/kg/day	0.2 {5.0}	
Manganese	µg/kg/day	1.0 {50.0}	
Molybdenum	µg/kg/day	0.25 {5.0}	
Iodide	µg/kg/day	1.0 {1.0}	
		Infants	Children >1 year
Calcium	mg/l	500–600	200–400
Phosphorus	mg/l	400–450	150–300
Magnesium	mg/l	50–70	20–40
Zinc	µg/kg/day	<3 mths: 250 >3 mths: 100	50–80 {5000}

Adapted from [3]
Key {} = Maximum total intake
* See explanation in text

ADMINISTRATION OF PN

A detailed account of the techniques of PN administration is available elsewhere [3, 29].

Vascular access

PN may be infused via a peripheral or scalp vein, or via a central venous catheter. Each route has advantages and disadvantages [41]. Peripheral lines are rarely associated with septicaemia and are useful in short term PN (7–10 days) where the fluid allowance is not restricted and where venous access is good. They are often used in neonates. One major disadvantage is the risk of thrombophlebitis caused by the hypertonic solutions used. A maximum concentration of glucose used with these lines is 12%. Infiltration is also a common problem: the peripheral line may penetrate the surrounding tissues resulting in leaking of the infusion. This leakage is known as extravasation which if undetected can cause tissue necrosis and severe scarring. Drip sites must be inspected frequently to avoid this. Drips that fail must be resited

quickly to avoid the risks of rebound hypoglycaemia and suboptimal nutritional intake.

Central venous catheters (Broviac/Hickman catheters) allow the infusion of more concentrated solutions than peripheral lines. These catheters are introduced into the superior vena cava via the subclavian vein and are burrowed under the skin. These silicone catheters have a lower sepsis rate and are less likely to block as they inhibit fibrin production. The catheters are tunnelled under the skin and have a subcutaneous Dacron cuff to help to hold them in place. A central line can remain in situ for months, if properly cared for, and allows for free arm movement; it

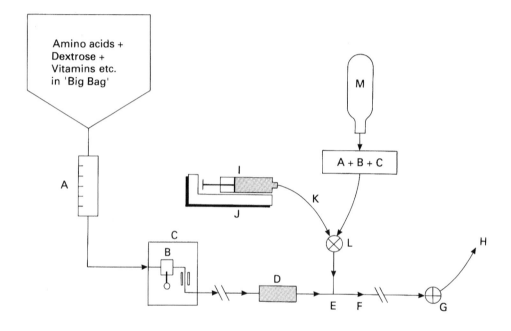

Key

A Burette administration set (used to monitor the volumetric accuracy of the pump)
B Cassette
C Volumetric pump
D Air-eliminating filter (0.2 μm) with an injection port below the filter
E Y-connector
F Fine bore extension tubing (allows freedom of movement)
G One way tap
H Short 25 cm extension tubing (permanently attached to the catheter and **G**)

I Syringe 60 ml, filled with fat emulsion
J Syringe pump
K Fine bore extension tubing
L One way tap
M Bottle of fat emulsion: alternative administration to **I** and **J** for older children, with larger volumes of fat

All connections are 'luer lock'

Note All apparatus **A** to **F** must be changed daily.

Adapted from [43]

Fig. 4.1 Equipment required for intravenous feeding

is more suitable for longer term PN. The major disadvantages of central venous catheters are the risks associated with insertion and catheter care. Catheter related sepsis is a life threatening complication; care of a central venous catheter is the most important factor in preventing this complication and only PN (not drugs) should be given via a single lumen catheter [3, 41]. The risk of infection increases with the number of times the system is accessed. If venous access is required for blood samples, blood products or medication, then separate venous access should be organised. Double lumen catheters are usually inserted when intravenous drug therapy and PN are required (as in bone marrow transplants).

DELIVERY METHODS

PN can be delivered by a variety of systems. Infants and children usually have a 'big bag' system in which the amino acids and dextrose are mixed and delivered over 24 hours. The fat emulsion is delivered from a separate container but mixes with the amino acid and dextrose solution as close as possible to the peripheral or central line. Some adult centres use 'all in one' mixes (containing amino acids, dextrose and lipids). There are now similar products available which can be used in paediatrics for children who are relatively stable, e.g. Kabimix 11. These products do not contain vitamins.

There are specialist computer-based programs available to ensure that the nutrient content of the bag is appropriate for the child's age, condition and biochemistry. They also help to ensure that nutrient stability is assessed and drug-nutrient interactions avoided [42].

PN is supplied in a premixed collapsible bag with an opaque cover to protect vitamins in the solution from photodegradation. When low rates of infusion are prescribed and the solution remains in the burette for long periods, light protective sets are also used.

EQUIPMENT

A steady flow rate should be maintained when infusing PN. Hyperglycaemia and hyperlipidaemia will result if infusions are delivered too quickly. If the line blocks or the infusion stops suddenly, hypoglycaemia may occur [3]. Volumetric pumps are sufficiently accurate for use in children; these deliver measured volumes via a cassette with a syringe mechanism

ensuring accuracy. Syringe pumps are used instead of volumetric pumps when small volumes are required. These have a linear drive mechanism and can be set to deliver as little as 0.5 ml per hour. Filters are needed to remove any bacterial or fungal contamination and prevent air embolism and entry of particulate matter. They must be inserted before the lipid enters the line as lipid emulsions cannot be filtered – the lipid molecules are larger than the filter pore size (0.2 µm). Figure 4.1 illustrates the equipment needed for PN.

REFERENCES

1 Evans TJ, Cockburn F Parenteral feeding. In: McLaren DS, Burman D (eds) *Textbook of Paediatric Nutrition*, 2nd edn. Edinburgh: Churchill Livingstone, 1990, 337–54.

2 Puntis JWL Update on intravenous feeding in children. Guidelines to regimes and techniques for TPN. *Brit J Int Care*, 1993, Aug, 299–305.

3 Milla PJ, Bethune K, Hill S, Long S, Meadows N, Pierro A, Thomas A *Current perspectives on paediatric parenteral nutrition*. A report by the working party for the British Association for Parenteral and Enteral Nutrition, Maidenhead, Berks, 2000.

4 Lifschitz CH Enteral feeding in children. *Annales Nestle*, 1988, **46** 73–81.

5 Hughes CA, Dowling RH Speed of onset of adaptive mucosal hypoplasia and hypofunction in the intestine of the parenterally fed rat. *Clin Sci*, 1980, **59** 317–27.

6 McClure RJ, Newell SJ Randomised controlled trial of trophic feeding and gut motility. *Arch Dis Childh, Fetal and Neonatal edn*, 1999, **80** F54–8.

7 Pierro A Cholestatic jaundice in newborn infants receiving parenteral nutrition. *Semin Neonatal*, 1996, 1 231–9.

8 Ball PA, Booth IW, Holden CE, Puntis JWL *Paediatric Parenteral Nutrition*. Milton Keynes: Pharmacia Ltd, 1998.

9 Maurer J, Weinbaum F, Turner J, Brady T *et al.* Reducing the inappropriate use of parenteral nutrition in an acute care teaching hospital. *J Parenter Enteral Nutr*, 1996, **20** 272–4.

10 Wesley JR Nutrition support teams; past present and future. *Nutr Clin Pract*, 1995, **10** 219–28.

11 Puntis JWL, Booth IW The place of a nutritional care team in paediatric practice. *Inter Ther Clin Mon*, 1990, 132–6.

12 Payne James J Cost effectiveness of nutrition support teams. Are they necessary? *Nutrition*, 1997, **13** 928–30.

13 Braunschweig CL, Wesley JR, Mercer N Rationale and guidelines for parenteral and enteral transition feeding

of the 3–30 kg child. *J Am Diet Assoc*, 1988, **88** 479–82.

14 Payne James J, Grimble G, Silk D Metabolic complications of parenteral nutrition. In: *Artificial Nutrition Support in Clinical Practice*, (ed. Jorgen Nordenstrom). London: Edward Arnold, 1995, pp. 343–58.

15 ESPGAN Committee on nutrition of preterm infants. Nutrition and feeding of preterm infants. *Acta Paediatr Scand*, 1987, (Suppl) **336** 1–14.

16 Wigglesworth JS Malnutrition and brain development. *Develop Med Child Neurol*, 1969, **11** 791–803.

17 Merritt RJ Cholestasis associated with total parenteral nutrition. *J Pediatr Gastroenterol Nut*, 1985, **5** 9–22.

18 Candy DCA Parenteral nutrition in paediatric practice a review. *J Hum Nutr*, 1980, **34** 287–96.

19 Puntis JWL, Booth IW A clinical trial of two parenteral nutrition solutions in neonates. *Arch Dis Childh*, 1990, **65** 559–64.

20 Bisset WM, Stapleford P, Long S, Chamberlain A, Sokal B, Milla PJ Home parenteral nutrition in chronic intestinal failure. *Arch Dis Childh*, 1992, **67** 109–14.

21 Nutritional Support Committee *Parenteral Nutrition Manual*, 4th edn. Childrens Hospital of Pittsburgh. One Childrens Place, 3705 Fifth Avenue, Pittsburgh PA, 1996.

22 Kerner JA, Parenteral nutrition In: Walker WA, Durie PA, (eds) *Paediatr Gastrointest Dis*, 1991, **41** 1645–75. New York: BC Decker Inc.

23 World Health Organisation *Energy and Protein Requirements*. Report of a joint FAO/WHO/UNN meeting. Geneva: WHO, 1985.

24 Goran MI Total energy expenditure in burned children using the doubly labelled water technique. *Am J Physiol*, 1990, **259** 576–85.

25 Palmblad J Intravenous lipid emulsions and host defence – a critical review. *Clin Nutr*, 1991, **10** 303–308.

26 Bresson JL, Narcy P, Putet G, Ricour C, Fachs C, Rey J Energy substrate utilisation in infants receiving total parenteral nutrition with different glucose fat ratios. *Paediatr Res*, 1989, **25** 645.

27 Phelps SJ, Cochrane EC, Kamper CA Peripheral venous line infiltration in infants receiving 10% dextrose, 10% dextrose/amino acids, 10% dextrose/aminoacids/fat emulsion. *Paediatr Res*, 1987, **21** (Abstract 67A).

28 Bresson JL Protein metabolism kinetics and energy substrate utilisation in infants fed parenteral nutrition solutions with different glucose–fat ratios. *Am J Clin Nutr*, 1991, **54** 370–76.

29 Menon G Parenteral nutrition for the neonate. Composition and administration of PN. *Brit J Int Care*, May/June, 1992, 185–92.

30 Taylor C, Nunn T, Rangecroft L Parenteral nutrition for infants and children. In: Grant A, Todd E, (eds) *Enteral and Parenteral Nutrition*, 2nd edn, Oxford: Blackwell Science, 1987.

31 Sower P *et al.* Substrate utilisation of newborn infants fed intravenously with or without a fat emulsion. *Paediatr Res*, 1984, **18** 804 (Abstract 46).

32 Andrew G, Chan G, Schiff D Lipid metabolism in the neonate. The effects of intralipid infusion plasma triglyceride and free fatty acid concentrations in the neonate. *J Pediatr*, 1976, **88** 273–8.

33 Park W *et al.* Impaired fat utilisation in parenterally fed low birthweight infants suffering from sepsis. *J Parent Ent Nutr*, 1986, **10** 627–30.

34 Friedman Z *et al.* Rapid onset of essential fatty acid deficiency in the newborn. *Paediatr*, 1976, **58** 640.

35 Scaglia F, Longo N Primary and secondary alterations of neonatal carnitine metabolism. *Semin Perinatol*, 1999, **23** 152–61.

36 Barum PR Carnitine in neonatal nutrition. *J Child Neurol*, 1995, **10** (Suppl. 2) S25–31.

37 Kumpf KJ. Parenteral Iron Supplementation. *Nutr Clin Prat*, Aug 1996, **11** 139–46.

38 Greene HL *et al.* Guidelines for the use of vitamins, trace elements, calcium, magnesium and phosphorus in infants and children receiving total parenteral nutrition: Report of the subcommittee on paediatric parenteral nutrient requirements from the committee on clinical practice issues of the American Society for Clinical Nutrition. *Am J Clin Nutr*, 1988, **48** 1324–42.

39 Allwood MC Compatability and stability of TPN mixtures in big bags. *J Clin Hosp Pharm*, 1984, **9** 181–98.

40 Taylor A Detection and monitoring of disorders of essential trace elements. *Ann Clin Biochem*, 1996, **33** 486–510.

41 Hansell D Intravenous nutrition: the central or peripheral route? *Int Ther Clin Mon*, 1989, **10** 184–90.

42 Cole D, Thickson N, Oruck J Computer assisted compounding of neonatal/pediatric parenteral nutrition solutions. *Can J Hosp Pharm*, 1991, **44** 229–33.

43 Grant A, Todd E *Enteral and Parenteral Nutrition*, 2nd edn. Oxford: Blackwell Science, 1987.

SECTION 3

Preterm and
Low Birthweight Nutrition

CHAPTER 5

Preterm Infants

DEFINITIONS

A preterm infant is one born before 36 weeks completed gestation. An infant born <2500 g is termed low birth weight (LBW) regardless of gestation, <1500 g very low birth weight (VLBW) and those <1000 g extremely low birth weight (ELBW). Categorisation of infants born smaller than expected is more contentious; however, they are often divided into small for gestational age (SGA) and intrauterine growth retarded (IUGR). SGA infants are usually <10th or 3rd percentile for weight at birth (depending on source of definition) and probably constitute a heterogeneous group, i.e. those destined to be born small due to genetic influences and those who are IUGR. The former group tends to be proportionally small. Those who are IUGR will have similarly low birth weight but may show head and/or length sparing depending on timing of intrauterine nutrient restriction. These infants are at high risk of perinatal problems [1].

The prevalence of IUGR is reported to be up to 7% of all deliveries [2]; however, this is made up by a disproportionally large number of preterm infants [3]. Early nutritional management may be vital to later outcome [4, 5], but it is hampered by immature or dysfunctional gastrointestinal tract and poor tolerance of parenteral nutrition.

NUTRITIONAL REQUIREMENTS

Preterm infants have limited stores of many nutrients as accretion occurs predominantly in the last trimester [6]. They are poorly equipped to withstand inadequate nutrition: theoretically endogenous reserves in a 1000 g infant are only sufficient for 4 days if unfed [7]. It is generally accepted that most infants <1500 g will need some parenteral nutrition while enteral feeds are gradually increased.

The following is a brief discussion of the requirements for the major nutrients, via the enteral route unless otherwise specified, as it is beyond the scope of this review to fully cover parenteral requirements; the most recent comprehensive review and recommendations, at the time of writing, are published in [8]. A summary of their recommendations is presented in Table 5.1. The interested reader is strongly advised to read this book for more information.

Fluid

During the initial phase of adaptation to extra-uterine life, fluid management is complicated as there is a delicate balance between matching high transcutaneous losses (although these should be minimised by nursing under plastic sheeting in a humidified atmosphere) and avoiding fluid overload due to renal immaturity. An extracellular fluid contraction is desirable over the first few days but this should not be excessive (i.e. more than 7% birth weight). Early fluid management to a large degree takes precedence over nutritional management, with extreme restrictions sometimes necessary. However, nutritional intakes should always be optimised within the fluid allowed.

Energy

The components contributing to energy requirements are summarised in Table 5.2 and demonstrate the wide range possible. As measurement of individual energy expenditure remains a research tool, energy intake should be adjusted according to indirect measures, i.e. growth and serum biochemistry. As

Table 5.1 Composition of preterm formulas. Correct at time of writing, please check company data

NUTRIENTS Per 100 ml	Recommendations by Tsang (1993) [8] Based on 80 kcal/100 ml	Cow & Gate NUTRIPREM	Farley's OSTERPREM	Milupa PREMATIL	SMA LBW
Energy (kcal/kJ)	80/335	80/335	80/335	80/335	82/415
Protein (g/kg) <1000 g >1000 g	3.6–3.8 3.0–3.6	—	—	—	—
Protein (g)		2.4	2.0	2.4	2.0
Fat (g) MCT (✔) LCP Linoleic acid (g) Linolenic acid (g)	3.5–4.8 (tentative) ns Conditionally essential 0.35–1.36 0.09–0.35	4.4 AA/DHA/GLA 0.57 0.06	4.6 DHA/GLA 0.54 0.06	4.4 AA/DHA/GLA 0.73 0.06	4.4 (✔) 15% total fat AA/DHA 0.7 0.07
Carbohydrate (g)	ns	7.8	7.6	7.8	8.6
Minerals Sodium (mg)	30–46	41	42	41	35
Potassium (mg)	52–80	80	72	80	85
Chloride (mg)	47–71	48	60	48	60
Calcium (mg)	80–154	100	110	100	80
Phosphorus (mg)	40–94	50	63	50	43
Ca:P ratio	ns	2:1	1.7:1	2:1	1.9:1
Magnesium (mg)	5–10	10	5	10	8
Iron (mg)	2.0 (mg/kg)	0.9	0.04	0.9	0.8
Zinc (mg)	0.7	0.7	0.9	0.7	0.8
Copper (µg)	80–100	80	96	80	83
Iodine (µg)	20–40	25	8	14	10
Manganese (µg)	5	10	3	8	10
Selenium (µg)	0.9	1.9	ns	ns	ns
Vitamins Vitamin A (µg)*	CLD: 450–840 No CLD: 210–450 µg/kg	227	100	108	74
Vitamin D (µg)*	2.4–6.4 (Min 10/day)	5.0	2.4	2.4	1.5
Vitamin E (TE) (mg)	2.7–5.4 (max 25 IU/d)	3.0	10	3.0	1.2
Vitamin K (µg)	5.3–6.7	6.6	7.0	6.6	8.0
Thiamin B$_1$ (mg)	0.12–0.16	0.14	0.1	0.14	0.12
Riboflavin B$_2$ (mg)	0.16–0.24	0.2	0.18	0.2	0.2
Niacin (mg)	2.4–3.2	3.0	1.0	2.5	1.3
Panthothenic Acid (mg)	0.8–1.2	1.0	0.5	1.0	0.45
Pyridoxine B$_6$ (mg)	0.1–0.14	0.12	0.1	0.12	0.07
Folic Acid (µg)	17–34	48	50	48	49
Vitamin B$_{12}$ (µg)	0.2	0.2	0.2	0.2	0.3
Biotin (µg)	2.4–4.0	3.0	2.0	3.0	2.4
Vitamin C (mg)	12–16	16	28	16	11
Choline (mg)	ns	10	5.6	10	13
Taurine (mg)	2.25–6.0	5.5	5.1	5.5	7.0
Inositol (mg)	16–54	30	3.2	30	4.5
Carnitine (mg)	ns	2.0	1.0	2.0	2.9
Nucleotides	ns	✔	✕	✕	✕
Beta-carotene (µg)	ns	40	24	ns	2.5
Osmolality (mOsmol/kg/H$_2$O)	ns	293	300	312	277
Est renal solute load (mOsmol/l)	ns	148	134	148	134

ns = not specified; CLD = chronic lung disease; MCT = medium chain triglycerides; AA = arachidonic acid; DHA = docosahexaenoic acid; GLA = gamma linolenic acid.
* Conversion factors vit A: µg ÷ 0.3 = IU; vit D: µg × 40 = IU.

Table 5.2 Energy requirements. Energy expenditure increases with age, intake and growth rate [8]

kcal/kg/day (*multiply by 4.18 for kJ*)	Acute phase	Intermediate phase	Convalescence
Resting energy expenditure (REE)[1]	45	50–60	50–70
Cold stress	0–10	0–10	5–10
Activity/handling[2]	0–10	5–15	5–15
Stool losses[3]	0–10	10–15	10–15
Specific dynamic action[4]	0	0–5	10
Growth	0	20–30	20–30
Total[5]	50–80	85–135	105–150

[1] The lower level applies to babies with normal REE, upper limit to those with diseases associated with increased REE, e.g. cardiac abnormalities/chronic lung disease
[2] Zero if paralysed/heavily sedated
[3] Zero if on TPN
[4] 10% of calories infused if on TPN
[5] Upper limit probably not physiological and should not be necessary

a rough guide Tsang *et al.* [8] suggest aiming for 80–90 non-protein kcal/kg parenterally and 110–120 kcal/kg enterally. Intakes above requirements will lead to higher weight gains but this will usually be due to fat deposition in excess of uterine accretion rates [8] and will lead to higher metabolic rates [9]. There are no advantages for lean body mass or skeletal growth even when protein is also increased (see next section). Energy requirements may be decreased in very sick infants whose growth is slowed due to the stress response as the energy cost of growth is normally a substantial part of total requirements [10, 11]. Higher nutrient requirements may be necessary for some IUGR babies. Again this will vary between individuals and can only be established by monitoring progress and adjusting prescribed nutrient intakes accordingly. Tsang *et al.* [8] point out that force-feeding these infants gives no advantages.

Protein

Tsang *et al.* [8] suggest protein intakes are stratified according to birthweight as *in utero* accretion rates decline with advancing gestation (<1000 g 3.6–3.8, >1000 g 3.0–3.6 g/kg/day). Between 27 and 35 weeks gestation daily accretion is around 2 g/kg. This can be achieved post-natally as long as the above protein intakes are accompanied by at least 110 kcal/kg/day

enterally or 80 non-protein kcal/kg parenterally. Protein gain increases in a linear fashion up to an intake of around 4 g/kg/day after which it is static at a little higher than *in utero* rates [8]. The capacity for protein gain above the intrauterine rate may be useful when catch-up growth is occurring. However, in other circumstances feeding over 4 g/kg/day puts an unnecessary metabolic stress on the vulnerable immature infant [12, 13] and may lead to adverse neurological sequelae [14].

Hepatic immaturity leads to the need for exogenous supplies of cysteine, glycine and taurine normally considered non-essential in older individuals.

Fat

The recommendation for fat intake varies from 4.4 to 6 g/100 kcal in formula for preterm infants. Of this the essential fatty acids linoleic and linolenic acid should provide 4–15% and 1–4% energy respectively [8]. Absorption will be variable but the more immature the infant the higher the risk for malabsorption due to low bile salt pools [15] and low pancreatic lipase [16]. Controversy exists on the provision of the longer-chain derivatives of linoleic and linolenic acids namely arachidonic (AA) and docosahexaenoic (DHA) acids. Although Tsang *et al.* [8] felt that definite recommendations could not be made, others have made them suggesting that both should be added to preterm formula [17]. There seem to be advantages with respect to visual and neurodevelopmental outcome for preterm infants [18, 19].

Theoretically medium chain triglycerides (MCT) should lead to improved fat absorption, although no consistent advantage with respect to fat [20] or nitrogen balance [21] has been found. In addition large amounts of MCT might interfere with DHA production [22]. VLBW and ELBW infants will develop essential fatty acid deficiency very rapidly and need an early supply of parenteral lipid. As little as 0.5 g/kg/day will suffice [23].

Carbohydrate

Lactase levels are low in preterm infants, although feeding a lactose containing milk will aid precocious development of lactase activity aiding tolerance [24]. Poor tolerance of intravenous glucose infusion is more common – see the section on parenteral nutrition later in this chapter.

Folic acid

Requirements for folic acid have been established [25] and preterm formulas are all fortified appropriately (17–34 μg/80 kcal) [8]. Many units still use a folic acid supplement, and although not seen as toxic, the appearance of unmetabolised folic acid in the serum may be undesirable, particularly in infants given a large weekly dose [26].

Fat soluble vitamins

A note of caution is warranted when interpreting studies on enteral fat soluble vitamin supplementation. Due to the relatively poor enteral fat digestion and absorption [15, 16] very high doses are often needed to normalise status. Digestive capacity appears to develop rapidly in term infants [27] and dietary fat supplementation can enhance gastric lipase in preterm infants [28].

Vitamin A

Many preterm infants are born with poor vitamin A stores [29] and there is some evidence that high dose enteral supplementation (5000 IU/day, 1500 μg/day) is needed to normalise serum levels [30]. There is renewed interest in appropriate vitamin A supplementation as it may help reduce risk of chronic lung disease (CLD) [31]. Tsang *et al.* [8] suggest higher doses once CLD is established to aid lung repair (CLD 450–840 μg/kg; no CLD 210–450 μg/kg), but future studies are likely to show that higher doses are needed earlier [31]. Until recently some commonly used parenteral infusion products were licensed for only a quarter of the recommended dose [32]; this has now been rectified and should improve early vitamin A status.

Vitamin D

A daily enteral intake of 10 μg to a maximum of 20 μg is recommended with a lower parenteral dose as the gut barrier is bypassed [8]. Previously higher enteral intakes had been thought necessary, but these have not been shown to improve outcome [33]. A recent study demonstrated that even a population from northerly latitudes, likely to have the lower range of vitamin D status at birth, did well on 10 μg/day [34].

Vitamin E

At least 0.68 mg vitamin E/g linoleic acid and 0.5 mg vitamin E/100 kcal up to a maximum of 17 mg/day should be provided [8]. In the past routine supplementation was not considered beneficial [35]. Some institutions in North America give pharmacological doses to infants with the first stages of retinopathy of prematurity to good effect with no excess levels of sepsis or necrotising enterocolitis (NEC) reported [36]. A call to re-evaluate vitamin E supplementation has been made [37].

Calcium, phosphorus and magnesium

The fetus acquires 80% of the normal term content of calcium during the last trimester [38] and preterm infants have high requirements for calcium and other minerals needed for bone formation. Tsang *et al.* [8] recommend 80–154 mg calcium and 40–94 mg phosphorus/80 kcal. Although a calcium : phosphorus ratio is not specified [8], all current preterm formulas fall between 1.7 : 1–2 : 1 complying with previous guidelines [39].

Iron

Iron stores are low in preterm infants and without supplementation will become depleted by 8 weeks [40]. Current recommendations are that supplements could start any time between birth and 8 weeks as either a supplemented formula or medicinal iron at a level of 2 mg/kg/day to a maximum of 15 mg/day [8]. Although the early anaemia of prematurity is not affected by iron supplementation there is some evidence that infants supplemented by 2 weeks had better iron status at discharge [41]. Despite high ferritins after blood transfusions this stored iron may not be available for haemopoiesis, therefore supplementation should continue regardless of transfusion status [8, 42]. In well infants a standard formula with 0.5 mg/100 ml iron seems to meet iron needs post-discharge, but more may be needed for those who were smaller at birth and have been sicker [43]. Due to the interactions of iron, copper and zinc during absorption, excessive amounts of each individual nutrient should be avoided.

Zinc

Zinc may be an important growth regulator during infancy. In a longitudinal study of preterm infants, length at 3 months was correlated only with length at birth and zinc intake [44]. Tsang *et al.* suggest 0.7 mg/80 kcal; others have suggested that more is necessary [45]. Renal losses may be high due to repeated acute phase protein responses and diuretic therapy [46, 47].

Selenium

Selenium status is low at birth in preterm infants [48] which is of concern as selenium is a component of the antioxidant enzyme glutathione peroxidase [49]. Enteral feeds should be supplemented to the levels recommended by Tsang *et al.* [8], i.e. 0.9 µg/80 kcal.

Iodine

There is risk of deficiency with unsupplemented preterm formulas [50], Tsang *et al.* recommend 20–40 µg/80 kcal [8].

β-carotene

No recommendations for the addition of β-carotene to preterm formula exist although its presence in human milk, its role as an antioxidant and its provitamin-A activity have prompted some manufacturers to add it. Beta-carotene comprises only approximately 25% of the total carotenoid activity of human milk and its levels vary greatly depending on time and number of lactations [51]. In adult studies supplementation has lead to adverse effects [52]. Intake should not be increased above that available from current formulas until evidence on outcome is available.

CONDITIONALLY ESSENTIAL NUTRIENTS

Nucleotides

Nucleotides may be conditionally essential for the gut and immune system during times of stress [53] and levels are high in human milk. Studies have been published describing reduction of diarrhoea in term infants [54] and improved growth in SGA infants [55]. Supplemented formula should be evaluated in the preterm population to assess the usefulness of this potentially beneficial nutrient.

Glutamine

Glutamine is an important fuel for the small intestine and immune system and possibly becomes rate limiting during increased demand [56]. Glutamine has been associated with improved outcome in both parenterally [57] and enterally fed preterm infants [58]. This may become an important supplement in the future.

PARENTERAL NUTRITION

With increased survival, preterm infants have become a major recipient of parenteral nutrition, usually in association with minimal enteral feeds [59]. Early initiation of parenteral nutrition has been shown to be well tolerated [60, 61, 62]. Due to high energy requirements up to 12 mg/kg/min glucose and 0.15 g/kg/hour lipid infusions are optimal. However, raised blood glucose and triglyceride levels are common in sick preterm infants. Insulin is often given, but should not be used to aid tolerance of >12 mg/kg/min of glucose. Reduction of lipid infusion due to lipaemia should be as brief as possible to minimise suboptimal energy, fat soluble vitamin and essential fatty acid intake. There is a high risk of bone disease of prematurity when solutions containing relatively insoluble inorganic calcium and phosphate are given. For this reason interest is growing in organic mineral salts such as glycerophosphate. The definitive guidelines for mineral and vitamin levels remain those of Greene *et al.* [32]. Parenteral solutions should be protected from the high light intensity often found on neonatal units to minimise photo degradation of susceptible nutrients and production of toxic hydroperoxides [63, 64 for further background reading].

ENTERAL NUTRITION

The advantages of early and minimal enteral feeding have been shown in many studies [65, 66, 67, 68]. The milk of choice is undoubtedly mother's own freshly expressed breast milk. Advantages include improved feed tolerance [69, 70], reduced risk of necrotising enterocolitis [68, 71] and reduced risk of sepsis [68, 70,

72]. The latter two studies showed a dose dependent reduction of risk. There may be long-term neurodevelopmental advantages in feeding human milk [73, 74]. Banked donor breast milk retains some immunological advantages [71], although heat labile vitamins, bile salt stimulated lipase and live cells are reduced or destroyed and it is recommend for initiation of feeds only in the absence of mother's own milk.

Human milk may be nutritionally adequate in many respects for infants >1500 g when fed in sufficient volumes, i.e. up to 220 ml/kg in well infants, although an iron supplement will be needed by 2 months. However <1500 g some nutrients may be limiting particularly protein and some minerals and vitamins. Serum phosphate should be kept above 1.5 mmol/l, but below serum calcium levels. When phosphate is <1.5 mmol/l a supplement is required; 0.5 mmol b.d. has been given successfully [75], but should be titrated according to serum biochemistry. Milk during the first 2–3 weeks lactation may have higher protein levels, although this is not a consistent finding and wide variations have been reported [76].

An indirect measure of protein intake may be the serum urea level. This was found to drop below 1.6 mmol/l in most cases when human milk protein intake fell <3 g/kg/day [77]. Protein fortification can be considered once serum urea reaches 2 mmol/l after a consistent fall. A commercially produced human milk fortifier has many advantages over supplementing with liquid formula, as this will allow use of full volumes of mother's milk. Although not all fortifiers have undergone sufficiently large trials one North American product supported growth and was well tolerated [78]. Choosing one which brings human milk nutritional composition to within the Tsang guidelines will negate the need for separate additions of most minerals, vitamins and protein. However, a separate iron supplement will still be necessary by 2 months of age (see Table 5.3 for a comparison of those currently available in the UK). Fortification should occur as close to feeding time as possible to avoid loss of immunological factors [79]. Supplementation of human milk with energy alone is not advised as this will reduce the protein:energy ratio to an unacceptably low level. Table 5.4 shows the composition of milk from mothers delivering preterm and mature milk. Occasionally expressing technique may need improving to ensure all the hind milk is removed at each expression thus avoiding a low fat and energy milk. Fortification should continue until the infant is feeding fully from the breast and thriving, or around

2.0–2.5 kg. There is no firm data to give guidance on the best weight at which to stop preterm formula; 2.5 kg may be optimal, allowing time for catch-up growth without the need to take very large feed volumes [80].

See [81] for further details on all practical aspects of enteral nutrition.

PRETERM FORMULAS

For those infants <2000 g birth weight who do not have access to human milk the feed of choice is a preterm formula. In addition, those infants whose mothers' milk supply is inadequate should be supplemented with preterm formula. However, it is not advisable to mix and store human milk and formula for prolonged periods (see the section 'Infants under 12 months' in Chapter 3, Enteral Feeding).

Preterm formulas are highly specialised milks designed to meet the increased nutritional needs of preterm infants without exceeding volume tolerance. Although they all generally follow ESPGAN [39] or Tsang *et al.* [8] guidelines they do still differ significantly in some aspects (see Table 5.1 for composition of those formulas currently available in the UK).

Of note are the differing levels of iron, fat soluble vitamins and some of the 'conditionally' essential nutrients, e.g. arachidonic acid, docosohexaenoic acid, nucleotides, inositol and β-carotene. Some formulas will need supplementing with fat soluble vitamins and iron in order to comply fully with the most recent guidelines, and although all contain sufficient folic acid many units appear to continue giving supplements. There is a wide variation between neonatal units as to the age and weight at which preterm formula is stopped. A suggested range is between 2000 and 2500 g.

Some infants born >2000 g <2500 g may benefit from a time on a nutrient enriched post-discharge formula, rather than a term formula. However, it is important to remember that at any age or weight each individual baby may need assessment to decide on an optimal formula.

METHOD OF ENTERAL FEEDING

Due to an immature suck-swallow-breathe pattern, preterm infants require tube feeding until around 35–37 weeks' gestation or longer. There are advantages and disadvantages to both bolus and continuous

Table 5.3 Composition of human milk and milk fortifiers. Correct at time of writing, please check with manufacturers

Composition of recommended dose	Nutriprem breast milk fortifier (Cow & Gate)	Eoprotin (Milupa)	Enfamil (Mead Johnson)	SMA breast milk fortifier (SMA)[1]	Mature[4] human milk	Preterm milk (5–18 days)
Recommended dose (g/100 ml)	3	3	4	4	—	—
Protein (g)	0.7[2]	0.6	0.7	1.0	1.3	1.8
Whey:Casein	60:40	60:40	60:40	100:0	60:40	70:30
Energy (kcal)[3] (4.18 = kJ)	10	11	13	15	69	71
Minerals (mmol)						
Ca	1.5	1.0	2.2	2.25	0.85	1.45
P	1.3	0.8	1.4	1.45	0.48	0.48
Mg	0.25	0.09	0.04	0.12	0.12	0.14
Na	0.3	0.8	0.3	0.8	0.65	1.08
K	0.1	0.06	0.4	0.6	1.48	1.85
Cl	0.2	0.45	0.5	0.5	1.18	2.37
Trace elements (μg)						
Zn	300	—	700	200	300	450
Cu	26	—	62	—	40	—
Mn	6	—	4.7	4.6	trace	—
I	11	—	—	—	7.0	—
Vitamins (μg)						
A (RE)	130	30	285	270	58	—
C (mg)	12	15	11.6	40	4	9
D	5	—	5.2	6.6	0.04	—
E (TE)	2600	330	4500	3000	0.34	0.83
K	6.3	0.2	4.4	11	—	—
Biotin	2.5	—	2.7	—	0.7	—
Folic Acid	50	—	2.5	—	5.0	—
Niacin (NE)	2500	—	3000	3600	200	—
B_{12}	0.2	—	0.18	0.3	trace	—
B_6	110	—	114	260	100	—
Riboflavin	170	—	210	260	300	—
Thiamin	130	—	141	220	200	—
Pantothenic Acid B_5	750	—	730	—	250	—
Presentation	1.5 g sachets	200 g tins	1 g sachets	2 g sachet	—	—

[1] Available on request to company
[2] Hydrolysed protein
[3] All contain carbohydrate only as energy source
[4] McCance and Widdowson: *The Composition of Foods*, 5th ed, Royal Soc. Chemistry 1991

gastric tube feeding. Boluses may aid gut maturation via cyclic production of gut hormones [82] and have been associated with less feed intolerance [68]. However, they may lead to a deterioration in respiratory function compared to continuous feeds due to gastric distension [83]. Continuous feeding of human milk can lead to excessive fat loss [84] and risk of sedimentation of added minerals. An alternative method has been shown to work well. This involves 2-hour slow infusion every 3 hours and has led to improved feed tolerance [85]. There is much evidence that rapid advancement of enteral feeds is associated with increased risk of necrotising enterocolitis (NEC) [86, 87]. A limit of 20 ml/kg/day increase has been suggested, particularly in those felt to be at high risk of NEC.

For some infants, particularly those who have been very unwell, the transition to nipple feeding is very difficult. Liaison with an experienced speech and language therapist is invaluable in these circumstances. Some mother-infant pairs benefit from specialist advice on establishing breast feeding, and with support, infants born at as young as 24 weeks can leave neonatal units fully breast feeding.

CHRONIC LUNG DISEASE

Chronic lung disease (CLD), previously known as bronchopulmonary dysplasia, is a disease first described following the survival of mechanically ventilated infants. Lung damage probably results from the barotrauma of ventilation and possibly oxygen toxicity. The result is a requirement for prolonged ventilatory support and possible discharge home on nasal prong oxygen. Some studies have found significantly poorer nutritional intake in those infants going on to develop CLD [88]. Others have found significantly higher energy expenditures (EE) once CLD is established [89, 90]. The elevation in EE was closely associated with respiratory status in one study [91], but not in another [92]. Using the doubly labelled water technique EE was not found to be raised but was far more variable in those with CLD [93]. Intervention studies have not been able to improve growth or respiratory outcome, despite increased energy intake [94, 95].

The increasing use of steroids to aid weaning from ventilatory support has had a major impact on growth and nutrition of infants with CLD. During treatment infants become catabolic with raised serum urea and amino acids [96]. Skeletal growth is arrested [97], despite apparently adequate nutrient intakes [98] and no increase in EE [99]. Weight gain is not as severely affected as length gain. Some have suggested that the babies continue putting on weight but as a relatively larger amount of fat which is less energy costly than accretion of lean body mass [100]. High fat formulas have been shown to reduce carbon dioxide production but not to improve respiratory function [101].

Optimal nutrition is seen as fundamental to the management of these infants [102]. However, many infants with CLD show growth failure resistant to nutritional intervention and other factors such as anaemia must be considered [103] or sodium depletion if on diuretics [104], and the effect of adequate oxygen therapy [105].

POST-DISCHARGE NUTRITION

All mothers should be encouraged to demand breast feed their infants wherever possible post-discharge. For those mothers who cannot comply, alternatives to term formulas have been developed. Nutrient enriched post-discharge formulas (NEPDF) are available for preterm infants who have been observed to take up to 300 ml/kg of term formula post-discharge [80]. Although limited, there is data showing improved growth, bone mineralisation and possibly neurodevelopment [18, 106, 107]. Some formulas also have the advantage of negating the need for separate iron and vitamin supplements post-discharge.

A NEPDF (e.g. Premcare) should be used until around 6–9 months or once catch-up growth has been achieved, whichever is sooner. However, it is always best to assess each infant's needs individually.

After NEPDF a term formula can be used up to 12–18 months. Iron status should be adequately maintained without supplements [43], although some infants with limited dietary intakes may need them. Infants breast feeding on discharge will need iron and a multivitamin supplement (containing vitamin D). When formula or breast milk is changed to unmodified cow's milk at 12–18 months the infant should be started on children's vitamin drops as per DH guidelines [108].

WEANING

Solids should not be introduced before 16 weeks post-delivery unless there are exceptional circumstances. A suggested upper limit is 7 months post-delivery. Concern has been voiced about the safety of introducing a preterm infant to solids before 16 weeks' post-due date (i.e. 40 weeks gestation). However, the introduction of milk feeds leads to a precocious development of the gastrointestinal tract with respect to digestion [24] and motility [109]. There is no evidence for increased risk of allergy [110] or of obesity, the latter theoretically as a result of passive overfeeding. On the other hand preterm infants seem to have a higher prevalence of behavioural feeding problems [111, 112]. This may be due to solids (particularly lumps) having been delayed beyond a critical period for their acceptance [113]. Once weaning has started it should proceed according to current guidelines [108]. (See [114] for further details on weaning preterm infants.)

REFERENCES

1 Teberg AJ, Hotrakitya S, Wu PY, Yeh SY, Hoppenbrouwers T Factors affecting nursery survival of very low birth weight infants. *J Perinat Med*, 1987, **15** 297–306.

2 Galbraith RS, Karchmar EJ, Piercy WN, Low JA The clinical prediction of intrauterine growth retardation. *Am J Obstet Gynecol*, 1979, **133** 281–6.

3 Sparks JW Human intrauterine growth and nutrient accretion. *Semin Perinatol*, 1984, **8** 74–93.

4 Powls A, Botting N, Cooke RW, Pilling D, Marlow N Growth impairment in very low birthweight children at 12 years: correlation with perinatal and outcome variables. *Arch Dis Childh Fetal Neonatal edn*, 1996, **75** F152–7.

5 Georgieff MK, Hoffman JS, Pereira GR, Bernbaum J, Hoffman Williamson M Effect of neonatal caloric deprivation on head growth and 1-year developmental status in preterm infants. *J Pediatr*, 1985, **107** 581–7.

6 Friss-Hanson B Body composition during growth: in-vivo measurements and biochemical data correlated to differential anatomical growth. *Pediatr*, 1971, **47** 264–74.

7 Heird WC, Driscoll JM Jr, Schullinger JN, Grebin B, Winters RW Intravenous alimentation in pediatric patients. *J Pediatr*, 1972, **80** 351–72.

8 Tsang RC, Lucas A, Uauy R, Zlotkin S Nutritional needs of the preterm infant: scientific basis and practical guidelines. New York: Caduceus Medical Publishers, 1993.

9 Brooke OG Energy balance and metabolic rate in preterm infants fed with standard and high-energy formulas. *Br J Nutr*, 1980, **44** 13–23.

10 Chwals WJ, Lally KP, Woolley MM, Mahour GH Measured energy expenditure in critically ill infants and young children. *J Surg Res*, 1988, **44** 467–72.

11 Chwals WJ Metabolism and nutritional frontiers in pediatric surgical patients. *Surg Clin North Am*, 1992, **72** 1237–66.

12 Raiha NCR, Heinonen K, Rassin DK, Gaull GE Milk protein quantity and quality in low birth weight infants: I metabolic responses and effects on growth. *Pediatr*, 1976, **57** 659–74.

13 Svenningsen NW, Lindroth M, Lindquist B Growth in relation to protein intake of low birth weight infants. *Early Hum Dev*, 1982, **6** 47–58.

14 Goldman HI, Goldman JS, Kaufman I, Liebman OB Late effects of early dietary protein intakes on low birth weight infants. *J Pediatr*, 1974, **85** 764–96.

15 Signer E, Murphy GM, Edkins S, Anderson CM Role of bile salts in fat malabsorption of premature infants. *Arch Dis Childh*, 1974, **49** 174–80.

16 Hamosh M Lipid metabolism in premature infants. *Biol Neonate*, 1987, **52** (Suppl 1), 50–64.

17 ESPGAN (European Society of Paediatric Gastroenterology and Nutrition) Comment on the content and composition of lipids in infant formula. *Acta Paed Scand*, 1991, **80** 887–96.

18 Carlson SE, Werkman SH, Peeples JM, Wilson WM Long-chain fatty acids and early visual and cognitive development of preterm infants. *Eur J Clin Nutr*, 1994, **48** 527–30.

19 Gibson RA, Makrides M The role of long chain polyunsaturated fatty acids (LCPUFA) in neonatal nutrition. *Acta Paediatr*, 1998, **87** 1017–22.

20 Hamosh M, Mehta NR, Fink CS, Coleman J, Hamosh P Fat absorption in premature infants: medium-chain triglycerides and long-chain triglycerides are absorbed from formula at similar rates. *J Pediatr Gastroenterol Nutr*, 1991, **13** 143–9.

21 Sulkers EJ, von Goudoever JB, Leunisse C, Wattimena JL, Sauer PJ Comparison of two preterm formulas with or without addition of medium-chain triglycerides (MCTs). I: Effects on nitrogen and fat balance and body composition changes. *J Pediatr Gastroenterol Nutr*, 1992, **15** 34–41.

22 Carnielli V, Rossi K, Baden T Medium chain triacylglycerols in formulas for preterm infants: effect on plasma lipids, circulating concentrations of medium chain fatty acids and essential fatty acids. *Am J Clin Nutr*, 1996, **64** 152–8.

23 Cook R, Yeh YY, Gibson D *et al.* Soybean oil emulsion administration during parenteral nutrition in the preterm infant: effect on essential fatty acid, lipid and glucose metabolism. *J Pediatr*, 1987, **111** 767–73.

24 Shulman RJ, Schanler RJ, Lau C, Heitkemper M, Ou CN, Smith EO Early feeding, feeding tolerance, and lactase activity in preterm infants. *J Pediatr*, 1998, **133** 645–9.

25 Ek J, Behncke L, Halvorsen KS, Magnus E Plasma and red cell folate values and folate requirements in formula fed premature infants. *Eur J Pediatr*, 1984, **142** 78–82.

26 Kelly P, McPartland J, Goggins M, Weir DG, Scott JM Unmetabolised folic acid in serum: acute studies in subjects consuming fortified food and supplements. *Am J Clin Nutr*, 1997, **65** 1790–95.

27 Manson WG, Dale E, Harding M, Coward WA, Weaver LT Functional capacity of the newborn to digest dietary fats. *J Pediatr Gastro Nutr*, 1996, **22** 427A.

28 Pereira GR, Barsky D, Hamosh M, Henderson TR, Armand M Dietary fat supplements enhances gastric lipase activity in premature neonates. *Pediatr Res*, 1995, 37 316A.

29 Mupanemunda RH, Lee DS, Fraher LJ, Koura IR, Chance GW Postnatal changes in serum retinol status in very low birth weight infants. *Early Hum Dev*, 1994, 38 45–54.

30 Landman J, Sive A, De V, Hesse H, Van der Elst C, Sacks R Comparison of enteral and intramuscular vitamin A supplementation in preterm infants. *Early Hum Dev*, 1992, 30 163–70.

31 Kennedy KA, Stoll BJ, Ehrenkranz RA, Oh W, Wright LL, Stevenson DK, Lemons JA, Sowell A, Mele L, Tyson JE, Verter J Vitamin A to prevent bronchopulmonary dysplasia in very-low-birth-weight infants: has the dose been too low? The NICHD Neonatal Research Network. *Early Hum Dev*, 1997, 49 19–31.

32 Greene HL, Hambidge KM, Schanler R, Tsang RC Guidelines for the use of vitamins, trace elements, calcium, magnesium, and phosphorus in infants and children receiving total parenteral nutrition: report of the Subcommittee on Pediatric Parenteral Nutrient Requirements from the Committee on Clinical Practice Issues of the American Society for Clinical Nutrition (published errata appear in *Am J Clin Nutr*, 1989, June 49(6) 1332 and 1989, Sept 50(3) 560). *Am J Clin Nutr*, 1988, 48 1324–42.

33 Evans JR, Allen AC, Stinson DA, Hamilton DC, St John BB, Vincer MJ, Raad MA, Gundberg CM, Cole DE Effect of high-dose vitamin D supplementation on radiographically detectable bone disease of very low birth weight infants. *J Pediatr*, 1989, 115 779–86.

34 Backstrom MC, Maki R, Kuusela AL, Sievanen H, Koivisto AM, Ikonen RS, Kouri T, Maki M Randomised controlled trial of vitamin D supplementation on bone density and biochemical indices in preterm infants. *Arch Dis Childh*, 1999, 80 F161–6.

35 Law MR, Wijardene K, Wald NJ Is routine vitamin E administration justified in very low birth weight infants? *Dev Med Child Neurol*, 1990, 32 442–50.

36 Johnson L, Quinn GE, Abbasi S, Gerdes J, Bowen FW, Bhutani V Severe retinopathy of prematurity in infants with birth weights less than 1250 grams: incidence and outcome of treatment with pharmacologic serum levels of vitamin E in addition to cryotherapy from 1985 to 1991. *J Pediatr*, 1995, 127 632–9.

37 Raju T, Langenberg P, Bhutani V, Quinn GE Vitamin E prophylaxis to reduce retinopathy of prematurity: a reappraisal of published trials. *J Pediatr*, 1997, 131 844–50.

38 Ziegler EE, O'Donnell AM, Nelson SE, Komon SJ Body composition of the reference fetus growth. *Growth*, 1976, 40 329–41.

39 ESPGAN (European Society of Paediatric Gastroenterology and Nutrition) Nutrition and feeding of preterm infants. *Acta Paed Scand*, 1987, Supp 336.

40 Olivares M, Llaguno S, Marin V, Hertrampf E, Mena P, Milad M Iron status in low-birth-weight infants, small and appropriate for gestational age. A follow-up study. *Acta Paediatr*, 1992, 81 824–8.

41 Yuen D, Kim J, Brazeau Gravelle P Early iron [Fe] supplementation of low birth weight [LBW] infants improves erythropoiesis. *Pediatr Res*, 1996, 39 322A.

42 Ehrenkranz RA Iron requirements of preterm infants. *Nutr*, 1994, 10 77–8.

43 Griffin IJ, Cooke RJ, Reid MM, McCormick KPB, Smith JS Iron nutritional status in preterm infants fed formulas fortified with iron. *Arch Dis Childh*, 1999, 81 F45–9.

44 Friel JK, Gibson RS, Kawash GF, Watts J Dietary zinc intake and growth during infancy. *J Pediatr Gastroenterol Nutr*, 1985, 4 746–51.

45 Friel JK, Andrews WL Zinc requirement of premature infants. *Nutr*, 1994, 10 63–5.

46 Askari A, Long CL, Blakemore WS Urinary zinc, copper, nitrogen, and potassium losses in response to trauma. *J Parenter Enteral Nutr*, 1979, 3 151–6.

47 Wester PO Tissue zinc at autopsy – relation to medication with diuretics. *Acta Med Scand*, 1980, 208 269–71.

48 Lockitch G, Jacobson B, Quigley G, Dison P, Pendray M Selenium deficiency in low birth weight neonates: an unrecognized problem. *J Pediatr*, 1989, 114 865–70.

49 Daniels LA Selenium metabolism and bioavailability. *Biol Trace Elem Res*, 1996, 54 185–99.

50 Ares S, Quero J, Duran S, Presas MJ, Herruzo R, Morreale de Escobar G Iodine content of infant formulas and iodine intake of premature babies: high risk of iodine deficiency. *Arch Dis Childh Fetal Neonatal edn*, 1994, 71 F184–91.

51 Patton S, Canfield LM, Huston GE, Ferris AM, Jensen RG Carotenoids of human colostrum. *Lipids*, 1990, 25 159–65.

52 Rowe PM Beta-carotene takes a collective beating, (news). *Lancet*, 1996, 347 249.

53 Rudolph FB Symposium: dietary nucleotides: a recently demonstrated requirement for cellular development and immune function. *J Nutr*, 1994, 124 1431S–2S.

54 Brunser O, Espinoza J, Araya M, Cruchet S, Gil A Effect of dietary nucleotide supplementation on diarrhoeal disease in infants. *Acta Paediatr*, 1994, 83 188–91.

55 Cosgrove M, Davies DP, Jenkins HR Nucleotide supplementation and the growth of term small for gestational age infants. *Arch Dis Childh Fetal Neonatal edn*, 1996, 74 F122–5.

56 Powell-Tuck J Glutamine, parenteral feeding, and intestinal nutrition. *Lancet*, 1993, 342 451–2.

57 Lacey JM, Crouch JB, Benfell K, Ringer SA, Wilmore CK, Maguire D, Wilmore DW The effects of glutamine-supplemented parenteral nutrition in premature infants. *J Parenter Enter Nutr*, 1996, **20** 74–80.

58 Neu J, Roig JC, Meetze WH, Veerman M, Carter C, Millsaps M, Bowling D, Dallas MJ, Sleasman J, Knight T, Auestad N Enteral glutamine supplementation for very low birth weight infants decreases morbidity. *J Pediatr*, 1997, **131** 691–9.

59 Berseth CL Neonatal small intestinal motility: motor responses to feeding in term and preterm infants. *J Pediatr*, 1990, **117** 777–82.

60 Murdock N, Crighton A, Nelson LM, Forsyth JS Low birthweight infants and total parenteral nutrition immediately after birth. II. Randomised study of biochemical tolerance of intravenous glucose, amino acids, and lipid. *Arch Dis Childh Fetal Neonatal edn*, 1995, **73** F8–12.

61 Gilbertson N, Kovar IZ, Cox DJ, Crowe L, Palmer NT Introduction of intravenous lipid administration on the first day of life in the very low birth weight neonate. *J Pediatr*, 1991, **119** 615–23.

62 Van-Goudoever J, Colen T, Wattimena JL, Huijmans JG, Carnielli VP, Sauer PJ Immediate commencement of amino acid supplementation in preterm infants: effect on serum amino acid concentrations and protein kinetics on the first day of life. *J Pediatr*, 1995, **127** 458–65.

63 King C *Neonatal Unit Parenteral Nutrition Policy*. Dietetics Department, Hammersmith Hospital, London, 1998.

64 MacMahon RA, Yu V Intravenous nutrition of the neonate. London: Arnold Publishing, 1992.

65 Dunn L, Hulman S, Weiner J, Kliegman R Beneficial effects of early hypocaloric enteral feeding on neonatal gastrointestinal function: preliminary report of a randomized trial. *J Pediatr*, 1988, **112** 622–9.

66 Meetze WH, Valentine C, McGuigan JE Gastrointestinal priming prior to full enteral nutrition in very low birth weight infants. *J Pediatr Gastroenterol Nutr*, 1992, **15** 163–70.

67 Ehrenkranz R, Younes N, Fanaroff AA *et al.* Effect of nutritional practices on daily weight gain in VLBW infants. *Pediatr Res*, 1996, **39** 308A.

68 Schanler RJ, Shulman RJ, Lau C, Smith EO, Heitkemper MM Feeding strategies for premature infants: randomized trial of gastrointestinal priming and tube-feeding method. *Pediatrics*, 1999, **103** 434–9.

69 Lucas A Aids and milk bank closures. *Lancet*, 1987, **i**, 1092–3.

70 Uraizee F, Gross SJ Improved feeding tolerance and reduced incidence of sepsis in sick very low birth weight (VLBW) infants fed maternal milk. *Ped Res*, 1989, **25** 298A.

71 Lucas A, Cole TJ Breast milk and neonatal necrotising enterocolitis. *Lancet*, 1990, **336** 1519–23.

72 Hylander MA, Strobino DM, Dhanireddy R Human milk feedings and infection among very low birth weight infants. *Pediatr*, 1998, **102** E38.

73 Lucas A, Morley R, Cole TJ Breast milk and subsequent intelligence quotient in children born preterm. *Lancet*, 1992, **339** 261–4.

74 Lucas A, Morley R, Cole TJ, Gore A randomised multicentred study of human milk vs formula and later development in preterm infants. *Arch Dis Childh*, 1994, **70** F141–6.

75 Holland P, Wilkinson A, Diez J, Lindsell D Prenatal deficiency of phosphate, phosphate supplementation and rickets in very low birth weight infants. *Lancet*, 1990, **335** 697–701.

76 Velona T, Abbiati L, Beretta B, Gaiaschi A, Flauto U, Tagliabue P, Gailli CL, Restani P Protein profiles in breast milk from mothers delivering term and preterm babies. *Pediatr Res*, 1999, **45** 658–63.

77 Polberger SKT, Axelsson IE, Raitia NCR Urinary and serum urea as indicators of protein metabolism in very low birth weight infants fed varying human milk protein intakes. *Acta Paed Scand*, 1990, **79** 737–42.

78 Lucas A, Fewtrell MS, Morley R Randomised outcome trial of human milk fortification and developmental outcome in preterm infants. *Am J Clin Nutr*, 1996, **64** 142–51.

79 Jocson MA, Mason EO, Schanler RJ The effects of nutrient fortification and varying storage conditions on host defense properties of human milk. *Pediatr*, 1997, **100** 240–43.

80 Lucas A, King F, Bishop NB Post discharge formula consumption in infants born preterm. *Arch Dis Childh*, 1992, **67** 691–2.

81 King C *Neonatal Unit Enteral Feeding Policy*, 1st edn, pp. 1–44. Nutrition and Dietetic Department, Hammersmith Hospital, London, 1999.

82 Aynsley-Green A, Adrian TE, Bloom SR Feeding and the development of enteroinsular hormone release in the preterm infant: effects of continuous intragastric infusion of human milk compared with intermittent boluses. *Acta Paediatr Scand*, 1982, **71** 379–83.

83 Macagno F, Demarini S Techniques of enteral feeding in the newborn. *Acta Paediatr* (Suppl), 1994, **402** 11–13.

84 Narayanan I, Singh B, Harvey D Fat loss during feeding of human milk. *Arch Dis Childh* 1984, **59** 475–7.

85 de Ville K, Knapp E, Al Tawil Y, Berseth CL Slow infusion feedings enhance duodenal motor responses and gastric emptying in preterm infants. *Am J Clin Nutr*, 1998, **68** 103–108.

86 Uauy RD, Fanaroff AA, Korones SB Necrotising enterocolitis in very low birth weight infants. Biodemographic and clinical correlates. *J Pediatr*, 1991, **119** 630–38.

87 McKeown RE, Marsh D, Amarnath U Role of delayed feeding and of feeding increments in necrotising enterocolitis. *J Pediatr*, 1992, **121** 764–70.

88 Wilson DC, McClure G, Halliday HL, Reid MM, Dodge JA Nutrition and bronchopulmonary dysplasia. *Arch Dis Childh*, 1991, **66** 37–8.

89 Kurzner SI, Garg M, Bautista DB, Bader D, Merritt RJ, Warburton D, Keens TG Growth failure in infants with bronchopulmonary dysplasia: nutrition and elevated resting metabolic expenditure. *Pediatr*, 1988, **81** 379–84.

90 Yunis KA, Oh W Effects of intravenous glucose loading on oxygen consumption, carbon dioxide production, and resting energy expenditure in infants with bronchopulmonary dysplasia. *J Pediatr*, 1989, **115** 127–32.

91 de Meer K, Westerterp KR, Houwen RH, Brouwers HA, Berger R, Okken A Total energy expenditure in infants with bronchopulmonary dysplasia is associated with respiratory status. *Eur J Pediatr*, 1997, **156** 299–304.

92 Kao LC, Durand DJ, Nickerson BG Improving pulmonary function does not decrease oxygen consumption in infants with bronchopulmonary dysplasia. *J Pediatr*, 1988, **112** 616–21.

93 Leitch CA, Ahlrichs JA, Karn CA, Denne SC Total energy expenditure is not increased in premature infants with bronchopulmonary dysplasia. *Pediatr Res*, 1995, **37** 313A.

94 Fewtrell MS, Adams C, Wilson DC, Cairns P, McClure G, Lucas A Randomized trial of high nutrient density formula versus standard formula in chronic lung disease. *Acta Paediatr*, 1997, **86** 577–82.

95 Moyer-Mileur L, Chan GM, Ammon BB, Ostrom KM Growth and tolerance of calorically dense, high fat feeding in infants with bronchopulmonary dysplasia (BPD). *Pediatr Res*, 1994, **35** 317A.

96 Williams AF, Jones M Dexamethasone increases plasma amino acid concentrations in bronchopulmonary dysplasia. *Arch Dis Childh*, 1992, **67** 5–9.

97 Gibson AT, Pearse RG, Wales JKH Growth retardation after dexamethasone administration assessment by kneemometry. *Arch Dis Childh*, 1993, **69** 505–9.

98 Weiler HA, Paes B, Shah JK, Atkinson SA Longitudinal assessment of growth and bone mineral accretion in prematurely born infants treated for chronic lung disease with dexamethasone. *Early Hum Dev*, 1997, **47** 271–86.

99 Leitch CA, Ahlrichs J, Brondyke A *et al.* Total energy expenditure in premature infants with bronchopul-

monary dysplasia on and off dexamethasone. *Pediatr Res*, 1994, **35** 316A.

100 Leitch CA, Ahlrichs J, Karn C, Denne SC Energy expenditure and energy intake during dexamethasone therapy for chronic lung disease. *Pediatr Res*, 1999, **46** 109–13.

101 Pereira GR, Baumgart S, Bennett MJ Use of a high fat formula for premature infants with BPD metabolic pulmonary and nutritional studies. *J Pediatr*, 1994, **124** 605–11.

102 Wilson DC, McClure G, Dodge JA The influence of nutrition on neonatal respiratory muscle function. *Intensive Care Med*, 1992, **18** 105–108.

103 Stockman JA, Clarke DA Weight gain: a response to transfusion in selected preterm infants. *Amer J Dis Childh*, 1984, **138** 828–30.

104 Chance CW, Raddle IC, Willis DM, Park E Postnatal growth of infants <1.3 kg birth weight: effects of metabolic acidosis, of caloric intake and of calcium, sodium and phosphorus supplementation. *J Pediatr*, 1977, **91** 787–93.

105 Groothuis JR, Rosenberg AA Home oxygen promotes weight gain in infants with bronchopulmonary dysplasia. *Am J Dis Childh*, 1987, **141** 992–5.

106 Lucas A, Bishop NJ, King FJ, Cole TJ Randomised trial of nutrition for preterm infants after discharge. *Arch Dis Childh*, 1992, **67** 322–7.

107 Bishop NJ, King FJ, Lucas A Increased bone mineral content of preterm infants fed a nutrient enriched formula after discharge from hospital. *Arch Dis Childh*, 1993, **68** 573–8.

108 COMA Department of Health *Weaning and the Weaning Diet*. London: The Stationery Office, 1994.

109 Berseth CL Effect of early feeding on maturation of the preterm infants small intestine. *J Pediatr*, 1992, **120** 947.

110 David TJ, Ewing CI Atopic eczema and preterm birth. *Arch Dis Childh*, 1988, **63** 435–6.

111 Douglas JE, Bryon M Interview data on severe behavioural eating difficulties in young children. *Arch Dis Childh*, 1996, **75** 304–308.

112 Martin M, Shaw NJ Feeding problems in infants and young children with chronic lung disease. *J Human Nutr*, 1997, **10** 271–5.

113 Illingworth RS, Lister J The critical or sensitive period with special reference to certain feeding problems in infants and children. *J Pediatr*, 1964, **65** 839–49.

114 King C *Neonatal Unit Weaning Policy*. Nutrition and Dietetic Department, Hammersmith Hospital, London, 2000.

SECTION 4

Diseases of Organ Systems

CHAPTER 6

The Gastrointestinal Tract

The gastrointestinal (GI) tract is one of the most interesting and challenging areas in paediatric dietetics. The medical conditions encountered are diverse and require an understanding of normal GI function before correct dietetic advice can be given. Problems as varied as diarrhoea, constipation and GI dysmotility can affect normal intake and absorption of nutrients. Manipulation of feeds and diet is often the primary treatment for the underlying condition and carers need careful explanation of the principles of the feed and diet prescribed.

NUTRITIONAL REQUIREMENTS

These vary according to the underlying disorder, with specific nutrient requirements discussed in this chapter. For GI disorders that do not result in malabsorption, normal requirements for most nutrients will suffice, with additional energy and protein required for catch-up growth.

When malabsorption is present requirements for all nutrients are raised to cover stool losses, particularly fluid, energy, protein and electrolytes. Most infants will have high to very high requirements. Careful monitoring of nutritional status, by anthropometric and biochemical means, is needed.

Table 6.1 can be used as a guide for requirements for infants with malabsorption fed enterally and are based on actual rather than expected weight.

FLUID AND DIETARY THERAPY OF ACUTE DIARRHOEA

Acute diarrhoea remains one of the leading causes of childhood morbidity and mortality in developing nations, with an estimated 5 to 18 million deaths attributed to this cause each year. In industrial nations

the mortality rate is much lower. Infants and children are particularly vulnerable to the effects of acute diarrhoea because of their greater relative fluid requirements and their susceptibility to faecal-oral agents.

The mechanisms in the GI tract causing acute diarrhoea are:

- Increased secretion
- Decreased absorption.

Often these coexist to produce an increased fluid load that exceeds the colonic absorptive capacity and results in diarrhoea. Both viral and bacterial pathogens can affect the gut in this way.

Transport of glucose and amino acids is an active process and requires the presence of a sodium gradient across the brush border membrane maintained by the Na^+-K^+ ATPase pump. The movement of water in the gut is a passive event driven by the movement of solute. The regulation of electrolye transport is controlled by several mediators and inhibition of these pathways results in poor absorption and active chloride secretion into the gut.

In infective diarrhoea decreased absorption is not necessarily due to reduced villous size. With increased cell loss immature epithelial cells replace fully differentiated, mature absorptive cells. These cells have defective electrolyte and nutrient transport and functional impairment may be severe. This situation is worsened by cycles of fasting and starvation commonly seen in infants and children with acute diarrhoea in developing countries.

Oral rehydration solutions

Oral rehydration therapy should be the cornerstone of treatment of dehydration seen in infective

Table 6.1 Suggested requirements for infants with malabsorption

Energy	High	130–150 kcal/kg/day (540–630 kJ/kg/day)
	Very high	150–220 kcal/kg/day (630–900 kJ/kg/day)
Protein	High	3–4 g/kg/day
	Very high	Maximum 0–6 months 6 g/kg/day, increasing to maximum of 10 g/kg/day by 1 year
Sodium	High	3.0 mmol/kg/day
Potassium	Very high	4.5 mmol/kg/day
Fluid	High	180–220 ml/kg/day

Table 6.2 Oral rehydration solutions (ORS) available in the UK

	mmol per litre			
	Na⁺	K⁺	Cl⁻	CHO
Diocalm Junior (SmithKline Beecham Healthcare)	60	20	50	111 (glucose)
Dioralyte (powder) (Rhône-Poulenc Rorer)	60	20	60	90 (glucose)
Electrolade (Eastern)	50	20	40	111 (glucose)
Rehidrat (Searle)	50	20	50	91 (glucose) 94 (sucrose)
Dioralyte Relief* (Rhône-Poulenc Rorer)	60	20	50	30 g (rice starch)
WHO Rehydration Salts	90	20	80	111 (glucose)

* Not recommended for use in infancy.
Effervescent and flavoured preparations are not suitable for young infants.

diarrhoea. The aim should be to correct dehydration and maintain hydration. The sodium-glucose coupled transport mechanism stimulates water and electrolyte transport and this process is preserved in acute diarrhoeal disorders.

Specific recommendations for the composition of oral rehydration solutions (ORS) for European children have been published by the European Society of Paediatric Gastroenterology and Nutrition (ESPGAN) [1]:

- Carbohydrate should be present as either monomeric glucose or glucose polymer at a concentration between 74 and 111 mmol/l. Cereal based ORS have been demonstrated to be more effective at reducing stool output than glucose based ORS. Rice should be used in preference to other cereals because of the risk of adverse reactions in young infants.
- To minimise the risk of hypernatraemia ORS in Britain should contain 60 mmol/l sodium, which is less than the 90 mmol/l recommended by the World Health Organisation (WHO) for developing countries.
- Potassium should be added to replace stool losses.
- The final osmolality should be low (200–250 mOsm/kgH₂0) to ensure optimal water absorption.

ORSs available in the UK are summarised in Table 6.2.

Feeding during acute diarrhoea

For many years it has been common practice not to give feeds during diarrhoeal episodes. There were concerns that decreased lactase activity chiefly associated with rotavirus gastroenteritis, one of the most common causes of acute diarrhoea in young children, would cause lactose malabsorption if milk feeds were introduced too early. It was also thought that food proteins could be transported across an impaired mucosal barrier and evoke sensitisation.

Bottle fed infants with gastroenteritis have traditionally been managed by feeding ORS alone for 24 hours before feed reintroduction. Some units start dilute feeds and increase the strength over 2–4 days. This advice, together with a decreased appetite, results in a reduced nutritional intake at a time when requirements are increased due to infection [2]. Mothers of breast fed infants have been advised to continue to breast feed and give supplemental feeds of ORS to replace stool losses.

A meta-analysis of randomised clinical trials published in 1994 showed that the routine dilution of milk feeds and use of lactose-free formula was not justified in the treatment of infants and children with acute diarrhoea [3]. A multicentre European study has shown that the complete resumption of a child's normal feeding after 4 hours of rehydration with ORS led to a significantly greater weight gain during hospitalisation and did not result in worsening or prolonged duration of diarrhoea, increased vomiting or lactose intolerance [4]. Many studies have demonstrated that rapid introduction of age appropriate feeds can have a beneficial effect on the outcome. This is especially important in developing countries where children may already be malnourished.

ESPGAN now recommends that management of gastroenteritis should consist of oral rehydration with a suitable ORS for 3–4 hours (100 ml/kg over 4–6 hours in moderately dehydrated patients), followed by rapid introduction of normal feeding [5]. Supplementation with ORS should continue to compensate for stool fluid and electrolyte losses while diarrhoea continues. As a guide 10 ml per kg body weight of ORS should be given for each liquid stool passed. This represents a change in current practice which will take time and education to be adopted by units. As recommended before, breast feeding should be continued at all times with supplementation of ORS.

There is no evidence to support the use of lactose reduced or cow's milk protein-free formula in infants and children with acute diarrhoea, even if the infective agent is rotavirus. A very small minority of patients who show signs of intolerance (worsening of diarrhoea with acidic stools containing >0.5% reducing substances) may need dietary manipulations and the temporary use of a lactose free-formula (Table 6.15).

CONGENITAL CHLORIDE LOSING DIARRHOEA

This is inherited as an autosomal recessive trait and is the consequence of a selective defect in intestinal chloride transport in the ileum and colon. As a result lifelong secretory diarrhoea occurs with high faecal chloride concentrations. It has been reported in most populations including Britain; however it is most commonly seen in Finland and the Arabian Gulf.

In the past it generally resulted in severe lethal dehydration. Watery diarrhoea is present from birth but often goes unnoticed as the fluid in the nappy is thought to be urine. Dehydration occurs rapidly followed by disturbances in electrolyte concentration causing hyponatraemia and hypochloraemia with mild metabolic acidosis.

Treatment

As the intestinal defect cannot be corrected treatment requires replacement of the diarrhoeal losses of chloride, sodium and water. Initially this may need to be given intravenously but this should gradually be changed to the oral route. Dietary manipulation is not required in this disorder other than to ensure a normal intake for age in conjunction with the prescribed electrolyte and fluid therapy.

PROTEIN INTOLERANCES

It is thought that the relatively high incidence of adverse reactions to food proteins seen in infancy is the result of an increased gut permeability to large molecules and the immaturity of local and systemic immune systems. These reactions can be immunologically mediated, defined as food protein allergy; or non-immunologically mediated, defined as food intolerances (p. 193). The most common organs to be affected are the skin, gut and respiratory tract. GI symptoms that can be caused by protein intolerances are summarised in Table 6.3.

Cow's milk protein intolerance

Cow's milk is the most common food to cause a reaction in infants and the incidence of cow's milk protein intolerance (CMPI) or allergy reported in developed countries is between 2 and 3%; 0.5% of breast fed infants are reported to be food allergic or intolerant, reacting to exogenous food proteins secreted into the mother's milk. There is no single diagnostic laboratory test so the diagnosis can often only be based on a clinical response to cow's milk protein withdrawal and challenge. When alternative infant formulas are tried it is necessary to persist with a feed for a reasonable length of time, observing symptoms carefully, before abandoning it in favour of a different feed.

Table 6.3 Gastrointestinal symptoms that can be caused by intolerance to dietary proteins

Gastro-oesophageal reflux
Vomiting
Enteropathy
Enterocolitis
Proctitis
Allergic colitis
Constipation
Diarrhoea
Coeliac disease

Delayed reactions to foods can occur several days after their ingestion.

Prognosis is good with remission in approximately 50% of infants by 1 year of age, 75% at 2 years and 90% at 3 years of age. Less than 1% of infants maintain a lifelong food intolerance [6].

Alternative infant formulas

It is vital that an infant is given a nutritionally complete milk substitute to replace a formula based on cow's milk protein. In breast fed infants the mother's diet needs to be modified, by the removal of cow's milk and any other foods allergenic to the infant, ensuring that the maternal diet continues to include adequate amounts of calcium, fluid, energy and protein. It has been found that breast fed infants can be sensitised to multiple allergens, including egg, soy, wheat and fish [7].

Mammalian milks

Mammalian milk is not suitable to be used as an infant feed without modification due to its high renal solute load and inadequate vitamin and mineral content. The proteins in goat's and sheep's milks share antigenic cross-reactivity with cow's milk proteins. Infant formulas based on these milks are not recommended for use in gastrointestinal food intolerances [8].

Soy protein based formulas

A soy protein based formula was used for the first time in 1929 to feed infants with cow's milk protein allergy. Today these feeds are based on a soy protein isolate supplemented with l-methionine to give a suitable amino acid profile for use in infancy. They are lactose free with the carbohydrate generally being present as glucose polymer; only one soy formula in the UK contains the disaccharide sucrose (Table 6.4). The fat is a mixture of vegetable oils which provide long chain fatty acids, including essential fatty acids. Feeding modern soy formulas to infants is associated with normal growth, protein status and bone mineralisation [9].

Soy protein has a very large molecular weight and after digestion can generate a large number of potential allergens. Severe gastrointestinal reactions to soy protein formula have been described for more than 30 years and include some reactions seen in CMPI such as enteropathy, enterocolitis and proctitis. It is suggested that an intestinal mucosa damaged by cow's milk allows increased uptake and increased immunologic reaction to soy protein. A reported 60% of infants with cow's milk protein induced enterocolitis are equally sensitive to soy. For these reasons soy protein based formulas should not be used in the management of cow's milk protein enteropathy or enterocolitis [9].

Infants with documented IgE-mediated allergy to cow's milk protein can do well on soy protein based formula [10, 11]. In other gastrointestinal manifestations of possible CMPI, such as constipation or vomiting where the mucosa is not damaged, soy feeds can be used. It should be remembered that soy formula has the benefit of being at least half the cost of hydrolysed protein formula and is much more palatable. Soy infant formulas available in the UK are summarised in Table 6.4.

Table 6.4 Composition of soy infant formula available in the UK, per 100 ml

Name and manufacturer	Dilution %	Energy (kcal)	Energy (kJ)	CHO (g)	Protein (g)	Fat (g)	Osmolality (mOsmol/kgH₂O)
InfaSoy (Cow & Gate)	12.7	66	277	6.7	1.8	3.6	200
Wysoy (SMA Nutrition)	13.3	67	280	6.9	1.8	3.6	214
Farley's Soya Formula (HJ Heinz)	13.7	70	294	7.0	2.0	3.8	N/A
Prosobee (Mead Johnson)	13.0	68	285	6.6	2.0	3.6	180
Isomil (Abbott)	13.0	68	285	6.9 (40% sucrose)	1.8	3.7	250

Table 6.5 Milk-free diet

Foods permitted	Foods to be excluded	Check ingredients
Milk substitute Vegetable oils Custard made with milk substitute, sorbet	All mammalian milks, cheese, yoghurt, fromage frais, ice cream, butter	Margarines
Meat, fish, eggs, pulses		Sausages, pies, foods in batter or breadcrumbs Baked beans
All grains, dry pasta, flour Bread, most breakfast cereals	Pasta with cheese or milk sauce, milk bread, nan bread Cream cakes, chocolate biscuits	Tinned pasta Bought cakes or biscuits
Fruit and vegetables		Instant mashed potato
Plain crisps, nuts		Flavoured crisps
Sugar, jam, jelly Marmite, ketchup	Milk chocolate, toffee	Plain chocolate Salad dressings, soups
Milk shake syrups and powder Pop, juice, squash	Malted milk drinks	

Milk-free diet

It is important that carers of infants requiring a cow's milk protein-free feed are given appropriate advice about excluding cow's milk from solids. The following ingredients indicate the presence of cow's milk in a manufactured food: casein, hydrolysed caseinates, whey, hydrolysed whey, lactose, milk solids, non-fat milk solids, butter fat. Parents should be taught to recognise these in lists of ingredients and exclude foods containing them from the diet. Milk-free dietary information is summarised in Table 6.5.

Feeds based on protein hydrolysates

Infants with severe CMPI and proven or suspected soy intolerance need an alternative type of formula. The allergenicity or antigenicity of a particular protein is a function of the amino acid sequences present and the configuration of the molecule. An epitope is the area of a peptide chain capable of stimulating antibody production. During the manufacture of a hydrolysate the protein is denatured by heat treatment and hydrolysed by proteolytic enzymes leaving small peptides and free amino acids. The enzymes are then inactivated by heat and, along with residual large peptides, are removed by filtration [12].

The proteins used to make a hydrolysate vary and production methods also differ between manufactur-

ers. The profile of peptide chain lengths between different feeds will not be identical, even when the initial protein is the same (Table 13.2).

Potential problems with hydrolysate formulas

Despite the rigorous conditions employed in the manufacture of these feeds there are still potential sequential epitopes present which can be recognised by sensitive infants. Extensively hydrolysed protein based feeds vary considerably in their molecular weight profile and hence in their residual allergenic activity (p. 195). Feeds with peptides of greater than 1500 daltons have been demonstrated to have residual allergenic activity [14, 15]. The degree of hydrolysis does not predict the immunogenic or the allergenic effects in the recipient infant. It has been recommended that dietary products for treatment of cow's milk protein allergy in infants should be tolerated by at least 90% of infants with documented cow's milk allergy [8]. In instances where an infant is not malnourished and fails to tolerate one hydrolysate formula, a second hydrolysate from a different protein source can be tried.

Table 6.6 shows the composition of extensively hydrolysed feeds available in the UK. All of these feeds are suitable to be used in infants with CMPI who are also intolerant to soy. Feed choice may be influenced by:

Table 6.6 Extensively hydrolysed infant feeds available in UK

Name and manufacturer		Dilution %	Energy (kcal)	(kJ)	CHO (g)[1]	Protein (g)	Fat (g)[2]	Na⁺ (mmol)	K⁺ (mmol)	Osmolality (mOsmol/kg H₂O)
Casein	Nutramigen (Mead Johnson)	13.5	68	284	7.4	1.9	3.4	1.4	1.9	290
	Pregestimil (Mead Johnson)	13.5	68	284	6.9	1.9	3.8 (55%)	1.4	1.9	330
Whey	Pepti-Junior (Cow & Gate)	12.8	66	276	6.6 trace lactose	1.8	3.6 (50%)	0.9	1.7	210
	Alfaré (Nestlé)	15	72	301	7.8 trace lactose	2.5	3.6 (50%)	1.9	2.3	220
Pork and soya	Prejomin (Milupa)	15	75	313	8.6	2.0	3.6	1.7	2.1	220–230
	Pepdite years (SHS)	15	71	297	7.8	2.1	3.5 (3%)	1.5	1.5	237
	MCT Pepdite 0–2 years** (SHS)	15	68	286	8.9	2.1	2.7 (83%)	1.5	1.5	277

[1] Carbohydrate is present as glucose polymers derived from different sources unless otherwise stated.

[2] Figures in parenthesis indicate the percentage of fat present as medium chain triglycerides (MCT).

** Patients who are receiving a significant proportion of their nutritional requirements from MCT Pepdite, may need to supplement their intake of essential fatty acids to meet UK dietary reference values 1991 [16] and ESPGAN guidelines 1991 (p. 114). This can be achieved with the addition of walnut oil to the feed [13].

SHS = Scientific Hospital Supplies

- Palatability, which is affected by the presence of bitter peptides. This is particularly important in infants older than 3 months of age
- Coexisting fat malabsorption, where a feed with some of the fat as medium chain triglycerides (MCT) may be indicated
- Cost, some hydrolysates being twice as expensive as others
- Religions, where parents do not wish their children to be given products derived from pork.

Feed introduction

Hydrolysate feeds should be introduced slowly to infants with severe gastrointestinal symptoms as they have a higher osmolality than normal infant formula. Feeds containing a high percentage of MCT should also be introduced gradually over 48 hours to ensure tolerance, the speed of introduction depending on clinical symptoms; a minimum of 12 hours on a half strength feed before the introduction of full strength formula is suggested. If the diarrhoea is very severe then it may be necessary to introduce quarter strength feeds initially, grading up to full strength feeds over 4 days. If severe diarrhoea is present in an older infant it is preferable to stop all solids while a new feed is being introduced, to ensure tolerance.

In an outpatient setting where feed tolerance is less of a problem, full strength formula can be introduced from the outset. However in infants older than 6 months there may be an advantage in initially mixing the hydrolysate with their usual formula to slowly introduce the new taste and encourage acceptance. A suggested regimen is shown in Table 6.7. Milk shake flavours at 2–4% concentration can also be used in this age group if sucrose is not contraindicated.

In clinical situations where an infant refuses to drink a hydrolysate a nasogastric tube needs to be passed to ensure adequate feed volumes. Where failure to thrive coexists, feeds can be fortified in the usual manner by the addition of fat, carbohydrate or an increase in formula concentration. All changes should be made slowly to ensure they are tolerated.

Pepti-Junior has a sodium content similar to standard infant formula which may not be sufficient for an infant with increased stool losses. Low urinary sodium (<20 mmol/litre) alongside a normal plasma sodium concentration can indicate sodium depletion and feed supplementation with sodium chloride may be required.

Introduction of solids

Weaning should take place at the recommended age, between 4 and 6 months. It is important to ensure that the diet offered is free of cow's milk protein. Other dietary proteins which may need to be excluded include egg, soy and wheat. In very sensitive infants it may be wise to introduce new foods singly.

In conditions where soy intolerance is present in addition to CMPI, foods containing soy and milk protein should be excluded from the diet (Table 6.8).

Vegetable or soy oils and soya lecithin are normally tolerated by individuals sensitive to soy protein and do not need to be excluded from the diet except in severely affected individuals.

Amino acid based infant formula

Only pure amino acid mixtures are considered to be non-allergenic as there are no peptide chains present to act as epitopes. In infants who fail to tolerate a hydrolysate this is the next logical step, so long as there is not a co-existing fat or carbohydrate intolerance. In these situations a modular feeding approach should be used (p. 84). At present there is only one such feed for infants in the UK, Neocate (Table 6.9). Studies have shown this to be effective in a number of clinical settings where protein hydrolysates have not been tolerated [15]. The sodium content of Neocate is relatively low for infants with chronic diarrhoea and may need further supplementation.

Feeds suitable for use for older children

In older children with food intolerances or allergy a suitable infant formula should be continued for as long as possible. In situations where a large percentage of the child's nutrition comes from a formula this will either need fortification to meet nutritional requirements or a feed designed for older children should be used. The feeds in Table 6.10 have been designed to meet the requirements of older children requiring hypoallergenic feeds. Other adult feeds based on soy or hydrolysed protein should be used with care in older children and may require modification or vitamin and mineral supplementation.

Table 6.7 Suggested plan for introducing hydrolysate feeds to older infants fed by mouth

Day number	Percentage own feed	Percentage new hydrolysate feed
1	75	25
2	50	50
3	25	75
4	0	100

Table 6.8 Foods containing soya protein

All soy based products including tofu and soy sauce Soy margarines	Texturised vegetable proteins	Breads, biscuits and cakes which contain soy flour	Baby foods containing soy protein

Table 6.9 Infant formula based on amino acids available in the UK per 100 ml

Name and manufacturer	Dilution %	Energy (kcal)	(kJ)	CHO (g)	Protein equivalent (g)	Fat (g)	Na+ (mmol)	K+ (mmol)	Osmolality (mOsmol/kg H$_2$O)
Neocate (Scientific Hospital Supplies)	15	71	298	8.1	2.0	3.5 (4.5% MCT)	0.8	1.6	360

Table 6.10 Hydrolysate and amino acid based feeds for older children per 100 ml

Name	Dilution %	Energy (kcal)	(kJ)	CHO[1] (g)	Protein equivalent (g)	Fat[2] (g)	Na+ (mmol)	K+ (mmol)	Osmolality (mOsmol/kg H$_2$O)
Hydrolysate feeds									
Pepdite 2+[†]	20	88	369	11.4	2.8	3.5 (35)	1.8	2.6	351
MCT Pepdite 2+[†][**]	20	91	380	11.8	2.8	3.6 (83)	1.8	2.6	389
Amino acid feeds									
Neocate Advance	25	100	420	14.6	2.5	3.5	2.6	3.0	636
Elemental O28□* (unflavoured)	20	76	323	14.1	2.0	1.3 (5)	2.2	2.4	496
Elemental O28□* Extra (unflavoured)	20	85	359	11	2.5	3.5 (35)	2.7	2.4	502
Emsogen □* (unflavoured)	20	88	370	11	2.5	3.3 (83)	2.6	2.4	539

[1]   All present as glucose polymer derived from different sources.
[2]   Figures in parenthesis show percentage fat present as MCT.
[†]   Should only be used in children 2 years or older.
□   Should not be used as the sole source of nutrition in children under the age of 5 years.
*   Flavoured versions of these feeds are also available.
**   Patients who are receiving a significant proportion of their nutritional requirements from MCT Pepdite 2+, may need to supplement their intake of essential fatty acids to meet UK DRVs 1991 [16] and ESPGAN guidelines 1991 (p. 114). This can be achieved with the addition of walnut oil to the feed [13].
All feeds manufactured by Scientific Hospital Supplies.

In children over the age of 2 years consuming a well balanced diet and tolerating soy protein, super-market 'adult' liquid soy milks can be given as an alternative to cow's milk, those with added calcium helping to ensure an adequate intake of this nutrient. For children intolerant to soy and cow's milk, rice or oat milks available in health food shops or some super-markets can be useful as a social replacement to cow's milk. These are currently not fortified with calcium which should be given as a supplement in amounts equivalent to the reference nutrient intake (RNI) for age [16]. Calcium intakes below the recommended intakes have been identified in a number of children limiting cow's milk in their diet, which may affect bone density [17].

COELIAC DISEASE

This is an autoimmune disease primarily affecting the proximal small intestine characterised by an abnormal small intestinal mucosa and associated with a perma-nent intolerance to gluten. There are at least two pre-requisites for developing coeliac disease (CD): a genetic predisposition and ingestion of gluten. More than one member of a family may be affected. The incidence has been estimated in England to be between 1 in 2000 and 1 in 6000, whilst in the west of Ireland it has been reported to be as high as 1 in 300. Recently there has been a trend towards a decrease in incidence in most European centres and an increase in the age at the time of diagnosis. The latter is possibly due to a change in weaning practices since the mid-1970s with a delayed introduction of gluten containing cereals, although the data available are contradictory [18, 19]. There is considerable vari-ation in the age of onset and in the mode of presen-tation, with patients now being diagnosed well into adulthood.

CD is an immunological disorder with local and systemic production of food antibodies and the pro-duction of autoantibodies against structural proteins

The Gastrointestinal Tract

77

of the small intestine mucosa. The presence of IgA antigliadin antibodies in the blood is not specific for small intestine damage. Antireticulin and anti-endomysial antibodies are more specific markers although these can also be raised in healthy first degree relatives with a normal small intestinal biopsy. Therefore the 'gold standard' for diagnosis remains a small intestinal biopsy demonstrating initial mucosal damage followed by a clinical response to gluten withdrawal [20]. It is important that patients with suspected CD continue on a normal diet until the diagnostic biopsy has been performed and a clear diagnosis made.

Treatment

CD is treated by excluding all dietary sources of gluten, a protein found in wheat, rye and barley. The gluten can be divided into four subclasses: gliadin, glutenins, albumins and globulins. In wheat the injurious constituent is the prolamin fraction of α-gliadin. The equivalent in rye is secalin and in barley hordein. Enzymatic degradation studies have suggested that the damaging fraction is an acidic polypeptide with a molecular weight of less than 1500 daltons.

The gluten free diet

All possible sources of wheat, rye and barley need to be excluded from the diet which, in true CD, needs to be followed for life (Table 6.11). Oat exclusion may also be needed. This excludes a number of staple foods such as bread, pasta, biscuits and cakes and parents need a great deal of support and help in finding suitable substitutes which the child will eat. Wheat flour is commonly used in processed foods as a binding agent, filler or carrier for flavourings and spices. Parents and children with CD need to be taught to identify sources of the offending cereals in lists of food ingredients. They should also be aware that, at present, manufacturers do not need to list the constituents of compound ingredients that form a small percentage weight of the final product, such as the flavourings used in snack foods.

Children tend to be the highest consumers of savoury snack foods and the processed foods that need to be excluded on this diet. The food list produced annually by the Coeliac Society and updated regularly using data from supermarkets and manufacturers is an important resource for all coeliacs. This helps to identify gluten free foods that would not be obvious from the label, for instance flavoured crisps. Increased variety of foods allowed will improve patient

Table 6.11 Gluten-free diet

Foods permitted	Foods to avoid	Check ingredients
Milk, butter, cream, cheese		Cheese spreads, yoghurts, custard
Meat, fish, eggs, pulses	Products with pastry, thickened gravies and sauces, breadcrumbs, batter	Sausages, tinned meats
Rice, corn (maize), buckwheat, millet, tapioca, soya, gram flour, arrowroot. Special gluten free flours, breads, biscuits and pasta	Wheat, rye, barley, Triticale. Oats*. Bread, crumpets, cakes, biscuits, crackers, crispbread, chapattis, nan bread, pasta, noodles, semolina, couscous	Baking powder
Corn and rice based cereals	Wheat based cereals e.g. Weetabix, Shredded Wheat	
Vegetables, potato, fruit and nuts	Potato croquettes	Flavoured potato crisps, dry roasted nuts
Sugar, jam, honey, some chocolates	Liquorice	Filled chocolates, boiled sweets
Tea, coffee, drinking chocolate, fizzy drinks, juice, squash	Malted milk drinks e.g. Horlicks and Ovaltine. Barley water, beer	

* Exclusion may be necessary.

compliance. Young children should be taught to check with parents before eating foods outside the home or offered by siblings or friends. Where possible meals should be prepared that are suitable for the whole family so that the child does not feel different. Children's parties are a source of concern to parents and the coeliac child should be sent with suitable foods of their own to eat.

Commercially produced gluten free foods

A large number of proprietary gluten free foods are available, often based on wheat starch. In ordinary manufactured foods containing wheat starch the latter is not pure enough to be included in a gluten free diet. However, specially manufactured foods that comply with the International Gluten Free Standard (WHO Codex Alimentarius 1981) are suitable for inclusion in the diets of most coeliacs. A number of the more basic food items have been passed as prescribable for patients with CD by the Advisory Committee on Borderline Substances (ACBS), while the more luxurious items such as fruit cakes can be purchased via pharmacies or health food shops.

A large number of companies produce such foods and a complete list can be found in the *British National Formulary* (BNF) or in the Coeliac Society's manufactured food list. Products vary and patients should be encouraged to try different food items to aid dietary compliance. Some of the larger companies will send newly diagnosed patients trial packs of their own products on application.

Oats

Traditionally oats have been excluded from the coeliac diet although this is now a point of controversy. Problems with earlier studies included small patient numbers, insensitive functional tests and small intestinal biopsies that were often difficult to interpret [21]. The Coeliac Society's Medical Advisory Council have published interim guidelines until further conclusive evidence is available. These state that moderate amounts of oats may be consumed by most adult coeliacs without risk, although the situation is less clear with children. Highly sensitised coeliacs should at present not be allowed oats and patients should be carefully followed up [22]. A further complicating factor is that oats can be contaminated with wheat at various stages of production:

in fields, transportation, storage, milling and processing. Care should therefore be taken to avoid contaminated sources. Oat products are now included in an appendix to the Coeliac Society's annual food list.

The Coeliac Society

This is an independent registered charity with free membership which all parents of children with coeliac disease should be encouraged to join. As well as the aforementioned food list the society publishes a biannual magazine, information for newly diagnosed coeliacs and a recipe book. It now has a web site with up-to-date information on diet and CD: www.coeliac.co.uk.

Gluten challenge

Transient gluten intolerance is recognised and, previously, ESPGAN insisted that all patients with CD underwent a gluten provocation test and repeat biopsy to confirm the diagnosis. Now it is felt necessary only to do this when there is some doubt at the time of initial diagnosis [20]. For challenge purposes gluten can be introduced into the diet in two forms, either as gluten powder that can be mixed in foods such as yoghurts, or as gluten containing foods. Both need to be given daily in sufficient amounts to ensure an adequate challenge. Two slices of bread a day for older children has been suggested by one author [20]. Our practice has been to put the children onto a normal diet for the duration of the challenge. Parents are often anxious that the inclusion of normal foods in the diet will make returning to the gluten free diet difficult if the diagnosis of CD is confirmed. Reassurance is required and an explanation of the procedure to the child is very important in ensuring its success.

Associated food intolerances

Although a secondary disaccharidase deficiency can be demonstrated at the time of diagnosis it is rarely necessary to exclude lactose from the diet of a newly diagnosed coeliac. However, some infants do seem to be intolerant of cow's milk protein and benefit from a temporary dietary exclusion in addition to gluten. They should be rechallenged with cow's milk 2–3 months after the commencement of the gluten free diet.

CARBOHYDRATE INTOLERANCES

Sugar malabsorption increases the osmotic load of GI fluid, draws water into the small intestine and stimulates peristalsis, resulting in diarrhoea. The severity depends on the quantity of ingested carbohydrate, the metabolic activity of colonic bacteria (which is reduced after antibiotic therapy) and the absorptive capacity of the colon for water and short chain fatty acids.

The infant is at a disadvantage compared to the adult as the small intestine is shorter and the reserve capacity of the colon to absorb luminal fluids is reduced. Because of a faster gut transit time there is less time for alternative paths of carbohydrate digestion to be effective, including the salvage of malabsorbed carbohydrate by colonic bacterial fermentation. The undigested sugar is either excreted unchanged or is fermented in the colon to short chain fatty acids and lactic acid.

Disaccharidase deficiencies

In the brush border of the small intestine there are four disaccharidase enzymes with the highest level of activity occurring in the jejunum (Table 6.12). Deficiencies of these enzymes can be primary in nature due to a congenital enzyme defect or can be secondary to some other GI insult.

Table 6.12 Brush border enzyme activity in the small intestine

Enzyme	Substrate	Product
Sucrase-isomaltase (accounts for 80% maltase activity)	Sucrose α1–6 glucosidic bonds in starch molecule (approx. 25%) Isomaltose Maltose Maltotriose	Glucose Fructose
Maltase-glucoamylase (accounts for 20% maltase activity)	Maltose Maltotriose Starch	Glucose
Lactase	Lactose	Glucose Galactose
Trehelase	Trehalose	Glucose

Congenital sucrase-isomaltase deficiency

Congenital sucrase-isomaltase deficiency (CSID) is an autosomal recessively inherited disease which is a rare but frequently misdiagnosed cause of chronic diarrhoea in infants and children. It is characterised by a complete lack of sucrase activity and a marked reduction, but not necessarily absence, of isomaltase activity. The heterogeneous nature of this results in differing degrees of dietary tolerance.

While being breast fed or given a normal infant formula the infant remains asymptomatic and thrives. The introduction into the diet of starch or sucrose in weaning foods or the change in formula to one containing glucose polymer or sucrose initiates symptoms. The clinical presentation of CSID is very variable. Chronic watery diarrhoea and failure to thrive are common findings in infants and toddlers. A delay in the diagnosis may be related to the empirical institution of a low sucrose diet by parents, which controls symptoms. Some children attain relatively normal growth with chronic symptoms of intermittent diarrhoea, bloating and abdominal cramps before diagnosis. In older children such symptoms may result in the diagnosis of irritable bowel syndrome. CSID has been diagnosed as late as in adulthood.

One retrospective study suggests that a change in infant feeding practices in the last 20 years has resulted in the delayed introduction and decreased ingestion of sucrose and isomaltose in infancy. This has modified the course and the symptoms of the disease resulting in milder forms of chronic diarrhoea which may not start until a few weeks after the introduction of solids compared to a more acute onset of symptoms previously observed [23].

Treatment

In the first year of life this generally requires the elimination of sucrose, glucose polymers and starch from the diet (Table 6.13). The lactose in normal infant formula, breast milk and cow's milk will be well tolerated. In the very rare case where cow's milk protein intolerance is thought to co-exist with CSID a modular feed with carbohydrate present as either lactose or monosaccharides would need to be given (p. 84).

Care needs to be taken to ensure an adequate vitamin intake and it may be beneficial to continue an infant formula after 1 year of age. All medications should be sucrose free; a suitable complete carbohydrate-free vitamin supplement is Ketovite liquid and tablets.

With age the tolerance of starch and the lower sucrose containing foods should improve until, by the age of 2–3 years, the restriction of starch should no longer be needed. Tolerance can be titrated against dietary intake; if the capacity to absorb carbohydrate is exceeded this will cause osmotic diarrhoea. Figures for the sucrose content of fruits are shown in Table 6.14. Fruits containing increasing amounts of sucrose can be added to the diet according to tolerance. Reducing the starch to the previously tolerated level will result in normal stools. If children have problems tolerating starch in reasonable quantities, soy flour can be used in recipes to replace wheat flour as it only contains 15 g starch per 100 g compared with 75 g per 100 g in wheat flour. Parents need reassuring that occasional dietary indiscretions will not cause long term problems.

Older children diagnosed as having this problem should initially be advised to avoid dietary sources of sucrose only. If this does not lead to a prompt improvement in symptoms then the starch content of the diet can be reduced, particularly those foods with a high amylopectin content such as wheat and potatoes. Advice needs to be given to increase energy from protein and fat to replace the loss in energy from carbohydrate. Glucose tablets and Lucozade may be included in the diet.

Enzyme substitution therapy has recently been applied to patients with CSID. Baker's yeast has been shown to improve sucrose tolerance in these patients although it is unpalatable and poorly accepted. A tasteless liquid preparation, sacrosidase, containing high concentrations of yeast derived invertase (sucrase) has been used with a similar result (Sucraid, Orphan Medical Inc). This may allow the consumption of a more normal diet by children with CSID and decrease the high incidence of chronic gastrointestinal complaints [26, 27].

Lactase deficiency

Congenital lactase deficiency is very rare, the largest group of patients being found in Finland. Severe diarrhoea starts during the first days of life, resulting in dehydration and malnutrition, and resolves when either breast milk or normal formula are ceased and a lactose-free formula is given (Table 6.15).

Table 6.13 Low sucrose, low starch solids (<1 g per 100 g)

Protein	Meat, poultry, egg*, fish
Fats	Margarine, butter, lard, vegetable oils
Vegetables	Most vegetables *except* potato, parsnip, carrot, peas, onion, sweet potato, sweetcorn, beetroot [24]
Fruits	Initially use fruits with less than 1 g sucrose per 100 g fruit (Table 6.14) Most fruits contain negligible amounts of starch
Milk	Breast milk, infant formula (free of glucose polymer and sucrose) Cow's milk, unsweetened natural yoghurt, cream
Others	Marmite, Bovril, vinegar, salt, pepper, herbs, spices, 1–2 teaspoons of tomato purée can be used in cooking, gelatine, essences and food colourings, sugar-free jelly, sugar-free drinks, fructose, glucose

* Soft eggs should not be given to babies under 1 year of age.

Table 6.15 Lactose free, cow's milk protein based formula available on prescription in the UK

Galactomin Formula 17 (Scientific Hospital Supplies)
AL 110 (Nestle)
Enfamil Lactofree (Mead Johnson)
SMA LF (SMA Nutrition)

Table 6.14 Sucrose content of some common fruits (per 100 g edible portion) [25]

<1 g sucrose	<3 g sucrose	<5 g sucrose
Bilberries, blackcurrants, cherries, damsons, gooseberries, grapes, lemons, loganberries, lychees, melon (except Gallia), pears, raisins, raspberries, redcurrants, rhubarb, strawberries, sultanas	Gallia melon, grapefruit, kiwi fruit, passion fruit, plums	Apples, apricots, oranges, clementines, satsumas

Primary adult type hypolactasia is found in a large proportion of the world's populations. Lactase levels are normal during infancy but decline to about 5–10% of the level at birth during childhood and adolescence. These population groups are common in East and South East Asia, tropical Africa and native Americans and Australians. The age of onset of symptoms varies but is generally about 3 years or later, and only if a diet containing lactose is offered. In the majority of Europeans lactase levels remain high and this pattern of a declining tolerance of lactose with age is not seen.

In other ethnic groups with this problem a moderate reduction of dietary lactose will be sufficient, using either lactose-free milks available from the supermarket or soy milks. It is important to ensure that children meet their requirements for calcium.

Secondary disaccharidase deficiency

Carbohydrate malabsorption can occur secondary to any insult causing damage to the GI mucosa. This can present at any age, with onset of symptoms occurring shortly after the primary injury, for instance in cow's milk protein enteropathy, rotavirus infection, Crohn's disease, short gut syndrome and immunodeficiency syndromes.

Lactase deficiency is the most common secondary enzyme deficiency to be seen, probably because it has a lower activity than the other intestinal enzymes and is located on the distal end of the villous tip making it more susceptible to damage. However, a secondary sucrase-isomaltase deficiency can also occur.

Treatment

Treatment is to eliminate the offending carbohydrates and treat the primary disorder causing the mucosal damage. Clinical course depends on the underlying disease but studies in infants with rotavirus infections have shown an incidence of 30–50% lactose intolerance which recovers 2–4 weeks after the infection.

Children requiring a lactose-free formula and diet can use either lactose-free, cow's milk protein based formula (Table 6.15) or soy formula (Table 6.4). A milk-free diet (Table 6.5) is necessary although mature cheese can be included. Medications need to be checked as these can contain lactose as a filler.

Monosaccharide malabsorption: glucose-galactose malabsorption

This is a congenital disorder resulting from a selective defect in the intestinal glucose and galactose/sodium co-transport system in the brush border membrane. It is extremely rare with an estimated 100 living cases worldwide. Glucose, galactose, lactose, sucrose, glucose polymers and starch are all contraindicated in this disorder. It presents in the neonatal period with the onset of severe watery, acidic diarrhoea leading to dehydration and metabolic acidosis. It is a heterogeneous condition in its expression and older children seem to have considerable variation in their tolerance of the offending carbohydrates.

Treatment

Initial intravenous rehydration is required. The use of ORS, all of which are glucose or starch based, is contraindicated. A fructose based complete infant formula, Galactomin 19, should be introduced slowly, initially as quarter and half strength formula with intravenous carbohydrate and electrolyte support, to avoid metabolic acidosis (Table 6.16).

Table 6.16 Composition of Galactomin 19 per 100 ml

Per 100 ml	Dilution %	Energy (kcal)	(kJ)	Protein (g)	CHO (g)	Fat (g)	Na^+ (mmol)	K^+ (mmol)	Osmolality (mOsmol/kg H_2O)
Galactomin 19 Fructose Formula (Scientific Hospital Supplies)	12.9	69	288	1.9	6.4	4.0	0.9	1.7	487

Once the infant is established on feeds and gaining weight, it is important to discuss with the child's doctor a suitable protocol for oral rehydration should the child become unwell. Plain water or a 2–4% fructose solution can be given, but this does not have the same effect on water absorption as ORS as fructose utilises a different transport mechanism to glucose. In severe infectious diarrhoea the infant may need intravenous fluids.

Fructose is available on prescription for this condition and can be used to sweeten foods for older children and as an additional energy source. It is important to ensure that all medicines are carbohydrate free.

Solid introduction

Initially weaning solids should contain minimal amounts of starch, sucrose, lactose or glucose (Table 6.17). Manufactured baby foods are not suitable because of the restrictive nature of the diet and it is necessary for weaning solids to be prepared at home. All foods should be cooked without salt and initially blended to a very smooth texture. To save time parents can prepare foods in advance and freeze in clean ice cube trays. Recipes are available for egg custard sweetened with fructose and for fructose meringues.

Table 6.17 Foods allowed in children with glucose-galactose malabsorption (<1 g glucose and galactose per 100 g)*

Protein	Meat, poultry, egg**, fish
Fats	Margarine, butter, lard, vegetable oils
Vegetables	Ackee (canned), asparagus, bamboo shoots, beansprouts (canned only), broccoli, celery, cucumber, endive, fennel, globe artichoke, lettuce, marrow, mushrooms, spinach, spring greens, steamed tofu, watercress, preserved vine leaves
Fruits	Avocado pear, rhubarb, lemon juice
Milk substitute	Galactomin 19 Formula
Others	Marmite, Bovril, vinegar, salt, pepper, herbs, spices, 1–2 teaspoons of tomato purée can be used in cooking, gelatine, essences and food colourings, sugar-free jelly, sugar free drinks, fructose

*   The lists of foods have been compiled calculating the amount of glucose and galactose as: g starch + g glucose + g lactose + $\frac{1}{2}$ g sucrose [24, 25].
** Soft eggs should not be given to babies under 1 year of age.

Infants and young children are very dependent on Galactomin 19 to meet their requirements for energy and vitamins and parents should be encouraged to continue this feed for as long as the child will take it. If sufficient formula is taken a vitamin supplement should not be needed.

With age children gradually begin to absorb more of the offending carbohydrates due to colonic salvage. The fruits and vegetables in Table 6.18 are grouped to allow a gradual increase in the amount of glucose and galactose in the diet. These lists can be used as a guide by parents. Small amounts of new foods can be introduced cautiously and increased as tolerated. Too much of these foods will exceed the individual's tolerance and cause diarrhoea. In this situation the child should return to the diet previously well tolerated and try introductions again a few months later.

FAT MALABSORPTION

Intestinal lymphangiectasia

This is characterised by dilated enteric lymphatic vessels which rupture and leak lymphatic fluid into the gut, leading to protein loss. The presentation is variable but diarrhoea and hypoproteinaemic oedema are commonly seen. Failure to thrive can also be a significant problem. Children generally present in the first 2 years of life although cases being diagnosed as late as 15 years of age are documented [28]. The diagnosis is definitively established by a small intestinal biopsy demonstrating the characteristic lymphatic abnormality, although because the lesion is patchy one negative biopsy does not exclude the diagnosis [29].

Treatment

Treatment is generally by diet unless the lesion is localised enough to allow surgical excision of the involved part of the intestine. A reduced long chain triglyceride (LCT) diet is needed to control symptoms. This reduces the volume of intestinal lymphatic fluid and the pressure within the lacteals. It is recommended that the amount of LCT should be restricted to between 5 and 10 g per day [29]. A very high protein intake may also be needed to maintain plasma levels of albumin. Intakes as high as 6 g protein/kg/day with sufficient energy to ensure

Table 6.18 Glucose and galactose content of foods (per 100 g edible portion [24, 25])

1–2 g glucose + galactose	2–3 g glucose + galactose	3–5 g glucose + galactose
Protein Quorn, all 'hard' cheeses, cream cheese, brie, camembert *Vegetables* Aubergine, beans – french and runner, brussel sprouts, cabbage, cauliflower, celeriac, courgettes, gherkins (pickled), leeks, okra, onions (boiled), green peppers, radish, spring onions, swede, tomatoes (including tinned), turnip *Fruits* Gooseberries, redcurrants *Other* Ordinary mayonnaise (retail) – not reduced calorie	*Vegetables* Carrots *Fruits* Apples – cooking (sweeten with fructose or artificial sweetener), blackberries, loganberries, melon (all types), pears, raspberries, strawberries *Other* Double cream	*Vegetables* Sugar snap peas, butternut squash, mange-tout *Fruits* Apricots, blackcurrants, cherries, clementines, grapefruit, nectarines, oranges, peaches, pineapple, satsumas, tangerines *Other* Whipping cream

Table 6.19 Composition of minimal fat, cow's milk protein-based infant formulas per 100 ml

Per 100 ml	Dilution %	Energy kcal	kJ	Protein g	CHO g	Fat g	Na$^+$ mmol	K$^+$ mmol	Osmolality mOsmol/kg H$_2$O
Monogen (Scientific Hospital Supplies)	17.5	74	310	2.0	12.0	2.0 (93% MCT) (7% LCT)	1.5	1.5	280
Caprilon (Scientific Hospital Supplies)	12.7	66	275	1.5	7.0	3.6 (75% MCT) (25% LCT)	0.8	1.7	233

proper utilisation may be required initially. Medium chain triglycerides (MCT) can be used as an energy source and to increase the palatability of the diet as these are absorbed directly into the portal system and not via the lymphatics.

Suitable feeds to use in infancy and early childhood are Monogen or Caprilon, the former being preferable due to its higher protein and energy content and lower LCT content (Table 6.19). Hydrolysates containing a high percentage of MCT such as MCT Pepdite 0–2 yrs or Pregestimil could also be used, although there is no advantage to these over a whole protein feed (Table 6.6). If additional protein needs to be given to maintain plasma albumin levels, this can be added to a complete feed as Maxipro HBV. The fat and electrolyte content of this product should be calculated in addition to the quantities supplied by the feed.

Minimal fat diet

Minimal fat weaning solids should initially be introduced and gradually expanded aiming to keep the total LCT intake below 10 g per day, certainly in the first two years of life. Details of minimal fat diets are given elsewhere (p. 190, 322). Attention may need to be given to protein intake and extra very low fat, high protein foods given.

As the problem is lifelong it is necessary to continue dietary restrictions, certainly until the end of the pubertal growth spurt, although maintaining such a low intake of fat becomes increasingly difficult as the child becomes older. There is no information about the degree of fat restriction required in older children and some relaxation of the diet should be possible so long as symptoms are controlled and growth is adequate. Nutritional supplements such as Build Up made with skimmed milk, Fortijuce, Enlive and Provide Xtra may be useful to ensure adequate protein intake in older children requiring very restricted diets (p. 144).

As the dietary restrictions are long term it is particularly important to ensure that the recommended amounts of essential fatty acids (EFAs) are included in the diet once the volume of complete infant formula is reduced. Walnut oil provides the most concentrated source of EFAs and can be given as a measured amount as a dietary supplement daily. Recommended amounts would be at least 0.1 ml per 56 kcal (234 kJ) provided from foods and drinks not supplemented with EFAs (pp. 188, 320); however, there is no data as to how well it would be absorbed in this disorder and it is prudent to give double the normal amount of walnut oil as a divided dose mixed with food or as a medicine. This needs to be included in the daily fat allowance.

Fat soluble vitamin supplements (A, D, E) to meet at least the RNI for age should also be given separately. However supplements mentioned in this chapter are fortified with these vitamins. Blood levels should be monitored at outpatient clinics.

MODULAR FEEDS FOR USE IN INTRACTABLE DIARRHOEA

Intractable diarrhoea can be defined as chronic diarrhoea in the absence of bacterial pathogens of greater than a 2 week duration with failure to gain weight. Some infants with severe enteropathy or short gut syndrome fail to respond to feed manipulation as previously described and a modular feed becomes the feed of choice [30]. This allows individual manipulation of ingredients resulting in a tailor-made feed for a child. Careful assessment and monitoring is important to prevent nutritional deficiencies and to evaluate the response to feed manipulation. This approach can also assist in the diagnosis of the underlying problem.

Theories as to why modular feeds work include:

- The omission of a feed ingredient which is poorly tolerated
- The very slow mode of introduction which allows time for gut adaptation to take place
- The delay in adding fat to the feed (traditionally the last ingredient to be added) which may alter the inflammatory response in the gut.

None of these theories have been proven but clinical experience has demonstrated the efficacy of the approach.

Feed ingredients

Some of the possible choices of feed ingredients are listed in Tables 6.20, 6.21, 6.22 and 6.23. Before starting, careful dialogue needs to take place with the referring physician to elucidate the preferred feed composition for an individual. Some of the advantages and disadvantages for different products are described in the tables. The aim is to produce a feed that is well tolerated and meets the infant's nutritional requirements.

The following parameters need to be considered:

- Total energy content and appropriate energy ratio from fat and carbohydrate
- Protein, both type used and quantity
- Essential fatty acid intake
- Full vitamin and mineral supplementation, including trace elements
- Suitable electrolyte concentrations
- Feed osmolality.

Practical details

- Accurate feed calculation and measurement of ingredients is required to make the small daily feed alterations. Scoop measurements may not be accurate enough and weighing ingredients on electronic scales is preferable.
- Before starting a modular feed it is necessary to assess the infant's symptoms and current nutritional support. If parenteral nutrition is not available feeds should be introduced more rapidly than suggested below to prevent long periods of inadequate nutrition.

Table 6.20 Protein sources for use in modular feeds

Product	Protein type	Suggested dilution (g/100 ml)*	Protein content of feed (g/100 ml)	Comments
Comminuted chicken** (Scientific Hospital Supplies)	Chicken	30	2.3	Not ready to feed. Contains some essential fatty acids and trace elements. Whole protein, low osmolality
Peptide Module (Code 767) □ (Scientific Hospital Supplies)	Hydrolysed pork and soya	2.5	2.2 (Protein equivalent)	Contains some electrolytes, but needs further addition of potassium
Complete Amino Acid Mix (Code 124) □ (Scientific Hospital Supplies)	l-amino acids	2.5	2.0 (Protein equivalent)	Amino acids increase feed osmolality

* This is a suggested dilution only. Quantities can be varied according to the desired protein intake, age of child and feed tolerance.
** In some countries (Canada, USA and Italy) lamb is used as a hypoallergenic whole protein source [31].
□ These products are not ACBS listed.

Table 6.21 Carbohydrate sources for use in modular feeds

Product	Suggested concentration (g/100 ml)	Comments
Glucose Polymer* e.g. Maxijul (Scientific Hospital Supplies) Polycal (Nutricia)	10–12	Carbohydrate of choice as has the lowest osmolality
Glucose	7–8	Use when glucose polymer intolerance is present. A combination of the two monosaccharides can be used to utilise two transport mechanisms.
Fructose	7–8	Monosaccharides will increase final feed osmolality

* Intolerance to glucose polymers has been documented in the literature [32]. This may be due to a deficiency of pancreatic α-amylase or of the disaccharidase α-glucoamylase. Monosaccharides become the carbohydrates of choice in this situation.

Table 6.22 Fat sources for use in modular feeds

Product	Suggested concentration (g/100 ml*)	Comments
Calogen (Arachis oil emulsion) (Scientific Hospital Supplies)	6–10	Contains linoleic acid (C18:2)
Solagen (Soy oil emulsion)□ (Scientific Hospital Supplies)	6–10	Contains linoleic acid (C18:2) + α-linolenic acid C18:3)
Liquigen (MCT emulsion) (Scientific Hospital Supplies)	4–8	MCT increases feed osmolality. Does not contain EFAs
Vegetable oils e.g. olive, sunflower □	3–5	Not water miscible. An emulsion can be prepared by mixing 50 ml oil with 50 ml water and liquidising with 1–2 g gum acacia

* The amount of fat used will depend on tolerance and also protein source used. Comminuted chicken contains 0.9% fat at suggested dilution.
□ These ingredients are not ACBS listed

Table 6.23 Vitamins and mineral supplements for use in modular feeds

Product	Comments
Metabolic Mineral Mixture (MMM) (Scientific Hospital Supplies) or Aminogran Mineral Mixture (UCB Pharma)*† + Ketovites, 5 ml liquid + 3 tablets (Paines and Byrne)	The minerals should be dissolved in the feed. These provide electrolytes. Vitamins should be given separately
Paediatric Seravit (Scientific Hospital Supplies)	Contains glucose polymer which may be contraindicated. Does not contain electrolytes. These need to be added separately to the feed or given medicinally

* MMM and Aminogran Minerals do not contain selenium, molybdenum or chromium. When being used with an artificial protein source such as amino acids or peptides, deficiency states can be induced. Paediatric Seravit plus added electrolytes should be used unless adequate trace minerals are present from solids.
† Minerals should be given as a dosage of 1 g per 100 ml up to a maximum of 8 g total. Greater than 1.5 g/kg body weight/day results in an excessive electrolyte intake.

Table 6.24 Suggested plan of introduction of a modular feed based on comminuted chicken

Time	Comminuted chicken	Maxijul	Calogen	MMM	Ketovite liquid + tablets	Volume*
Day 1–4	Quarter strength increasing to full strength	5%	Nil	Quarter strength increasing to full strength	✔ Unless on full TPN vitamins	As prescribed
Day 5–10	Full strength	Increase in 1% increments to 10%	Nil	Full strength	✔	No change
Day 11–16	Full strength	10%	Add in 1% increments to 6%	Full strength	✔	No change
Day 16 onwards	Full strength	10%	6%	Full strength	✔	Increase volume if required

* If the child is having total parenteral nutrition (TPN) 10–20 ml/kg/day of feed should be given until a full energy feed is established, after which the feed volume can be increased in 2–5 ml/kg daily increments and the parenteral nutrition reduced in tandem.

- In the absence of intravenous glucose the carbohydrate content of the feed should never be less than 4 g per 100 ml because of the risk of hypoglycaemia. A higher percentage of energy from fat than from carbohydrate may result in excessive ketone production.
- Infants with protracted diarrhoea will better tolerate frequent small feeds as one to two hourly bolus feeds or continuous feeds via a nasogastric tube, rather than larger bolus feeds. Comminuted chicken is a suspension of chicken meat in water and may prove difficult to deliver for feeding continuously (p. 105). The other protein sources are more soluble and can be fed by continuous infusion.

- Attention needs to be given to the combination of ingredients chosen as these will affect the osmolality of the final feed. The smaller the molecular size the greater the osmotic effect. Most hospital laboratories will analyse feed osmolality on request.
- Infants requiring a modular feeding approach will have high requirements for all nutrients.

Introduction of modular feeds

The model of introduction of a comminuted chicken based feed (Tables 6.24 and 6.25) can be applied to other protein sources. Suggested incremental changes take place every 24 hours; however, if well tolerated

Table 6.25 Example of a full strength modular feed using comminuted chicken

Per 100 ml	Energy (kcal)	(kJ)	Protein (g)	CHO (g)	Fat (g)	Na+ (mmol)	K+ (mmol)	Osmolality (mOsmol/kg H$_2$O)
30 g comminuted chicken	17	71	2.3		0.9	0.1	0.4	
10 g Maxijul	38	156		9.5				
6 ml Calogen	27	243			3.0			
1 g Metabolic Mineral Mixture						1.7	2.1	
Ketovites (given separately)								
Final Feed/100 ml	82	470	2.3	9.5	3.9	1.8	2.5	247

this process can be accelerated. The infant's response to each change of feed should be assessed daily before making any further alterations. Avoid making more than one change at a time.

Teaching for home

To ease teaching parents for home feed, ingredients need to be converted into scoop measurements using the minimum number of different scoops possible to avoid confusion. In the case of comminuted chicken, half or whole jar measurements should be used. If scales are to be used these should have an accuracy to 1 g increments. A 24-hour recipe should be given and it is important to demonstrate the method for making the feed to the infant's carers on at least one occasion before discharge. If a feed based on comminuted chicken is not decanted from mixing jug to bottle immediately, the chicken fibres settle to the bottom. The feed should be thoroughly stirred each time before pouring into bottles. Similarly bottles of feed need to be shaken before feeding.

Not all the suggested ingredients for modular feeds are ACBS listed. A separate letter to the child's general practitioner may be needed to arrange a supply of the product or a supply of these items may need to be given from the hospital.

Introduction of solids

Solids should be introduced after the infant or child is established on a nutritionally complete feed. The restrictions imposed will depend on the underlying diagnosis. Sometimes it is necessary to introduce food items singly to determine tolerance of different foods.

INFLAMMATORY BOWEL DISEASE

Crohn's disease

Crohn's disease (CrD) is caused by a chronic transmural inflammatory process that may affect any part of the gastrointestinal tract from the mouth to the anus. It is an extremely heterogeneous disorder with great anatomical and histological diversity. The small intestine is involved in 90% of cases. The aggressive inflammatory process can cause fibrosis of the small bowel, stricture formation and ulceration leading to fistula formation. The aetiology of CrD is not yet fully understood but is now thought to be the result of an inappropriate immune response to the antigens of the normal bacterial flora in a genetically susceptible individual [33].

The presentation of CrD in children depends largely on the location and extent of the inflammation. In most cases it is insidious in onset with non-specific gastrointestinal symptoms and growth failure often leading to an initially incorrect diagnosis [34]. It can also be associated with other inflammatory conditions affecting the joints, skin and eyes.

Over time the disease causes nausea, anorexia and malabsorption. The mean energy intake of patients with active CrD has been found to be up to 420 kcal (1.75 MJ) per day lower than in age matched controls [35]. The energy and protein deficit is reflected as weight loss and a decreased height velocity [36]. Weight loss occurs in up to 87% of children presenting with CrD and may be as great as 6 kg in magnitude. Specific nutrient deficiencies such as calcium, magnesium, zinc, iron, folate, B$_{12}$ and fat soluble

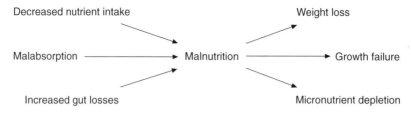

Fig. 6.1 Features associated with the undernutrition seen in Crohn's disease

vitamins are common findings. During periods of active inflammation there is often enteric leakage of protein resulting in hypoalbuminaemia. Accompanying this is retarded bone mineralisation and development and delayed puberty [37, 38].

The features associated with the undernutrition seen in CrD are shown in Fig. 6.1 [36].

Treatment

CrD is a chronic and as yet incurable disease and its management requires a combination of nutritional support, judicious use of drugs and appropriate surgery.

Enteral feeds as primary therapy

Nutrition as a treatment modality for CrD was discovered in the 1970s. Since then many controlled trials have been completed with the aim of elucidating its efficacy as a primary therapy. These have compared enteral feeds with corticosteroids, a pharmacological treatment known to be effective in the treatment of CrD, as a treatment to induce disease remission and compared the effectiveness of different feed types (elemental, hydrolysate and polymeric) as a treatment in active CrD.

Two meta-analyses of the studies published between 1984 and 1994 have been completed and the conclusions reached that steroids were more effective than enteral nutrition in the treatment of active CrD, although the latter was effective in inducing disease remission in a significant number of patients; and that there is no evidence to support an advantage of elemental formula, the traditional feeds used in CrD, over polymeric (whole protein) feeds [39, 40].

Criticisms have been levelled at the trials completed. Most of the studies have used adult patients, in some the patient numbers are small and in virtu-

ally all a Crohn's disease activity index has been used to assess clinical response to treatment. These indices are based on a combination of clinical and biochemical data and it is known that steroids will favour the clinical index because they cause a feeling of well-being in patients [33].

Although it is agreed that enteral feeds work for a significant number of patients their mode of action is not understood. Hypotheses include:

- Alterations in intestinal microbial flora
- A reduction in food allergens presented to the gut
- Nutritional repletion in a malnourished patient
- A reduction in the intestinal synthesis of inflammatory mediators secondary to the low LCT content of some feeds used
- An as yet misunderstood immunomodulatory effect of enteral feeds [36].

A new feed, Modulen IBD, has recently been launched for patients with CrD. This has reported immunomodulatory effects due to the presence of transforming growth factor (TGF) β, an anti-inflammatory cytokine present in casein. There are no published trials to date comparing this feed with other polymeric feeds.

The current evidence for enteral feeds as a treatment in active CrD is far from clear [36]. However, most paediatric centres use enteral feeds as a primary therapy despite the increased cost compared to steroids and the potential difficulty following the treatment prescribed. As children with CrD are often chronically malnourished enteral feeds are important for nutritional repletion. Feeds are also preferable as a first line of treatment because of the deleterious effect of steroids on growth. A better outcome in terms of lean body mass and linear growth is seen when enteral nutrition is used [41].

Protocol for enteral feeding in CrD

Although there is convincing evidence that polymeric feeds are as effective as hydrolysate or elemental feeds in the treatment of CrD, our current protocol uses two different feed types, the use of which is decided by a history of atopy in either the patient or first degree relatives. For those patients with no history suggestive of possible food allergy, a polymeric, whole protein, casein based feed is used, while, in the atopic individuals a feed based on hydrolysed protein is used. Polymeric feeds have the advantage of being more palatable and cheaper than the elemental alternatives.

For all feeds the following protocol can be applied:

- Feeds should be gradually introduced over 3–5 days depending on symptoms
- The enteral feed should provide complete nutrition for a 4–8 week period
- All solid food should be stopped for the duration of the treatment
- Clear fluids, boiled sweets and chewing gum are allowed orally to improve compliance.

As patients with CrD are generally adolescents they find this particularly difficult and require a high degree of support and motivation to complete the treatment. Despite this feeds are well tolerated by most patients and the full 6 weeks generally adhered to, with 72% of patients in one study reporting it as a preferred treatment or as acceptable as steroid therapy [42].

A hospital admission of 3–5 days is generally required to establish a suitable feeding regimen that is tolerated by the individual, unless the patient is sure that they will be able to manage orally at home. Once the feed type allowed and volumes to be prescribed have been decided the aim is to give as much control to the patient as possible. Feeds should be tried orally with different flavourings and the volume required daily explained carefully. Patients are given the option of drinking the feed or using a nasogastric tube. If the former is decided on it is important that they understand that the prescribed volume needs to be completed every day as compliance can become an issue. If a tube is chosen patients are taught to pass this each night and remove it in the morning to cause minimum inconvenience to their daily routine. Some patients choose to drink full volumes of even hydrolysate feeds, others opt for a combination approach (a percentage orally and the remainder via the tube) and some for solely nocturnal nasogastric feeds.

Nutritional requirements and monitoring

Most studies have failed to show increased basal energy requirements in patients with CrD unless the patient has a fever [37, 41]. The initial aim should be to provide the estimated average requirement (EAR) for age for energy and RNI for protein from the full feed, checking that all vitamins and minerals are present in amounts at least equivalent to the RNI [16]. If feed volume is a problem some of the energy requirements can be met with glucose polymer which can be added to drinks throughout the day.

On discharge patients should be weighed weekly and monitored by telephone. A follow-up appointment is arranged 2–3 weeks after discharge to ensure that the patient is responding to treatment and that weight gain is being achieved. Occasionally additional energy is required to achieve the latter and this can be given as increased feed volume or by increasing the energy density of the feed.

Introduction of foods and discontinuation of feeds

There is no agreement about the best methods of food introduction to patients completing a period of enteral feeds and the possibility of food intolerances causing CrD has always been a consideration. In the UK two main centres have published data with conflicting results. The East Anglian study found that a large number of patients were food intolerant, the most common foods cited as causing problems being corn, wheat, yeast, egg, potato, rye, tea and coffee [43]. This trial has been criticised as patients only completed 2 weeks of an elemental diet before foods were introduced, which was not long enough to allow full disease remission, only a resolution of symptoms. Foods were also introduced daily which would not identify delayed reactions. More recently this approach has been modified and a reduced allergen, low fat, low fibre diet devised to be introduced at the end of the 2–3 week period of enteral feeds with subsequent food reintroductions [44].

Pearson at Northwick Park Hospital used a 4–8 week period on elemental diet before introducing foods singly over 5 day periods. Suspect foods were reinvestigated with open and, when possible, double blind challenges; 48% of patients identified food sensitivities, with 24% having a recurrence of symptoms with open rechallenge. Food sensitivities could only be identified in 7% of the patients by double blind challenge. Most importantly, there was no significant difference in the duration of remission between patients who did or did not identify food sensitivities [45].

Beattie and Walker-Smith concluded that neither study confirmed that intolerance to foodstuffs is seen in CrD and that no particular foods are known to exacerbate symptoms in a large group of patients [46].

Until there is further evidence it would appear prudent to reduce feed volume over a period of 3–4 weeks and gradually introduce foods into the diet, ensuring that continued weight gain is maintained. Single food introductions do not seem worthwhile in the majority of patients and merely prolong the resumption of a normal diet. Patients found to be atopic requiring a hydrolysate feed should be advised to continue a milk-free diet, ensuring an adequate energy and calcium intake. Patients with a tight stricture in the ileum may require a low fibre diet to control symptoms until the stricture is surgically removed.

Some patients require continued nutritional support either by nasogastric tube, gastrostomy or orally if appetite remains poor. It has also been reported that continued use of nocturnal feeds in addition to a normal diet is associated with prolonged periods of disease remission and improved linear growth [42].

Ulcerative colitis

Like CrD, ulcerative colitis (UC) is a chronic, relapsing, inflammatory disease of the intestine which is confined to the colonic and rectal mucosa. It also has an unknown aetiology with evidence for an inherited predisposition to the disease alongside other, possibly environmental, factors. Tissue injury is most likely a result of non-specific activation of the immune system with some evidence that this has an autoimmune aetiology.

Drug therapy is used to induce and maintain disease remission. There is no evidence to support the use of enteral nutrition as a primary therapy in UC. The nutritional problems found in CrD are not as severe in UC because of the lack of involvement of the small intestine [38].

Nutritional support is needed if there is growth failure or weight loss and this can generally be given as a high energy diet and oral sip feeds.

DISORDERS OF ALTERED GUT MOTILITY

Gastro-oesophageal reflux

Gastro-oesophageal reflux (GOR) refers to the inappropriate opening of the lower oesophageal sphincter (LOS) releasing gastric contents into the oesophagus. An estimated 20% of infants have problems with regurgitation (seen as posseting and vomiting) during the first year of life. Regurgitation can, in the majority of children, be considered as an uncomplicated self-limiting condition which spontaneously resolves by 12–15 months of age.

More severe forms of this problem are found when an infant with regurgitation does not respond to simple treatment and when it is associated with other symptoms such as failure to thrive, haematemesis, respiratory symptoms, apnoea, irritability, feeding disorders and iron deficiency anaemia. GOR is also a common finding in infants with neurological problems.

Treatment

Parental reassurance is very important and may preclude the need for any other measures. However recurrent symptoms of inconsolable crying or irritability, feeding or sleeping difficulties, persistent regurgitation or vomiting may lead to unnecessary parental distress and recurrent medical consultations, and may need further treatment.

Postural treatment of infants has been demonstrated to help and a prone elevated position at 30° is the most successful in reducing GOR [47]. This is now difficult to recommend because of the publication of several studies showing an increased risk of sudden infant death syndrome (SIDS) in the prone sleeping position. It also means the purchase of a special cot in which the baby has to be tied up to keep in place, which is not always possible [48]. A more practical approach is to avoid positions which exacerbate the situation. Young infants tend to slump when placed in a seat, which increases pressure on the stomach and makes the reflux worse. It is better to place them in a seat that reclines or to lie them down.

It is important to ensure that the infant is not being overfed and is being offered an age-appropriate volume of milk. Small, more frequent feeds may also be beneficial by reducing gastric distension, e.g. 150 ml of formula/kg/day as 6–7 feeds. However, in practice frequent feeds may be difficult for parents to manage and reduced feed volumes may cause distress in a hungry baby.

The use of feed thickeners has been proven to reduce the vomiting in infants, although the effects on the incidence of reflux episodes have been found to be inconsistent with pH monitoring [49]. They are generally well tolerated with very few side effects reported and should be used as a first line treatment in infants with regurgitation [48]. A variety of manufactured feed thickeners are on the market in the UK, based either on carob seed or modified maize starch (Table 6.26). Of the former, Instant Carobel has an advantage over Nestargel in that it thickens the feed without the need to be cooked. The complex carbohydrates in both products are non-absorbable and can lead, in a minority of infants, to the passage of frequent loose stools. Both products have the added flexibility of being mixed as a gel and fed from a spoon before breast feeds.

Where failure to thrive is a problem a starch based thickener should be used to provide extra energy. The lowest amount of thickener recommended should be added initially and the amount gradually increased to the maximum level if there is no resolution of symptoms. Feeding through a teat with a slightly larger hole, or a variable flow teat, is recommended. Ordinary cornflour can also be used as a thickening agent for infant feeds but has the inconvenience of requiring cooking. This should be done in approximately half the volume of water required for the final feed recipe and cooled before the formula is added. Such feeds generally require sieving before use.

Enfamil AR is a nutritionally complete pre-thickened formula available on prescription (ACBS) which contains a high-amylopectin, pre-gelatinised rice starch. The EC Scientific Committee for Food has accepted the addition of starch to a maximum of 2 g/100 ml in infant formula. The feed is made up at a standard dilution using water that has been cooled to room temperature to avoid lumps forming. The bottle then requires rolling between the hands to ensure proper mixing. The viscosity of the feed increases when exposed to the acid pH of the stomach. Recent recommendations suggest that labelling should make it clear that 'AR' stands for 'Anti-Regurgitation' and not for 'Anti-Reflux'. Such feeds should be used as a therapeutic intervention only and their over-use avoided [50].

Omneo Comfort 1 and 2 are thickened infant and follow-on formulas made from partially hydrolysed whey protein and contain prebiotic oligosaccharides. They are designed for bottlefed babies with minor feeding problems. These are new products on the market and it remains to be seen whether they are beneficial in the treatment of this condition.

In more complicated GOR which fails to respond to simple treatment, a therapeutic change of formula should be considered as it has been demonstrated that GOR can be secondary to food allergy. Two studies have demonstrated that 30–40% of infants with GOR resistant to treatment have cow's milk allergy, with symptoms significantly improving on a cow's milk protein-free diet [51, 52]. The use of either soy or hydrolysate feeds in these infants for a trial

Table 6.26 Feed thickeners available in the UK

Product	Thickening agent	Suggested dilution (g/100 ml)	Added energy per 100 ml (kcal)	(kJ)	ACBS prescribable
Instant Carobel (Cow & Gate)	Carob seed	1–3	3–8	13–33	✔
Nestargel[†] (Nestle)	Carob seed	0.5–1	Negligible		✔
Thick and Easy (Fresenius)	Pre-cooked	1–3	4–12	17–50	✔
Thixo-D (Sutherland Health Ltd)	maize starch				
Vitaquick (Vitaflo Ltd)					
Cornflour*[†]	Maize starch	1–3	4–12	17–50	✘

* Product can be purchased from supermarkets
[†] Product requires cooking before use

period should therefore be considered as a treatment option.

Medications that can be used to treat GOR range from antacids to H₂ antagonists, such as ranitidine, which reduce gastric acid secretion and domperidone, which elevates the lower-oesophageal sphincter pressure and increases gastric emptying. A combination of these is often given to control symptoms.

In extreme cases which do not respond to the above treatments surgery may be needed to correct the problem. A fundoplication which wraps the fundus of the stomach around the LOS creates an artificial valve and prevents GOR (p. 100). Generally a gastrostomy is inserted for venting gas from the stomach and occasionally feeding purposes. There is considerable morbidity associated with this operation.

Feeding problems in GOR

Feeding difficulties are common in this disorder and are characterised by oral motor dysfunction, episodes of dysphagia and negative feeding experiences by both mother and baby. Infants with GOR are significantly more demanding and difficult to feed and have been found to ingest significantly less energy than matched infants without GOR [53]. These problems often persist after medical or surgical treatment with the aversive behaviour being caused by associating pain with previous feeding experiences.

Where there are severe feeding problems it may be necessary to instigate feeding via a nasogastric tube or gastrostomy to ensure an adequate nutritional intake. Wherever possible an oral intake, however small, should be maintained to minimise later feeding problems. The child's feed should be administered as oral or bolus day feeds with continuous feeds overnight at a slow rate which ensures no feed aspiration. The feed volume may need to be reduced below that recommended for age to ensure tolerance and feeds fortified in the usual way to ensure adequate nutrition for catch-up growth. If using a fine bore nasogastric tube to administer bolus feeds, thickening agents should be kept to the minimum concentration recommended to prevent the tube blocking and an inappropriate length of time being taken to administer the feed. There is no evidence that reduced fat feeds promote gastric emptying and reduce GOR in these infants [50].

The requirement for tube feeding can continue for prolonged periods of time, as long as 36 months

in one study [54]. Parents of infants with feeding problems secondary to GOR need a great deal of support. Optimal management should employ a multidisciplinary feeding disorder team including a psychologist with experience of children with these problems, a paediatrician, a dietitian and a speech therapist.

Idiopathic constipation

Constipation is a symptom rather than a disease and can be caused by anatomical, physiological or histopathological abnormalities. Idiopathic constipation is not related to any of these and is thought to be most often due to the intentional or subconscious withholding of stool after a precipitating acute event. Constipation has been found to account for 3% of visits to general paediatric outpatient clinics and 10–25% of visits to a paediatric gastroenterologist, and so it is a sizeable problem.

Average stool frequency has been estimated to be four stools per day in the first week of life, two per day at 1 year of age, and decreasing to the adult pattern of between three per day and three per week by the age of 4 years. Within these patterns there is a great variation and constipation can be described as the infrequent passage of dry, hardened faeces, often accompanied by straining and pain.

In idiopathic constipation prolonged stretching of the anal walls associated with chronic faecal retention leads to an atonic and desensitised rectum which perpetuates the problem as large volumes of stool must be present to initiate the call to pass a stool. Encopresis or soiling is mostly as a result of chronic faecal retention and rarely occurs before the age of 3 years.

Treatment

Treatment typically involves three phases: disimpaction, laxative use to stimulate daily bowel motions and reduce the chronically large rectal vault size, and a high fibre diet that will encourage the regular passage of soft stools.

Dietary fibre can be classified into water-soluble and -insoluble forms. The former includes pectins, gums and mucilages which can be fermented by colonic bacteria to produce short chain fatty acids. This has been shown to increase stool water content and volume. Insoluble fibre mainly acts as a bulking agent in the stool by trapping water in the intestinal tract and acting like a sponge. Both soften and enlarge the stool and reduce GI transit times.

Surveys have shown that constipated children often eat considerably less fibre than their non-constipated counterparts. Even when advised to increase their fibre intake by a physician the fibre intake was only half the amount of the control population. It appears that families can only make the necessary changes with specific dietary counselling [55]. Children with chronic constipation have also been shown to have lower energy intakes and a higher incidence of anorexia. It is difficult to know if this existed previously and predisposed to the condition or whether it is caused by early satiety secondary to constipation [56].

In infancy and childhood it is important to ensure that adequate fluids are taken. In babies the addition of carbohydrate to feeds can induce an osmotic softening of the stool, but is not to be encouraged as a general public health message. Once solids are introduced these should include fruit and vegetables, with wholegrain cereals being introduced after the age of 6 months. Bran should not be used in infancy and with caution in older children.

In a select group of children with constipation which fails to respond to conventional treatment, cow's milk protein-free diets have been shown to be beneficial [57]. Motility studies in these patients have indicated that the delay in faecal passage is a consequence of stool retention in the rectum and not of a generalised motility disorder [58]. It has therefore been proposed that all children with chronic constipation that fail to respond to normal treatment as outlined above should be considered for a trial of a cow's milk-free diet, especially if they are atopic [59].

Gut motility disorders

Integration of the digestive, absorptive and motor functions of the gut is required for the assimilation of nutrients. In the mature and adult gut, motor functions are organised into particular patterns of contractile activity which have several control mechanisms.

After swallowing, a bolus of milk or food is propelled down the oesophagus by peristalsis; this action differs from the motility of the rest of the intestine in that it can be induced voluntarily. The LOS relaxes to allow food or fluid to pass into the stomach which acts as a reservoir and also initiates digestion. It has a contractile action which grinds food to 1–2 mm particle size. Gastric emptying can be modulated by feed components via hormonal secretion. Long chain triglycerides have been found to inhibit gastric emptying. Different dietary proteins also have an effect with whey hydrolysates emptying more rapidly than whole protein feeds [60].

In the small intestine, motor activity is effected by smooth muscle contraction which is controlled by myogenic, neural and chemical factors. In the fasting state the gut has a contractile activity which keeps the luminal bacteria in the colon. Abnormalities of this phasic activity can result in bacterial overgrowth of the small intestine and malabsorption. Post-prandial activity is initiated by hormones and food eaten to produce peristalsis in the gut, relaxation of the muscle coats below and contraction above the bolus of food through the intestine.

Disturbances in this co-ordinated system can occur at all levels.

Toddler diarrhoea

Toddler diarrhoea, also known as chronic non-specific diarrhoea, is the most frequent cause of chronic diarrhoea in children between the ages of 1 and 5 years of age. Symptoms include frequent watery stools containing undigested foodstuffs in a child who is otherwise well, gaining weight and growing satisfactorily. Despite the children generally presenting in a good nutritional state, parental anxiety is high. The diarrhoea ceases spontaneously, generally between 2 and 4 years of age.

Proposed mechanisms

A primary problem has still not been identified. Children with this disorder are known to have a rapid gut transit time and intestinal motility is generally thought to be abnormal, although it is unsure whether this is due to a reduced colonic transit time or a disturbance of small intestinal motility.

Carbohydrate malabsorption, particularly of fructose, has been extensively investigated in this disorder. Fructose is known to be slowly absorbed in the small intestine and is often present in large amounts in fruit juice. In recent years the diets of children in this age group have undergone changes with an increase in the amount of squash and fruit juices and a decrease in water taken as drinks [61]. As apple juice particularly has been implicated as causing toddler diarrhoea, studies have been completed using hydrogen breath tests to measure carbohydrate malabsorption. What now seems to be evident is that non-absorbable monosaccharides and oligosaccharides such as galacturonic acid are produced by enzymatic treatment of the fruit pulp in clear fruit juices, including apple, grape and bilberry juices. It is thought that these may cause problems in sensitive individuals, rather than fructose [62].

Treatment

All sources agree that parental reassurance is of primary importance. However the role of diet in this disorder is controversial [29, 63]. It would appear prudent to give advice to correct any dietary idiosyncracies. Excessive fluid intake, particularly of fruit juices and squash, should be discouraged. Fibre intake has frequently been reduced by parents in an attempt to normalise stools, therefore increasing this to normal levels should be recommended. Fat intake may also have been reduced, either due to the excessive consumption of high carbohydrate fruit drinks or for health reasons, and should be increased to 35–40% of total dietary energy. Often parents have tried excluding foods from the child's diet, mistakenly believing the problems to be due to food intolerance. Once the diagnosis is established these foods should be reintroduced.

Chronic idiopathic pseudo-obstruction disorder

This term embraces a heterogeneous group of disorders that cause severe intestinal dysmotility with recurrent symptoms of intestinal obstruction in the absence of mechanical occlusion. Gut transit time is generally in excess of 96 hours. The cause is usually an enteric myopathy or neuropathy which can also affect the urinary tract. It is an extremely rare disorder with a high morbidity and mortality.

Nutritional support is vital for these children. In one series of 44 patients, 72% required parenteral nutrition for a relatively long period of time, 7 children dying of TPN related complications with a further 10 remaining dependent on long term home parenteral nutrition [64].

Full enteral nutrition is possible to achieve in some patients but generally needs to be started slowly, with a gradual decrease in parenteral nutrition volume as the enteral nutrition is increased. Particular attention needs to be paid to fluid and electrolyte requirements. Many of the children have an ileostomy to decompress the gut. The loss of sodium rich effluent through the stoma generally results in high sodium requirements (up to 10 mmol/kg/day) which are not met by the enteral feed alone. Enteral feed can often be pooled in the intestine for a prolonged period of time before passing through the stoma, resulting in a lack of appreciation of the relatively high fluid requirements of these children.

Treatment

The following suggestions for the nutritional management of these patients have proved beneficial:

- Liquids are easier for the dysmotile gut to process than highly textured foods. Aim to give full requirements from the feed or parenteral nutrition, or a combination of the two, to minimise intake of solids.
- Enteral feeds are more likely to be tolerated as a continuous infusion than as bolus feeds.
- Whey hydrolysates have been found to empty more rapidly from the stomach and form the mainstay of treatment (pers. comm.).
- Care should be taken to ensure that enteral feeds are made as cleanly as possible to prevent the introduction of organisms into the gut, which could contribute to bacterial overgrowth. In older children the use of sterile feeds is preferable.
- Fluid and sodium requirements should be accurately assessed and supplements given as needed.
- Where solids are taken these should be low in fibre so as not to cause obstruction. Semi-solid or bite-dissolvable consistencies such as purées, mashed potato and Rice Krispies will be more easily digested.

Weight measurements on these children are not always accurate due to distended loops of gut pooling large quantities of fluid. They should be used in conjunction with other anthropometric measurements such as mid-arm circumference or skinfold thicknesses to assess nutritional state.

REFERENCES

1 Recommendations for Composition of Oral Rehydration Solutions for the Children of Europe. Report of an ESPGAN Working Group. *J Pediatr Gastroenterol Nutr*, 1992, **14** 113–15.

2 Kaila M *et al*. Treatment of acute diarrhoea in practice. *Acta Paediatr*, 1997, **86** 1340–44.

3 Brown KH *et al*. Use of non-human milks in the dietary management of young children with acute diarrhoea: a meta-analysis of clinical trials. *Pediatr*, 1994, **93** 17–27.

4 Sandhu BK *et al*. Early feeding in childhood gastroenteritis. A multicente study on behalf of the European Society of Paediatric Gastroenterology and Nutrition working group on acute diarrhoea. *J Pediatr Gastroenterol Nutr*, 1997, **24** 522–7.

5 Walker-Smith JA *et al*. Recommendations for feeding in childhood gastroenteritis. European Society of Paediatric Gastroenterology and Nutrition. *J Paediatr Gastroenterol Nutr*, 1997, **24** 619–20.

6 Wyllie R Cow's milk protein allergy and hypoallergenic formulas. *Clin Pediatr*, 1996, **35** 497–500.

7 de Boissieu D *et al*. Multiple food allergy: a possible diagnosis in breastfed infants. *Acta Paediatr*, 1997, **86** 1042–46.

8 Host A *et al*. Dietary products used in infants for treatment and prevention of food allergy. Joint statement of the ESPACI Committee on allergenic formulas and the ESPGAN Committee on nutrition. *Arch Dis Childh*, 1999, **81** 80–84.

9 American Academy of Pediatrics Committee on Nutrition Soy protein-based formulas: recommendations for use in infant feeding. *Paediatr*, 1998, **101** 148–53.

10 Zeiger RS *et al*. Soy allergy in infants and children with IgE-associated cow's milk allergy. *J Pediatr*, 1999, **134** 614–22.

11 Businco L *et al*. Allergenicity and nutritional adequacy of soy protein formulas. *J Pediatr*, 1992, **121** S21–8.

12 Lee YH Food processing approaches to altering allergenic potential of milk based formula. *J Pediatr*, 1992, **121** S47–50.

13 SHS International Ltd. www.shsweb.co.uk

14 Wahn U *et al*. Comparison of the residual allergenic activity of six different hydrolyzed protein formulas. *J Pediatr*, 1992, **121** S80–84.

15 Vanderhoof JA *et al*. Intolerance to protein hydrolysate infant formulas: an under-recognised cause of gastrointestinal symptoms in infants. *J Pediatr*, 1997, **131** 741–4.

16 The Department of Health Report on Health and Social Subjects No. 41, Dietary Reference Values for Food Energy and Nutrients for the United Kingdom. London: The Stationery Office, 1991.

17 Madsen CD, Henderson RC Calcium intake in children with positive IgG RAST to cow's milk. *J Paediatr Child Health*, 1997, **33** 209–12.

18 Challacombe DN *et al*. Changing infant feeding practices and declining incidence of coeliac disease in West Somerset. *Arch Dis Childh*, 1997, **77** 206–209.

19 Ascher H *et al*. Influence of infant feeding and gluten intake on coeliac disease. *Arch Dis Childh*, 1997, **76** 113–17.

20 Revised criteria for diagnosis of coeliac disease. Report of working group of ESPGAN. *Arch Dis Childh*, 1990, **65** 909–11.

21 Schmitz J Lack of oats toxicity in coeliac disease. *Brit Med J*, 1997, **314** 159–60.

22 The Coeliac Society Guidelines on coeliac disease and oats. High Wycombe: Coeliac Society, 1998.

23 Baudon JJ *et al*. Sucrase-isomaltase deficiency: changing pattern over two decades. *J Pediatr Gastroenterol Nutr*, 1996, **22** 284–8.

24 Holland B *et al*. Vegetables, herbs and spices. The fifth supplement to McCance & Widdowson's *The Composition of Foods*, 4th edn. Cambridge: Royal Society of Chemistry, MAFF, 1991.

25 Holland B *et al*. Fruit and nuts. The first supplement to McCance & Widdowson's *The Composition of Foods*, 5th edn. Cambridge: Royal Society of Chemistry, MAFF, 1992.

26 Treem WR Congenital sucrase-isomaltase deficiency. *J Pediatr Gastroenterol Nutr*, 1995, **21** 1–14.

27 Treem WR *et al*. Sacrosidase therapy for congenital sucrase-isomaltase deficiency. *J Pediatr Gastroenterol Nutr*, 1999, **28** 137–42.

28 Vardy PA *et al*. Intestinal lymphangiectasia: a reappraisal. *Pediatr*, 1975, **55** 842–51.

29 Walker Smith J, Murch S *Diseases of the Small Intestine in Childhood*, 4th edn. New York: Isis Medical Media Ltd, 1999.

30 Walker-Smith JA Nutritional management of enteropathy. *Nutr*, 1998, **14** 775–9.

31 Weisselberg B *et al*. A lamb-meat based formula for infants allergic to casein hydrolysate formulas. *Clin Pediatr*, 1996, **35** 491–5.

32 Fisher SE *et al*. Chronic protracted diarrhea: intolerance to dietary glucose polymers. *Pediatrics*, 1981, **67** 271–2.

33 Beattie M *et al*. Childhood Crohn's disease and the efficacy of enteral diets. *Nutr*, 1998, **14** 345–50.

34 Walker-Smith JA Management of growth failure in Crohn's disease. *Arch Dis Childh*, 1996, **75** 351–4.

35 Thomas AG *et al*. Dietary intake and nutritional treatment in childhood Crohn's disease. *J Pediatr Gastroenterol Nutr*, 1993, **17** 75–81.

36 Griffiths AG Inflammatory bowel disease. *Nutr*, 1998, **14** 788–91.

37 Hyams JS Crohn's disease in children. *Pediatr Clin N Amer*, 1996, **43** 255–77.

38 Boot AM *et al*. Bone mineral density and nutritional status in children with chronic inflammatory bowel disease. *Gut*, 1998, **42** 188–94.

39 Fernandez-Banares F *et al.* How effective is enteral nutrition in inducing clinical remission in active Crohn's disease? A meta-analysis of the randomized clinical trials. *J Parent Ent Nutr*, 1995, **19** 356–64.

40 Griffiths AM *et al.* Meta-analysis of enteral nutrition as a primary treatment of active Crohn's disease. *Gastroenterol*, 1995, **108** 1056–67.

41 Azcue M *et al.* Energy expenditure and body composition in children with Crohn's disease: effect of enteral nutrition and treatment with prednisolone. *Gut*, 1997, **41** 203–208.

42 Wilschanski M *et al.* Supplementary enteral nutrition maintains remission in paediatric Crohn's disease. *Gut*, 1996, **38** 543–8.

43 Riordan AM *et al.* Treatment of active Crohn's disease by exclusion diet: East Anglian multicentre controlled trial. *Lancet*, 1993, **342** 1131–4.

44 Woolner JT *et al.* The development and evaluation of a diet for maintaining remission in Crohn's disease. *J Human Nutr Dietetics*, 1998, **11** 1–11.

45 Pearson M *et al.* Food intolerance and Crohn's disease. *Gut*, 1993, **34** 783–7.

46 Beattie RM, Walker-Smith JA Treatment of active Crohn's disease by exclusion diet. *J Pediatr Gastroenterol Nutr*, 1994, **19** 135–6.

47 Orenstein SR *et al.* Positioning for prevention of infant gastroesophageal reflux. *J Paediatr*, 1983, **103** 534–7.

48 Vandenplas Y *et al.* Current concepts and issues in the management of regurgitation of infants: a reappraisal. *Acta Paediatr*, 1996, **85** 531–4.

49 Orenstein SR *et al.* Thickening of infant feedings for therapy of gastroesophageal reflux. *J Pediatr*, 1987, **110** 181–6.

50 Vandenplas Y *et al.* Dietary treatment for regurgitation – recommendations from a working party. *Acta Paediatr*, 1998, **87** 462–8.

51 Cavataio F *et al.* Clinical and pH-metric characteristics of gastro-oesophageal reflux secondary to cow's milk protein allergy. *Arch Dis Childh*, 1996, **75** 51–6.

52 Cavataio F *et al.* Gastroesophageal reflux and cow's milk allergy in infants: a prospective study. *J Allergy Clin Immunol*, 1996, **97** 822–7.

53 Mathisen B *et al.* Feeding problems in infants with gastro-oesophageal reflux disease: a controlled study. *J Paediatr Child Health*, 1999, **35** 163–9.

54 Dellert SF *et al.* Feeding resistance and gastroesophageal reflux in infancy. *J Pediatr Gastroenterol Nutr*, 1993, **17** 66–71.

55 McClung HJ *et al.* Constipation and dietary fiber intake in children. *Pediatr*, 1995, **96** 999–1000.

56 Roma E *et al.* Diet and chronic constipation in children: the role of fiber. *J Pediatr Gastroenterol Nutr*, 1999, **28** 169–74.

57 Iacona G *et al.* Intolerance of cow's milk and chronic constipation in children. *New England J Med*, 1998, **339** 1100–104.

58 Shah N *et al.* Cow's milk and chronic constipation in children (letter). *New England J Med*, 1999, **340** 891–2.

59 Loening-Baucke V Constipation in children. *New England J Med*, 1998, **339** 1155–6.

60 Tolia V *et al.* Gastric emptying using three different formulas in infants with gastroesophageal reflux. *J Pediatr Gastroenterol Nutr*, 1992, **15** 297–301.

61 Petter LPM *et al.* Is water out of vogue? A survey of the drinking habits of 2–7 year olds. *Arch Dis Childh*, 1995, **72** 137–40.

62 Hoekstra JH Toddler diarrhoea: more a nutritional disorder than a disease. *Arch Dis Childh*, 1998, **79** 2–5.

63 Kneepekens CMF, Hoestra JH Chronic non-specific diarrhoea of childhood, pathophysiology and management. *Paediatr Clin N Am*, 1996, **43** 375–90.

64 Heneyke S *et al.* Chronic intestinal pseudo-obstruction: treatment and long term follow up of 44 patients. *Arch Dis Childh*, 1999, **81** 21–7.

FURTHER READING

Walker Smith J, Murch S *Diseases of the Small Intestine in Childhood*, 4th edn. Oxford: Isis Medical Media Ltd, 1999.

Walker WA *et al.* *Pediatric Gastrointestinal Disease. Pathophysiology, Diagnosis and Management*, 2nd edn, vols 1 & 2. Philadelphia: BC Decker Inc, 1996.

USEFUL ADDRESSES

Coeliac Society
PO Box 220, High Wycombe, Bucks HP11 2HY

CICRA (Children with Crohn's and Colitis)
Parkgate House, 356 West Barnes Lane, Motspur Park, Surrey KT3 6NB

GMD Support Network (For children with gut motility disorders)
7 Walden Rd, Sewards End, Saffron Walden, Essex CB10 2LE

Half PINNT (For children on intravenous and nasogastric feeding)
PO Box 3126, Christchurch, Dorset BH23 2XS

CHAPTER 7

Anatomical Abnormalities of the Gastrointestinal Tract

There are a number of congenital malformations requiring surgery in the neonatal period. These malformations affect the oesophagus, stomach, duodenum and the small and large intestines. The type of feed and the method by which it is given will be governed by the area of gut affected and the surgery performed to correct the defect.

OESOPHAGEAL ATRESIA AND TRACHEO-OESOPHAGEAL FISTULA

Oesophageal atresia occurs in about 1 in 3000 births [1]. The oesophagus ends blindly in a pouch so that there is no continuous route from the mouth to the stomach. This means that at birth the infant cannot swallow saliva and is seen to froth at the mouth. Aspiration of this saliva causes choking and cyanotic attacks. The obstruction usually occurs 8–10 cm from the gum margin. Approximately 85% of neonates with oesophageal atresia will also have a distal tracheo-oesophageal fistula (TOF) where the proximal end of the distal oesophagus is confluent with the trachea (Fig. 7.1). In this case any reflux of stomach contents will enter the trachea and, hence, the lungs. Oesophageal atresia is associated with other anomalies. Myers *et al.* reviewed 618 patients over a 44 year period and found the most common associated anomalies in oesophageal atresia to be: cardiac (20.7%), urinary (21.6%), gastrointestinal (22.7%), orthopaedic (15.7%); lesser associations were with the central nervous system, eye and chromosomal anomalies [2]. Similar incidences are found in reports from other authors [3, 4]. In Myers' most recent review of the 5 year period to 1988, survival in babies with oesophageal atresia reached 100% (though 9 of the 72 babies were not operated on because they had other lethal anomalies) [5]. Mortality is most commonly associated with major congenital cardiac malformations and very low birth weight (<1500 g) [6].

Obviously, the infant cannot be fed via the enteral route until the lesion is corrected surgically and will, therefore, require parenteral nutrition initially. Treatment of oesophageal atresia, whether associated with TOF or not, is undertaken as soon as possible after birth. It involves the repair of the oesophagus by anastomosing the upper and lower ends, after closing any TOF if present, so that both the oesophagus and trachea are separate and continuous. This is possible in about 90% of affected babies.

Feeding the baby with oesophageal atresia and TOF

When the proximal and distal ends of the oesophagus can be joined in one procedure, once the lesion has been repaired these infants can be feeding orally within 48–72 hours of birth, ideally being breast fed, or receiving expressed breast milk or infant formula. In Puntis and co-workers' study, 50% of infants undergoing a primary anastomosis were breast fed for a median period of three months [7]. Contrast studies prior to feeding will show whether the oesophagus is intact.

If it is technically impossible to join the upper and lower ends of the oesophagus, so-called long gap oesophageal atresia, a staged procedure is required. The oesophagus is temporarily abandoned and a cervical oesophagostomy may be formed to allow the infant to swallow saliva. The oesophagus is left for 3–6 months before attempting to join the upper and lower ends. Although cervical oesophagostomy prevents growth in the upper pouch of the oesophagus, the lower pouch hypertrophies and shortens the dis-

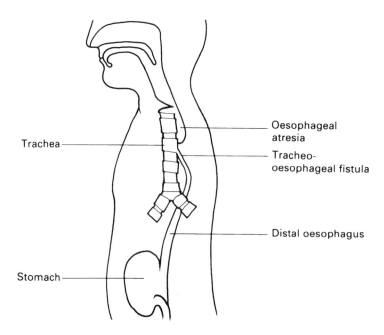

Trachea

Oesophageal atresia

Tracheo-oesophageal fistula

Distal oesophagus

Stomach

Fig. 7.1 Oesophageal atresia and tracheo-oesophageal fistula

tance between the two ends. Alternatively, the upper oesophagus is left intact with a double lumen Replogle tube in situ for 6–8 weeks, through which continuous low pressure suction can be applied to remove accumulating saliva; the upper pouch probably lengthens in this case and hypertrophies. A gastrostomy is formed to allow enteral feeding to proceed. If a TOF is present it must be disconnected and the defect in the trachea closed. Feeding these babies undergoing a staged repair presents more of a challenge.

The gastrostomy feed will be either expressed breast milk (EBM) or infant formula and should be given at the same volume and frequency as the infant would receive orally. In order for the baby to experience normal oral behaviour, sham feeding should begin as soon as possible. To allow for normal development and co-ordination, the sham feed should be of the same volume as the gastrostomy feed, and the feed should be of the same duration and frequency so that the baby learns to associate sucking with hunger and satiety. It is also important that a similar taste is offered in the sham feed as that being put into the gastrostomy so that there is no refusal of feeds on the grounds of taste once the infant later has an intact gut. The sham feed seeps out of the

oesophagostomy, along with saliva and is usually dealt with by wrapping a towel or other absorbent material around the baby's neck (Fig. 7.2). Puntis *et al.* report that 38% of babies with oesophagostomies were breast fed for a median duration of 2.5 months [7]. It is now more regular practice for mothers who wish to give their babies breast milk to express their milk so that this can be given via the gastrostomy; the baby would be given infant formula by mouth for the sham feed. There are, however, problems with sham feeding:

- It is difficult to co-ordinate holding the baby, feeding from a bottle and mopping up feed from the oesophagostomy while giving a gastrostomy feed. This event may defeat nursing staff let alone the mother coping single-handedly at home
- One third of babies with oesophageal atresia suffer from cardiovascular complications and may need ventilating, making sham feeding impossible
- The baby may tire quickly and not be able to suck for long enough to take the same volume orally as is going through the gastrostomy
- Many babies have small stomachs and initially require small volumes of gastrostomy feed very frequently, e.g. 2 hourly, making it difficult to

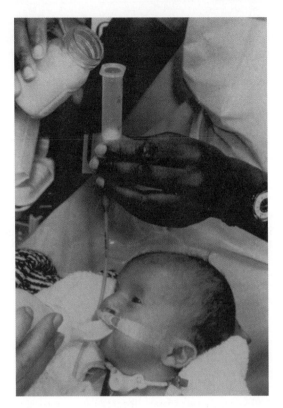

Fig. 7.2 Infant with tracheo-oesophageal fistula and cervical oesophagostomy receiving oral sham feeds whilst being fed via a gastrostomy tube. The infant also has a tracheostomy and cleft palate and takes oral feeds from a Rosti bottle

co-ordinate sham with gastrostomy feeding. However, this problem rapidly corrects itself if the feed volume is increased.

There may be no route for sham feeding if an oesophagostomy has not been formed as part of the initial corrective surgical procedure. Infants deprived of oral feedings for the first weeks to months of life can experience great difficulty in establishing sucking. This should not be a major problem if oral feeding is established within 2–3 months of life, but if oral feeding is delayed any longer than this, it is associated with gagging and vomiting; the baby may avert its head at the very sight of the bottle or push out the teat with the tongue. Desensitisation to this oral aversion is a long, slow process. It is important to remember that feeding is not just a process of pro-

viding nutrition; babies are very alert at feeding time and develop cognitive and motor abilities while feeding.

Babies with oesophageal atresia with or without TOF can grow well on breast milk and normal infant formulas if adequate volume of feed is taken. If there is a problem with weight gain, feeds can be concentrated and supplemented or commercial nutrient-dense feeds may be indicated (p. 13).

Weaning

In order to promote normal development, these babies should be weaned at the appropriate age, though it has been observed that weaning in babies that have undergone a primary anastomosis is delayed to 6 months of age and the introduction of lumpy solids to 12 months of age [7]. Weaning solids should be sham fed if the oesophagus has not yet been joined up. There is controversy over what should go down the gastrostomy tube at this stage. A nutritionally adequate feed should be given in preference to weaning solids. In order to get strained weaning foods of the right consistency to go down the tube they have to be watered down, so diluting their energy and nutrient content. If this practice is continued in the long term, drastic failure to thrive results. In the study conducted by Spitz *et al.*, of 148 children with oesophageal atresia, 27% of the patients were below the 3rd centile for height and weight at 6 months and 5 years [4]. A contribution to this could well have been the practice of inappropriate solids being administered down gastrostomy tubes, as was common practice until very recently. If gagging is experienced when sham weaning solids are introduced, oral intake may be reduced to just tastes of food rather than giving large boluses in order to dispel the association between solid food and gagging. Both mother and child need to build up confidence about eating.

Feeding the older child

The attempt to join the oesophagus to the rest of the gastrointestinal tract may occur as early as 6 months of life, but may occur as late as 3–4 years in others. Until joined up, sham feeding of age appropriate foods should continue with nutritionally adequate feeds through the gastrostomy. Fortified baby milks, such as concentrated infant formula, high energy formulas (SMA High Energy, Infatrini), may safely be used up to the age of one year or so, but will need to be replaced by a more nutritionally dense feed such as Paediasure or Nutrini to maintain good growth in the older child (Table 3.2).

There are various methods of replacing the atretic oesophagus: gastric transposition involves pulling the stomach up into the chest and joining the end of the oesophagus to the fundus of the stomach; colonic interposition involves removing a piece of the colon and transplanting it between the oesophagus and the stomach. Oesophagostomies, if present, are closed at this time. A feeding jejunostomy may be formed as a route for nutrition while the child is sedated post-surgery for gastric transposition as the pre-existing gastrostomy can no longer be used. Oral nutrition is introduced as soon as possible, but supplementary overnight jejunostomy feeds may be indicated until an adequate intake is taken by mouth. Both oesophageal replacement procedures have their problems when feeding recommences. The advantage of the gastric transposition is that there is only one join in the gastrointestinal tract, but the stomach is now sited in a much smaller place in the thorax than it usually occupies in the abdomen. The volume of feed or meals that can be taken comfortably may be greatly reduced, imposing a feeding regimen of little and often. The problem with colonic interposition is that two areas of the gut have undergone surgery and joining. The transplanted colon makes a rather 'baggy' oesophagus because of the nature of its musculature, and the repaired oesophagus may not have normal peristaltic function. The colon may suffer temporary dysfunction because of surgical trauma and malabsorption may ensue, necessitating a change to a hydrolysed feed (Table 6.6). A third method of achieving oesophageal continuity is to perform a gastric tube oesophageal replacement procedure; a tube is formed from the greater curve of the stomach, using staples, which is then joined to the lower pouch of the oesophagus. The end result of surgery may be oesophageal continuity, but not necessarily normal oesophageal function.

Problems with oesophageal function following repair

Gastro-oesophageal reflux (GOR) is common following repair, with an incidence of at least 25% [8]. It may respond to medical management, e.g. thicken-ing fluids (Table 6.26), positioning the baby appropriately after feeding or the administration of drugs such as metoclopromide and domperidone. These are dopamine antagonists which stimulate gastric emptying and small intestinal transit, and enhance the strength of oesophageal sphincter contraction. H_2 receptor antagonists, Cimetidine or Ranitidine, may be administered. If GOR is severe and unresolved by these methods, surgical correction may be required by performing a Nissen fundoplication.

This anti-reflux procedure involves mobilising the fundus of the stomach and folding it behind the oesophagus, thus fashioning a loose wrap. Between 18% and 45% of children undergoing repair for oesophageal atresia have significant GOR, leading to life threatening aspiration of feed, and require such anti-reflux surgery [4, 9]. Following unsuccessful medical management of GOR, 45% of the 31 babies described by Curci and Dibbins required Nissen fundoplication [9]. Together with children with neurological dysfunction, infants and children who have a repaired oesophageal atresia and TOF comprise the majority of patients needing such a procedure.

The change from receiving full nutrition from a gastrostomy/jejunostomy feed to maintaining an adequate intake orally is slow and there is often a long period where the child needs supplementary tube feeds while learning to eat normally. Prior to being joined up, the child has not experienced the sensation of a bolus of food passing the entire length of the oesophagus. Although the child should have been exposed to sham feeding, this method of feeding does not always lead to successful swallowing. Therefore, many children panic when offered any food other than in liquid form and the establishment of normal feeding has to proceed through stages of gradually altering the consistency of foods from purées to finely minced and mashed foods and then to the normal diet.

After repair, whether the child has undergone a primary repair in the first few days of life or whether a staged procedure has been performed, a circular scar will form where the upper and lower segments of the oesophagus are sutured together. With perfect healing the scar will have the same diameter as the oesophagus and will grow with the child. However, if the gap between the upper and lower pouches is greater than 2 cm the two ends of the oesophagus have to be stretched to meet and this puts the repair under tension. This reduces the blood supply to the forming scar tissue, causing the tissue to shrink and form a stricture. Stricture occurs in about 20% of children and the normal passage of food is impeded. Bread, meat and poultry, apple and raw vegetables are the foods most often cited as getting stuck.

If there is reflux of stomach contents up into the oesophagus the acid will inflame the healing scar, which may also lead to stricture formation. Sometimes, the anastomosis joining the ends of the oesophagus leaks and this also causes a stricture to form. Anastomotic leaks occurred in 21% of infants receiving a primary repair in Spitz and co-workers' study [4]. Children with these problems will show difficulty in feeding and a reluctance to swallow. These strictures require repeated dilatations to soften the scar tissue and allow the easier passage of solid food. The oesophagus may also go into spasm at the site of the join and particulate foods like mince and peas get stuck.

The frightening experience of repeated choking leads to fraught mealtimes that both parents and children come to dread. One third of parents of babies with primary repair in Puntis *et al.*'s study reported problems with choking or coughing, 17% with vomiting and 20% with feed refusal at feeding times at least twice a day in the first year of life [7]. A similar frequency was seen in children after closure of oesophagostomy. The introduction of solids in these delayed repair children was significantly later than in both controls and children with primary repair, solid foods being introduced at 12 months and lumpy foods as late as 18 months. It is often easier to abandon the feeding of solids and go back to a completely liquid diet. If this is not supervised, the diet can quickly become very poor nutritionally.

Children often become bored with food; if foods are liquidised to stop them getting stuck in the throat there is the danger that every meal will end up looking the same brown unappetising mush. This can be improved by liquidising the foods separately so that tastes and colours can be distinguished. Mealtimes can become very anti-social; choking and vomiting are common at meals and children may need hefty pats on the back or turning upside down to dislodge food that has stuck. Eating can be a very slow process for the child as foods have to be thoroughly chewed before swallowing can be attempted. Parents understandably feel inhibited about eating out of the home, which curtails the social experience of the child. It is often difficult for parents and carers to understand the problems with swallowing following repair of oesophageal atresia and force feeding the child may be a temptation.

Adequate nutrition can usually be achieved with small frequent meals that are energy-dense, and the provision of fluids at mealtimes to help wash down the food. Such are the problems associated with eating that families need help, advice and encouragement from all professionals with appropriate experience, including dietitians, speech therapists and clinical psychologists as well as the medical and nursing professions. The Tracheo-Oesophageal Fistula Support Group (TOFS) is a self-help organisation where carers of these children can share their experiences and offer advice.

Dysphagia may remain a problem for many years after repair, but improves with time. Half of the children in Puntis *et al.*'s study experienced feeding difficulties at the age of 7 years [7]. Anderson *et al.* looked at the long term follow-up of children undergoing either colonic interposition or gastric tube interposition to see if one method of oesophageal replacement had an advantage over the other [10]. Most of the children fell at or below the 10th percentile for height and weight, half needed to eat slowly and to avoid certain meats, and dysphagia was rare. There was no apparent difference between the two groups. More recently Davenport *et al.* have studied the long term effects of gastric transposition in 17 children who had undergone the procedure more than 5 years previously [11]. They concluded that gastric transposition is compatible with life and allowed satisfactory growth and nutrition for the majority of subjects. They suggest that all children should have oral iron supplementation after the procedure to correct or prevent any defect in iron absorption since low ferritin levels were found in all children tested; one third were anaemic. Iron absorption is facilitated by the presence of acid in the stomach, and the high incidence of hypochlorhydria seen in some adults after gastric transposition suggests this as a mechanism for defective iron absorption.

Chetcuti and co-workers interviewed 125 adults born with oesophageal atresia with or without TOF before 1969 to see how their congenital disease had affected their quality of life. Dysphagia and symptoms of gastro-oesophageal reflux was present in over half the adults, but most enjoyed a normal diet provided they drank fluids with their meals. Their social achievements and failures matched that of the rest of the population [12].

Dumping following oesophageal replacement and Nissen fundoplication

Dumping syndrome is often seen in infants and young children following gastric transposition and is most probably due to rapid gastric emptying [13]. Ravelli *et al.* studied gastric emptying in 12 children who had undergone gastric transposition using electrical impedance tomography [14]. Gastric emptying was normal in one patient, delayed in seven and accelerated in four. Like the repaired oesophagus the transposed stomach does not behave normally. The stomach retains its function as a reservoir but its emptying is extremely irregular. Spitz found that the dumping experienced in the early post-operative period was short-lived, although it lasted for as long as 6 months in some children and recurred periodically in one child [13].

Dumping can occur in children following Nissen fundoplication for severe GOR. Gastric emptying can be accelerated, with the result that hyperosmolar foodstuffs leave the stomach very rapidly and hence draw large quantities of fluid into the small bowel. This produces the 'early' symptoms of distension, discomfort, nausea, tachycardia and pallor. This may be associated with hyperglycaemia. 'Late' symptoms may occur from 1 to 4 hours later as a result of hypoglycaemia and may be indistinguishable from early symptoms [15].

There are no large studies on children with dumping syndrome and most of the published papers are case histories; all workers regard it as difficult to treat. Various dietary manoeuvres have been tried to overcome the symptoms of dumping and no one treatment is recommended. The aim is to avoid swings in blood sugar levels. Some children respond to a combination of treatments. In summary these are:

- Giving small frequent meals [13, 15]
- Taking fluids separately from solid foods [13, 16]
- Avoiding a high glucose intake [13, 16]
- Adding uncooked cornstarch to feeds at a concentration of 3.5–7% [16] or 50 g/litre of feed [17]
- Adding pectin to the diet: 5–10 g (<12 years) or 10–15 g (>12 years) divided into six doses [16]
- Administering continuous feeds with added fat (both long chain and medium chain fats are used) or small frequent meals enriched with fat [17, 18, 19].

Borovoy *et al.* described eight children with dumping syndrome fed by gastrostomy and found that uncooked cornstarch controlled glucose shifts, resolved most of the symptoms, allowed bolus feedings and enhanced weight gain [20]. A guideline for the administration of uncooked cornstarch could be taken from the treatment of glycogen storage disease (p. 299).

DUODENAL ATRESIA

Duodenal atresia is a common cause of congenital intestinal obstruction. Intestinal obstruction has an incidence of 1 in 1500. Duodenal atresia presents as significant vomiting after the first oral feed is given; the vomitus is usually bile-tinged as secreted bile cannot pass down the intestine. The obstruction is corrected by one of three surgical procedures: side-to-side duodenoduodenostomy, side-to-side duodenojejunostomy or diamond-shaped duodenoduodenostomy. The former procedure seems to be favourable in terms of allowing earlier feeding and discharge from hospital [21]. There are other anomalies associated with this atresia: Down's syndrome, oesophageal atresia, imperforate anus and cardiac malformations occur in over 50% of babies with duodenal atresia. Mortality is related to the severity of the associated anomalies. Mooney and co-workers report an improval in survival from 72% in 1973 to 100% in 1983 [22].

Total parenteral nutrition is used routinely to feed these babies in the first days of life. Once the amount of bile aspirate decreases (indicating that the lower gut is patent) and bowel sounds return, oral feeding can be commenced. The feeding problems following repair of duodenal atresia are usually associated with the motility of the duodenum. In utero, the duodenum proximal to the atresia is stretched because ingested material cannot get past the atretic area of gut. The musculature does not function properly once the obstruction is removed, resulting in a baggy proximal duodenum. The infant may feed normally, but milk will accumulate in the lax duodenum rather than continuing its passage down the gut. This can result in huge vomits, up to 200 ml at a time. Feeds need to be small and frequent to overcome this problem.

A transanastomotic tube may be passed in the early days post-surgery to help in the delivery of feeds, though jejunal feeding tubes are associated with perforation and are easily dislodged. Mooney *et al.* found that transanastomotic tubes prolonged the time until oral feeding was tolerated by 10 days: babies without the tube tolerated oral feeds at 5.3 days; babies with the tube at 15.7 days [22]. Breast milk or normal infant formula should be used for feeding and, if administered correctly should provide adequate nutrition. If weight gain is poor the usual methods of feed fortification can be used. If GOR is present, feeds can be thickened and the baby should be positioned correctly after feeding. As the gut grows and matures with the infant, problems should resolve so that the older child will feed normally.

SHORT BOWEL SYNDROME

Small intestinal obstruction in the infant requires surgical resection to remove the obstruction and restore a continuous tract. Obstruction may be due to small intestinal atresias (either jejunal or ileal), or duplications, or malrotation with or without volvulus. Intestinal resection may be necessary for necrotising enterocolitis, which occurs predominantly in premature infants. Other conditions that may require resection of the small intestine are given in Table 7.1. The surgical correction reduces the length of the bowel and thus its absorptive area. This will affect the absorption of water and nutrients and cause a diarrhoeal state. The degree of malabsorption will depend on how much of the small intestine is removed (or perhaps more importantly how much of the small intestine remains). Massive intestinal resection is defined as a resection of more than 30% of small intestine [23]. The clinical effects of such surgery are known as the short bowel syndrome. Sur-

vival of the infant will be determined by the remaining length of bowel; Wilmore reports a survival rate of 90% if more than 40 cm of small intestine remains after corrective surgery, 50% survival if 15–40 cm remains, and a remaining length of less than 15 cm to be incompatible with life [24].

Absorptive function of the small intestine

The site of the resection will determine how well the gut will function post-operatively. The absorptive functions of the jejunum and the ileum are given in Table 7.2. The jejunum has long villi and presents a large absorptive surface for nutrients. However, resection of the jejunum does not usually cause any long term significant malabsorption because the ileum can adapt and is able to absorb carbohydrates, protein, fat, and the minerals and vitamins that are normally dealt with by the jejunum. The ileum has shorter villi and normally has less absorptive capacity for nutrients than the jejunum. However, the ileum is important for the absorption of fluid and electrolytes, vitamin B_{12} and bile salts. Resection of the ileum has profound results as the proximal jejunum cannot develop the mechanisms for absorbing fluid, vitamin B_{12} and bile acids. This may result in depletion of the bile acid pool and, hence, malabsorption of fat with resultant steatorrhoea; megaloblastic anaemia will be apparent

Table 7.1 Causes of small intestinal obstruction requiring resection in infants

Small intestinal atresia – jejunal or ileal
Malrotation with or without volvulus
Meconium ileus
Necrotising enterocolitis
Intussusception
Duplication of intestine
Colonic aganglionosis
Inflammatory bowel disease
Long segment Hirschsprung's disease

Table 7.2 Absorptive functions of the jejunum and the ileum

Jejunum	Ileum
Glucose	Vitamin B_{12}
Disaccharides	Bile salts
Protein	Fluid
Fat	Electrolytes
Calcium	
Magnesium	
Iron	
Water-soluble vitamins:	
thiamin	
riboflavin	
pyridoxine	
folic acid	
ascorbic acid	
Fat-soluble vitamins:	
vitamin A	
vitamin D	

once body stores of vitamin B_{12} are depleted. Massive resection of the jejunum and ileum will result in the malabsorption of all nutrients and water. Diarrhoea and electrolyte loss are the immediate consequences, followed by a dramatic growth failure.

The presence or absence of the ileocaecal valve (ICV) after resection will have an effect on final outcome; if present it slows gut transit time thereby minimising fluid and electrolyte losses and maximising absorption time. If this valve is removed, transit time is quickened. A review by Galea *et al.* considers that if the ileocaecal valve is intact, infants with a remaining segment of small bowel of 20cm are salvageable. However, if the ICV is removed, more than 30cm of small intestine needs to remain to provide enough absorptive area for the infant to survive [25]. Loss of the ICV may also be related to bacterial colonisation of the small bowel as the barrier to reflux of bacteria from the colon is lost, which will worsen the pre-existing diarrhoea.

Small bowel transit time is also affected by gut hormones and nutrients in the gut. Gut hormones that affect small bowel motility e.g. glucagon and peptide YY (PYY) are produced in the ileum and are thought to slow gut motility and reduce gastric emptying. Ileal resection will reduce the levels of circulating hormones; the resultant more rapid gastric emptying and intestinal motility may contribute to the large fluid losses seen in small bowel syndrome. Fat in the ileum has an antimotility effect as it is a potent stimulus for the release of these gut hormones [26]. This effect of fat in the ileum is known as the 'ileal brake' and has a role in slowing motility so that absorption can take place in the small bowel [27]. In the absence of the ileal brake in short bowel syndrome transit of nutrients from mouth to the end of the small bowel is rapid. In a study of adults with short bowel Nightingale *et al.* have shown evidence for a 'colonic brake'. They found that the preservation of the colon after major small bowel resection slows entry of nutrients into the shortened small intestine so that the time for absorption is maximised; they suggest that the mechanism may be humoral as the colon also produces enteroglucagon and PYY [28].

Dietetic management

Whatever the cause of the primary lesion, infants and children with the short bowel syndrome need the same management: adequate nutrition within the confines of a gut that has lost the majority of its absorptive capacity. After resection the remaining gut will go into a state of ileus and total parenteral nutrition (TPN) is needed to stabilise fluid and electrolyte status and to provide nutrition while the gut is in ileus. Once the ileus resolves, profuse watery secretions high in electrolyte content (especially sodium) are produced and fluid losses through the ileostomy are large. TPN may be required for at least 2–3 months following massive intestinal resection. Georgeson and Breaux have reviewed 52 neonates with short bowel syndrome and report a mean duration of some parenteral nutrition (not TPN) for a period of 16.6 months [29]. The duration of the parenteral nutrition was related to the presence or absence of the ICV: those with an intact ICV were fed parenterally for a mean duration of 7.2 months; those without an ICV required parenteral support for a mean of 21.6 months.

Enteral feeding

There are differing views as to when enteral feeding should be introduced: as soon as the ileus has resolved or after 1–2 months of gut rest [23, 30]. Early introduction of enteral feeding will lessen the mucosal hypoplasia seen when enteral feeding is withheld. Continuous enteral feeding is much better tolerated than bolus feeds and should be commenced at very small volumes. Enteral feeding provides the stimulus for intestinal adaptation. Tolerance of enteral feeds reduces the need for TPN and reduces the associated risks of line infections and TPN-related liver disease (the major complication for children with short bowel syndrome). Intermittent parenteral nutrition, e.g. given overnight, may decrease the risk of liver complications [29]. A hydrolysed formula, with the protein present as peptides, will be better absorbed than the amino acids found in elemental feeds. The digestion of long chain fat may present a problem because of bile salt deficiency, and feeds with a significant proportion of the fat as medium chain triglycerides (MCT) may be advantageous. However, the osmotic effect of these shorter chain triglycerides in the gut may favour a mixture of LCT and MCT fat. Disaccharides should be avoided because of the reduced disaccharidase activity in the shortened gut.

The better absorbed feeds will be Pregestimil,

MCT Pepdite 0–2, Alfare and Pepti-Junior. Intolerance of glucose polymer may increase the diarrhoea associated with a shortened gut in the early days and carbohydrate may have to be given in the form of monosaccharides. A modular feed (p. 84) allows greater flexibility of feed design for the individual baby. The source of protein can be whole protein, e.g. comminuted chicken meat; peptides, e.g. Peptide Module 767; or amino acids, e.g. Complete Amino Acid Mix 124. Carbohydrate may best be given as a mixture of glucose and fructose. Any increase in steatorrhoea can be dealt with by the partial substitution of the LCT in Calogen with the MCT emulsion Liquigen. The osmotic effects of using monosaccharides and MCT in the feed may restrain their use. It is important to include some LCT in the feed as this form of fat is the most potent stimulus for mucosal adaptation, and also provides a source of essential fatty acids [30]. The 'chix' feed settles out on standing but may be administered continuously by thickening the suspension with Nestargel at a concentration of 0.5%.

The process of enteral feed introduction is a very slow one. It is advisable to change only one constituent of the feed at a time, e.g. volume or concentration, so that any worsening diarrhoea can be more easily traced to the change in feed composition. Throughout this period adequate fluids and nutrition will be supplied by parenteral nutrition. Codeine may be given to help control the diarrhoea. The gastric hypersecretion which may follow resection lowers duodenal pH and therefore can further impair absorption by the inactivation of pancreatic digestive enzymes. Treatment with H_2 receptor antagonists, e.g. ranitidine, may be necessary [31]. It is unusual, however, for acid hypersecretion to occur in children and is more common in adults. Loperamide hydrochloride is used to slow transit time and reduce secretion. Cholestyramine may improve diarrhoea by binding bile acids but will further deplete the bile salt pool.

The remaining ileum has the capacity to adapt after resection. Within a couple of months of resection hormonal changes and luminal nutrition cause significant changes in the lining of the ileum. There is mucosal hyperplasia so that the ileum has an increased number of cells that perform the normal digestive and absorptive function of the small bowel. Enteroglucagon is thought to be the major trophic hormone involved in this ileal adaptation [32]. As a result of this adaptation the gut is able, with time, to digest and absorb some of the more normal constituents of the diet.

Goulet *et al.* have shown that the time taken for adaptation to be completed is dependent on the length of the residual bowel [33]. In 31 infants with less than 40 cm of bowel, adaptation was complete 27.3 months after resection. In the 51 infants who had 40 to 80 cm of remaining bowel, adaptation was completed at 14 months.

Some degree of malabsorption will, however, continue throughout the first year or two post-resection and a balance needs to be made between enteral and parenteral nutrition to prevent the child from failing to thrive and suffering from the conditions caused by the malabsorptive state, e.g. rickets (vitamin D, calcium and magnesium deficiency), neurological abnormalities (vitamin E deficiency). Serum levels of calcium, magnesium and the fat-soluble vitamins need to be checked regularly to see if further supplementation of these nutrients is necessary.

Oral feeding

Although enteral nutrition is best absorbed by continuous feeding, the oral route must not be ignored. The infant needs oral stimulation and experience of feeding if later feeding problems are to be averted. Weaning should be started when the infant is old enough and well enough. Initially the diet should be free of disaccharides, and it is usual practice to avoid milk, egg and gluten. A typical weaning diet is given in Table 7.3. Diarrhoea will gradually decrease with time as the gut adapts, but it may take up to a year for the child to obtain adequate nutrition from the enteral route. Along with the weaning diet, the child should be tentatively tried with bolus oral feeds rather than receiving only continuous enteral feeds. If continuous

Table 7.3 Weaning diet – milk, egg, gluten and disaccharide free

Breakfast	Milk-free baby rice mixed with milk substitute
Lunch	Purée chicken, meat, fish
	Potato, rice, gluten-free pasta
	Low sucrose vegetables e.g. cabbage, cauliflower, courgette, marrow, spring greens
Tea	Custard made with cornflour and milk substitute
	'Milk pudding' made with milk substitute and rice, sago or tapioca
	Sweeten with glucose

enteral feeds are necessary the family should be provided with a portable pump to give some mobility. For those infants and children who are tube feed dependent, gastrostomy feeding should be offered to replace the nasogastric route.

As diarrhoea subsides, previously avoided foods can gradually be tried in the toddler's diet to assess tolerance. Gluten and egg may be introduced first; then disaccharides in the form of sucrose-containing vegetables and, later, fruit. Milk (and lactose) are tried last of all. Most children by this time will be able to tolerate a normal diet, though a degree of fat malabsorption may remain. Matsuo *et al.* reviewed eight children over a period of 2–19 years and found abnormal absorption of fat in those with a residual small intestine of less than 45 cm [34]. Ohkohchi *et al.* found similar results: nine infants were followed up for 1.5 to 14.6 years and severe steatorrhoea was noted in those with a bowel length of less than 50 cm [35].

There are some children in whom the adaptive process is less successful and they may become susceptible to abnormal water and electrolyte losses during intercurrent illness, especially a gastroenteritis. They may need intravenous fluids at these times to maintain fluid and electrolyte balance. Other children never achieve tolerance of a normal diet and need some degree of long term dietary modification to keep their malabsorptive diarrhoea in abeyance.

Infants requiring massive small intestinal resection have had improved survival rates with advances in surgical technique, TPN and dietetic management in the last 20 years. Dorney *et al.* quote survival rates before 1972 at 27%, rising to 69% after 1972 [36]. Weber *et al.* have looked at the survival rates and quality of life of 16 children with short bowel syndrome over a period of 2–10 years and found a 94% rate of survival [37]. They conclude that the advent of home parenteral and enteral nutritional support has not only improved survival, but allowed these children to enjoy a much improved psychosocial environment. These findings are echoed by Goulet *et al.* who quote an overall 90% survival rate in children with less than 40 cm of small bowel [33]. Survival has improved dramatically since the introduction of home TPN, with survival at 65% before 1980, and at 95% in those born after 1980 when home TPN became available.

Normal growth can be expected with proper nutritional management [33, 34]. The long term problems that may be encountered include renal

calculi, cholelithiasis and fractures [34]. Long term steatorrhoea may lead to low serum levels of vitamin D, total cholesterol and disruption of bile acid absorption. Nutritional supplements to offset this chronic fat malabsorption are probably necessary [35].

New treatments for short bowel syndrome

Feed supplements

It may take many years for gut adaptation to be complete in the child with short bowel syndrome. This has prompted studies of the addition of nutrients to enteral feeds to promote this adaptive process. There is very little published in the literature about supplementing feeds in humans and no practice can be recommended. A summary of these treatments is given by Booth [38].

Pectin is a water soluble dietary fibre that has been added to the diet of rats who have undergone 80% small bowel resection. Pectin promoted intestinal adaptation, increasing villus height, crypt depth and mucosal thickness in the ileum. Pectin (1 g/ 100 ml) has been added to the feeds of a 3 year old boy with only 18 cm of jejunum remaining. Gut transit time was increased and nitrogen absorption improved.

Glutamine is a non-essential amino acid that is the preferred metabolic fuel for the epithelial cells of the small intestinal mucosa. When added to parenteral nutrition fluids it has been shown to reduce the gastrointestinal atrophy seen when receiving parenteral nutrition. In a study where glutamine content of an enteral feed was increased from the usual 4–10% of total amino acids to 25%, an enhanced hyperplasia of the mucosa of the jejunum and ileum was seen. Other studies have not found any trophic effect of glutamine on intestinal adaptation.

Short chain fatty acids (SCFAs) are the byproducts of colonic bacterial degradation of unabsorbed starch and non-starch polysaccharide. These SCFAs provide a major source of energy for the gut mucosa and the colon has a role of salvaging energy that would otherwise be lost in patients with short bowel syndrome [39]. SCFAs have also been shown in the rat to promote intestinal mucosal growth. Rats with 60% small bowel resection which have been given a feed where part of the carbohydrate has been replaced with short chain triglycerides (providing 40% of non-protein energy) had significantly greater mucosal weight and protein content in the jejunum and colon than rats fed on medium chain fat or low fat feeds.

Surgery

A number of surgical interventions have been employed to alter intestinal transit and promote intestinal adaptation in children with small bowel syndrome [31]. These include: intestinal plication where there is small bowel dilatation resulting in stasis and defective peristalsis; insertion of a short length of colon into the small bowel to prolong intestinal transit and hence improve nutrient absorption; formation of an intestinal valve. These techniques carry risks and may compromise the remaining functioning gut so are only recommended if there are serious complications associated with long term parenteral nutrition or if there is no evidence of continuing intestinal adaptation and hence enteral feeding cannot be fully established.

The major breakthrough in the management of children with small bowel syndrome who require long term parenteral nutrition has been intestinal transplantation. The use of FK506 as an immunosuppressant agent has made transplantation an option for those children with severe parenteral nutrition-related liver disease. The survival rate of transplantation is 50% in at least 100 reported operations. It is not presently justified to offer small bowel transplantation to those children who are successfully managed on TPN [40].

HIRSCHSPRUNG'S DISEASE

Hirschsprung's disease describes a total absence of ganglion cells in the affected part of the large intestine. It has an incidence of 1 in 5000 infants [1]. Some 80–90% of cases present as complete intestinal obstruction, bilious vomiting and profound abdominal distension in the neonate, with a delayed passage of meconium. Surgery aims to clear the obstruction either by fashioning a colostomy as the initial procedure, followed by a pull-through procedure at a later date; or by performing a primary pull-through. Some children present later with intractable constipation alternating with diarrhoea which may be treated symptomatically with a high fibre diet. In long-

segment Hirschsprung's disease there is small intestinal involvement; resection of aganglionic bowel will be necessary, leaving the infant with a shortened length of bowel. The dietary management is as described for short bowel syndrome.

EXOMPHALOS AND GASTROSCHISIS

These conditions are not abnormalities of the gastrointestinal tract, but are abdominal wall defects involving the exposure of the infant's intestine to the outside world. There is an incidence of 1 in 5000 to 10 000 births [1]. An exomphalos can be small or large and occurs when the lateral folds of the abdominal wall fail to meet *in utero*. Not only bowel, but also solid viscera like the liver are exposed, covered by a translucent membrane. Sometimes the bowel can be placed back inside the abdomen in one operation, but if it is a large exomphalos this is not possible. The exomphalos sac is covered with either a Prolene or Silastic prosthesis to protect it and the abdominal cavity is left to grow so that it will accomodate the bowel in stages.

In gastroschisis, a rupture of the umbilical cord *in utero* allows the intestine to escape outside the abdominal wall. Again the bowel is put back inside the abdomen in one go, if possible, or may need a staged procedure, tightening the prosthetic sac gradually [41]. Both Silastic and Prolene prostheses and primary fascial closure are considered acceptable procedures; the primary closure has the advantage of avoiding additional operations [42].

The pressure of the prosthetic sac or the closed abdominal wall forces the intestine back into the abdomen, but this continual pressure will upset its normal function and the gut may suffer a prolonged paralytic ileus. Most of these infants will need TPN for several weeks or months before bowel function returns and the use of TPN is of major importance in the survival of these infants [43]. Adam *et al.* found that delayed closure of the abdomen in exomphalos leads to more readily established enteral feeding [44]. However, Sauter *et al.* found no difference in the time taken to establish enteral feeding in babies with gastroschisis and exomphalos whether they underwent primary repair or a delayed procedure [42].

When bowel sounds return enteral feeding can be considered. Expressed breast milk or infant formula is usually tolerated if given as small frequent bolus feeds. Large boluses are not tolerated as the intestinal tract is under contant pressure and cannot accomodate a large amount of fluid at once. If the baby can be handled normally and does not need to be nursed flat, breast feeding is possible. If there is malabsorption, then a hydrolysed feed is indicated.

Exomphalos and gastroschisis were fatal abnormalities prior to the 1970s. The advent of TPN and temporary prosthetic sacs, which allow delayed abdominal closure, has allowed the good survival rates seen today [41].

A study of 40 patients published in the early 1990s shows 90% of babies with gastroschisis surviving [45]. Davies and Stringer followed up 23 survivors of gastroschisis who were born between 1972 and 1984 [46]. They found that despite experiencing intrauterine growth retardation children with uncomplicated gastroschisis eventually achieve relatively normal growth. Other authors have shown that catch-up growth occurs throughout childhood, mostly within the first 5 years. Most babies surviving infancy after repair of gastroschisis can expect to become healthy adults [46].

REFERENCES

1 Spitz L Surgical emergencies in the first few weeks of life. In: Milla PJ, Muller DPR (eds.) *Harries' Paediatric Gastroenterology*, 2nd edn. Edinburgh: Churchill Livingstone, 1988.

2 Myers NA *et al*. Oesophageal atresia and associated anomalies: a plea for uniform documentation. *Pediatr Surg Int*, 1992, 7 97–100.

3 Chittmittrapap S *et al*. Oesophageal atresia and associated anomalies. *Arch Dis Childh*, 1989, **64** 364–8.

4 Spitz L *et al*. Esophageal atresia: five year experience with 148 cases. *J Pediatr Surg*, 1987, **22** 103–108.

5 Myers NA Evolution of the management of oesophageal atresia from 1948–1988. *Pediatr Surg Int*, 1991, 6 407–11.

6 Spitz L *et al*. Oesophageal atresia: at-risk groups for the 1990s. *J Pediatr Surg*, 1994, **29** 723–5.

7 Puntis JWL *et al*. Growth and feeding problems after repair of oesophageal atresia. *Arch Dis Childh*, 1990, **65** 84–8.

8 Spitz L Esophageal atresia and tracheoesophageal fistula in children. *Current Opinion Pediatr*, 1993, **5** 347–52.

9 Curci MR, Dibbins AW Problems associated with a Nissen fundoplication following tracheoesophageal fistula and esophageal atresia repair. *Arch Surg*, 1988, **123** 618–20.

10 Anderson KD *et al*. Long-term follow-up of children with colon and gastric tube interposition for esophageal atresia. *Surgery*, 1992, **111** 131–6.

11 Davenport M *et al*. Long term effects of gastric transposition in children: a physiological study. *J Pediatr Surg*, 1996, **31** 588–93.

12 Chetcuti P *et al*. Adults who survived repair of congenital oesophageal atresia and tracheo-oesophageal fistula. *Brit Med J*, 1988, **297** 344–6.

13 Spitz L Gastric transposition for esophageal substitution in children. *J Pediatr Surg*, 1992, **27** 252–9.

14 Ravelli AM *et al*. Gastric emptying in children with gastric transposition. *J Pediatr Gastroenterol Nutr*, 1994, **19** 403–409.

15 Rivkees SA *et al*. Hypoglycaemic pathogenesis in children with dumping syndrome. *Pediatr*, 1987, **80** 937–42.

16 Samuk I *et al*. Dumping syndrome following Nissen fundoplication, diagnosis and treatment. *J Pediatr Gastroenterol Nutr*, 1996, **23** 235–40.

17 Khoshoo V *et al*. Nutritional manipulation in the management of dumping syndrome. *Arch Dis Childh*, 1991, **66** 1447–8.

18 Veit F *et al*. Dumping syndrome after Nissen fundoplication. *J Paediatr Child Health*, 1994, **30** 182–5.

19 De Vries TW *et al*. Dumping syndrome in a young child. *Eur J Pediatr*, 1995, **154** 624–6.

20 Borovoy J *et al*. Benefit of uncooked starch in the management of children with dumping syndrome fed exclusively by gastrostomy. *Am J Gastroenterol*, 1998, **93** 14–18.

21 Weber TR *et al*. Duodenal atresia: a comparison of techniques of repair. *J Pediatr Surg*, 1986, **21** 1133–6.

22 Mooney D *et al*. Newborn duodenal atresia: an improving outlook. *Am J Surg*, 1987, **153**(4) 347–9.

23 Walker-Smith J, Murch S Short bowel syndrome and small intestinal transplantation. In: *Diseases of the Small Intestine in Childhood*, 4th edn. Oxford: Isis Medical Media, 1999.

24 Wilmore DW Factors correlating with a successful outcome following extensive intestinal resection in newborn infants. *J Pediatr*, 1972, **80** 88.

25 Galea MH *et al*. Short-bowel syndrome: a collective review. *J Pediatr Surg*, 1992, **27** 592–6.

26 Vanderhoof JA Short bowel syndrome in children. *Current Opinions Pediatr*, 1995, **7** 560–68.

27 Vanderhoof JA Short bowel syndrome. In: Walker WA, Watkins JB (eds.) *Nutrition in Pediatrics*, 2nd edn. Hamilton: BC Decker Inc., 1997.

28 Nightingale JMD *et al*. Disturbed gastric emptying in the short bowel syndrome. Evidence for a 'colonic brake'. *Gut*, 1993, **34** 1171–6.

29 Georgeson KE, Breaux CW Jnr Outcome and intestinal adaptation in neonatal short-bowel syndrome. *J Pediatr Surg*, 27 344–8.

30 Milla PJ The management of massive intestinal resection. *Maternal Child Health*, 1986, **11** 59–64.

31 Stringer MD, Puntis JWL Short bowel syndrome. *Arch Dis Childh*, 1995, **73** 170–73.

32 Sager GR *et al*. The effect of altered luminal nutrition on cellular proliferation and plasma concentrations of enteroglucagon and gastrin after small bowel resection in the rat. *Br J Surg*, 1982, **69** 14–18.

33 Goulet OJ *et al*. Neonatal short bowel syndrome. *J Pediatr*, 1991, **119** 18–23.

34 Matsuo Y *et al*. Massive small bowel resection in neonates – is weaning from parenteral nutrition the final goal? *Surg Today*, 1992, **22** 40–45.

35 Ohkohchi N *et al*. Evaluation of the nutritional condition and absorptive capacity of 9 infants with short bowel syndrome. *J Pediatr Gastroenterol Nutr*, 1986, 5(2) 198–206.

36 Dorney SFA *et al*. Improved survival in very short small bowel of infancy with use of long-term parenteral nutrition. *J Pediatr*, 1985, **107** 521–5.

37 Weber TR *et al*. Short-bowel syndrome in children. Quality of life in an era of improved survival. *Arch Surg*, 1991, **126** 841–6.

38 Booth IW Enteral nutrition as primary therapy in short bowel syndrome. *Gut*, 1994, Suppl S69–S72.

39 Nordgaard I *et al*. Colon as a digestive organ in patients with short bowel. *Lancet*, 1994, **343** 373–6.

40 Kelly DA, Buckels JAC The future of small bowel transplantation. *Arch Dis Childh*, 1995, **72** 447–51.

41 Randolph J Omphalocele and gastroschisis: different entities, similar therapeutic goals. *South Med J*, 1982, **75** 1517–19.

42 Sauter ER *et al*. Is primary repair of gastroschisis and omphalocele always the best operation? *Am Surg*, 1991, 57 142–4.

43 Hoffman P *et al*. Omphalocele and gastroschisis: problems in intensive treatment. *Zentralb Chir*, 1986, **111** 448–56.

44 Adam AS *et al*. Evaluation of conservative therapy for exomphalos. *Surg Gynecol Obstet*, 1991, **172** 395–6.

45 Stringer MD *et al*. Controversies in the management of gastroschisis: a study of 40 patients. *Arch Dis Childh*, 1991, **66** 34–6.

46 Davies BW, Stringer MD The survivors of gastroschisis. *Arch Dis Childh*, 1997, **77** 158–60.

USEFUL ADDRESS

The Tracheo-Oesophageal Fistula Support Group (TOFS)
St George's Centre, 91 Victoria Road, Netherfield, Nottingham NG4 2NN.

CHAPTER 8

The Liver and Pancreas

THE LIVER

Liver disease in children differs greatly from that in adults. Klein *et al.* have summarised the differences [1]:

- Liver disease in paediatrics is rare
- The causes of disease are more diverse
- There is a greater prevalence of inborn errors of metabolism, biliary tract disease, primary infections and autoimmune disorders
- The higher anabolic needs for growth plus catabolic effects of liver disease may result in more nutritional deficiencies.

The nutritional management of an infant or child will depend on whether the liver disease is acute, chronic or metabolic. Potential problems warranting nutritional attention occur when there is a disturbance in the usual metabolic functions of the liver. These include glucose homeostasis, protein synthesis, bile salt production, lipid metabolism and vitamin storage.

Dietary therapy is usually aimed at the presenting symptoms including:

- Hypoglycaemia from poor glycogen storage
- Fat malabsorption as a result of poor bile production or flow
- Reduction in protein synthesis especially albumin, exacerbating ascites (Fig. 8.1).

Specific inborn errors of metabolism within the liver, however, require more specific dietary treatment. These include tyrosinaemia, fatty acid oxidation disorders, urea cycle defects, glycogen storage disease, galactosaemia and fructosaemia (Section 5).

Infants tend to present with symptoms of biliary tract disorders that can progress to a chronic condition. Acute presentations are usually due to poisoning,

or as a result of an inborn error of metabolism. An acute presentation in an older child may be due to hepatitis infection, ingestion of a toxic substance or to decompensation of an underlying chronic liver disease which has been 'silently' progressing over time, such as Wilson's disease or autoimmune liver disease.

MECHANISMS FOR MALNUTRITION

Potential causes of malnutrition in liver disease can be summarised as:

- Inadequate intake
  - anorexia, nausea, vomiting associated with liver disease
  - early satiety as a result of tense ascites, enlarged liver/spleen
  - behavioural feeding problems
  - hospitalisation related depression
  - unpalatable diet/feeds
- Impaired nutrient digestion and absorption
  - bile salt deficiency
  - pancreatic insufficiency
  - portal hypertension related enteropathy
  - malnutrition related villous atrophy
- Increased nutritional requirements
  - hypermetabolism (during stress such as infection)
  - accelerated protein breakdown
  - insufficient protein synthesis.

NUTRITIONAL ASSESSMENT

Routine nutritional assessment is the basis for identification and management of malnutrition in liver

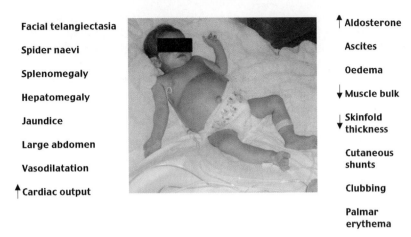

Facial telangiectasia

Spider naevi

Splenomegaly

Hepatomegaly

Jaundice

Large abdomen

Vasodilatation

↑Cardiac output

↑Aldosterone

Ascites

Oedema

↓Muscle bulk

↓Skinfold thickness

Cutaneous shunts

Clubbing

Palmar erythema

Fig. 8.1 Liver disease in children

disease. Difficulty arises as the severity of malnutrition does not always correlate with measurable biochemical markers such as liver function tests or vitamin and mineral status [2]. Plotting length/height can indicate chronic malnutrition over long time periods [3] but is not a very sensitive marker in the short term. Weight measures can be useful initially but become meaningless with organomegaly and ascites [4]. Many other measures, biochemical in particular, are not useful in liver disease [5]. Serial measures of upper arm muscle circumference and triceps skinfold thickness are essential parameters [6] on which to rely for assessment of body fat and muscle stores [7, 8].

As well as serial anthropometric measures, assessment should include observation of physical signs of vitamin deficiencies, dietary intake, degree of early satiety and any self-imposed restrictions. It is important to consider any nutrition related problems such as nausea, vomiting, diarrhoea or anorexia.

ACUTE LIVER DISEASE

Acute liver failure describes severe impairment of liver function in association with hepatocellular necrosis, where there is no underlying chronic liver disease. The term fulminant is usually used when acute liver disease is associated with encephalopathy [9]. However, children often do not exhibit encephalopathy.

Causes of acute liver disease

- Infective, e.g. viral
- Inborn errors of metabolism including haemochromatosis
- Toxins/drugs including chemotherapy
- Irradiation
- Ischaemic, e.g. Budd-Chiari syndrome
- Infiltrative such as leukaemia
- Autoimmune
- Trauma from abuse or seat belt laceration in a road traffic accident.

If presentation is rapid, infants and children are often well nourished, so management is based on maintaining nutritional status until there is some improvement. If onset is dramatic there is a possibility of the critical life-threatening complication of cerebral oedema, so patients are often treated in intensive care. If the child survives, liver function should return to near normal.

If the definition of fulminant hepatic failure is strictly adhered to, a problem arises. It is difficult to distinguish between disease that is actually acute and that which is (undiagnosed) chronic disease, manifesting as acute. The two conditions can appear the same. A thorough investigation of all possible causes is necessary. In particular, mitochondrial disorders of metabolism should be excluded.

Developments in treatment

Present developments in the treatment of extreme cases of acute liver disease include auxiliary liver transplantation. A live donor may be used, but this is rarely necessary. A lobe of liver is transplanted and used in addition to the child's native liver. This can provide a temporary back up in the acute situation. The obvious benefits are that the native liver is not removed, but allowed to get better. If this happens the transplanted liver is removed by surgery or destroyed by weaning down the immunosuppressive drugs. The immediate disadvantage is that the child may have a longer crisis and convalescence period due to the presence of the necrotic native liver and the addition of immunosuppression.

Auxiliary transplantation is also useful in the case of an inborn error of metabolism that originates from a defective enzyme in the liver, in that it provides a source of the required enzyme. It may be that genetic engineering will eventually supercede the need for transplantation so that the transplanted auxiliary liver could be removed, negating the need for lifelong immunosuppression. Mitochondrial-based defects however are not organ specific and will eventually result in multisystem failure. There is no cure at present for these disorders and liver transplantation is not indicated.

Dietetic management in acute liver failure

On presentation one of the liver related inborn errors of metabolism may be suspected, e.g. galactosaemia, fatty acid oxidation defect.

Step 1 – emergency regimen

An emergency type regimen should be started as soon as possible, as intravenous (IV) dextrose with additional potassium if the child is having diuretic therapy. Enteral feeding should be established by the addition of glucose polymer (i.e. lactose/fructose-free source of carbohydrate) to either oral rehydration solution or water. Additional sodium/potassium supplements are necessary. The child should be fed continuously over 24 hours.

The aim of treatment initially is to meet glucose oxidation rates to prevent protein/fat catabolism. Guidelines for glucose requirements (p. 296):

- Infants 8–9 mg/kg/min
- Toddlers 7 mg/kg/min
- Adolescents 4 mg/kg/min.

The amount of glucose given can be increased slowly according to tolerance. Infants often tolerate 18 g glucose/kg/day, i.e. 12.5 mg/kg/min. A modular feed is then developed.

Step 2 – addition of protein

Twenty to 48 hours after onset (or sooner) protein should be added to the feed. The protein source should be lactose-free if galactosaemia has not yet been excluded and fat-free if fatty acid oxidation defects have not been excluded. Essential Amino Acid Mix (SHS) is a suitable lactose and fat-free source of protein. A child with any inborn error, including those of protein metabolism, should tolerate some protein which contains all amino acids.

Infants should be given 1.5–1.9 g protein/kg dry weight/day and children 0.8–1.0 g protein/kg dry weight/day, based on the minimum protein requirements (World Health Organisation) [10]. If more protein is required, a tyrosine, methionine, phenylalanine free amino acid mix, XPTM Tyrosidon, (fat-free, lactose-free) should be used until tyrosinaemia is excluded.

Any protein should be added gradually in increments of 0.5 g/kg/day. It is important not to over-restrict protein, which could result in endogenous ammoniagenesis from protein catabolism. If galactosaemia is excluded, Maxipro (which contains traces of lactose) may be used as the protein source.

Step 3 – addition of fat

Small quantities of walnut oil are needed to provide essential fatty acids (EFAs): 1 ml per 100 kcal (420 kJ) is recommended in the treatment of liver disease. Additional fat, however, will be necessary to meet energy requirements.

Long chain triglyceride (LCT) and/or medium chain triglyceride (MCT) fat emulsion (Calogen/Liquigen) can be added slowly as the condition of the child is monitored. Increments of 1 g fat/kg/day are recommended. A complete vitamin and mineral supplement will be necessary, such as Paediatric Seravit. It is essential to meet basal protein and energy requirements as soon as possible to prevent catabo-

Table 8.1 An example of a modular feed for the treatment of acute liver disease. Infant weight = 5 kg; Fluid allowance = 100 ml/kg

	Energy kcal/kg (kJ/kg)	Protein g/kg	CHO %	Fat %
Step 1				
Fluids = 500 ml/day				
Glucose oxidation: 8 mg/kg/min				
= 8 × 5 × 60 × 24 mg/day				
= 58 g glucose/day (12 g/kg/day)				
Day 1 12 g glucose/kg	48 (201)	0	11	0
60 g Maxijul + water up to 500 ml				
Step 2				
Day 2 18 g glucose/kg	74 (309)	0.5	17	0
90 g Maxijul + 3 g Ess AA mix* + water up to 500 ml				
Day 3 90 g Maxijul + 6 g Ess AA mix* + water up to 500 ml	76 (318)	1.0	17	0
Day 4 90 g Maxijul + 9 g Ess AA mix* + water up to 500 ml	78 (326)	1.5	17	0
Step 3				
Day 5 90 g Maxijul + 9 g Ess AA mix* + 10 ml fat emulsion + water up to 500 ml	87 (364)	1.5	17	1
Day 6 90 g Maxijul + 9 g Ess AA mix* + 20 ml fat emulsion + water up to 500 ml	96 (401)	1.5	17	2
Day 7 90 g Maxijul + 9 g Ess AA mix* + 30 ml fat emulsion + water up to 500 ml	105 (439)	1.5	17	3

Sodium, potassium, vitamins, minerals can be added from day 1.
* Ess AA mix = Essential Amino Acid Mix (SHS) 1 g contains 0.8 g protein.

lism and the build up of lethal metabolites as well as to preserve muscle and fat stores (working example in Table 8.1).

Older children and adolescents in particular are less likely to have an undiagnosed inborn error of metabolism than are infants, with the exception of Wilson's disease. A standard enteral feed may be introduced and hence full nutritional requirements will be met far more rapidly.

Branched chain amino acids

Abnormal amino acid profiles are seen in liver disease. Plasma concentrations of aromatic amino acids increase and the branched chain amino acids (BCAAs) valine, leucine and isoleucine rapidly decrease [11]. The extent of these changes is thought to correlate with the degree of encephalopathy [12]. A review by Morgan [13] concludes that the use of BCAAs as a supplement is ineffective as a treatment for encephalopathy. However, BCAAs are preferentially used in catabolism and as a result, supplementation may allow a higher protein intake without deterioration in mental state [14]. Unfortunately, there have been no randomised controlled trials in paediatrics on the use of BCAAs in acute liver failure.

CHRONIC LIVER DISEASE

There are many causes of chronic liver disease, some of which are more likely than others to have an early presentation. Some diseases may not be recognised until the child is in adolesence.

Disorders presenting in infancy

- Metabolic disorders
- Infections
- Biliary malformations including atresia
- Vascular lesions

- Toxic and nutritional disorders including hypervitaminosis A and total parenteral nutrition (TPN)
- Cryptogenic disorders, e.g. neonatal hepatitis.

Disorders presenting in children and adolescents

- Inherited metabolic disorders, e.g. cystic fibrosis (CF)
- Infections and inflammatory, e.g. sclerosing cholangitis
- Biliary malformations such as choledochal cyst
- Toxic, nutritional, cryptogenic including malnutrition.

Cirrhosis

This represents the end-stage of any chronic liver disease. The chronic disease may initiate a repetitive sequence of cell injury and repair. The consequence of this is cyclical necrosis and fibrogenesis can lead to irreversible damage superimposed onto the original disease process [15]. The liver can compensate for the damage such that the cirrhosis is asymptomatic. Decompensated cirrhosis occurs when damage within the liver causes blood flow to be impaired resulting in symptoms such as portal hypertension, ascites and varices.

Symptoms that can necessitate nutritional intervention

Jaundice

Jaundice is classified as either conjugated or unconjugated. Conjugated bilirubin is made water-soluble by the addition of glucuronide in the liver and enters the bile. If bile flow from the liver is reduced the stools will lack pigment. In this case the (conjugated) bilirubin glucuronide passes into the serum and is then excreted in urine. Conjugated hyperbilirubinaemia occurs when the total serum bilirubin is raised and more than 20% of the bilirubin is conjugated (normally <5% is conjugated). This type of jaundice, with pale stools and dark urine, represents significant hepatobiliary disease and is described as cholestatic liver disease.

Unconjugated hyperbilirubinaemia is characterised clinically by jaundice without bile in the urine.

This may be physiological in the newborn and is not usually an indication for dietetic intervention. Many of the infants seen in a specialist liver centre present with conjugated hyperbilirubinaemia and the diagnosis of its cause is made later. Most of the possible diagnoses for conjugated hyperbilirubinaemia are given later (p. 120).

If the bile flow from the liver into the gut is limited, fat emulsification and digestion is reduced. This leads to malabsorption of fat, fat soluble vitamins and some minerals. Steatorrhoea, growth failure and rickets are common clinical consequences [16–18].

Fat malabsorption

To ensure an energy dense diet is given, fat should not be restricted but given to tolerance. In infants, for whom fat is a more significant energy source, a proportion of fat should be given as MCT [19], which is independent of bile acids for absorption. Many infants compensate for the loss of energy due to fat malabsorption by taking increased volumes of formula. Intakes can be as much as 2–3 times normal fluid requirements. For this reason, an MCT rich formula (containing adequate amounts of EFAs) should be introduced to provide a form of fat and energy that can be absorbed and hence feed volume can be reduced to normal fluid requirements (150–180 ml/kg) (Table 8.2).

Breast fed babies with cholestasis tend to demand huge quantities of milk without thriving due to fat malabsorption. A significant proportion of their requirements should be met by an MCT rich formula (100–120 ml/kg), with breast feeds used as a top up, at least until bile flow recovers. Alternatively an energy supplement of MCT oil or Liquigen (combined with glucose polymer, e.g. Maxijul if better tolerated) can be given before each breast feed. The amount of this energy supplement given will depend on growth. Care is needed to ensure adequate amounts of breast milk are still being taken to provide all other nutrients. All infants should be given some fat containing LCT, either as breast milk or prescribed formula, to provide a source of EFAs.

However, the amount of EFAs needed, as a percentage of total energy intake, is unclear in children with liver disease as deficiency may still occur in those who have received supplementation [20]. Recommendations from the European Society for Paediatric Gastroenterology and Nutrition (ESPGAN) [21] are that infant formulas (including those used for malab-

Table 8.2 Specialised products containing MCT fats and their EFA content

Product	% fat as MCT	EFAs as % energy		
		Linoleic acid	α linolenic acid	Ratio
Caprilon (SHS)	75	6.0	0.8	7.5
Pregestimil (Mead Johnson)	55	10.1	0.6	16.8
MCT Pepdite 0–2 (SHS)	83	3.9	0.02	195
Pepti-Junior (Cow and Gate)	50	12.8	0.2	64
Monogen (SHS)	93	1.1	0.2	5.5
Calogen (SHS)*	0	20	1.0	20
Solagen (SHS)*	—	53	7.5	7.1
Liquigen (SHS)*	100	0	0	0
Duocal (SHS)*	35	9.2	0.2	45
Liquid Duocal (SHS)*	30	16.7	0.3	60
MCT Duocal (SHS)*	83	4.8	0.1	48
15% Caprilon + 5% Duocal	67	6.8	0.65	10.3
Generaid Plus (SHS)**	35	8.3	0.15	55
Frebini (Fresenius)**	45	9.9	1.4	6.9
Emsogen (SHS)**	83	3.7	—	—
Nutrison MCT (Nutricia)	67	5.3	0.7	7.6
ESPGAN [21] recommendations		4.5–10.8		5–15

* These are energy supplements not infant formulas
** Products used as comparison but are not infant formulas

sorption) should contain 4.5–10.8% energy as linoleic acid and that the ratio of linoleic:alpha-linolenic is between 5 and 15 (Table 8.2). It may be assumed that the aim should be to meet the upper limit as a significantly greater amount will be required in a state of fat malabsorption.

Children over 1 year of age will often tolerate more fat as LCT than infants do. An energy dense diet is encouraged to meet the necessary increased requirements. Glucose polymers are useful energy supplements when a maximum fat intake is reached. There are MCT rich feeds that are suitable for older children, e.g. Frebini, Emsogen, Nutrison MCT. Some products do not contain a suitable proportion of EFAs, supported by clinical data [22], unless taken with an additional source of fat from solids or walnut oil. Up to 2 ml walnut oil per 100 kcal (420 kJ) may need to be added to meet the upper limit of EFAs depending on the levels already provided by the feed.

Pancreatic enzyme insufficiency

Some types of liver disease, including Alagille's syndrome, progressive intra-hepatic cholestasis and choledochal cysts, may be accompanied by pancreatic enzyme deficiency which aggravates malabsorption. Since bile salts are required to activate pancreatic lipase a functional deficiency may be present in cholestasis. Finding a low stool elastase may support a deficiency. In these cases, pancreatic enzymes should be started and continued if a clinical benefit is seen. It is unwise to use doses above 10 000 units lipase/kg/day.

Hypoglycaemia

The liver is essential for glucose homeostasis. It stores glycogen and during fasting mobilises glucose. Infants and children with liver disease commonly become hypoglycaemic due to impairment of this function. Muscle glycogen homeostasis is also disrupted in liver disease. In infants, more frequent feeds may need to be offered, as well as ensuring an adequate volume of intake. Overnight continuous feeds may be indicated if the infant does not wake for feeds during the night. It may be necessary to add carbohydrate in the form of a glucose polymer to the infant formula feeds. Initially 1–3 g/100 ml feed is added and may be gradually increased to 6 g/100 ml if needed. Caution is necessary when feeds contain large amounts of glucose as hypoglycaemia may result from a rebound effect, particularly as the feed is discontinued.

In children, regular complex carbohydrate in meals and snacks is encouraged. Sugary foods and glucose drinks can also be encouraged as long as the intake is divided into regular portions to avoid the rebound effect. It may be necessary to provide a continuous overnight feed, or evening doses of uncooked cornstarch (p. 299) to ensure blood glucose is maintained throughout the night. An IV infusion of dextrose may be the only way of controlling blood sugar initially while a feeding routine is established and is a more accurate way of determining the quantity of sugar required to maintain adequate blood sugar levels.

Failure to thrive

Failure to thrive is very common in children with liver disease as energy requirements are increased [23, 24] and intake is unlikely to be adequate without intervention. A diet high in energy and protein is encouraged but utilisation of nutrients may be poor [25]. Additional supplements may be necessary but often, if appetite is poor, nasogastric (NG) feeding during the day or overnight is indicated.

As liver function diminishes muscle wasting increases, especially in decompensated liver disease. The value of BCAAs as a protein source is a subject of discussion. Chin [26] showed an improvement in height and weight in children with end stage liver disease when supplemented with a BCAA formula compared to an isocaloric, isonitrogenous standard formula. This is possibly because BCAAs are metabolised outside the liver and are preferentially utilised by skeletal muscle.

Generaid Plus (SHS) is a formula feed containing BCAAs (37% of the protein) that is sometimes used. However palatability is poor. Flavourings can be successfully added, or NG tube feeding may be required. Although Generaid Plus is not a complete feed and is not prescribable for children under 1 year, it has been successfully used in infants from 4–6 months when the diet would normally include mixed solids; adequate monitoring is necessary.

Ascites and hepatomegaly

The greatest significance of ascites and hepatomegaly on nutritional status is the associated loss of appetite due to a reduced abdominal capacity for feeds and/or food. The aim is to give smaller, more frequent and nutrient dense meals and snacks. Supplementary NG feeding is often required. Ascites is a feature of decompensated liver disease and is managed aggressively with restriction of sodium and fluid intake. Diuretics are used in preference to fluid restriction to allow an adequate nutritional intake; however, resistant ascites may warrant fluid restriction of 60–80% normal requirements. In extreme cases it may be that the infant self-restricts fluid intake to a greater extent than that imposed. A reduction in fluid volume will necessitate the need for a concentrated feed, preferably with a low sodium content (1.2–1.5 mmol/kg/day). Generaid Plus can be used and concentrated to as much as 2 kcal (8 kJ)/ml (44% dilution) if this is done slowly and to tolerance. An MCT based infant formula such as Caprilon can be concentrated and an energy supplement, e.g. Duocal, added, although sodium intakes may then be too high and protein intake inadequate.

A modular feed system based on Maxipro, glucose polymer and LCT and MCT fat emulsions may be used to meet all specific requirements. Sodium content can then be altered by the addition of sodium chloride. Such a modular feed will need vitamin and mineral supplementation. Examples of suitable feeds are given in Table 8.3 for comparison.

Modular feeds can be patient specific allowing flexibility in energy and protein contents, MCT to LCT ratio, electrolyte concentration and fluid volume. If increased cautiously modular feeds can be given at a density of 2 kcal (8 kJ)/ml (as with Generaid Plus), which is advantageous if nutritional requirements are high or fluid tolerance is poor. Care is needed when teaching parents to prepare feeds, particularly when more than two ingredients are used. At home parents will always need to ensure that they have an adequate supply of each ingredient.

All fluids given within the daily allowance should be nutritious, with proprietary supplements used if necessary. The discouragement of salty foods can help to reduce natural thirst as well as enforcing a sodium restriction (p. 164). A rigid sodium restriction is difficult to impose in children and often results in a corresponding reduction in appetite and energy intake and should therefore be avoided.

Portal hypertension and malabsorption

Cirrhosis can obstruct blood flow to the liver causing portal hypertension associated with an enteropathy and malabsorption, possibly secondary to increased pressure in the mesenteric venous system, i.e. oedema of the mucosa of the small intestine. In this case the malabsorption can be very difficult to control. Dietary treatment is not universal and depends on the extent of malabsorption. More frequent (if not continuous) feeds may increase absorption. Semi elemental feeds may be required (p. 74). However, in extreme cases TPN (preferably with some minimal enteral feeding to preserve a functioning gut mucosa) may be necessary.

Oesophageal varices

The presence of varices is not normally a contraindication to NG tube feeding, or to continuing a normal diet. Occasionally, in end-stage liver disease, the huge varices that frequently bleed give rise to a high level of caution such that TPN has been warranted. Clear fluids and progression onto a soft diet are introduced only 16–24 hours after sclero-therapy.

Table 8.3 Examples of feeds suitable for infants with chronic liver disease

Modular feed

		Energy (kcal)	(kJ)	Protein (g)	Fat (g)	% MCT	CHO (g)	Sodium (mmol)	Potassium (mmol)	Calcium (mmol)
25 g	Maxipro (SHS)	98	416	20	1.5		1.2	1.4	3.0	3.1
125 g	Maxijul (SHS)	475	2019				119	1.1	0.2	
25 ml	Calogen (SHS)	113	463		12.5			0.1		
40 ml	Liquigen (SHS)	180	740		20			0.5		
14 g	Paediatric Seravit (SHS)	42	179				10.5	0.1		9.0
0.8 ml	30% Sodium chloride (50 mmol in 10 ml)							4.0		
5 ml	Potassium chloride (20 mmol in 10 ml)								10.0	
Sterile water up to a total of 900 ml										
Total		908	3817	20	34		130.7	7.2	13.2	12.1
Per 100 ml		101	424	2.2	3.8	59	14.5	0.8	1.5	1.3

Concentrated Caprilon and Duocal

		Energy (kcal)	(kJ)	Protein (g)	Fat (g)	% MCT	CHO (g)	Sodium (mmol)	Potassium (mmol)	Calcium (mmol)
15 g	Caprilon (SHS)	78	328	1.8	4.2		8.3	0.9	2.2	1.6
5 g	Duocal (SHS)	25	103		1.1		3.6			
Sterile water up to a total of 100 ml										
Per 100 ml		103	431	1.8	5.3	68	11.9	0.9	2.2	1.6

*Generaid Plus

		Energy (kcal)	(kJ)	Protein (g)	Fat (g)	% MCT	CHO (g)	Sodium (mmol)	Potassium (mmol)	Calcium (mmol)
22 g	Generaid Plus (SHS)									
Sterile water up to a total of 100 ml										
Per 100 ml		101	428	2.4	4.2	35	13.6	0.7	2.6	1.7

*Frebini

		Energy (kcal)	(kJ)	Protein (g)	Fat (g)	% MCT	CHO (g)	Sodium (mmol)	Potassium (mmol)	Calcium (mmol)
Per 100 ml		100	420	2.5	4.0	45	13.5	2.6	2.6	1.5

* Feeds not infant formulas but used with caution when fluid volume is restricted in older infants and when sodium balance can be monitored

Chronic encephalopathy

Restriction of protein is an accepted method of initially treating encephalopathy and reducing ammonia producing gut flora [9]. This can have a deleterious effect on the nutritional status of the child. The degree of encephalopathy must be assessed to determine the level of restriction. Ideally energy intake should be increased to decrease the protein : energy ratio and prevent protein breakdown for energy. Sodium benzoate may permit tolerance of a higher protein intake. The use of BCAAs in encephalopathy has been discussed elsewhere (p. 113).

ENTERAL FEEDING

Nasogastric tube feeding

The use of fine bore polyurethane/silicone tubes is well tolerated and is associated with low risk of variceal haemorrhage [27]. Feeds may be administered as boluses, top up feeds, continuous feeds over 24 hours, or overnight infusion via a pump. Overnight feeds are particularly useful as an addition to the usual daytime regimen. The continuous delivery of feeds is often the only route tolerated in cases of extreme malabsorption or hypoglycaemia.

Gastrostomy

The placement of gastrostomies is contraindicated in liver disease, particularly if the child has ascites. It may also create potential problems with access to the abdominal cavity (due to adhesions) during liver transplantation. There is also a possibility of variceal formation at the stoma site. The enlarged liver/spleen creates a greater risk of puncture if undergoing endoscopic placement of gastrostomy.

However, gastrostomies have been placed in exceptional circumstances (Alagille's, cystic fibrosis) when portal hypertension is not too advanced.

WEANING

Weaning is encouraged as normal from 4–6 months, with progression to nutrient-dense foods. Dried baby foods can be mixed with formula, otherwise extra energy can be added in the form of household ingredients (butter/oil/cheese) or energy supplements.

Progression in texture should be encouraged as quickly as possible. Failure to give solids regularly during the normal stage of development when chewing is learned (about 6–7 months) may have profound effects in terms of feeding behaviour later. Advice from speech therapists, play therapists, psychologists and health visitors can help, particularly if they are involved at an early stage.

VITAMINS, MINERALS AND ESSENTIAL FATTY ACIDS

All infants and children with cholestatic liver disease require additional fat soluble vitamins. Good levels may be achieved with a complete vitamin supplement daily, e.g. 5 ml Ketovite liquid, three Ketovite tablets and a separate vitamin K supplement (1 mg IV preparation given orally), at least until cholestasis resolves. There are no studies to assess whether these children are water-soluble vitamin deficient, but it is likely that there is a greater need for B vitamins with their increased energy requirements.

Fat-soluble vitamin deficiencies are a feature of cholestatic and long standing severe liver disease. Cholestyramine is prescribed to increase gall bladder contraction and impairs absorption of fat-soluble vitamins. The general supplement is continued in these cases. Adequate monitoring of fat-soluble vitamin levels is essential and separate oral vitamin doses should be given and adjusted accordingly if necessary. In severe malabsorption, adequate levels become difficult to achieve and this can highlight the need for the vitamins to be given as intra-muscular (IM) injections.

Increased mineral requirements may include iron if bleeding has been a problem; zinc if vitamin A deficiency occurs; and calcium and phosphate if vitamin D deficient rickets is found. Selenium deficiency is associated with EFA deficiency.

EFA deficiencies may be seen in children with severe fat malabsorption or those who have been on very low fat diets for long periods. Additional supplements of these may also be required. Walnut oil provides the ideal ratio of linoleic to alpha-linolenic acid (p. 320).

NUTRITIONAL SUPPORT PRE-TRANSPLANTATION

As decompensation occurs, a good nutritional state becomes more and more difficult to maintain in the child with chronic liver disease. Fortunately earlier liver transplantation offers a future for the majority at this stage. Although donor matching is based on blood type only, waiting time on the list is unpredictable. The advancement in live related transplantation is likely to lead to fewer fatalities while waiting.

A decline in nutritional status despite maximal nutritional support often highlights the need for transplantation, as malnutrition adversely affects the outcome of liver transplantation [28]. With transplantation as the particular aim, both patients and carers show increased willingness for aggressive nutritional support. Sometimes the struggle to maintain nutritional status necessitates a combination of enteral and parenteral nutrition.

PRESCRIBING PARENTERAL NUTRITION

Prescriptions must consider fluid and sodium restrictions. Fat is usually provided as long chain triglycerides directly into the circulation, with due monitoring of lipid clearance by measuring plasma triglycerides. Fan *et al.* [29] demonstrated however that lipid clearance can improve when using an LCT/MCT blend.

BCAAs have been given intravenously, though as with enteral administration, the evidence that they are beneficial is controversial. There may be a benefit in avoiding preterm amino acid solutions (e.g. Primene) as they contain higher levels of aromatic amino acids which are already elevated in liver disease. Manganese should be avoided as it is not cleared from the liver when bile flow is impeded and as such is toxic to hepatocytes. Manganese may also be deposited in the brain.

NUTRITIONAL SUPPORT POST-ORTHOTOPIC LIVER TRANSPLANTATION

Immediately post-transplantation

Liver transplantation in children is technically more difficult than in adults. The liver is cut down to size match, sometimes just using the right or left, or part of the left lobe. As a result of the higher incidence of biliary tract disease as an indication for transplant in children, and the increased use of cut-down donor livers, it is unusual for the bile duct to remain intact. In a child who has not previously required a Kasai operation (p. 120), a Roux loop will be fashioned from

the intestine, through which the bile will drain from the transplanted liver. This reconstruction delays enteral feeding for 4–5 days.

For children who have had a previous Kasai procedure, enteral feeds may start on the third day. Feeds are gradually increased thereafter as tolerated. Total parenteral nutrition should be considered when enteral feeds are delayed, but is not routine and depends on the nutritional status of the child. Double lumen enteral tubes are used in adults for gastric aspiration alongside jejunal feeding. Such tubes, however, are not available for children due to the variation in size requirements. It is not usual practice to insert two tubes; hence, adequate enteral nutrition may be delayed until gastric stasis resolves. Normal age appropriate feeding is introduced gradually over a couple of days. A good dietary intake can be expected 7 days post-transplantation.

Generally children with nutritional problems pre-transplantation continue to have problems post-transplantation, particularly those previously nasogastrically fed. Usually the appetite returns quickly for those who had good intakes prior to transplantation.

The clearing of long-standing jaundice and the introduction of high dose steroids (as anti-rejection treatment) play an important role in promoting a good appetite post-transplant. It can be surprising how many children begin to eat well, including those previously reliant on tube feeds with little solid intake. Taste preferences can alter dramatically post-transplantation, possibly due to taste perception altered by cyclosporin (an anti-rejection drug). Parents are encouraged to offer new foods and to expect taste changes alongside an increased willingness to eat.

Possible complications

Chylous-ascites may develop as a result of damage to lymph vessels during transplant surgery. This resolves but needs treatment for up to 2 weeks on a low LCT diet, using an MCT-based formula to provide energy, e.g. Monogen or Emsogen (p. 115).

During periods of sepsis or rejection, bile flow may temporarily become limited, again necessitating the use of an MCT formula. Hepatic artery thrombosis may require retransplantation. Intestinal perforation will require gut rest. In both situations enteral feeds are further delayed and TPN may be needed.

Immunosuppression

Basic food hygiene rules using common sense should be encouraged. The commonly used anti-rejection drugs, tacrolimus and cyclosporin, present nutritional challenges. Tacrolimus absorption is affected by food and should ideally be given 1 hour before or after food. This can substantially reduce the hours available for feeding an infant. Both cyclosporin and tacrolimus cause low serum magnesium. Levels need to be monitored and extra magnesium given, as much as 0.5–1.0 mmol/kg/day. These supplements are not well tolerated and can cause diarrhoea. Grapefruit (including juice) needs to be avoided when on tacrolimus, as it may induce toxicity.

LIVER DISEASES IN YOUNG CHILDREN REQUIRING NUTRITIONAL MANAGEMENT

Infantile conjugated hyperbilirubinaemia is the most common presentation for an infant with hepatobiliary disease. It is not a diagnosis but a symptom and needs further investigation. Several tests (e.g. blood tests, ultrasound, biopsy) will be required to find the diagnosis and at this stage an inborn error of metabolism may be considered. Galactosaemia needs to be excluded (although in some parts of the UK screening for galactosaemia is routinely done on the Guthrie card at birth).

Galactosaemia

The urine is tested for reducing substances using a Clinitest tablet and for glucose using a dip stick. Galactosaemia is unlikely if the urine is negative for reducing substances and negative for glucose. There can be a false negative result if the infant has not been fed lactose recently. Confirmation is via the measurement of blood galactose-1-phosphate uridyl transferase level (p. 303). If there is any doubt while awaiting confirmation, a lactose-free formula should be started and breast feeding discontinued (mothers should be encouraged to express their breast milk). Pregestimil is a suitable formula as it also contains some MCT fat.

Biliary atresia

Biliary atresia (BA) is a progressive disease which is defined as the complete inability to excrete bile due to obstruction, destruction or absence of the extra hepatic bile ducts. This leads to bile stasis in the liver with progressive inflammation and subsequent fibrosis. Bile drainage can be restored by the 'Kasai' operation which bypasses the blocked ducts. It should be performed as soon as possible after birth. Late Kasai operations, i.e. after 8 weeks of age, are associated with a poor prognosis [30].

Prior to the giving of feeds with a high MCT content post-Kasai, the majority of children did not thrive [19]. It is now routine to advise a feed high in MCT, preferably up to 1 year of age. Occasionally, infants do well on breast feeding alone but a walnut oil supplement is recommended to ensure adequate EFAs (p. 114). Additional vitamins orally and IM are prescribed. As BA is a progressive condition, despite having the Kasai procedure, all but about 10% of children will require liver transplantation at some point in the future. Hence, nutritional monitoring is essential and further intervention may well be necessary.

Alpha-1-antitrypsin deficiency

The genetic deficiency of the glycoprotein alpha-1-antitrypsin can cause various degrees of liver disease in infancy and can present with cholestasis. The exact physiological role of alpha-1-antitrypsin is not known. The liver disease is thought to be secondary to the uninhibited action of proteases which are critical in the inflammatory response (although the explanation is unlikely to be as simple as this). The severity of this condition, degree of liver involvement and nutritional management vary significantly. Some children require no nutritional intervention and are clinically well whereas others will need intense nutritional support and may come to transplantation before the age of 1 year. Initially fat malabsorption is the main problem but as damage progresses other symptoms of decompensated liver disease will require other dietary therapy.

Alagille's syndrome

This syndrome is diagnosed on a collection of features including intra-hepatic biliary hypoplasia (paucity of the intra-hepatic bile ducts), and cardiovascular, skeletal, facial and ocular abnormalities. It is a rare condition. Chronic cholestasis predominates clinically [31], although some have cyanotic heart disease as their main problem. Conjugated hyper-bilirubinaemia presents followed by pruritus and finally, if severely affected, xanthelasma which usually appears by 2 years of age. This is possibly the most challenging condition in terms of nutritional management. Frequent problems include:

- Poor growth and failure to thrive
- Appalling appetite
- Pancreatic insufficiency and malabsorption
- Vomiting
- Severe itching thought to be exacerbated by improved nutrition.

In those severely affected children who suffer with xanthelasma there is no evidence at present that restricting dietary cholesterol and saturated fats helps reduce their cholesterol levels. The majority that are severely affected are NG fed and warrant all possible nutritional intervention. Indeed malnutrition and severe itching may be the main considerations for the need for transplantation, providing that the associated heart disease is not a compounding factor.

Choledochal cysts

Choledochal cysts are dilatations of all or part of the extra-hepatic biliary tract. They may occur in infants (and can be detected in utero) and children. They may remain undiagnosed for years. Ursodeoxycholic acid is a drug used in this situation to improve bile flow and may enable a small cyst to disappear requiring no further treatment. However, cysts often require surgical removal. Indeed some are so large and invasive that the extra-hepatic bile ducts have to be removed and a Kasai procedure is performed (see above). Dietetic intervention is indicated when bile flow is affected and fat malabsorption occurs. Post-surgery, any required catch-up growth should occur quickly negating further nutritional intervention.

Haemangioma

These are benign vascular tumours of the liver and there are two types: they may undergo spontaneous regression by thrombosis and scarring, or they may grow rapidly. If large the tumours are supplied by wide blood vessels taking a large proportion of the cardiac output. Initially spontaneous regression will be awaited. However, if cardiac failure develops in a young infant, hepatic artery ligation is essential to cut off the blood supply to the tumour. Nutritional intervention is often not needed at all.

In rare cases, the child may require liver transplantation, if for some reason ligation cannot be performed. These cases are dramatic presenting with a huge liver, worsening cardiac function and a very small capacity for feeds. Continuous NG feeds will almost certainly be needed with restricted volume and sodium. A modular type feed or Generaid Plus may be the most useful formula (Table 8.3).

Cystic fibrosis

Cystic fibrosis can present in the newborn as conjugated hyperbilirubinaemia.

Neonatal hepatitis

The cause of the hepatitis is unknown. The severity varies and rarely results in cirrhosis. Usually bile flow resolves in time. In these cases fat malabsorption is treated with dietary intervention until bile flow and adequate growth resume.

Inspissated bile syndrome

This is conjugated jaundice caused by a plug of thick bile blocking the bile duct and hence affecting bile flow. Resolution may occur naturally with time, or with the help of ursodeoxycholic acid (enhancing bile flow), or under percutaneous transhepatic cholangiography (PTC), or in rare cases it requires surgical excision. Nutritional intervention with an MCT-containing formula may be necessary until this time. The syndrome often occurs in infants who have been nil by mouth, e.g. after surgery and long courses of TPN.

TPN induced cholestasis

The exact pathogenesis is unknown. Opinions are divided as to whether the TPN is a direct insult to the liver or whether the damage to the immature liver is caused by infections from lines and sepsis from gut bacterial translocation. There are several suggested measures [32] that appear to minimise effects on liver function. These include:

- Starting minimal enteral feeds if possible, preferably with some bolus feeds to stimulate bile flow
- Starting ursodeoxycholic acid to improve bile flow
- Minimising sepsis through line care
- Rotational antibiotics to prevent gut bacterial overgrowth
- Reducing the number of hours or days on TPN where possible.

Minimising lipids is possibly helpful but only when adequate alternative energy can be provided.

TPN induced cholestasis is often associated with infants with short guts. The difficulty is providing adequate nutrition while the gut is given time to grow without necessitating a liver transplant from irreversible damage from TPN. Desperate measures have included gut lengthening surgery to decrease gut adaptation time, use of novel substrates (glutamine, growth hormone, fish oils, probiotics e.g. Yakult), as well as continuous enteral feeding of adequate volumes to promote gut adaptation (p. 104).

COMMON PRESENTATIONS OF LIVER DISEASE IN OLDER CHILDREN

Auto-immune hepatitis

This rarely necessitates dietetic intervention, unless associated with inflammatory bowel disease (IBD). If dietetic input is required, management of the presenting symptoms will be needed, which may range from failure to thrive and malabsorption, to obesity aggravated by steroid therapy.

Wilson's disease

This is an inborn error of metabolism resulting in defective copper metabolism. It leads to an accumulation of copper in the liver, brain, kidney and cornea. Accumulation can take years and hence presentation is delayed. Oral chelating agents (e.g. penicillamine) bind dietary copper and have negated the need for a strict low copper diet although avoiding foods with a high copper content is sensible: offal, particularly liver, and animals/fish eaten whole which thus contain the liver, e.g. shellfish. Other foods with a high copper content include cocoa and mushrooms but these are unlikely to be eaten in the quantity required to warrant a restriction. In advanced disease,

or acute onset, liver transplant may be the only option due to the poisonous nature of copper.

Cystic fibrosis related liver disease

Significant portal hypertension and associated malnutrition are characteristics of the liver disease related to CF. Jaundice is rarely seen. Liver function tests are not reliable markers for disease severity. Assessment and treatment needs to take into account:

- Usual weight for height percentages used in the nutritional assessment of CF are not useful due to ascites and organomegaly (p. 111). Anthropometry of the upper arm is more reliable.
- An increase in malabsorption with progressive liver disease in CF is most likely to be as a result of portal hypertension enteropathy. Increases in pancreatic enzyme replacement therapy above 10000 units lipase/kg are thus unlikely to be helpful.
- Large volumes of feeds are not tolerated well due to organomegaly and ascites.
- Restrictions in sodium may not be needed as requirements are greater in CF.

An elemental feed containing MCT fat, Emsogen, may be beneficial and does not require an increase in the dose of enzyme supplements. The feed may be concentrated into small volumes and fed overnight. Hyperosmolar feeds tend to be well tolerated in CF. Early data [33] suggests that:

'Aggressive nutritional support providing 50% estimated average requirement (EAR) for energy for age, via overnight NG feeding, does improve nutritional status prior to tranplantation, using mid upper arm anthropometry as a measure' [33].

Liver tumours

These tumours rapidly infiltrate the liver whether benign or malignant. Medical management includes the use of steroids and chemotherapy to reduce the tumour size. Resection may then be possible allowing the liver to regenerate, otherwise transplant may be the only option. Nutritional support and monitoring will be required throughout the course of treatment.

Bone marrow transplantation – immune deficiency disorders

Immune deficiency causing liver destruction has led to a need for bone marrow transplantation followed by liver transplantation, in some cases. The main nutritional complications have included severe vomiting and diarrhoea, requiring nutritional support in the form of enteral and parenteral nutrition throughout the critical course of treatment.

THE PANCREAS

CONGENITAL ANOMALIES

The incidence of congenital anomalies is uncertain. Children are often asymptomatic and anomalies are found incidentally. They include annular ectopic pancreas, pancreatic agenesis, hypoplasia and dysplasia, and ductal abnormalities. Some anomalies are complicated, e.g. the common channel syndrome, whereby the common bile duct and pancreatic duct are seen together for a longer segment than usual, and is implicated in the pathogenesis of choledochal cysts and development of pancreatitis [34]. In childhood this can present with jaundice, cholangitis and pancreatitis and may well require surgery. Abnormalities can be so severe that they result in pancreatic insufficiency and require enzyme replacement.

HEREDITARY DISORDERS

These include:

- Cystic fibrosis (Chapter 10)
- Schwachman's syndrome
- Johanson-Blizzard syndrome
- Exocrine pancreatic insufficiency with refractory sideroblastic anaemia
- Isolated enzyme deficiencies.

Many inherited disorders result in pancreatic insufficiency and fat malabsorption necessitating enzyme replacement therapy. Required dosage is usually the greatest in CF.

ACQUIRED DISORDERS

Malnutrition has been associated with decreased pancreatic enzyme production [35] though enzyme activity usually returns with adequate nutrition [36]. Surgical resection of the pancreas, e.g. in the treatment of Nesidioblastosis (which is a cause of hyperinsulinaemia and hypoglycaemia in infancy) may result in insufficient pancreatic function. Tumours are rare in children, but if found may also require surgical resection. Enteropathies (e.g. coeliac disease) are associated with pancreatic insufficiency [37]. Pancreatic replacement therapy will be required.

ACUTE PANCREATITIS

Injury to the liver and pancreas is the most common cause of acute pancreatitis. Abdominal trauma may be as a result of child abuse, handle bars on bicycles and seat belts in road traffic accidents, or sporting injuries from ball games, contact sports or even horse riding. Infections, gallstones and vasculitis are also possible causes. Hereditary forms of recurrent acute pancreatitis are recognised.

Current management

This is based on the concept of resting the pancreas. The fasting state results in a decrease in pancreatic enzymes, while gastric secretions are removed via an NG tube. The necessity for gut rest depends on the severity of the pancreatitis. If the symptoms of pancreatitis include vomiting and paralytic ileus, little argument can be made against gastric decompression.

The nutritional management of acute pancreatitis is controversial. Klein *et al.* review the treatment in adults with acute pancreatitis [1]:

- Additional nutritional support as either enteral nutrition or TPN has no beneficial effect on clinical outcome in patients with mild or moderate pancreatitis.
- Patients with severe disease or complications often require nutritional support.
- Enteral feeding can be safely administered. Jejunal tube feeding is often tolerated in mild to moderate pancreatitis and those who have had surgery.

Whether to use the NG, duodenal or jejunal route remains uncertain, as well as the choice of feed. Polymeric, elemental and low fat feeds have all been used.

- While IV lipids have been associated with pancreatitis [38], where TPN is needed they are considered safe to use provided hypertriglyceridaemia is avoided.

Recent randomised trials in adults [39, 40] have also concluded that enteral feeding is beneficial compared to parenteral in acute pancreatitis. However, there are no patient-controlled randomised trials which have evaluated potential benefits of nutritional therapy for acute pancreatitis in paediatrics.

CHRONIC PANCREATITIS

This condition is characterised by the recurrence of abdominal pain with development of pancreatic insufficiency and/or diabetes mellitus. As mentioned, this may be the result of inherited pancreatic conditions, or anomalies within the pancreas or associated with metabolic disease (alpha-1-antitrypsin deficiency, Wilson's disease).

Malnutrition and growth failure may result from food avoidance, abdominal pain, nausea, vomiting and increased losses of fat. A high energy diet, with adequate fat intake, is required to achieve normal growth. Enteric coated pancreatic enzymes should be used and the dose tailored to the individual child. Additional fat soluble vitamins may be necessary. When diabetes mellitus is a feature, control of associated symptoms is not easily achieved on diet therapy alone. This is particularly hard to achieve when trying to improve energy intake. Treatment with insulin may be necessary but the amounts needed are often low (p. 129).

REFERENCES

1 Klein S *et al.* Nutritional support in clinical practice. Review of published data and recommendations for future research directions. *J Parent Ent Nutr*, 1997, **21** 133–54.
2 Chin SE *et al.* The nature of malnutrition in the children with end stage liver disease awaiting orthotopic liver transplantation. *Am J Clin Nutr*, 1992, **56** 164.
3 Goulet OJ *et al.* Preoperative nutritional evaluation and support for liver transplant in children. *Transplant Proc*, 1987, **4** 3249.
4 Sokol RJ, Stall C Anthropometric evaluation of children with chronic liver disease. *Am J Clin Nutr*, 1990, **52** 203.
5 Novy MA, Schwarz KB Nutritional considerations and management of the child with liver disease. *Nutrition*, 1997, **13** 177–84.
6 Hehir DJ *et al.* Nutrition in patients undergoing orthotopic liver transplant. *J Parent Ent Nutr*, 1985, **9** 695–700.
7 Frisancho AR Triceps skinfold and upper arm muscle size norms for assessment of nutritional status. *Am J Clin Nutr*, 1974, **27** 1052.
8 Frisancho AR New norms of upper limb fat and muscle areas for assessment of nutritional status. *Am J Clin Nutr*, 1981, **34** 2540–45.
9 Mowat AP *Liver Disorders in Childhood*, 3rd edn. London: Butterworths, 1994.
10 World Health Organisation *Energy and protein requirements*. Report of a Joint FAO/WHO/UNU Meeting. Geneva. WHO Technical Report Series, 1985, 724.
11 Weisdorf SA *et al.* Amino acid abnormalities in infants with extrahepatic biliary atresia and cirrhosis. *J Pediatr Gastroenterol Nutr*, 1987, **6** 860.
12 Morgan MY, Milsom JP, Sherlock S Plasma ratio valine, leucine, and isoleucine to phenylalanine and tyrosine in liver disease. *Gut*, 1978, **19** 1068.
13 Morgan MY The treatment of chronic hepatic encephalopathy. *Hepato-Gastroenterology*, 1991, **38** 377–87.
14 Keohane PP *et al.* Enteral nutrition in malnourished patients with hepatic cirrhosis and acute encephalopathy. *J Parent Ent Nutr*, 1987, **7** 346–50.
15 Walker WA, Drurie PR, Hamilton JR, Walker-Smith JA, Watkins JB *Pediatric Gastrointestinal Disease – Pathophysiology, Diagnosis, Management*, vol. 2, 1st edn. Philadelphia/Toronto: BC Decker Inc, 1991.
16 Glasgow JFT *et al.* Fat absorption in congenital obstructive liver disease. *Arch Dis Childh*, 1973, **48** 601.
17 Gourley GR *et al.* Essential fatty acid deficiency after hepatic portoenterostomy for biliary atresia. *Am J Clin Nutr*, 1982, **36** 1194.
18 Andrews WS *et al.* Fat soluble vitamin deficiency in biliary atresia. *J Pediatr Surg*, 1981, **16** 284.
19 Cohen MI, Gartner LM The use of medium chain triglycerides in the management of biliary atresia. *J Paed*, 1971, **79** 379–84.
20 Yamashiro Y *et al.* Docosahexaenoic acid status of patients with extrahepatic biliary atresia. *J Pediatr Surg*, 1994, **29** 1455.
21 Aggett PJ *et al.* ESPGAN Committee Report On Nutrition; Comment on the content and composition of lipids in infant formulas. *Acta Paediatr Scanda*, 1991, **80** 887–96.
22 Kaufmann SS *et al.* Influence of Portagen and Pregestimil on essential fatty acid status in infantile liver disease. *Pediatr*, 1992, **89** 151–4.

23 Pierro A *et al*. Resting energy expenditure is increased in infants and children with extrahepatic biliary atresia. *J Pediatr Surg*, 1989, **24** 534.

24 Dolz C *et al*. Ascites increases the resting energy expenditure in liver cirrhosis. *Gastroenterol*, 1991, **100** 738–44.

25 Schneeweiss B *et al*. Energy metabolism in patients with acute and chronic liver disease. *Hepatology*, 1990, **11** 387.

26 Chin SE *et al*. Nutritional support in children with end stage liver disease: a randomised crossover trial of a branched chain amino acid supplement. *Am J Clin Nutr*, 1992, **56** 1–6.

27 Chin SE *et al*. Pre-operative nutritional support in children with end-stage liver disease accepted for liver transplantation: an approach to management. *J Gastroenterol Hepatol*, 1990, **5** 566.

28 Shepherd RW Pre- and post-operative nutritional care in liver transplantation in children. *J Gastro Hepatology*, 1996, **11** s7–10.

29 Fan ST *et al*. Metabolic clearance of fat emulsion containing medium chain triglycerides in cirrhotic patients. *J Parent Ent Nutr*, 1992, **16** 279–83.

30 Mieli-Vergani G *et al*. Late referral for biliary atresia – missed opportunities for effective surgery. *Lancet*, 1989, **1** 421–3.

31 Alagille D Management of paucity of interlobular bile ducts. *J Hepatol*, 1985, **1** 561.

32 Meadows N Monitoring and complications of parenteral nutrition. *Nutr*, 1998, **14** 806–808.

33 Bartlett FM *et al*. Enteral feeding improves nutritional status in cystic fibrosis patients, with liver disease. *Netherlands J Medicine*, 1999, **54** s66.

34 Kato O, Hattori K, Suzuki T, Tachio F, Yuasa T Clinical significance of anomalous pancreaticobiliary union. *Gastrointest Endosc*, 1983, **29** 94–8.

35 Pitchumoni CS Pancreas in primary malnutrition disorders. *Am J Clin Nutr*, 1973, **26** 374–9.

36 Barbezat GO, Hansen JDL The exocrine pancreas and protein energy malnutrition. *Pediatr*, 1968, **42** 77–92.

37 Bustos Fernanez L *et al*. Exocrine pancreas insufficiency secondary to gluten enteropathy. *Am J Gastroenterol*, 1970, **53** 564–9.

38 Lashner BA, Kirsner JB, Hanauer SB Acute pancreatitis associated with high concentrated lipid emulsion during total parenteral nutrition therapy for Crohn's disease. *Gastroenterol*, 1986, **90** 1039.

39 Windsor AC *et al*. Compared with parenteral nutrition, enteral feeding attenuates the acute phase response and improves disease severity in acute pancreatitis. *Gut*, 1998, **42** 431–5.

40 Kalfarentzos F *et al*. Enteral nutrition is superior to parenteral nutrition in severe acute pancreatitis: results of a randomized prospective trial. *Br J Surg*, 1997, **84** 1665–9.

USEFUL ADDRESS

Children's Liver Disease Foundation
AXA Equity & Law House, 35–37 Great Charles Street, Queensway, Birmingham B3 3JY.

CHAPTER 9

Diabetes Mellitus

The incidence of type 1 diabetes mellitus in children is increasing at the rate of 2% per annum, and in Scotland currently stands at 25 per 100 000 population per year in the under 14 year old age group [1]. It is primarily a hormone deficiency disease, due to autoimmune destruction of the pancreatic islet β–cells.

It is preferable for these children to attend a specialist children's diabetes clinic and be cared for by a paediatric multidisciplinary diabetes team [2]. This team should include the paediatrician, diabetes nurse specialists and a paediatric dietitian, and should have access to psychological services and social workers in addition to services offered in primary care. The team should work collaboratively to educate and support the children and their families, while empowering them to manage diabetes on a day to day basis.

The parents of a child who is diagnosed as having a chronic disease (including a newly diagnosed diabetic child) are initially shocked and devastated. Parents can also feel a sense of guilt: they may feel that their child has developed diabetes because they have permitted him or her to eat sweets excessively. Since diabetes is partly genetic, parents feel guilty about passing on 'bad genes', a feeling enhanced if there is a family history.

An effective, family-based dietary education programme which is going to result in the modification of a child's eating habits can only begin when parents are allowed to grieve and come to terms with the diagnosis of diabetes in their child. It is vital to develop a rapport with the family so that a high quality of consistent dietetic care can be provided. Frequent and short teaching sessions are preferable, with the entire family if appropriate. Unlike insulin, blood sugars and hypoglycaemia, food is familiar to all, so it may be beneficial to commence the teaching process with food and diet-related topics before the nursing and medical staff begin detailed teaching. Conducting the teaching sessions in the family's own home has many advantages: less disruption, familiar surroundings, the child's usual food and exercise pattern is maintained, first hand knowledge of the domestic set-up and the session may become more learner centred. The disadvantages are that these sessions are costly in terms of travelling time and resources.

THE EATING PLAN FOR A CHILD WITH DIABETES

Aims of the eating plan

(1) To meet the child's nutritional requirements

Children with diabetes have the same basic nutritional needs as their non-diabetic counterparts. It can be emphasised that the eating plan recommended is 'healthy eating' for the entire family.

(2) To contribute towards optimising blood sugar levels and hence HbA1c (glycosylated haemoglobin) results, avoiding swings between hyper- and hypoglycaemia.

The distribution of carbohydrate throughout the day is important and should balance the effects of the injected insulin. A pre-prandial blood glucose of 4–6 mmol/l is ideal; however, a target of obtaining 80% of the blood sugars in the range 4–10 mmol/l is probably more realistic. It is imperative to aim to maintain blood glucose concentrations close to the normal range to decrease the frequency and severity of long term microvascular and cardiovascular complications [3]. Recurrent episodes of hypoglycaemia are undesirable, particularly in young children where the developing brain may be particularly susceptible.

(3) Dietary modifications must ensure normal growth and development

Dietary energy should be sufficient for growth and allow for variable exercise patterns, but should not provoke obesity. Growth should be plotted at regular intervals using standard height and weight charts. Growth velocity charts and body mass index are useful for anticipating the onset of obesity or stunting. Growth can be a useful indicator of diabetic control, as poor physical development may be a consequence of inadequate diabetic management. Obesity is less of a problem in diabetic children than in diabetic adults, but if children do gain weight disproportionately to their height, suitable dietetic advice should be given at a very early stage. Particular care should be taken to monitor the weight of adolescent girls, as this group is most prone to obesity [4] because they reach adult stature before their peers and generally take less exercise.

(4) the diet should minimise the development of diabetic complications such as cardiovascular and microvascular disease.

If insufficient carbohydrate is allowed then children will tend to compensate by eating more protein and fat, which is undesirable.

(5) To inculcate good dietary habits for good health.

RECOMMENDATIONS

Two documents have published recommendations for people with diabetes. The British Diabetic Association's 1980 document [5], updated in 1992, *Dietary Recommendations for People with Diabetes: An Update for the 1990s* [6], recommends that at least 50% of the dietary energy should be derived from carbohydrate, mainly fibre rich polysaccharides. More specifically *Dietary Recommendations for Children and Adolescents with Diabetes* were made in 1989 by the British Diabetic Association [7]. These suggest that dietary carbohydrate should never be restricted below the usual family intake (40–45% energy). They also recognise that the energy distribution between carbohydrate, fat and protein will differ depending on age: breast fed infants will obtain approximately 55% energy from fat, 5% from protein and 40% from carbohydrate, whereas a 5 year old may derive 35% energy from fat, 15% from protein and 50% from carbohydrate. Tra-

ditional dietary regimens have emphasised only the carbohydrate component. Present day practice adopts a more holistic dietary approach.

An increase in carbohydrate, particularly from high fibre sources, and a reduction in fat is recommended. In addition the energy content of the diet should be tailored to the individual. This is of major importance in order to minimise the risk of chronic degenerative disease such as obesity and coronary heart disease.

Carbohydrate

The current recommendation for the child with diabetes is that carbohydrate provides more than 40% energy. The formula: 120 g carbohydrate + 10 g for every year of life reflects current thinking and provides a baseline of daily carbohydrate that should provide at least 40% energy from carbohydrate. For example, this formula suggests that a 2 year old boy should have 120 g + 20 g (140 g) carbohydrate daily. His estimated average energy requirement is 1190 kcal, hence a minimum of 47% energy should be derived from carbohydrate.

It should be noted however that the dietary reference values for food energy [8] were not designed for the individual but for groups. Allowance should be made for the child's body weight and activity. A boy growing along the 3rd centile for weight will weigh 14.4 kg, while a boy growing along the 97th centile will weigh 23.2 kg. Both are growing within normal limits, yet their weights vary by 8.8 kg. These two boys will require different energy and carbohydrate intakes.

Fibre (non-starch polysaccharide)

Dietary fibre is an integral part of any healthy diet. The British Diabetic Association recommends a fibre intake of 2 g/100 kcal/day [7], but admits that this will mean a large change for some children and their families, and that an intake of 1 g/100 kcal is a reasonable first step. Both cereal fibre and soluble dietary fibre have small hypoglycaemic effects in people with diabetes [9]. Soluble fibre and the similar leguminous fibre also improves blood lipids, reducing LDL- and VLDL-cholesterol, while maintaining HDL-cholesterol [10]. Gradual changes in fibre intake are necessary to minimise colic, flatulence and abdominal distension. High intakes can impair the absorption of calcium, iron and zinc due to the high level of phytate in high fibre foods, although it can be argued that these foods themselves, being less refined, have a higher vitamin and mineral content than lower fibre foods.

High fibre foods are less energy-dense than refined carbohydrate ones, therefore the child's total energy intake may be compromised if the diet contains large quantities of fibre. However, children can safely include a number of high fibre foods in their diet, e.g. wholemeal bread, high fibre breakfast cereals, baked beans and high fibre baked goods. A large proportion of children will eat at least one portion of fruit each day; many do not like vegetables, but will take them when included in soups and stews. Often raw vegetables will be taken in preference to those that are cooked.

High fibre pulses appear to be particularly beneficial for blood sugar control and many children will eat them in the form of baked beans, peas, sweetcorn, kidney beans or lentil soup.

Fat

Fat is necessary in children's diets to provide adequate energy, fat-soluble vitamins and essential fatty acids. However, if an older child's fat intake is higher than 35% energy or rapid weight gain is a problem at any age, the following advice can be given to reduce dietary fat:

- Take grilled and oven-baked foods in preference to fried foods
- Cut off visible fat on meat
- Take fish and poultry instead of red meat
- Cut down on the quantity of crisps eaten to 2–3 bags per week (often a compromise of a maximum of one bag per day has to be conceded); use reduced fat crisp varieties
- Take reduced-fat cheeses or varieties that are lower in fat (cottage cheese is not popular with children, so it seems more realistic to limit the amount of high fat cheese and encourage lower fat varieties such as Edam or half-fat hard cheese)
- Use semi-skimmed or skimmed milk, provided appetite is good and an adequate energy intake can be maintained. A supplement of vitamins A and D should be considered for children under the age of 5 years who are taking skimmed milk.

Finding out any family history of coronary heart disease is important. Patients with diabetes are prone to dyslipidaemia so attention to dietary fat intake is as important as good metabolic control.

Protein

Children with diabetes should have protein intakes no higher than those taken by other children. In the diets of most children, protein provides 15% of dietary energy, although actual requirements are considerably lower than this [8].

Sugar

School children take 20–30% of their carbohydrate as added simple sugars. Replacing these with polysaccharides high in fibre in a diabetic child's diet results in a considerable increase in the bulk of food eaten. For this reason it is hard for diabetic children to increase the proportion of energy eaten as dietary carbohydrate if it is to come from high fibre sources.

It is now recognised that the use of sugar taken as part of a mixed meal does not have a detrimental effect on blood sugar control in well-controlled insulin dependent diabetics who are not obese [11, 12]. It is also recognised that the rate of absorption of carbohydrates depends on a great many factors, and the idea that sucrose always causes a rapid rise in blood sugar is perhaps too simplistic. Rapidly absorbed carbohydrate such as a chocolate biscuit can be included in the dietary allowance at the end of a main meal, when the glycaemic response will be lower. The inclusion of a controlled amount of 'sugary' foods has a number of benefits:

- It makes the child feel that his diet is not too different from that of his peers
- It may increase dietary compliance
- It increases palatability and variety
- It discourages the use of diabetic products.

Exercise

Exercise has the effect of lowering blood glucose levels by increasing the non-insulin dependent uptake of glucose by the cells and increasing insulin sensitivity. Insulin doses can be reduced before periods of heavy exercise, but a child's energy expenditure is so variable from day to day and hour to hour that it is more practical, in most instances, to cover additional activity with extra carbohydrate. Additional carbohydrate given need not be in the form of simple sugars, although the child often favours these. Sugar based refined carbohydrate, e.g. a fun size bar, should be given prior to exercise to minimise the risk of hypoglycaemia. If more than 10 g of carbohydrate is required the sugary carbohydrate should be mixed with a more unrefined source, e.g. a chocolate wheaten biscuit. The amount required varies from individual to individual and is also dependent on the amount and type of 'work' done and the insulin regimen.

During prolonged strenuous exercise it will be necessary to 'top up' blood sugar during the exercise period, and this is most practically achieved by using rapidly absorbed simple sugars such as a glucose drink or sweet food. It is particularly important to avoid hypoglycaemia during potentially hazardous activities such as swimming or skiing, where altered concentration or consciousness could have serious consequences. Families need to be made aware that post-exercise hypoglycaemia may occur several hours after strenuous exercise, even during the night, and extra unrefined carbohydrate should be eaten at bedtime following an active day. Families and children themselves become the experts on how much and what type of carbohydrate to have. This comes with experience after trial and error, and with frequent blood sugar monitoring.

Low sugar and diabetic products

Low calorie drinks are extremely valuable in the diet of a child with diabetes. Other low sugar products marketed for the general population can also be useful, for instance reduced-sugar jams, fruit canned in natural juice, low sugar desserts. Diabetic products, however, have no place in the diet for the child with diabetes. They are expensive, can be unpalatable and in addition may contain sorbitol. The child should be encouraged to regard the diet as one of 'sensible eating' and not one which relies on the need to eat different or 'special' foods.

Sweeteners

Sorbitol is a sweetener with a similar energy value to carbohydrate. It is poorly absorbed and can cause osmotic diarrhoea, particularly in children, who have a lower body mass than that of the adult, for whom the products are designed. Fructose has no advantage over sucrose in terms of taste as a sweetener and gives less satisfactory results in baking. Although it does not require insulin for its metabolism it has a glucose-sparing effect in the body and causes a rise in blood sugar if large quantities are taken.

Non-nutritive sweeteners can be useful in drinks and desserts and to sprinkle on breakfast cereals. However many people find that saccharin has a bitter aftertaste. Aspartame, which many find more palatable, has a limited use because sweetening power is lost when it is subjected to prolonged heating. Acesulfame K is another non-nutritive sweetener that is currently not widely used but may gain popularity in the future as it is heat resistant and without aftertaste.

RECOMMENDING AN EATING PLAN

A dietary assessment is essential on diagnosis, so that the child's normal intake and meal pattern can be ascertained. The carbohydrate or energy allowance and distribution can then be tailored to the home situation. Providing the child is not overweight, the usual energy intake prior to the onset of diabetic symptoms can be used as a basis for deciding the diet. Carbohydrate should provide 40–50% of energy, and fat should be kept as low as practical, depending on the child's age.

Recommendations for dietary management must take into consideration the child's current insulin regimen. Regimens include:

- Single dose of isophane insulin injection daily (no longer commonly used)
- Twice a day injections (one before breakfast and one before evening meal) of mixed soluble and isophane insulin or mixed insulin analogue and isophane insulin
- Multiple injection therapy – three, four or five injections per day. Soluble insulin or insulin analogue is given before breakfast, lunch (if on four/five a day) and evening meal, and isophane insulin before bed and possibly before breakfast if on analogue insulin.

Isophane/soluble and isophane mixed insulin

It is important for children to take carbohydrate at regular intervals so that hypoglycaemia may be avoided and hyperglycaemia prevented. Meals should be consumed 30 minutes after an insulin injection (unless low blood sugar dictates otherwise) in order to optimise post-prandial blood sugar profiles. Carbohydrate in excess of 50–60 g given at any one time may also produce an inappropriately raised post-prandial blood sugar. A meal pattern of three meals and three snacks each day is appropriate for most children, although very young children and adolescents may need more snacks. Carbohydrate should be distributed throughout the day taking account of the peak periods of insulin action.

Analogue and isophane mixed insulins

The above applies to these mixes, except that meals can be eaten directly after injecting.

Insulin analogue used in multiple injection therapy

There is no requirement to wait 30 minutes between injecting and eating because of analogue's fast onset of action, and most children appreciate this. The additional advantage of insulin analogue is that, because of its short period of action, snacks between meals are not always necessary. This is useful for teenagers trying to lose weight (especially girls) and those who find eating snacks a real bind.

Multiple injection therapy

This offers more flexibility with regard to mealtimes – there is no need to adhere to rigid meal and snack times as short-acting insulin is injected prior to food.
   Figure 9.1 shows commonly used insulins and their action times. Table 9.1 shows a typical day's diet with carbohydrate distributed according to insulin regimen (Fig. 9.2).

Teaching approaches

It is important to give the family practical dietary advice which is age related, and the child should be involved as soon as they become old enough. The information should be delivered at a rate which considers the social, intellectual and cultural background of the child. Verbal instructions should be reinforced with appropriate written information and other resources should be used where possible, e.g. video, web site (see further reading and information, at the end of this chapter).

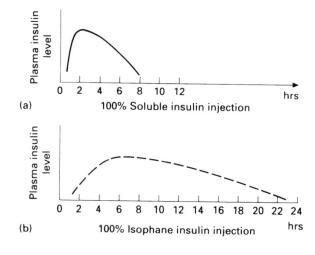

(a) 100% Soluble insulin injection

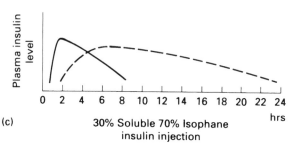

(b) 100% Isophane insulin injection

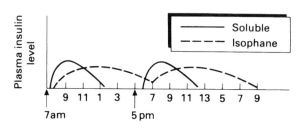

(c) 30% Soluble 70% Isophane insulin injection

Fig. 9.1 (a) 100% Soluble insulin injection
          (b) 100% Isophane insulin injection
          (c) 30% Soluble 70% isophane insulin injection

Fig. 9.2 Twice daily therapy of premixed 30% soluble 70% isophane insulin

Whether quantitative or qualitative methods should be adopted continues to be a controversial subject. Most dietitians (88%) who provide a service to children with diabetes use quantitative methods [13].

Table 9.1 A 12 year old boy is on a BD regime of premixed 30% soluble and 70% isophane insulin and has a daily allowance of 240 g of carbohydrate (see Fig. 9.2)

Insulin injection (7.00 AM)			gCHO
Breakfast (7.30 AM)	40 g	2 Weetabix	20 g
		1/3 pint semi-skimmed milk	10 g
		1/2 large slice of wholemeal toast and polyunsaturated spread	10 g
Mid morning (10.00 AM – school break time)	30 g	Apple	10 g
		1 plain biscuit	10 g
		1 small box raisins	10 g
Lunch (12.30 PM)	50 g	2 wholemeal rolls with chicken and salad	40 g
		1 carton of diet fruit yoghurt	10 g
		Low calorie drink	
Mid afternoon (2.30 PM – school break time)	20 g	Wholemeal scone and reduced sugar jam	20 g
(3.45 PM – after school)	10 g	1 packet crisps	10 g
		Low calorie drink	
Insulin injection (5.00 PM)			
Dinner (5.30 PM)	50 g	Bowl of lentil soup	10 g
		Wholemeal pasta; bolognaise sauce; side salad	30 g
		1 scoop of ice cream	10 g
		Low calorie drink	
Mid evening (7.30 PM)	20 g	1 glass semi-skimmed milk	10 g
		1 banana	10 g
Bedtime (9.00 PM)	20 g	1 large slice wholemeal toast with polyunsaturated spread	20 g
		Cup of tea	

Table 9.2 A brief list of 10 g carbohydrate exchanges

Bread		
Wholemeal or white	=	1/2 large slice/1 small slice
Rolls, baps	=	1/2 roll
Breakfast cereals		
All Bran, Branflakes	=	5 tablespoons
Cornflakes	=	5 tablespoons
Weetabix	=	1 biscuit
Porridge	=	7 tablespoons
Rice and pasta		
Brown or white rice cooked	=	3 tablespoons
Spaghetti	=	10 long strands
Pasta e.g. macaroni	=	3 tablespoons
Spaghetti – tinned	=	1/3 small tin
Biscuits		
Oatcakes	=	1 large
Crackers	=	2
Crispbread (wholewheat rye)	=	2
Digestive	=	1
Potatoes		
Boiled	=	1 small
Mashed	=	1 scoop
Baked	=	1 medium
Chips	=	5 average sized
Crisps	=	1 small packet
Beans		
Baked in tomato sauce	=	5 tablespoons
Dried uncooked	=	2 tablespoons
Fruit		
Apple	=	1
Banana	=	1
Grapes	=	10
Orange	=	1
Pear	=	1
Milk		
Semi-skimmed, whole, skimmed	=	1 glass (1/3 pint)
Natural/diet fruit yoghurt	=	1 carton
Fruit sweetened yoghurt	=	1/2 carton
Others		
Jelly	=	3 tablespoons
Soup	=	1 ladle
Ice cream	=	1 scoop

NB All tablespoon measures are level

Quantitative method

The child and his carers must have an understanding of the nutritional content of foods. At present the 10 g carbohydrate system (using handy measures) offers the best system for children, where a daily allowance of carbohydrate is given along with a suggested distribution of carbohydrate at each meal and snack time. This, however, may need revising when more is known about the glycaemic index of different foods or meals. A brief list of 10 g carbohydrate portions, or exchanges, is given in Table 9.2.

Qualitative diet

Alternative methods of dietary advice which do not involve measuring or estimating the carbohydrate value of individual foods include the 'plate model' used by the Swedish Diabetic Association [7]. In this type of diet a meal or snack of approximately equal carbohydrate is given at regular intervals; the meal as a whole is assessed by eye and no attempt is made to quantify individual foods. The exact amount of carbohydrate is less important than the type, and the diet is high in fibre, which slows the absorption of carbohydrate from the gut. This method is widely used in the treatment of adult diabetes but there is controversy over its use in childhood, particularly for very young children who may be erratic eaters and who may not accept or tolerate a high fibre diet [14]. A compromise may be to teach a measured diet initially on diagnosis, as many parents feel more secure using the 10 g exchange system, then to move onto an unmeasured diet when appropriate.

Hypoglycaemia

Causes of hypoglycaemia include:

- Exercise, without additional food or reduction in insulin dose
- Insufficient carbohydrate eaten, or being late for or missing a meal or snack
- Too much insulin/dose given at the wrong time
- Food not absorbed, e.g. vomiting and diarrhoea
- Alcohol.

Symptoms are similar to those seen in the adult and mild hypo symptoms include pallor, mood swings, irritability, headache, hunger and fatigue. Children often find it difficult to describe their own symptoms, but might experience shaky/wobbly legs or a 'funny' feeling.

If the hypo is moderate the child may be unaware of it, but confused and unco-operative. In severe hypoglycaemia the child is unconscious and may be fitting. Regular episodes of hypoglycaemia indicate that the diet and insulin are out of balance and that the whole regimen needs assessing. The possibility of surreptitious extra insulin administration should also be considered. Treatment depends on the severity of the hypoglycaemic episode.

Mild hypoglycaemia

For mild hypoglycaemia 10 g of rapidly absorbed carbohydrate should be sufficient to alleviate the symp-

toms. Examples include 3 glucose tablets, 50 ml of glucose drink like Lucozade, or 2 teaspoons of ordinary jam, honey or syrup. If the response is not adequate more can be administered after 10–15 minutes. Ordinary sweets and sweet drinks should be used with caution as a routine treatment since children may fake hypoglycaemia in order to have these 'forbidden foods'. The suggestion of doing additional blood sugar testing at the time of a suspected hypoglycaemia is often enough to act as a deterrent. If hypoglycaemia occurs just prior to a meal, then sufficient quick-acting carbohydrate should be given to alleviate symptoms and the meal or snack given soon after. If the next food is not due for an hour or more it is important to use a back-up of slower acting carbohydrate such as a digestive biscuit or piece of fruit in order to prevent blood levels dropping before the next meal.

Moderate hypoglycaemia

At the stage of moderate hypoglycaemia the child will need help to take a sugary drink or food and Hypostop can be most useful. Hypostop, which is available on prescription, is a rapidly absorbed glucose gel in a tube packaging which can be squeezed into the mouth if the child is unco-operative. This should be followed up with starchy carbohydrate once the child has recovered.

Severe hypoglycaemia

Most centres advise that parents keep an emergency supply of a GlucaGen Kit for severe hypoglycaemia. This is a glucagon injection to use at home if the child is unconscious or fitting or if they are unable to resolve hypoglycaemic symptoms.

Illness

Children often do not wish to eat during periods of illness and infection. Blood sugars are likely to be high at these times, so it is important that insulin injections are continued. A change in the insulin regimen to several doses of a rapidly acting insulin may be advised. Carbohydrate must be given to prevent the body using fat reserves as a source of fuel and producing ketones. Carbohydrate intake must not be cut to control the blood sugars. Blood sugars should be controlled by the insulin therapy.

If the usual diet is refused it is not essential to completely replace all the carbohydrate. A realistic aim is to give 70–80% of the normal intake. Small frequent doses of rapidly absorbed carbohydrate, preferably as a liquid, are often best tolerated. For example, if the usual diet provides 180g carbohydrate, distributed 40.20.40.20.40.20, then the aim would be to provide 35–40g carbohydrate as hourly drinks between the usual breakfast and lunch times, 45–50g between the usual lunch and evening meal and 50–55g during the evening and night. Low calorie/sugar-free drinks should be encouraged to prevent dehydration. During recovery the child should return gradually to foods normally eaten.

DIET THROUGHOUT CHILDHOOD

Regular and continued dietetic input is essential in order that the dietary advice is appropriate for the child's continuing and changing needs.

Babies

Adequate nutrition to promote growth is of major importance during the early months of life. Infants with diabetes should have their carbohydrate allowance based on requirement for milk feeds, which are the principal source of nutrition. The feeding pattern of infants is one of frequent and regular feeds and this is ideal for the diabetic regimen. If at the time of diagnosis the infant is breast fed the mother should be encouraged to continue. However, many mothers are anxious about hypoglycaemia if they are uncertain of the amount being consumed at each feed and will need reassurance. Whether breast or bottle fed, a baby's fluid requirement is 150–200 ml per kg per day; 150 ml breast or infant formula contains approximately 10 g carbohydrate. Providing growth and development is normal, the daily carbohydrate intake can be based on the baby's usual feeding pattern with the insulin dose adjusted accordingly. As with all infants, breast milk or infant formula should be the milk of choice until the child is 12 months old.

Weaning

Weaning can start at the usual time at around 4–6 months of age. Non-carbohydrate foods may be used initially (e.g. 1–2 teaspoons puréed vegetables) as these will not alter the carbohydrate intake. This allows the baby to become accustomed to the different taste and texture of solids without any anxiety being generated by food refusal. Once the baby has become familiar with spoon-feeding and the amount taken increased to 1–2 tablespoons, carbohydrate exchanges may be introduced. At first, 5 g carbohydrate exchanges are useful when only small quantities of food are being taken (e.g. half a rusk, 25 g potato, 5 g baby rice). The amount of mixed feeding will gradually increase and by the time the baby is 1 year old he will probably be having about 90 g carbohydrate as solids, the remainder of his carbohydrate intake coming from milk. Water and dilute low sugar squashes can be given as an additional drink.

Weaning is an anxious time for any parent and this anxiety is heightened if a dietary modification has to be observed. Tension about food must be relieved as a baby may refuse solids completely if his mother is fussing or worrying.

The Department of Health recommendations for vitamin supplements for infants and young children [15] also apply to the child with diabetes. The first year of life is the period of most rapid growth. Dietary intake is constantly changing due to the child's progression through normal feeding and developmental milestones. It is essential that the dietitian is in frequent contact with the family to offer advice.

Hypoglycaemia is a real fear for parents and can be hard to recognise in babies. It may only be noted when parents are routinely checking blood sugars. Advice should be given on how to recognise and treat symptoms. Extra milk, with or without additional sugar, or Super Soluble Maxijul, Ribena or sweetened fruit juice may be used. Usually 10g carbohydrate given as 150 ml baby milk or 75 ml baby milk plus one teaspoon of Maxijul is sufficient to treat hypoglycaemia. It may be necessary to introduce a cereal-based weaning food (e.g. baby rice) earlier than 3 months of age if there is a problem with regular hypoglycaemia. Nocturnal hypoglycaemia is a concern of parents, and milk and a cereal can be given before the baby settles for the night if he is no longer having night feeds and blood sugars are dropping overnight.

Toddlers

After 1 year of age the child can drink cow's milk and from 2 years semi-skimmed milk can be introduced as long as the child is taking a nutritionally adequate diet. Fully skimmed milk, however, contains too little fat (and hence energy) for the under fives and is not usually recommended. The introduction of skimmed milk over the age of five is a useful way to reduce the overall fat content of the diet. There is little fibre in the diets of children in their first year of life, but this can gradually increase from weaning. Some forms of fibre, such as Weetabix, raisins, bananas and baked beans, are popular with children; vegetable fibre and wholemeal bread need to be encouraged.

Small children do not understand the importance of their diet, so parents and health professionals must be flexible and compromise as much as is practical. Food strikes are common in children between 2 and 4 years of age. Rigid meals and snacks often do not work and well presented finger foods can be offered throughout the day. Most families manage to cope with the 'food refusal syndrome' without being manipulated, but the toddler with diabetes poses a real problem: with hypoglycaemia always a possibility, food refusal can become a powerful weapon. Parents are torn between maintaining good glycaemic control with the accompanying risk of hypoglycaemia, and allowing the blood sugars to be a little raised. Advice should be given not to force feed, nor to offer numerous alternatives, and to avoid fuss around mealtimes. Simply rely on the child's falling blood sugar to cause hunger and a desire to eat. In a small minority of cases toddlers' food refusal can be a persistent and unremitting problem causing parents enormous worry about hypoglycaemia. One practical solution is to allow the child to eat meals with no fuss and when the meal is over to give an appropriate dose of insulin analogue to cover the amount of food consumed.

In addition to food strikes, some young children with diabetes complain of incessant hunger. This may occur if control is poor and sugar is being lost in the urine or if the child is using food as a means to seek attention. Measurements of height, weight and dietary intake should be done regularly to reassure parents that adequate nutrition is being maintained.

This can prove to be a challenging stage when it is often difficult to achieve good glycaemic control and the families need plenty of support from their diabetes team.

Schoolchildren

While at school the teacher becomes one of the child's main carers and must know about the condition and in particular how to recognise and treat hypoglycaemia. The British Diabetic Association's publication, *Children with Diabetes Guidance for Teachers and School Staff*, offers a good explanation and should be given to each child's teacher. The dietitian and/or the diabetes nurse specialist may offer to visit the school to provide advice. Children with diabetes are advised to carry a hypo remedy (glucose tablets) at all times. The teacher should be equipped with glucose tablets and/or a glucose drink in case of hypoglycaemia.

Physical education teachers should be aware of the need for extra carbohydrate before exercise and to check that children are carrying extra carbohydrate during periods of prolonged exercise. School lunches can, but should not, present a problem; it is not always possible for children to go home and they may prefer to go to school lunch with their friends. Older children with a good grasp of their diet can choose their own meal and the cafeteria-style canteen allows a flexible choice of food. The organisation and provision of school meals can vary from area to area; it is not desirable for the child to have a 'special diet' away from his friends or at a different time from them. A normal main course should be suitable, with the dessert or pudding being replaced by fresh fruit or diet yoghurt. Discussion with the school cooks as well as teachers should help smooth problems. Advice can be given to parents about suitable packed lunches.

Children frequently eat sweets in the school playground and it is tempting for a child with diabetes to eat sweets also. Other less sweet snacks such as fruit, bread, low sugar cereal bars, raisins and sugar-free chewing gum should be suggested as alternatives. The best attitude is to use positive reinforcement when the child is doing well and to recommend that the best time for sweets is prior to exercise or after a main meal. If habitual bingeing is causing a problem the services of a child psychologist may be needed; bingeing suggests underlying stress.

Adolescents

Adolescence is often a period of rebellion and diabetes treatment is one more thing to rebel about. Snacking and eating out in the evening is common. Advice about alcohol and its hypoglycaemic effect will be necessary for teenagers.

Adolescent girls have a tendency to become obese and appropriate advice is needed. Occasionally weight control can be achieved by simply cutting out crisps and fried foods and exercising. The amount of carbohydrate in the diet should only be reduced after very careful examination of the diet as a whole, as this may cause an increase in consumption of fat and protein. In order to get the message across, it is useful to point out the energy content of some of the carbohydrate portions, e.g. one packet of crisps provides 10 g carbohydrate and 150 kcal; one apple also contains 10 g carbohydrate but only 50 kcal. Teenagers soon become aware of the fact that poor control can result in weight loss. A number will omit insulin as a method of weight control. The benefits of weight loss achieved by healthy lifestyle (eating and exercise) should be reinforced and the risks associated with poor control outlined.

Some teenagers, both male and female, can have a distorted view of their weight. Eating disorders can present just as in the non-diabetic population, such as bingeing, anorexia nervosa and bulimia. Diabetes may increase the risks of eating disorders as there is a greater focus on food, on weight (weighing people at each clinic visit, rapid weight gain with insulin) and a fear of hypoglycaemia often coupled with low self-esteem. Young adults suffering from an eating disorder need careful monitoring and intervention by the diabetes team and the psychiatrist/psychologist.

Parties and eating out

Parties are highlights in a child's life and advice is required to ensure that children with diabetes can enjoy the party as much as everyone else. They can eat most of the party fare and it is important to ensure that sufficient carbohydrate is eaten to compensate for extra activity and excitement. The host can help by providing low calorie drinks for everyone.

Many of the fast food eating places publish the carbohydrate content of their foods. Children should be educated about their diet as soon as possible so that they are able to manage it independently, with support from parents as necessary. All children are different, but most children from the age of about eight should be actively encouraged to have a full understanding of their diet. Parents may need encouragement gradually to hand over responsibility of treatment to the child.

Travel

Travel should pose no problems with a little extra planning. Carbohydrate foods, i.e. sandwiches, fruit or biscuits, should be carried to cover inevitable delays, as should a hypo remedy. Activity holidays will mean that more food is required and possibly a reduction in the insulin dose too to prevent hypoglycaemia. When travelling abroad advice should be given on how to avoid food poisoning and as always the children should wear some form of identification, e.g. SOS Talisman or Medicalert.

Parents may feel isolated and need much support and reassurance from the diabetes team. The British Diabetic Association has a role to play by producing useful publications and updates about food, and organising children's holiday camps and parent-child weekends. A local parents' group allows families in a similar situation to meet. Youngsters with diabetes should have an optimal quality of life in which a suitably tailored eating plan is an essential part.

The dietitian has a unique role to play in the management of childhood diabetes, and nutritional assessment and support must be an integral part of initial and continuing education programmes. Compliance is rarely ideal but this does not detract from the importance of balanced nutrition in this serious chronic disease.

REFERENCES

1 Patterson CC *et al.* Geographical variation in the incidence of diabetes mellitus in Scottish children during the period 1977–1983. *Diabetic Medicine*, 1988, **5** 160–65.
2 St Vincent Joint Task Force for Diabetes. *The Report.* Department of Health/British Diabetic Association, 1995, **4.04** 10–11.
3 The Diabetes Control and Complications Trial Research Group The effect of intensive treatment of diabetes on the development and progression of long–term complications in insulin-dependent diabetes mellitus. *N England J Med*, 1993, **329** 977–86.
4 Jackson R Growth and maturation of children with insulin dependent diabetes. *Pediatric Clinics N Am*, 1984, **31** 545–67.
5 Report of the Nutrition Sub-committee of the Medical Advisory Committee of the British Diabetic Association. Dietary Recommendations for diabetics for the 1980s. *Hum Nutr: Appl Nutr*, 1982, **36A** 378–94.
6 Nutrition Subcommittee of the British Diabetic Association's Professional Advisory Committee. Dietary recommendations for people with diabetes: an update for the 1990s. *Diabetic Medicine*, 1992, **9** 189–202.
7 Nutrition Subcommittee of the Professional Advisory Committee of the British Diabetic Association. Dietary recommendations for children and adolescents with diabetes. *Diabetic Medicine*, 1989, **6** 537–47.

8 Department of Health Report on Health and Social Subjects No 41. *Dietary Reference Values for Food Energy and Nutrients for the United Kingdom*. London: The Stationery Office, 1991.

9 Karlstrom B *et al*. Effect of four meals with different kinds of dietary fibre on glucose metabolism in healthy subjects and non-insulin diabetic patients. *Europ J Clin Nutr*, 1988, **42** 519–26.

10 Vinik A, Jenkins DJA Dietary fibre in the management of diabetes. *Diabetic Care*, 1988, **11** 160–73.

11 Mann J What carbohydrate foods should diabetics eat? *Brit Med J*, 1984, **288** 1025–6.

12 Slama G, Haardt M, Joseph P *et al*. Sucrose taken during mixed meal has no additional hyperglycaemic action over isocaloric amounts of starch in well controlled diabetics. *Lancet*, 1984, 12 July 122–4.

13 Waldron S, Swift P, Raymond N, Botha J A survey of the dietary management of children's diabetes. *Diabetes Medicine*, 1997, **14** 698–702.

14 Taitz LS, Wardley BL *Handbook of Child Nutrition*. Oxford: Oxford University Press, 1990.

15 Department of Health and Social Security Report on Health and Social Subjects No 32. *Present Day Practice in Infant Feeding, Third Report*. London: The Stationery Office, 1988.

FURTHER READING/INFORMATION

Best Ideas for Diabetes – Dietary Information. Alison Johnston. Available from Diabetes Service, Royal Hospital for Sick Children, Glasgow G3 8SJ, and on website http://www.childdiabetes-scotland.org

Childhood diabetes website http://www.childdiabetes-scotland.org

Infant diabetes (age 0–4) video, Childhood diabetes (age 5–11) video, Teenage diabetes video, available from Royal Hospital for Sick Children, Glasgow G3 8SJ.

A Guide to Life. Leaflets formatted to fit in a CD cover written by Yorkhill Diabetes Team and produced by Beckton and Dickinson, Cowley, Oxford OX4 3LY.

British Diabetic Association. *Children with Diabetes Guidance for Teachers and School Staff*. 1999 London: BDA.

USEFUL ADDRESS

Diabetes UK (formerly British Diabetic Association), 10 Queen Anne Street, London W1M 0BD

CHAPTER 10

Cystic Fibrosis

Cystic fibrosis (CF) is the commonest recessively inherited genetic disease in Caucasian populations. It has an incidence of 1 in 2415 live births in the UK [1] and 1 in 25 of the population are carriers [2]. The incidence in non-Caucasians is lower, with estimates around 1 in 20000 in black populations and 1 in 100000 in Oriental populations [3]. It is almost unknown in Japan, China and black Africa [4].

There is widespread dysfunction of exocrine glands with disturbances of ion and fluid movement resulting in abnormally thick and dehydrated secretions. This leads to multiorgan obstructive lesions including:

- Chronic obstructive lung disease with predominant airway obstruction and recurrent, persistent infections
- Exocrine pancreatic insufficiency with steatorrhoea
- Intestinal obstruction in neonates and older patients
- Infertility, especially in males
- Abnormally high levels of sodium chloride sweat, resulting from the failure of salt reabsorption in sweat gland ducts [5].

Gastrointestinal involvement is present in 85–95% of all cases and hepatobiliary complications in 5–15% [6] (Table 10.1). Most patients develop initial symptoms before the age of 2 years.

In 1989, the gene responsible for CF was localised to the long arm of chromosome 7 [7]. This gene encodes a protein called the CF transmembrane conductance regulator (CFTR). Its main role is as a cAMP regulated channel controlling secretions in sweat glands, respiratory, gastrointestinal and reproductive tracts [8]. More than 800 mutations of the gene have been identified and they are categorised into five classes on the basis of CFTR alterations [9]. The most predominant mutation, which accounts for approximately 70% of all the CFTR genes worldwide, is F508, but there is geographical variation and it is less common in non-white races.

The life expectancy of those with CF has increased in many countries, probably as the result of increased availability of medication, overall rigorous care with the development of specialist treatment centres, and diagnosis of the milder forms of the disease [10]. Where previously this disease was considered lethal in childhood, the median survival for newborns in the 1990s is predicted to be 40 years of age [11]. Survival is largely dependent on the severity and progression of lung disease and more than 90% of the mortality is due to chronic bronchial infections and their complications [2]. Patients with pancreatic insufficiency have a worse prognosis in terms of growth, pulmonary function and long term survival. The mortality of females is generally greater than that of males [1, 12]. As early as 1979 [13], an accelerated deterioration rate in pulmonary function was reported in females. This correlated with weight centiles and poorer survival. Even social class has been shown to be an important determinant of life expectancy in CF [14].

CLINICAL FEATURES

Most patients present with symptoms before the age of 2 years, but occasionally if the disease is mild it may be undiagnosed for many years.

Chronic respiratory disease

The lungs are normal at birth, but may become affected within a few weeks of life. Due to the

Table 10.1 Clinical features of CF

Intestine	Abdominal pain
	Rectal prolapse
	Distal intestinal obstruction syndrome
	Steatorrhoea/diarrhoea
	Abdominal distention
	Failure to thrive/growth failure
	Intussusception
	Gastrointestinal reflux
	Colonic strictures
	Digestive cancer
Pancreas	Pancreatic failure
	Pancreatitis
	Glucose intolerance
	Diabetes mellitus
Liver	Hepatomegaly
	Cirrhosis
	Portal hypertension
Gall bladder	Cholecystitis
	Cholelithiasis
	Obstructive jaundice
Lungs	Repeated respiratory infections
	Asthma/wheezing
	Nasal polyps
	Bronchiectasis
	Hyperinflation
	Clubbing of fingers
	Haemoptysis
	Pneumothorax
	Cor pulmonale
	Aspergillosis
	Sinusitis
Other	Growth failure/failure to thrive/weight loss
	Delayed puberty
	Salt depletion
	Male sterility
	Arthritis
	Fat-soluble vitamin deficiency
	Psychological (child and family)

abnormal secretions and resulting mucus there is obstruction in the small airways, with secondary infection which is progressive and destructive. Common cultured organisms from the lung are *Staphylococcus aureus*, *Haemophilus influenzae* and subsequently *Pseudomonas* species. This leads to damage of the bronchial wall, bronchiectasis and abscess formation [15]. The child has a persistent, loose cough productive of purulent sputum. On examination there is hyperinflation of the chest due to air trapping, coarse crepitations, or respiratory rhonchi.

A major objective of respiratory management is to control infection and remove thickened bronchial secretions, thereby maintaining respiratory function and delaying rate of lung damage. This is achieved by:

- Antibiotic therapy administered either intermittently, continuously or by aerosol
- Regular chest physiotherapy
- Use of bronchodilators, other anti-asthma treatment and oral steroids.

Frequent follow-up and routine bacterial surveillance are essential. General measures including avoidance of tobacco smoke, viral and other infections are important.

Gastrointestinal symptoms

Pancreatic insufficiency

This is the most common gastrointestinal defect in CF. It develops when more than 90% of acinar function is gone. Damage begins *in utero* with ongoing destruction and eventual replacement of the acini with fibrous tissue and fat [16]. As a result of pancreatic damage, the secretion of digestive enzymes and bicarbonate is disrupted, resulting in malabsorption of fat, protein, nitrogen, bile, fat-soluble vitamins and vitamin B_{12}.

It is estimated that up to 90% of CF patients have pancreatic insufficiency. In the other 10% of patients, although enzyme secretions are diminished, it is still adequate for digestion and absorption of nutrients without the necessity for pancreatic enzyme supplementation [17]. Pancreatic sufficiency is genetically determined by one or two mild CFTR mutations.

Meconium ileus

Meconium ileus can occur in up to 15% of infants with CF seen *in utero* with polyhydramnios, or within 48 hours of birth as abdominal obstruction [18]. This is caused by the blockage of the terminal ileum by highly proteinaceous meconium. 'Meconium ileus equivalent' or 'distal intestinal obstruction syndrome' (DIOS) may occur in childhood or adult life.

Abdominal pain

Abdominal pain has been reported in up to 11% of CF patients [19]. It is particularly common in children with poorly controlled malabsorption, but may be due to many other disorders, which may or may not be related to CF including intussusception, appendicitis, constipation and Crohn's disease.

Gastro-oesophageal reflux (GOR)

Gastro-oesophageal reflux has been frequently reported in CF and it has been estimated that as many as one in five newly diagnosed infants with CF have pathological GOR [20]. Although the mechanism of GOR in CF is unclear, there is evidence that it is mainly due to inappropriate relaxation of the gastro-oesophageal sphincter [21]. Postural drainage chest physiotherapy increases the risk of GOR [22]. GOR is more prevalent in young CF children, but improves with increasing age. It may adversely affect lung disease by aspiration and reflex bronchospasm [23].

Colonic strictures (fibrosing colonopathy)

The development of fibrotic strictures and ulceration of the ascending colon in some children with CF is known as fibrosing colonopathy. It is an irreversible lesion that usually requires surgery (frequently ileostomy and colectomy) for control. It was first reported in 1994 [24]. The pathogenesis of this disorder is unknown, but there is an association with high-dose enteric coated pancreatic enzyme supplements [25] or pancreatic enzyme coating [26].

Other gastrointestinal problems

Other problems include rectal prolapse, acute pancreatitis, duodenal ulcer, coeliac disease, Crohn's disease and cow's milk protein enteropathy. There is also evidence that the risk of digestive cancer is significantly elevated and incidence will increase with increased longevity [27].

Effect on growth

Chronic malnutrition with significant weight retardation and linear growth failure have long been recognised as a general problem among most CF populations. Patients have poor height and delayed puberty, and the eventual weight size of those surviving to adulthood is commonly below average [28]. Bone age and onset of menarche may be delayed [6, 29] and pubertal delay can occur despite good clinical state [6]. Nutritional impairment is noted at birth, with CF infants having an average birth weight of about 0.5 standard deviations (SD) lower than that of the normal populations [30]. Head circumference has also been shown to be 1.0 SD below normal at 4 years of age [31].

Reported growth patterns are similar. In a cross-sectional study of UK CF clinics, the mean body weight in boys is between −0.25 and −0.5 SD until the age of 10 years, and in girls approximates −0.5 SD below the population mean during the same period with body mass index (BMI) decreasing from the age of 5 years. Post-pubertal stature and weight maintenance in the CF population shows substantial deficits [32]. In children 5 years and under, no differences have been noted between screened and non-screened patients [33].

In a further cross-sectional survey of 223 patients attending a CF centre in Denmark, BMI was approximately 98% of normal in the younger patients, but declined to 90% in adult men and 83% in adult women with CF. All patients had a normal height, although the final height was achieved a little later than healthy controls [12]. In the US, the heights and weights of 13 116 children with CF aged from 0 to 18 years were reported; children had subnormal growth at all ages. Mean and median height and weight for age were found to be at the 30th and 20th percentiles in children with CF. Malnutrition (height or weight for age <5th percentile) was particularly pronounced in infants (47%) and adolescents (37%) and patients with newly diagnosed CF (47%) [34]. Comparison of growth data between Canada and the US demonstrated suboptimal growth in both countries, although Canadian patients had better weight and height scores [35].

Growth hormone has been used to improve growth in small groups of patients with CF with some success [5, 36].

Other clinical problems

Diabetes mellitus

Prevalence and incidence of diabetes mellitus (DM) in CF patients is high, varies according to CF genotype and increases with age. Using the World Health Organisation (WHO) criteria for the diagnosis of DM [37], the prevalence of impaired glucose tolerance and diabetes mellitus range from 14 to 36% and 5 to 24% respectively in three European centres [38, 39, 40]. The prevalence of DM in CF patients aged 10, 20 and 30 years is reported to be 1.5%, 13%, and 50% [41].

The diabetes is non-ketotic, has a slow onset [42], but is usually insulin dependent. An insidious decline in overall clinical status often occurs before diagnosis of diabetes is made [43]. The reason for the development of the DM in CF is not fully understood, but there is thought to be insulin deficiency as well as relative insulin resistance. Although the DM is considered mild, the frequency of serious secondary complications, e.g. microangiopathy and nephropathy is increasing [44, 45, 46]. Careful control of diabetes is important; identifying patients who are at risk is desirable and it is recommended that annual screening with oral glucose tolerance tests be carried out in all CF patients over the age of 10 years [47].

Liver disease

The prevalence of liver disease among CF patients ranges between 9% and 37%, depending on the definition of liver disease [48] and peaks during adolescence [49]. There is some evidence that it may occur more commonly in patients with pancreatic insufficiency [50]. Children with CF exhibit a spectrum of liver abnormalities, with intermittent rises in serum transaminases a common early finding. Abnormalities range from hepatic steatosis to focal biliary cirrhosis and eventually multilobular cirrhosis with portal hypertension. Variceal bleeding may occur. Clinical signs of cirrhosis occur late even when the disease is advanced. Patients are also at increased risk of developing gallstones with complications of cholecystitis, cholangitis, pancreatitis or complete obstruction of the biliary tree [49]. There is a 3.4% mortality rate from liver complications [51]. Liver transplantation has been successful in patients with advanced liver disease [52]. Prompt recognition of liver disease is important as there is evidence that ursodeoxycholic acid, a bile acid found in very low concentrations in humans, may prevent progression of CF-related liver disease [53], but long term benefit has still to be determined.

DIAGNOSIS

The sweat test remains the most reliable diagnostic laboratory test [54]. Sweat sodium, chloride and potassium concentrations are all raised but measurement of potassium is less reliable. When performed correctly, sweat testing has a low false-negative rate of less than 2%. If possible, it should be done in combination with DNA analysis [55].

Neonatal screening for CF has been implemented in some areas for 25 years [56]. Its benefits remain controversial and it is not routinely performed throughout the UK. Immunoreactive trypsin (IRT) is 2–5 times higher in neonates with CF and is measured from dried blood spots on Guthrie cards in the UK. It has a poor sensitivity and it should be used in combination with DNA analysis and sweat testing [15].

NUTRITIONAL MANAGEMENT

A variety of complex organic and psychological factors contribute to malnutrition in CF and will vary considerably between patients depending on their disease expression, clinical state, age and sex. Malnutrition has several adverse effects including poor growth, impaired muscle function [57], decreased exercise tolerance, increased susceptibility to infection and decreased ventilatory drive. Studies indicate that BMI strongly correlates with lung function [58], but the exact mechanism of this relationship has not been fully determined. Achieving optimum nutrition and growth may minimise the progressive decline in pulmonary function commonly seen in CF. Corey *et al.* [3] in a comparative study between patients in Toronto and Boston concluded that the longer survival of the patients in Toronto was due mainly to the aggressive nutritional support given in this centre. Good survival figures have also been reported in other CF centres with aggressive nutritional support programmes [12].

Causes of malnutrition

The nutritional problems in CF are determined by three factors: energy losses, increased energy expenditure and low energy intake.

Energy losses

Malabsorption Because pancreatic exocrine secretions contain less enzymes and bicarbonate, have a lower pH and are of a smaller volume, the physical properties of proteins and mucus within the lumen are affected. This results in obstruction to the small ducts and secondary damage to pancreatic digestive enzyme secretions causing malabsorption. Other problems such as gastric hypersecretion, reduced duodenal bicarbonate concentration and pH, disorders of bile salt metabolism, disordered intestinal motility and permeability, liver disease, and short bowel syndrome after intestinal resection in the neonatal period, may all contribute to malabsorption. The severity of malabsorption is variable; there can be significant malabsorption of protein and fat-soluble vitamins despite adequate use of enzyme supplements. Murphy *et al.* [59] have estimated that stool energy losses account for 11% of gross energy intake in CF patients, three times higher than normal.

Other losses Energy may be lost due to vomiting following coughing, physiotherapy or GOR. Diabetes mellitus if undiagnosed or poorly controlled may increase energy losses due to glycosuria. Further substantial nutrient losses may occur in the sputum. Nitrogen losses in the sputum can reach 10 g per day during severe acute pulmonary exacerbation, especially from *Pseudomonas aeruginosa* [60]. Sputum is particularly rich in amino acids [61].

Increased energy expenditure

Resting energy expenditure (REE), an estimate of basal metabolic rate, is 10–20% greater than in healthy controls and may contribute to energy imbalance [62, 63]. Increased REE appears to be closely associated with declining pulmonary function [62, 64] and subclinical infection [63]. Bronchial sepsis leads to local release of leukotrienes, free oxygen radicals and cytokines including tumour necrosis factor alpha (TNFα) [65]. Antibiotics have been shown to reduce energy requirements of moderately ill patients with chronic *Pseudomonas aeruginosa* [66].

Abnormal pulmonary mechanics may increase REE. Continuous injury to the lungs leads to progressive parenchymal fibrosis and airway obstruction with probable increased oxygen cost and work of breathing [65]. Even long term bronchodilator therapy with drugs such as salbutamol [67] and feeding has been shown to increase REE.

Controversy remains over the effect of genotype on REE. Patients homozygous for the mutation delta F508 have been found to have a higher REE than those with other genotypes [68], whereas more recent studies have shown no genotype-dependent differences in REE in asymptomatic or pre-symptomatic CF infants, children and adults when confounding variables such as body composition, lung function and nutritional status are taken into account [64, 69, 70].

Data is also conflicting on total energy expenditure [69, 71] with evidence that patients with moderate lung impairment adapt to an increased REE by reducing their activity levels, thereby maintaining total energy expenditure levels with controls [69].

Low energy intake

Although dietary assessments in CF children demonstrate that energy intake is greater than controls, it rarely exceeds 111% of requirements and growth and weight gain is suboptimal [72, 73, 74, 75] (Table 10.2). Healthy controls tend to under-report their dietary intake whereas CF patients often overestimate theirs to be in agreement with the nutritional advice they are usually receiving [60].

Factors associated with a reduced appetite include:

- Chronic respiratory infection and other complications of CF such as DIOS, abdominal pain, GOR resulting in oesophagitis, pain and vomiting
- Behaviour feeding problems in pre-school and school age children
- Media pressure to eat a healthy low fat, low sugar diet
- Inappropriate concepts regarding body image
- Depression
- Eating disorders in teenagers
- Poor use of dietary supplements
- Dislike of high energy foods
- Poverty.

Behaviour feeding difficulties and poor child–parent interactions at mealtimes are a particular problem and have received much attention. Mealtimes are the most frequently reported area of difficulty for parents of pre-school children. Abnormal eating behaviours in toddlers and school children include excessively long

Table 10.2 Energy intake and growth of CF patients

	Stark et al. 1995 [74]		Kawchak et al. 1996 [72]				Stark et al. 1998	Anthony et al. 1998 [73]
		Year 0	Year 1	Year 2	Year 3			
Age y	2–5	7.8	8.9	9.8	10.7	6–13	7–12	
No. of children with CF	32	24	18	23	16	28	25	
Controls	Healthy peers	Healthy peers	Healthy peers	Healthy peers	Healthy peers	Healthy peers	Healthy siblings	
Energy % RDA: CF	95%	107%	100%	101%	128%	100%	107%	
Controls	84%	94%	93%	90%	86%	95%	92%	
Ht Z score: CF		−0.3	−0.3	−0.4	−0.797	−0.33	−0.4	
Controls		0.1	0.4	0.3	0.371	0.48	0.3	
Wt Z score: CF		−0.3	−0.3	−0.4	−0.811	−0.25	−0.4	
Controls		0	0	−0.1	−0.528	0.36	−0.2	

RDA = recommended daily allowance

meals, delay tactics, food refusal and spitting out food [75, 76]. Toddlers with more feeding difficulties have lower energy intakes [76].

Aims of nutritional management

There are three main aims of nutritional management:

- To achieve optimal nutritional status
- To achieve normal growth and development
- To maintain normal feeding behaviour.

Energy

Crude estimates have suggested that patients may require 120–150% of the recommended daily allowance or estimated average requirement (EAR) for age and sex. More specific recommendations for energy intake taking into account REE, physical activity and disease severity have been published by a North American Consensus Committee but still have to be validated [77]. Reilly *et al.* [78] tested the accuracy of both these methods; errors in estimation of energy requirements for individuals were large.

The heterogeneity of these patients, including presence of respiratory infection, activity and nutritional status, make it difficult to give universal recommendations for energy requirements. Each individual's energy requirements will vary depending on clinical condition and activity levels. The only practical method to gauge adequate nutrition is by closely monitoring weight gain and growth. Some children will grow normally by consuming no more than the EAR for energy, whereas those with advanced pulmonary disease may need 50–60% more energy than normal. A useful guideline to follow is to assess the existing energy intake and increase this value by a further 20–30% if weight gain or growth is poor.

Protein

Exact protein requirements are unclear; it is generally accepted that the protein intake should be increased to compensate for excessive loss of nitrogen in the faeces and sputum and increased protein turnover in malnourished patients [79]. Protein should provide 15% of the total energy intake. In practice, the vast majority of CF patients have no difficulty in achieving this level of intake.

Fat

Fat is the most concentrated source of energy in the diet and the only source of essential fatty acids. It is now widely accepted that fat should be encouraged liberally and should provide 35–40% of the total energy intake. Some clinics have developed novel techniques to improve fat intake, including setting targets for daily fat intake [80]. Perhaps with the exception of severe liver disease, medium chain triglyceride (MCT) replacement of dietary fat has little role in CF. Theoretically with MCT oil, there is less dependence on intraluminal mechanisms of digestion. However, MCT oil has not been shown to improve growth, may result in essential fatty acid deficiency and may indirectly increase energy requirements as it requires more oxygen than carbohydrate to be oxidised in the liver. There is some parental concern about the effects of a high fat diet on blood lipid levels but in studies on adults with pancreatic insufficiency total cholesterol and lipid levels are normal to low [81].

Carbohydrate

A high carbohydrate intake should be encouraged to provide 45–50% of the total energy intake. Carbohydrates are well tolerated as pancreatic amylase deficiency is compensated for by salivary amylase and, to a lesser degree, intestinal glucoamylase [60]. However, antibiotics can reduce the ability of colonic flora to ferment carbohydrate and lead to a less salvageable energy. Starchy foods such as bread, potatoes and pasta as well as simple sugars should be encouraged, the latter providing a valuable energy source. Disaccharide intolerance may be a problem following surgery for meconium ileus.

Fibre

The traditional high fat, high sugar diet for children with CF is low in dietary fibre. Reports of fibre intake confirm this and there is evidence that children with low intakes of fibre suffer from more abdominal pain and take higher doses of pancreatic enzymes [82]. It is possible that lack of fibre may compromise colonic function, causing stasis of substrate, constipation and abdominal pain. Furthermore, fatty acids, derived from unabsorbed fibre, provide the colon with its major source of nutrition [25]. A malnourished colon may be at greater risk of developing complications such as DIOS and fibrosing colonopathy. Further work is needed on the role of fibre in CF.

NUTRITIONAL SUPPORT

Three levels of nutritional support are provided in cystic fibrosis:

- A high energy/high protein diet
- Dietary supplements
- Enteral feeding.

High energy/high protein diet

Energy intake from ordinary foods should be maximised. A good variety of energy rich foods should be encouraged, such as full cream milk, cheese, meat, full cream yoghurt, milk puddings, cakes and biscuits. Extra butter or margarine can be added to bread, potatoes and vegetables. Frying foods or basting in oil will increase energy density. Extra milk or cream can be added to soups, cereal, desserts or mashed potatoes and used to top tinned or fresh fruit. Regular snacks are important. Malnourished children achieve higher energy intake when more frequent meals are offered [83]. However, it is necessary that parents establish a good routine for meals and snacks and do not permit children to substitute sweets and chocolate for savoury food at mealtime.

Although this advice is simple, dietetic input should be intensive and dietary goals must be achievable and agreed in consultation with the child and parents at each clinic visit. Attention should be given to psychological, social, behavioural and developmental aspects of feeding. A meta-analysis of differing treatment interventions to promote weight gain in CF demonstrated that a behavioural approach was just as effective in promoting weight gain as invasive medical procedures [84].

Parents are encouraged to adopt normal feeding routines, limit meal times to a maximum of 30 minutes, develop consistent feeding strategies and above all, remain positive if food is refused. If simple dietary advice and reassurance fails, enlisting the help of a psychologist with an interest in feeding problems is invaluable.

Dietary supplements

Dietary supplements are useful and should be given if there is:

- Weight loss
- Decline in height or weight z score (providing weight z score is no more than 1 SD above height)
- Nutrient intake below dietary reference values
- Acute chest infection.

There is surprisingly little data to support efficacy of dietary supplements in CF. However, any benefit appears to directly relate to acceptability and patient compliance.

Rettammel *et al.* [85] studied a supplement designed for patients with CF that contained energy, fat, linoleic acid and fat soluble vitamins. Mean adherence to the supplement was 69% (range 26–100%). Those who consistently took the supplement had an increased total energy intake, indicating that the supplement did not replace food intake. They also gained weight. However, weight and mean energy intake for the groups as a whole was unchanged before and after the intervention. In contrast, in a study on an energy-protein powder supplement (Scandishake), compliance was good and mean energy intake and weight gain improved in a group of 26 children and adults with CF [86].

Guidelines for using dietary supplements in CF

The following is a useful guide:

1–3 years – 200 kcal (840 kJ)
4–5 years – 400 kcal (1680 kJ)
6–11 years – 600 kcal (2520 kJ)
over 12 years – 800 kcal (3360 kJ)

- Dietary supplements should be given two to three times daily after meals or at bedtime.
- No more than 20% of the EAR should be given as dietary supplements except during an acute infection or if the patient is being considered for enteral feeding. Excessive supplementation will impair appetite and decrease nutrient intake from normal foods.
- Dietary supplements should not be used to replace food at mealtimes; they are best accepted if served cold.
- Parents or children should be encouraged to prepare their own home-made milk shakes.
- Care should be used when using high protein supplements (>6.0 g protein/100 ml) in children under 5 years. The nutrient profile of these products is not designed for young children.
- Pancreatic enzyme supplements are needed with milk shake supplements.

Suitable dietary supplements for children with CF are given in Table 10.3.

Table 10.3 Useful dietary supplements in CF, suitable for 1–16 years

	Energy kcal	Energy kJ	Protein g	Fibre g
Fortified milk shakes (per 100 ml)				
Paediasure	101	424	2.5	—
Paediasure with fibre	100	420	2.5	0.5
Fresubin	100	420	2.5	—
Clinutren 1.5	150	630	5.6	—
Clinutren ISO	100	420	3.8	—
Complan	108	454	3.8	—
Fortisip	150	630	5.0	—
Resource Shake	170	714	5.1	—
Fortified juice drinks (per 100 ml)				
Enlive	125	525	4.0	—
Fortijuce	125	525	4.0	—
Provide Xtra	125	525	3.75	—
Fortified semi-solid supplements (per 100 g)				
Formance	176	739	4.8	—
Glucose polymer powders (per 100 g)				
Super soluble Maxijul	380	1596	—	—
Caloreen	400	1680	—	—
Polycal	380	1596	—	—
Vitajoule	380	1596	—	—
Glucose polymer drinks (per 100 ml)				
Liquid Polycal	247	1037	—	—
Liquid Maxijul	200	840	—	—

Enteral feeding

Approximately 5% of CF patients require enteral feeding [87]; the majority of these are teenagers reflecting the deterioration in nutritional status which occurs in adolescence. Enteral feeding should be considered if:

- Child is persistently less than 85% expected weight for height
- Child has failed to gain weight over a 3–6 month period
- Height and weight are below 2nd percentile.

Enteral feeding is associated with improvements in body fat, height, lean body mass and muscle mass, increased total body nitrogen, improved strength and development of secondary sexual characteristics. Improvement in weight precedes improvement in height [88]. If pulmonary function is poor (i.e. FEV_1 – forced expired volume in less than 1 second – less than 40% predicted) at the start of enteral feeding, there may be little improvement in nutritional status [89]. However some studies have documented stabilisation [90] or improvement in pulmonary function in CF with enteral feeding [89, 91].

To produce lasting benefit, numerous studies have demonstrated that enteral feeding should be continued long term [90, 91, 92]. However, Dalzell and co-workers demonstrated significantly greater height and weight scores in a group of 10 cystic fibrosis children 4 years after cessation of tube feeding of only 1 year duration [93].

Types of enteral feed

Many types of preparations have been used for enteral feeding in CF. These include elemental, semi-elemental and polymeric feeds. There is little published data comparing the efficacy of these feeds.

Polymeric feeds

Polymeric feeds are tolerated by most patients with CF and are the first feed of choice in most CF centres. Patients over 1 year will usually tolerate a 1.5 kcal/ml (6.3 kJ/ml) paediatric or adult (dependent on age or weight) standard feed. They have several advantages: they are cheap, prescribable (Advisory Committee on Borderline Substances (ACBS)), have a low osmolality and are available in ready-to-hang packs. No difference in fat malabsorption, nitrogen absorption and weight gain has been observed when polymeric together with enzyme replacement therapy, and semi-elemental feeds, have been compared [94].

Elemental feeds

Some centres in the UK prefer to routinely use an elemental formula for enteral feeding in CF. In theory, elemental feeds have a good buffering effect on gastric acidity at night and are low in fat. Some centres do not give pancreatic enzymes with elemental feeds, but this could be disputed as they contain a mixture of long chain as well as medium chain triglyceride fats. They are expensive, have a high osmolality and a low

energy density. In adult practice it is common to supplement elemental formula with glucose polymer and a medium chain triglyceride fat emulsion, and concentrations of 2.6 kcal/ml have been tolerated [95].

High fat feeds

The role of high fat feeds in CF is uncertain. Fitting's work has suggested that low carbohydrate, high fat feeds are not necessary for nutritional support in patients with chronic obstructive lung disease [96]. However, Kane and Hobbs have demonstrated that giving the high fat feed Pulmocare resulted in lower CO_2 production (VCO_2) and respiratory quotient in CF patients with moderate to severe pulmonary disease, than did feeding with a high carbohydrate feed [97].

In addition, high carbohydrate feeds have been shown to cause hyperglycaemia in glucose-intolerant adult CF patients [98] and high fat, low carbohydrate feeds may be preferable. There is only one high fat feed available in the UK, Pulmocare. It is not ACBS prescribable.

Administration of feed

The route used for feed will be influenced by the duration of feeding and by the preference of the patient, relatives and physician. Nasogastric, gastrostomy and jejunostomy feeds have all be used in CF and each method has merits and drawbacks (Table 10.4).

Percutaneous endoscopic gastrostomy (PEG) is now probably the preferred channel in children for long term feeding. It has been made more acceptable by the development of the gastrostomy button which can replace the PEG tube after 2–3 months. Gastrostomy feeding has been shown to improve weight gain, presumably due to better compliance and less loss of feeding time due to complications [99]. Problems associated with the nasogastric route include problems of inserting the tube, particularly with nasal polyps, nasal irritation, tube displacement with coughing or vomiting and the potential risk of aspiration. Other complications include nasopharyngeal sepsis and oesophageal erosion [95].

It is common practice to give enteral feeding for 8–10 hours overnight with a 1 or 2 hour break before

Table 10.4 Problems with enteral feeding in CF

Nasogastric feeding
Nasogastric tube displacement
Gastro-oesophageal reflux
Nasal irritation
Insertion of nasogastric tube with nasal polyps

Gastrostomy feeding
Gastrostomy tube blockage
Leakage around gastrostomy site
Dislodgement of gastrostomy catheter

Gastrointestinal and tolerance
Nausea
Abdominal distention
Diarrhoea
Feed intolerance during pulmonary exacerbations
Feed aspiration
Hyperglycaemia

Growth and body image
Inhibition of oral feeding
Slow improvements in linear growth
Failure to improve body image in adolescent girls

the first physiotherapy session in the morning. Allowing teenagers to have one or two nights off the feed each week helps compliance. At least 40–50% of the EAR for energy is usually given via the tube, with weight and growth being regularly reviewed. Hyperglycaemia is a potential problem and blood glucose should be monitored when receiving enteral feeding.

It is not known how best to give pancreatic enzymes with tube feeds, and practices vary widely. There is some suggestion that it may be better to give them at the beginning of the feed and just before the patient goes to sleep [100]. Dosage of pancreatic enzymes with enteral feeds is arbitrary but can be estimated by using the amount of pancreatic enzymes required for a normal meal and adjusting the quantity in accordance with the fat composition of the feed.

VITAMIN AND MINERAL SUPPLEMENTS

Fat-soluble vitamins

Deficiencies of vitamins A, D, E and K are well documented. Biochemical deficiency is not always manifested clinically but it is reasonable to correct deficiency when demonstrated.

Vitamin A

Low serum vitamin A levels are commonly reported in CF and documented clinical features of vitamin A deficiency include night blindness, conjunctival and corneal xerosis, dry thickened skin and abnormalities of bronchial mucosal epithelialisation. Vitamin A status is difficult to assess, owing to lack of a reliable marker, and serum levels of retinol do not adequately mirror the concentration of vitamin A in the liver. Although some researchers found liver stores of vitamin A in CF to be 2.5 times higher than those in control subjects, despite lower serum levels of retinol and retinol binding protein [101], this has not been supported by other studies [102].

Vitamin E

A neuropathy due to vitamin E deficiency has been widely reported in adult CF patients. Symptoms and signs include absent deep tendon reflexes, loss of position sense and vibration sense in lower limbs, dysarthria, tremor, ataxia and decreased visual activity. Vitamin E may also be important in controlling the progression of lung disease in CF. The antioxidant function of vitamin E and the scavenger role of both vitamins A and E may protect the lungs from oxygen-radical damage during the inflammatory response to infection. Both water-miscible and fat-soluble preparations of vitamin E are effective in achieving normal serum levels [103]. In one case report ursodeoxycholic acid appears to aid absorption in the presence of liver disease and pancreatic insufficiency [104].

Vitamin D

Decreased bone mineral density and osteopenia associated with low 25-hydroxyvitamin D levels have been described in patients with CF [105, 106], but may be related to poor nutritional status [107] and delayed puberty [108]. Rickets is rarely seen. Shaw *et al.* [108] demonstrated that 16 of 24 individuals with CF, aged from 3 to 29 years, had a bone mineral density below the mean, with six individuals having values more than two standard deviations below the mean. Only four patients had evidence of suboptimal vitamin D status. In contrast, in well-nourished patients with CF, bone mineral content has been shown to be normal [109]. Although the exact factors contributing to decrease in bone mineralisation are unclear, every effort should be made to optimise nutritional status, vitamin D and calcium intake.

Vitamin K

The true prevalence of vitamin K deficiency is unknown and there is no consensus on routine vitamin K supplementation. Studies of vitamin K status in CF patients have produced conflicting and inconclusive results, but recent evidence suggests it is as high as 78% in pancreatic-insufficient patients [110]. There is now a suggestion that routine vitamin K supplementation should be considered in all patients with pancreatic insufficiency and particularly for patients with severe non-cholestatic and cholestatic liver disease, major small bowel resection and following prolonged antibiotic treatment. More studies are needed on the dosage and frequency of vitamin K supplementation in CF [110, 111].

Dosage of fat soluble vitamin supplementation

The ideal dosage of each vitamin has not been adequately established and there is considerable variation in the dosages given worldwide. Current dosages of vitamin supplementation are given in Table 10.5 [87, 112, 113]. Brands of vitamin supplements are given in Table 10.6. Regimens combine a preparation containing vitamins A and D and an additional vitamin E supplement.

Compliance with vitamin therapy in CF is poor. A new multivitamin preparation specially formulated for CF containing vitamins A, D, E and K (ADEK®) was found to improve plasma vitamin A and E concentrations in children over 10 years. However, in children 7–10 years old, vitamin E concentrations were too high [114].

Minerals

Sodium

Normally there appears to be no need to recommend additional sodium, but salt depletion can occur in hot weather through physical exercise, causing increasing sweating, and in infancy when a normal low electrolyte formula such as SMA Gold (SMA Nutrition) or Premium (Cow & Gate) is being fed. Anorexia and poor growth may result from chronic salt depletion.

Table 10.5 Dosage of vitamin supplementation commonly given in CF

Vitamin		Dose per day
A		4000–8000 iu (1500–3000 µg)
D		400–800 iu (10–20 µg)
E	Infants	50 mg
	Children	100 mg
	Teenagers	200 mg

Table 10.6 Composition of vitamin preparations used in CF

Multivitamin preparations	Standard dose	Vitamin A (iu)	Vitamin D (iu)	Vitamin E (mg)
Abidec liquid (Warner Lambert Ltd)	0.6 ml	4000	400	—
Dalivit liquid (Eastern Pharmaceuticals)	0.6 ml	50000	400	—
Multivitamins BPC capsule or tablet	1	25000	300	—
Multivitamins tablet (Unichem)	1	2600	200	—
A and D capsule	1	4000	400	
Ketovite Tablets Ketovite Liquid (Paines and Byrne)	3 5 ml	2500	400	5

Significant hyponatraemia may be accompanied by vomiting. The amount given is arbitrary, but the following guidelines may be useful:

0–1 year	2 mmol/kg sodium in the form of sodium chloride solution (1 ml = 1 mmol sodium)
1–5 years	2 × 300 mg sodium chloride tablets (10 mmol sodium)
6–10 years	2 × 600 mg sodium chloride tablets (20 mmol sodium)
11 years +	(3–4) × 600 mg sodium chloride tablets (30–40 mmol sodium).

ESSENTIAL FATTY ACID DEFICIENCY

Essential fatty acid deficiency is frequently reported in CF, but particularly in infancy before a diagnosis is made [115]. Clinical features include increased water permeability of the skin, increased susceptibility to infection, impaired wound healing [116], growth retardation [117], thrombocytopenia and reduced platelet aggregation. It is characterised by a deficiency of linoleic acid with either low or normal arachidonic acid concentrations and increased concentrations of saturates and monounsaturates (such as palmitic, palmitoleic acid and eicosatrienoic acid).

The cause of essential fatty acid deficiency is debatable and has been demonstrated in both well-nourished young cystic fibrosis patients and undernourished patients [118]. It has been linked to both underlying defects of fatty acid metabolism, low fat diets and increased metabolic usage in undernourished patients. Possible causes include increased lipid turnover in cell membranes, defects in desaturase activity, increased oxidation of fatty acids for energy source, increased production of eicosanoids, increased peroxidation of polyunsaturated fatty acids or disorders of lipoprotein metabolism. Although linoleic acid supplements have been shown to be beneficial in CF and for children with recurrent respiratory infections [119], routine supplementation is not advocated.

INFANT FEEDING IN CYSTIC FIBROSIS

Screened and non-screened infants have been shown to have nutritional problems at diagnosis. Failure to thrive, anaemia, tocopherol deficiency [120], hypoalbuminaemia [121] and even kwashiorkor [122] are seen in unscreened infants. Nutritional deficits in screened infants are more subtle, but include reduced body mass, length, total body fat, total body potassium and low levels of linoleic acid [123], serum retinol, 25-hydroxyvitamin D [124] and plasma carnitine [125]. Delayed catch-up growth following diagnosis has been seen in screened [126] and non-screened infants [127].

Energy requirements

The energy requirements depend on age and clinical and nutritional state at the time of diagnosis. There is some evidence that infants with CF have increased energy expenditure compared with normal infants of the same age [71, 128]. Most infants with pancreatic insufficiency will thrive on a normal energy intake of 100–130 kcal (420–540 kJ) per kg in conjunction with pancreatic enzymes. If weight gain is less than

expected or if a meconium ileus has resulted in surgery and bowel resection, the energy requirements may be as high as 150–200 kcal (630–836 kJ)/kg/day.

Breast milk

Breast milk in conjunction with pancreatic enzyme supplements is widely advocated for the baby with cystic fibrosis [129, 130]. Infants on breast milk and pancreatic supplements grow and gain weight appropriately with near zero z scores [131]. Breast milk has several theoretical advantages over formula:

- It contains long chain polyunsaturated fatty acids
- It provides immunological protection against infection
- It contains taurine
- It contains optimal essential amino acids
- Breast feeding is better psychologically for the mother.

There are two concerns with breast feeding:

(1) *Electrolyte depletion* Breast milk is low in sodium. It is recommended that routine sodium supplements are given to all breast fed babies with CF (p. 147). Urinary and sodium electrolytes should be checked if a breast-fed baby has poor weight gain.
(2) *Successful establishment of breast feeding* The distress and anxiety associated with the diagnosis may lead to initial difficulties in production of breast milk. However, with good advice, encouragement and patience from health professionals, these will usually be resolved.

Normal infant formulas

Infants with CF have been shown to thrive satisfactorily on normal infant whey or casein based formula and pancreatic enzymes. Normal formula milks are low in sodium and there has been one report of four infants who had a total of six episodes of electrolyte depletion between them when fed normal formula milk [132].

High energy formulas

High energy formulas (Infatrini (Nutricia); SMA High Energy (SMA Nutrition)) are necessary if there is failure of catch-up weight, weight loss or decline in weight z score. High energy formulas are preferable to giving energy supplemented normal formulas as they have a better energy/protein ratio, a more concentrated micronutrient profile and are associated with improved growth (in boys) [133].

Protein hydrolysate formulas

Although protein hydrolysate formulas are commonly favoured in the USA, no advantages have been proven for their use in the routine care of newly diagnosed infants with CF [127]. They are also less palatable, more expensive and still need pancreatic enzymes administered with them. They should only be used in CF if an infant develops temporary disaccharide intolerance after surgery for meconium ileus.

Pancreatic enzyme supplements: administration in infants

Neither pancreatic powders nor enteric-coated microsphere enzyme preparations are designed for administration with breast milk or infant formulas.

Pancreatin powders

Pancreatin powders are now rarely used. They have several disadvantages: they taste unpleasant and enzyme on the outside of the infant's lips causes local skin irritation in the infant and of the mother's nipples. Pancreatin powders should be mixed with a little expressed breast milk or infant formula and given from a spoon. If the powder is added to a bottle of formula milk it will start digesting the milk and the powder may also get stuck in the hole of the teat.

Enteric coated microsphere enzyme preparations

The enteric coated microspheres can be mixed with a little expressed breast milk or formula and then given to a baby from a spoon or given on a wetted finger, but there is a tendency for granules to become lodged in the gums or cause choking. The most practical method of administering these enzymes is to mix them with a small amount of fruit purée (which will hold the enzymes in a gel) and give them from a spoon at the beginning of each feed.

Weaning

There is no need for early weaning in CF; any time between 4–6 months is recommended. Early weaning may significantly decrease the volume of breast milk or infant formula taken so there is little benefit in this practice. Parents are encouraged to introduce home-cooked or commercial weaning foods in the normal way. If the dried commercial baby foods are used, they can be made up with infant formula instead of water. From 6 months, adult yoghurt and milk puddings can be introduced, though cow's milk should not replace infant formula milk or breast milk for the first year of life.

It is important that parents are encouraged to persist with trying to introduce more texture into the diet after the first 6 months. Often CF infants, like normal infants, will refuse to take lumpy or mashed weaning foods but will readily accept strained or puréed food. Parents will tend to continue with the strained consistencies as they feel that at least their infant is eating something. However, failure to introduce more texture and encourage chewing may lead to later feeding problems.

TODDLERS AND BEHAVIOURAL FEEDING PROBLEMS

Excessive focus on food, feeding and weight gain can lead to abnormal feeding patterns and negative feeding behaviour in children with CF. Many factors may precipitate food refusal including parental anxiety about food, acute infections, frequent disruptions due to hospital admissions, and vomiting and gagging associated with coughing spasms. Reports of prolonged mealtimes, vomiting and gagging, constant parental nagging and force-feeding indicate that additional support on feeding behaviour management is needed.

The following simple guidelines are helpful when advising parents:

- Encourage parents to sit down at the table and eat together as a family so that mealtime becomes a social event. A lack of structure to mealtimes can lead to both poor routine and poor eating habits. Offer small regular meals.
- Advise parents not to make a fuss or push their child to eat food. If children are forced to eat, they will soon learn how to control the situation by being even more difficult.

- Initially offer foods that the child will readily accept, and gradually increase the variety. A microwave oven is useful to prepare small amounts of favourite food quickly. Favourite foods can be stored in a freezer so they are readily available.
- Remind parents to praise children if they eat anything, even if it is only a small amount. Uneaten food should be taken away without comment.
- Encourage parents to offer small portions of food. Second helpings can easily be given. Desserts served in small containers are particularly helpful.
- Remind parents that likes and dislikes may change from day to day and to keep offering foods even if they were previously refused. Avoid food for which the child has an obvious strong dislike.
- Advise parents not to rush children when eating – but do not let mealtimes drag on, otherwise one meal quickly runs into the next. It may be helpful to set a time limit of no more than 30 minutes.
- Ask parents not to use sweet foods as a bribe and keep these out of sight until savoury foods have been eaten at mealtimes.
- Ask parents not to discuss the child's feeding behaviour in front of them.
- If problems persist the involvement of a psychologist with an interest in feeding problems is indicated.

PANCREATIC ENZYME REPLACEMENT THERAPY

Most CF centres predominantly use enteric-coated microspheres (10 000) for all infants and children, either administered as granules or in a gelatine capsule. The most common preparations include Creon 10 000 (Solvay) and Pancrease (Cilag). These comprise pH sensitive enteric-coated microspheres contained within a capsule. The enteric coating protects the enzymes from stomach acid inactivation, disintegrating to release the enzyme only when pH rises above 5.5 in the duodenum [113]. The administration of enteric-coated microspheres should achieve at least 90% fat absorption if given in appropriate dosages. Several studies have demonstrated that enteric-coated microspheres are more effective then conventional pancreatic powder and enteric-coated capsules. The newer, smaller Creon 10 000 capsules are popular and effective with children [134]. The composition of common pancreatic enzymes available in the UK is given in Table 10.7.

Table 10.7 Pancreatic enzyme preparations available in the UK

Product (manufacturer)	Composition (per g powder/granules or per capsule/tablet BP units)		
	Lipase	Protease	Amylase
Powder			
Pancrex V® (Paines & Byrne)	25 000	1 400	30 000
Capsules			
Pancrex V '340 mg® (Paines & Byrne)	8 000	430	9 000
Pancrex V '125 mg® (Paines & Byrne)	2 950	160	3 300
Tablets			
Enteric-coated tablets			
Pancrex V® (Paines & Byrne)	1 900	110	1 700
Pancrex V Forte® (Paines & Byrne)	5 600	330	5 000
Enteric-coated microspheres			
Pancrease® (Cilag)	5 000	350	3 000
Creon 10 000® (Solvay)	10 000	600	8 000
Nutrizym GR® (Merck)	10 000	650	10 000
Creon 25 000® (Solvay)	25 000	1 000	18 000
Enteric-coated minitablets			
Pancrease HL® (Cilag)	25 000	1 250	22 500
Nutrizym 10® (Merck)	10 000	500	9 000
Nutrizym 22® (Merck)	22 000	1 100	19 800
Granule microspheres in sachets			
Creon® (Solvay)	20 000 per sachet	1 125 per sachet	22 500 per sachet

Several factors may affect the effectiveness of pancreatic enzymes: the buffering action of food may cause premature dissolution within the stomach leading to the destruction of the released enzyme; duodenal pH may be abnormally acid since pancreatic bicarbonate production is low and gastric hypersecretion is high [135].

High lipase pancreatic enzymes

In 1993, the UK Committee on Safety of Medicines recommended that Pancrease HL, Nutrizym 22 and Panzytrat 25 000 were contraindicated in CF for children aged 15 years and under. Most high lipase pancreatic enzymes containing 22 000–25 000 units of lipase per capsule are associated with the development of fibrosing colonopathy, although its precise aetiology remains uncertain. After the first reports in Liverpool similar cases were reported elsewhere in the UK [136, 137, 138], Ireland [139], Denmark [140] and the USA [141].

Fibrosing colonopathy should be considered in patients with CF who have evidence of obstruction, bloody diarrhoea or chylous ascites, or a combination of abdominal pain, distention with continuing diarrhoea and/or poor weight gain. Patients at higher risk include those less than 12 years of age, on high dosages of pancreatic lipase [142, 143], who have a history of meconium ileus [144] or DIOS, and those who have had any intestinal surgery or have a diagnosis of inflammatory bowel disease [145]. However, not all high strength products (i.e. Creon 25 000 (Solvay)) have been found to be associated with colonic strictures. Preparations linked with colonic strictures in the UK are all minitablets, which contain Eudragit-L, a co-polymer based on methylacrylic acid and ethyl acrylate in their coating (e.g. Pancrease HL (Cilag); Nutrizym 22 (Merck)). These compounds have been shown to have a toxic effect on the gut of experimental animals and may be a causal factor in the aetiology of fibrosing colonopathy [26]. This theory is supported by the observation of two cases of two younger children developing fibrosing colonopathy on the lower strength preparation, Nutrizym GR (Merck), which contains the methylacrylic copolymer [146]. The USA have found no relationship between coating and fibrosing colonopathy, although their interpretation of statistics has been criticised [147].

Dosage of pancreatic enzymes

It is recommended by the Committee on Safety of Medicines (CSM) that a maximum of 10 000 units lipase/kg/day is given from pancreatic enzyme preparations, irrespective of formulation [148]. The dosage depends on residual pancreatic function, enzyme supplement properties, amount of fat and protein consumed and patho-physiological factors [113]. Dosage is often determined by stool output (frequency/colour/consistency) and presence of abdominal pain, and by faecal fat studies. Before the recommendations by the CSM, it was not uncommon for many patients to be on much higher dosages of pancreatic enzymes. However it has been demonstrated that dosage can be reduced to acceptable

Table 10.8 Maximum daily dosage of pancreatic enzyme preparation to provide 10 000 units of lipase/kg/day

Weight	Creon 10 000	Pancrease
5 kg	5	10
10 kg	10	20
15 kg	15	30
20 kg	20	40
25 kg	25	50
30 kg	30	60
35 kg	35	70

Table 10.9 General guidelines for the use of pancreatic enzyme preparations

Give with every meal at the beginning and during the meal rather than all before or after

It may be necessary to give extra enzymes with fatty meals

Give enzymes with snacks, e.g. milk, crisps and chocolate biscuits. There is no need to give with squash, lemonade, fruit, boiled or jelly sweets

Give enzymes with supplemented milk shake drinks

Creon 10 000 and Pancrease capsules can be swallowed whole. Where swallowing is difficult, they may be opened and the contents taken with liquids or mixed with jam or honey. They should not be crushed or chewed

Do not mix with hot food or food with a pH of more than 5.5

intakes for many patients without deterioration in growth and acceptable coefficient of fat absorption [149, 150].

A guideline for the maximum number of pancreatic enzymes, using standard preparation per kg body weight, is given in Table 10.8.

Administration of pancreatic enzymes

Pancreatic enzymes should be administered with all meals and protein and fat-containing snacks (Table 10.9). There is evidence that pancreatic enzymes should be spread throughout the meal to optimise mixing and minimise partitioning of the pancreatin with the liquid phase of the meal, which empties more rapidly than the solid phase [151]. Young children should be encouraged to swallow the whole capsules as soon as possible, usually from 4–5 years of age. Until then, there is little option but to give the granules out of the capsule. However, some toddlers may chew the granules or hold them in their mouth for considerable periods of time, thus releasing the enzymes and predisposing to mouth ulcers. In addition, they are particularly unpopular in toddlers and enzyme refusal, coughing, choking and even vomiting is common. As the amount of food eaten by toddlers will vary from meal to meal, it is recommended to spread the pancreatic enzymes throughout the meal.

Adjunctive therapy to pancreatic enzymes

Histamine (H_2) receptor antagonists such as cimetidine have been used as an adjunct to pancreatic enzymes. They aim to reduce both the volume and the acid concentration of gastric secretion and thereby prevent acid/peptic inactivation of the enzymes. They may help increase efficiency of enteric-coated enzymes and are worth considering if patients have uncontrolled symptoms on large doses of pancreatic enzymes. Alternatives are proton pump inhibitors (e.g. omeprazole) which suppress gastric acid secretions.

DIETARY MANAGEMENT OF DIABETES IN CHILDREN WITH CF

No clear guidelines have been issued on ideal dietary management for patients with both cystic fibrosis and diabetes, although advice should be tailored according to the severity of the cystic fibrosis. Although the aim is to achieve normoglycaemia, the provision of optimal nutrition is still of paramount importance and any dietary restriction should be minimised.

Guidelines

- Encourage some complex carbohydrates at each meal and at bedtime
- Recommend regular snacks
- Sugar-containing foods can be eaten, e.g. chocolate, puddings, cakes and sweets, but preferably following complex carbohydrate
- Give sugar-free drinks instead of sugar-containing squashes and fizzy drinks
- Substitute glucose polymer supplements for milk containing supplements

- Biscuits, crisps, milk, cereals and cake are useful snacks
- Fat should not be restricted
- Nutritional status and blood glucose should be monitored closely.

Poor diabetic control should be improved by alterations in insulin therapy rather than imposing dietary restrictions that may adversely affect nutritional status. When treating the child with CF and diabetes it may be necessary to involve the expertise of the diabetic team who need to fully understand and support the rationale for the different dietary approach.

REFERENCES

1 Dodge JA, Morison S, Lewis PA, Coles EC, Geddes D, Russell G, Littlewood JM, Scott MT (the UK Cystic Fibrosis Survey Management Committee) Incidence, population, and survival of cystic fibrosis in the UK, 1968–1995. *Arch Dis Childh*, 1997, **77** 493–6.
2 Jackson A Clinical guidelines for cystic fibrosis care. *J Royal Coll Phys*, 1996, **30** 305–308.
3 Corey M, McLaughlin FJ, Williams M, Levinson H A comparison of survival, growth and pulmonary function in patients with cystic fibrosis. *J Clin Epidemiol*, 1988, **41** 583–91.
4 Forstner G, Durie P Nutrition in cystic fibrosis. In: Grand RJ, Sutphen JL, Dietz WH (eds) *Pediatric Nutrition. Theory and Practice*. Boston: Butterworths, 1987.
5 Alemzadeh R, Upchurch L, McCarthy V Anabolic effects of growth hormone treatment in young children with cystic fibrosis. *J Am Coll Nutr*, 1998, **17** 419–24.
6 Johannesson M, Gottlieb C, Hjelte L Delayed puberty in girls with cystic fibrosis despite good clinical outcome. *Pediatr*, 1997, **99** 29–34.
7 Kerem B–S, Rommens JM, Buchanan JA *et al.* Identification of the cystic fibrosis gene: genetic analysis. *Science*, 1989, **245** 1073–80.
8 Anthony H, Paxton S, Catto–Smith A, Phelan P Physiological and psychological contributors to malnutrition in children with cystic fibrosis: review. *Clin Nutr*, 1999, **18** 327–35.
9 Jaffé A, Bush A, Geddes DM, Alton EWFW Prospects for gene therapy in cystic fibrosis. *Arch Dis Childh*, 1999, **80** 286–9.
10 WHO/ICF (M) A Therapeutic approaches to cystic fibrosis: Memorandum from a joint WHO/ICF (M) A meeting. *Bulletin of the World Health Organisation*, 1994, **72** 341–52.

11 Elborn JS, Shale DJ, Britton JR Cystic fibrosis. In: Prasad SA, Hussey J (eds) *Paediatric Respiratory Care*. London: Chapman and Hall, 1991, pp. 159–75.

12 Nir M, Lanng S, Johansen HK, Koch C Long term survival and nutritional data in patients with cystic fibrosis treated in a Danish centre. *Thorax*, 1996, **51** 1023–7.

13 Guritz D, Francis P, Crozier M, Levison H Perspectives in cystic fibrosis. *Pediatr Clin North Am*, 1979, **26** 603–15.

14 Schechter MS, Margolis PA Relationship between socioeconomic status and disease severity in cystic fibrosis. *J Pediatr*, 1997, **132** 260–64.

15 Couriel J Respiratory disorders. In: Lissauer T, Clayden G (eds) *Illustrated Textbook of Paediatrics*. Mosby, London, 1997, pp. 157–71.

16 Kopito LE, Shwachman H, Vawter GF, Edlow J The pancreas in cystic fibrosis: chemical composition and comparative morphology. *Pediatr Res*, 1976, **10** 742–9.

17 Sokol RJ The GI system and nutrition in cystic fibrosis. *Pediatr Pulmonol*, 1990, (Suppl 5) 81–3.

18 Littlewood JM Gastrointestinal investigations in cystic fibrosis. *J Roy Soc Med*, 1992, (Suppl 18) **85** 13–19.

19 Littlewood JM Abdominal pain in cystic fibrosis. *J Roy Soc Med*, 1996, (Suppl 25) **88** 9–17.

20 Heine RG, Button BM, Olinsky A, Phelan PD, Catto-Smith AG Gastro-intestinal reflux in infants under 6 months with cystic fibrosis. *Arch Dis Childh*, 1998, **78** 44–8.

21 Cucchiara S, Santamaria F, Andreotti MR *et al.* Mechanisms of gastro-oesophageal reflux in cystic fibrosis. *Arch Dis Childh*, 1991, **66** 617–22.

22 Button BM, Heine RG, Catto-Smith AG *et al.* Postural drainage and gastro-oesophageal reflux in infants with cystic fibrosis. *Arch Dis Childh*, 1997, **76** 148–50.

23 Stringer DA, Sprigg A, Juodis E, Corey M, Daneman A, Levison HJ, Durie PR The association of cystic fibrosis, gastro-esophageal reflux, and reduced pulmonary function. *Can Assoc Radiol J*, 1988, **39** 100–102.

24 Smith RL, van Velzen D, Smyth AR, Lloyd DA, Heaf DP Strictures of ascending colon in cystic fibrosis and high strength pancreatic enzymes. *Lancet*, 1994, **343** 85–6.

25 Dodge JA The aetiology of fibrosing colonopathy. *Postgrad Med J*, 1996, (Suppl 2) **72** S52–5.

26 Van Velzan D, Ball LM, Dezfulian AR, Southgate A, Howard CV Comparative and experimental pathology of fibrosing colonopathy. *Postgrad Med J*, 1996, (Suppl 2) **72** 39–48.

27 Schoni MH, Maisonneuve P, Schöni-Affolter F, Lowenfels AB Cancer risk in patients with cystic fibrosis. *J Roy Soc Med*, 1996, (Suppl 27) **89** 38–47.

28 Bell SC, Bowerman AR, Davies CA, Campbell IA, Shale DJ, Elborn JS Nutrition in adults with cystic fibrosis. *Clin Nutr*, 1998, **17** 211–15.

29 Dodge JA The nutritional state and nutrition. *Acta Paediatr Scand*, 1985, (Suppl 317) 31–7.

30 Goodchild MC Nutritional management of cystic fibrosis. *Digestion*, 1987, **37** (Suppl 1) 61–7.

31 Ghosal S, Taylor CJ, Pickering M, McGaw J Head growth in cystic fibrosis following early diagnosis by neonatal screening. *Arch Dis Childh*, 1996, **75** 191–3.

32 Morison S, Dodge JA, Cole TJ, Lewis PA, Coles EC, Geddes D, Russell G, Littlewood JM, Scott MT Height and weight in cystic fibrosis: a cross sectional study. *Arch Dis Childh*, 1997, **77** 497–500.

33 Chatfield S, Owen G, Ryley HC *et al.* Neonatal screening for cystic fibrosis in Wales and the West Midlands: clinical assessment after 5 years of screening. *Arch Dis Childh*, 1991, **66** 29–33.

34 Lai H-C, Kosorok MR, Sondel SA, Chen S-T, FitzSimmons S, Green CG, Shen G, Walker S, Farrell PM Growth status in children with cystic fibrosis based on the national cystic fibrosis patient registry data: evaluation of various criteria used to identify malnutrition. *J Pediatr*, 1998, **132** 478–85.

35 Lai H-C, Corey M, FitzSimmons S, Kosorok MR, Farrell PM Comparison of growth status of patients with cystic fibrosis between the United States and Canada. *Am J Clin Nut*, 1999, **69** 531–58.

36 Huseman CA, Colombo JL, Brooks MA, Smay JR, Greger NG, Sammut PH, Bier DM Anabolic effect of biosynthetic growth hormone in cystic fibrosis patients. *Pediat Pulmonol*, 1996, **22** 90–95.

37 WHO Study Group Diabetes mellitus. World Health Organisation. *Tech Rep Ser*, 1985, **727** 1–113.

38 Lanng S, Hansen A, Thorsteinsson B, Nerup J, Koch C Glucose tolerance in patients with cystic fibrosis: 5 year prospective study. *Brit Med J*, 1995, **311** 655–9.

39 Robert JJ, Grasset E, de Montalembert M, Chevenne D, Deschamps I, Boitard C, Lenoir G Research of factors for glucose intolerance in mucoviscidosis (in French). *Arch Fr Pediatr*, 1992, **49** 17–22.

40 De Luca F, Arigo T, Nibali SC, Sferlazzas C, Gigante A, di Cesare E *et al.* Insulin secretion, glycosylated haemoglobin and islet cell antibodies in cystic fibrosis children and adolescents with different degrees of glucose tolerance. *Horm Metab Res*, 1991, **23** 495–8.

41 Lanng S, Thorsteinsson B, Lund-Andersen C, Nerup J, Schiøtz PO, Koch C Diabetes mellitus in Danish cystic fibrosis patients: prevalence and late diabetic complications. *Acta Paediatr*, 1994, **83** 72–7.

42 Cucinotta D, Arrigo T, De Luca F, Benedetto AD, Lombardo F Metabolic and clinical events preceding diabetes mellitus onset in cystic fibrosis. *Eur J End*, 1996, **134** 731–6.

43 Lanng S, Thorsteinsson B, Nerup J, Koch C Influence of the development of diabetes mellitus on clinical status in patients with cystic fibrosis. *Eur J Pediat*, 1992, **151** 684–7.

44 Sullivan MM, Denning CR Diabetic microangiography in patients with cystic fibrosis. *Pediatr*, 1989, **84** 642–7.

45 Allen JL Progressive nephropathy in a patient with cystic fibrosis and diabetes. *N Engl J Med*, 1986, **315** 764.

46 Dolan TF Microangiography in a young adult with cystic fibrosis and diabetes mellitus. *N Engl J Med*, 1986, **314** 991–2.

47 Lanng S, Hansen A, Thorsteinsson B, Nerup J, Koch C Glucose tolerance in patients with cystic fibrosis: 5 year prospective study. *Brit Med J*, 1995, **311** 655–9.

48 Wilschanski M, Rivlin J, Cohen S, Augarten A, Blau H, Aviram M, Bentur M, Bentur L, Springer C, Vila Y, Branski D, Karem B, Karem E Clinical and genetic risk factors for cystic fibrosis-related liver disease. *Pediatr*, 1999, **103** 52–7.

49 Sharp HL Cystic fibrosis liver disease and transplantation. *J Pediatr*, 1995, **127** 944–6.

50 Colombo C, Apostolo MG, Ferrari M *et al.* Analysis of risk factors in the development of liver disease in CF. *J Pediatr*, 1994, **124** 393–6.

51 FitzSimmons SC The changing epidemiology of cystic fibrosis. *J Pediatr*, 1993, **122** 1–9.

52 Mack DR, Traystman MD, Colombo C *et al.* Clinical denouement and mutation analysis of patients with cystic fibrosis undergoing liver transplantation for biliary cirrhosis. *J Pediatr*, 1995, **127** 881–7.

53 Colombo C, Battezzati PM, Podda M, Bettinardi N, Giunta A & Italian Group for the study of ursodeoxycholic acid in cystic fibrosis Ursodeoxycholic acid for liver disease associated with cystic fibrosis: a double-blind multicentre trial. *Hepatology*, 1996, **23** 1484–90.

54 Gibson LE, Cooke RE A test for concentration of electrolytes in sweat in cystic fibrosis of the pancreas utilising pilocarpine by iontophoresis. *Pediatr*, 1959, **23** 545–9.

55 Hill CM *Practical Guidelines for Cystic Fibrosis Care.* London: Churchill Livingstone, 1998.

56 Waters DL, Wilken B, Irwig L, Van Asperen P, Mellis C, Simpson JM, Brown J, Gaskin KJ Clinical outcomes of newborn screening for cystic fibrosis. *Arch Dis Childh Fetal Neonat*, 1999, **80** F1–F7.

57 De Meer K, Gulmans AM, van der Laag Peripheral muscle weakness and exercise capacity in children with cystic fibrosis. *Am J Respir Crit Care Med*, 1998, **159** 748–54.

58 Thomson MA, Quirk P, Swanson CE, Thomas BJ, Holt TL, Francis PJ, Shepherd RW Nutritional growth retardation is associated with defective lung growth in cystic fibrosis: a preventable determinant of progressive pulmonary dysfunction. *Nutrition*, 1995, **11** 350–54.

59 Murphy JL, Wootton SA, Bond SA, Jackson AA Energy content of stools in normal healthy controls and patients with cystic fibrosis. *Arch Dis Childh*, 1991, **66** 495–500.

60 Turck D, Michaud L Cystic fibrosis: nutritional consequences and management. *Baillière's Clin Gastr*, 1998, **12** 805–22.

61 Barth AL, Pitt TL The high amino-acid content of sputum from cystic fibrosis patients promotes growth of auxotrophic *Pseudomonas aeruginosa. J Med Microbiol*, 1996, **45** 110–19.

62 Vaisman N, Pencharz PB, Corey M, Cann GY, Hahn E Energy expenditure of patients with cystic fibrosis. *J Pediatr*, 1987, **111** 496–500.

63 Buchdahl RM, Cox M, Fulleylove C, Marchant JL, Tomkins AM, Brueton MJ, Warner JO Increased resting energy expenditure in cystic fibrosis. *J App Phys*, 1988, **64** 1810–16.

64 Fried MD, Durie PR, Tsui L-C, Corey M, Levinson H, Pencharz PB The cystic fibrosis gene and resting energy expenditure. *J Pediatr*, 1991, **119** 913–16.

65 Bell SC, Saunder MJ, Elborn JS, Shale DJ Resting energy expenditure and oxygen cost of breathing in patients with cystic fibrosis. *Thorax*, 1996, **51** 126–31.

66 Steinkamp G, Drommer A, von der Hardt H Resting energy expenditure before and after treatment for *Pseudomonas aeruginosa* infection in patients with cystic fibrosis. *Am J Clin Nutr*, 1993, **57** 685–9.

67 Vaisman N, Levy LD, Pencharz PB *et al.* Effect of salbutamol on resting energy expenditure in patients with cystic fibrosis. *J Pediatr*, 1987, **111** 137–9.

68 O'Rawe A, McIntosh J, Dodge JA, Brock DJH, Redmond AOB, Ward R, Macpherson AJ Increased energy expenditure in cystic fibrosis is associated with specific mutations. *Clin Sci*, 1990, **82** 71–6.

69 Spicher V, Roulet M, Schutz Y Assessment of total energy expenditure in free living patients with cystic fibrosis. *J Pediatr*, 1991, **118** 865–72.

70 Zemel BS, Kawchak DA, Cnaan A *et al.* Prospective evaluation of resting energy expenditure, nutritional status, pulmonary function, and genotype in children with cystic fibrosis. *Pediatr Res*, 1996, **40** 578–86.

71 Shepherd RW, Holt TL, Vasquez-Velasquez L, Prentice AM Increased energy expenditure in young children with CF. *Lancet*, 1988, **i** 1300–1303.

72 Kawchak DA, Zhao H, Scanlin MF, Tomezsko JL, Cnaan A, Stallings VA Longitudinal, prospective analysis of dietary intake in children with cystic fibrosis. *J Pediatr*, 1996, **129** 119–29.

73 Anthony H, Bines J, Phelan P, Paxton S Relation between dietary intake and nutritional status in cystic fibrosis. *Arch Dis Childh*, 1998, **78** 443–7.

74 Stark LJ, Jelalian E, Mulvihill MM, Powers SW, Bowen AM, Spieth LE, Keating K, Evans S, Creveling S, Harwood I, Passero MA, Hovell MF Eating in preschool children with cystic fibrosis and healthy peers: behavioral analysis. *Pediatr*, 1995, **95** 210–15.

75 Stark LJ, Mulvihill MM, Jelalian E, Bowen AM, Powers SW, Tao S, Creveling S, Passero MA, Harwood I, Light M, Lapey A, Hovell MF Descriptive analysis of eating behavior in school-age children with cystic fibrosis and healthy control children. *Pediatr*, 1997, **99** 665–71.

76 Crist W, McDonnell P, Beck M, Gillespie CT, Barrett P, Mathews J Behavior at mealtimes and nutritional intake in the young child with cystic fibrosis. *Dev Behav Pediatr*, 1994, **15** 157–61.

77 Ramsey BW, Farrell PM, Pancharz P & Consensus Committee Nutritional assessement and management in cystic fibrosis. *Am J Clin Nutr*, 1992, **55** 108–16.

78 Reilly JJ, Evans TJ, Wilkinson J, Paton JY Adequacy of clinical formulae for estimation of energy requirements in children with cystic fibrosis. *Arch Dis Childh*, 1999, **81** 120–24.

79 Shepherd RW, Holt TL, Johnson LP, Quirk P, Thomas BJ Leucine metabolism and body cell mass in cystic fibrosis. *Nutr*, 1995, **11** 138–41.

80 Collins CE, O'Loughlin EV, Henry RL Fat gram target to achieve high intake in cystic fibrosis. *J Paediatr Child Health*, 1997, **33** 142–7.

81 Slesinski MJ, Gloninger MF, Costantino JP, Orenstein DM Lipid levels in adults with cystic fibrosis. *J Am Diet Assoc*, 1994, **94** 402–408.

82 Gavin J, Ellis J, Dewar AL, Roles CJ, Connett GJ Dietary fibre and the occurrence of gut symptoms in cystic fibrosis. *Arch Dis Childh*, 1997, **76** 35–7.

83 Brown KH, Sanchez-Grinan M, Perez F, Peerson JM, Ganoza L, Stern JS Effects of dietary energy density and feeding frequency on total daily energy intakes of recovering malnourished children. *Am J Clin Nutr*, 1995, **62** 13–18.

84 Jelalaian E, Stark LJ, Reynolds L, Seifer R Nutrition intervention for weight gain in cystic fibrosis: a meta analysis. *J Pediatr*, 1998, **132** 486–92.

85 Rettammel AL, Marcus MS, Farrell PM, Sondel SA, Koscik RE, Mischler EH Oral supplementation with a high-fat, high-energy product improves nutritional status and alters serum lipids in patients with cystic fibrosis. *J Am Diet Assoc*, 1995, **95** 454–9.

86 Skypala IJ, Ashworth FA, Hodson ME, Leonard CH, Knox A, Hiller EJ, Wolfe SP, Littlewood JM, Morton A, Conway S, Patchell C, Weller P, McCarthy H, Redmond A, Dodge J Oral nutritional supplements promote significant weight gain in cystic fibrosis patients. *J Hum Nutr Diet*, 1998, **11** 95–104.

87 MacDonald A Nutritional management of cystic fibrosis: personal practice. *Arch Dis Childh*, 1996, **74** 81–7.

88 Rosenfield M, Casey S, Pepe M, Ramsey BW Nutritional effects of long-term gastrostomy feedings in children with cystic fibrosis. *J Am Diet Assoc*, 1999, **99** 191–4.

89 Walker SA, Gozal D Pulmonary function correlates in the prediction of long-term weight gain in cystic fibrosis patients with gastrostomy tube feedings. *J Pediatr Gastroenterol Nutr*, 1998, **27** 53–6.

90 Boland MP, Stoski DS, MacDonald NE, Saucy P, Patrick J Chronic jejunostomy feeding with a non-elemental formula in undernourished patients with cystic fibrosis. *Lancet*, 1986, **I** 232–4.

91 Shepherd RW, Holt TL, Thomas BJ *et al.* Nutritional rehabilitation in cystic fibrosis: controlled studies of effects of nutritional growth retardation, body protein turnover and cause of pulmonary disease. *J Pediatr*, 1986, **109** 788–94.

92 Steinkamp G, von der Hardt H Improvement of nutritional status and lung function after long-term nocturnal gastrostomy feeding in cystic fibrosis. *J Pediatr*, 1994, **106** 223–7.

93 Dalzell AM, Shepherd RW, Dean B, Cleghorn GJ, Holt TL, Francis PJ Nutritional rehabilitation in cystic fibrosis: a 5 year follow-up study. *J Pediatr Gastroenter Nutr*, 1992, **15** 141–5.

94 Erskine JM, Lingard CD, Sontag MK, Accurso FJ Enteral nutrition for patients with cystic fibrosis: comparison of a semi-elemental and non-elemental formula. *J Pediatr*, 1998, **132** 265–9.

95 Williams SGJ, Ashworth F, McAlweenie A, Poole S, Hodson ME, Westaby D Percutaneous endoscopic gastrostomy feeding in patients with cystic fibrosis. *Gut*, 1999, **44** 87–90.

96 Fitting JW Nutritional support in chronic obstructive lung disease. *Thorax*, 1992, **47** 141–3.

97 Kane RE, Hobbs PJ, Black P Comparison of low, medium and high carbohydrate formulas for night time enteral feedings in cystic fibrosis patients. *J Parent Ent Nutr*, 1990, **14** 47–52.

98 Milla C, Doherty L, Raatz S, Schwarzenberg SJ, Regelmann W, Moran A Glycemic response to dietary supplement in cystic fibrosis is dependent on the carbohydrate content of the formula. *J Parent Ent Nutr*, 1996, **20** 182–6.

99 Morton A, Conway S Enteral feeding by gastrostomy is more effective than by nasogastric route in patients with cystic fibrosis. X11th International Cystic Fibrosis Congress – I.C.F. (M)A, Jerusalem (abstract), 1996.

100 Patchell CJ, Desai M, Smyth RC, Bush A, Collins SA, Gilbody JS, Weller PH Creon 10000 vs Creon 8000 – a preference study. Presented at 23rd European CF Conference, The Hague (abstract), 1999.

101 Smith FR, Underwood BA, Denning CR, Varma A, Goodman DW Depressed plasma retinol-binding protein levels in cystic fibrosis. *J Lab Clin Med*, 1972, **80** 423–33.

102 Lindblad A, Diczfalusy U, Hultcrantz R, Thorell A, Strandvik B Vitamin A concentration in liver decreases with age in patients with cystic fibrosis. *J Ped Gastroenterol Nutr*, 1997, **24** 264–70.

103 Winklhofer-Roob BM, van't Hof MA, Shmerling DH Long-term oral vitamin E supplementation in cystic fibrosis patients: *RRR*-α-tocopherol compared with all-*rac*-α-tocopheryl acetate preparations. *Am J Clin Nutr*, 1996, **63** 722–8.

104 Thomas PS, Bellamy M, Geddes D Malabsorption of vitamin E in cystic fibrosis improved after ursodeoxy-cholic acid. *Lancet*, 1995, **346** 1230–31.

105 Henderson RC, Madsen CD Bone density in children and adolescents with cystic fibrosis. *J Pediatr*, 1996, **128** 28–34.

106 Donovan DS Jr, Papdopoulos A, Staron RB, Addesso V, Schulman L, McGregor C, Cosman F, Lindsay RL, Shane E Bone mass and vitamin D deficiency in adults with advanced cystic fibrosis lung disease. *Am J Respir Crit Care Med*, 1998, **157** 1892–9.

107 Laursem E, Mølgaard C, Michaelsen KF, Koch C, Müller J Bone mineral status in 134 patients with cystic fibrosis. *Arch Dis Childh*, 1999, **81** 235–40.

108 Shaw N, Bedford C, Heaf D, Carty H Osteopenia in adults with cystic fibrosis. *Am J Med*, 1995, **99** 690–91.

109 Salamoni F, Roulet M, Gudinchet F, Pilet M, Thiébaud D, Burckhardt P Bone mineral content in cystic fibrosis patients: correlation with fat-free mass. *Arch Dis Childh*, 1996, **74** 314–18.

110 Rashid M, Durie P, Andrew M, Kalnins D, Shin J, Corey M, Tullis E, Pencharz PB Prevalence of vitamin K deficiency in cystic fibrosis. *Am J Clin Nutr*, 1999, **70** 378–82.

111 Beker LT, Ahrens RA, Fink RJ, O'Brien ME, Davidson KW, Sokoll LJ, Sadowski JA Effect of vitamin K$_1$ supplementation on vitamin K status in cystic fibrosis patients. *J Ped Gastroenterol Nutr*, 1997, **24** 512–17.

112 Peters SA, Rolles CJ Vitamin therapy in cystic fibrosis – a review and rationale. *J Clin Pharm Ther*, 1993, **18** 33–8.

113 Leonard CH, Knox AJ Pancreatic enzyme supplements and vitamins in cystic fibrosis. *J Hum Nutr Diet*, 1997, **10** 3–16.

114 Leonard CH, Ross-Wilson C, Smyth AR, Polnay J, Range SP, Knox AJ A study of a single high potency multivitamin preparation in the management of cystic fibrosis. *J Hum Nutr Diet*, 1998, **11** 493–500.

115 Pencharz PB, Durie PR Nutritional management of cystic fibrosis. *Ann Rev Nutr*, 1993, **13** 111–36.

116 Jeppesen PB, Christensen MS, Høy CE, Mortensen PB Essential fatty acid deficiency in patients with severe fat malabsorption. *Am J Clin Nutr*, 1997, **65** 837–43.

117 van Egmond AWA, Kosorok MR, Koscik R, Laxova A, Farrell PM Effect of linoleic acid intake on growth of infants with cystic fibrosis. *Am J Clin Nutr*, 1996, **63** 746–52.

118 Parsons HG, Oloughlin EV, Forbes D, Cooper D, Gall DG Supplemental calories improve essential fatty acid deficiency in cystic fibrosis patients. *Pediatr Res*, 1998, **24** 353–6.

119 Venuta A, Spano C, Laudizi L, Bettelli F, Beverelli A, Turchetto E Essential fatty acids: the effects of dietary supplementation among children with recurrent respiratory infections. *J Int Med Res*, 1996, **24** 325–30.

120 Swann IL, Kendra JR Case Report. Anaemia, vitamin E deficiency and failure to thrive in an infant. *Clin Lab Haem*, 1998, **20** 61–3.

121 Bines JE, Israel EJ Hypoproteinemia, anemia and failure to thrive in an infant. *Gastroenterol*, 1991, **101** 848–56.

122 Phillips RJ, Crock CM, Dillon MJ, Clayton PT, Curran A, Harper JH Cystic fibrosis presenting as kwashiorkor with florid skin rash. *Arch Dis Childh*, 1993, **69** 446–8.

123 Marcus MS, Sondel SA, Farrell PM *et al*. Nutritional status of infants with cystic fibrosis associated with early diagnosis and intervention. *Am J Clin Nutr*, 1991, **54** 578–85.

124 Sokol RJ, Reardon MC, Accurso FJ *et al*. Fat-soluble vitamin status during the first year of life in infants with cystic fibrosis identified by screening of newborns (1989). *Am J Clin Nutr*, 1989, **50** 1064–71.

125 Lloyd-Still JD, Powers C Carnitine metabolites in infants with cystic fibrosis. *Acta Univ Carol (Med) (Praha)*, 1990, **36** 78–80.

126 Greer R, Shepherd R, Cleghorn G, Bowling FG, Holt T Evaluation of growth and changes in body composition following neonatal diagnosis of cystic fibrosis. *J Pediatr Gastroenterol Nutr*, 1991, **13** 52–8.

127 Ellis L, Kalnins D, Corey M, Brennan J, Pencharz P, Durie P Do infants with cystic fibrosis need a protein hydrolysate formula? A prospective, randomized, comparative study. *J Pediatr*, 1998, **132** 270–76.

128 Girardet JP, Tounian P, Sardet A *et al*. Resting energy expenditure in infants with cystic fibrosis. *J Pediatr Gastroenterol Nutr*, 1994, **18** 214–19.

129 Green MR, Buchanan E, Weaver LT Nutritional management of the infant with cystic fibrosis. *Arch Dis Childh*, 1995, **72** 452–6.

130 Anthony H, Catto-Smith A, Phelan P, Paxton S Current approaches to the nutritional management of cystic fibrosis in Australia. *J Pediatr Child Health*, 1998, **34** 170–74.

131 Holliday KE, Allen KJ, Walters DL, Gruca MA, Thompson SM, Gaskin KJ Growth of human milk-fed and formula fed infants with cystic fibrosis. *J Pediatr*, 1991, **118** 77–9.

132 Laughlin JJ, Brady MS, Eigen H Changing feeding trends as a cause of electrolyte depletion in infants with cystic fibrosis. *J Am Diet Assoc*, 1981, **87** 1353–6.

133 Clark S, MacDonald A, Booth IW Impaired growth and nitrogen deficiency in infants receiving an energy-

supplemented standard infant formula. Proceedings of the 2nd Annual Spring Meeting, Royal College of Paediatrics and Child Health, p. 75 (abstract), 1998.

134 Patchell CJ, MacDonald A, Weller PW Pancreatic enzymes with enteral feeds – how should we give them? 22nd European CF Conference, Berlin, p. 104 (abstract), 1998.

135 Barraclough M, Taylor CJ Twenty-four hour ambulatory gastric and duodenal pH profiles in cystic fibrosis: effect of duodenal hyperacidity on pancreatic enzyme function and fat absorption. *J Pediatr Gastroenterol Nutr*, 1996, **23** 45–50.

136 Oades PJ, Bush A, Ong PS, Breton RJ High-strength pancreatic enzyme supplements and large-bowel stricture in cystic fibrosis (letter). *Lancet*, 1994, **343** 109.

137 Campbell CA, Forrest J, Musgrove C High-strength pancreatic enzyme supplements and large-bowel stricture in cystic fibrosis (letter). *Lancet*, 1994, **343** 109.

138 Briars GL, Griffiths DM, Moore IE, Williams PH, Johnson K, Rolles CJ High-strength pancreatic enzymes. *Lancet*, 1994, **343** 600.

139 Mahoney MJ, Corcoran M High-strength pancreatic enzymes. *Lancet*, 1994, **343** 599–600.

140 Knabe N, Zak M, Hanson A *et al.* Extensive pathologic changes of the colon in cystic fibrosis and high-strength pancreatic enzymes. *Lancet*, 1994, **343** 1230.

141 Frieman JP, FitzSimmons SC Colonic strictures in patients with cystic fibrosis: results of a survey of 114 cystic fibrosis care centers in the United States. *J Pediatr Gastroenterol Nutr*, 1996, **22** 153–6.

142 Smyth RL, Ashby D, O'Hea U, Burrows E, Lewis P, van Velzen D, Dodge J Fibrosing colonopathy in cystic fibrosis: results of a case-control study. *Lancet*, 1995, **346** 1247–51.

143 FitzSimmons SC, Burkhart GA, Borowitz D, Grand RJ, Hammerstrom T, Durie PR High-dose pancreatic-ensyme supplements and fibrosing colonopathy in children with cystic fibrosis. *N Engl J Med*, 1997, **336** 1283–9.

144 Stevens JC, Maguiness KM, Hollingsworth J, Heilman DK, Chong SKF Pancreatic enzyme supplementation in cystic fibrosis patients before and after fibrosing colonopathy. *J Pediatr Gastroenterol Nutr*, 1998, **26** 80–84.

145 Borowitz DS, Grand RJ, Durie PR & Consensus Committee Use of pancreatic enzyme supplements for patients with cystic fibrosis in the context of fibrosing colonopathy. *J Pediatr*, 1995, **127** 681–4.

146 Jones R, Franklin K, Spicer R, Berry J, van Velzen D Colonic strictures in children with cystic fibrosis on low-strength pancreatic enzymes. *Lancet*, 1995, **346** (8973) 499–500.

147 Prescott P Pancreatic enzymes and fibrosing colonopathy. Correspondence. *Lancet*, 1999, **354** 250.

148 Committee on the Safety of Medicines *Report of the Pancreatic Enzymes Working Party*. London. Committee on the Safety of Medicines: Medicines Control Agency, 1995.

149 Lowden J, Goodchild MC, Ryley HC, Doull IJM Maintenance of growth in cystic fibrosis despite reduction in pancreatic enzyme supplementation. *Arch Dis Childh*, 1998, **78** 377–8.

150 Beckles-Willson N, Taylor CJ, Ghosal S, Pickering M Reducing pancreatic enzyme dose does not compromise growth in cystic fibrosis. *J Hum Nutr Diet*, 1998, **11** 487–92.

151 Taylor CJ, Hillel PG, Ghosal S, Frier M, Senior S, Tindale WB, Read N Gastric emptying and intestinal transit of pancreatic supplements in cystic fibrosis. *Arch Dis Childh*, 1999, **80** 149–52.

USEFUL ADDRESS

Cystic Fibrosis Trust,
11 London Road, Bromley, Kent BR1 1B7

CHAPTER 11

The Kidney

ACUTE RENAL FAILURE

Acute renal failure (ARF) can be described as a sudden decrease in renal function with retention of nitrogenous wastes and disturbance of water and electrolyte homeostasis. It is usually associated with oliguria (urine output <1 ml/kg body weight/hr in the young child), but occasional patients may have polyuria, e.g. when urinary obstruction is relieved following treatment of posterior urethral valves.

The causes of ARF in children can be categorised into pre-renal, e.g. cardiac failure; renal, e.g. haemolytic uraemic syndrome (HUS); or post-renal, e.g. posterior urethral valves, and are different from those in adult patients [1]. In newborns there are further considerations and causes [2]. The commonest cause of ARF in childhood in the UK is HUS. It typically follows a preceding bloody diarrhoeal illness often in association with *E. coli* 0157 infection [3]. Anorexia and vomiting often accompany and complicate the nutritional management, particularly in children who have colitis.

Management of ARF

ARF requires close attention to fluid balance and monitoring of electrolytes and blood pressure. Some children may be conservatively managed, i.e. without dialysis. In such patients a greater need for fluid restriction can complicate the nutritional prescription whereas dialysis should allow the removal of fluid and uraemic toxins, thereby providing more 'nutritional space' and greater flexibility in nutritional regimens. Indications for dialysis include:

- Hyperkalaemia
- Fluid overload
- Rapidly rising plasma urea and creatinine levels with oliguria
- Metabolic abnormalities, e.g. acidosis, hyperphosphataemia
- Creation of 'nutritional space'
- Removal of specific poisons.

Dialysis and ARF

Peritoneal dialysis is the dialysis technique generally favoured in children [4] as it avoids the need for access to blood vessels and is a continuous, 'gentler' form of dialysis. Haemodialysis or haemofiltration are implemented when peritoneal dialysis is complicated by leaks into the pleural cavity because of abdominal surgery or severe colitis. Various types of haemofiltration are often used in intensive care areas to remove excess fluid.

Nutritional management of ARF

The paediatric dietitian should be involved at the onset as the dietary prescription may change with alterations in clinical management and stage of the illness [5]. Adequate nutrition will help prevent catabolism, control metabolic abnormalities and hopefully alleviate clinical symptoms and hasten recovery [6].

Dietary principles of ARF

The basic aims are an energy supplemented, moderated protein diet (Table 11.1). A potassium, sodium and phosphate restriction is usually necessary. Those children with persistent diarrhoea may tolerate a semi-elemental feed in preference to parenteral nutrition. Fluid allowance depends on overall fluid balance and whether the patient is being dialysed. Daily interpretation of the biochemical parameters should be

Table 11.1 Nutritional guidelines for the child in acute renal failure (ARF)

	Energy* (kcal/kg body wt/day)	Protein (g/kg body wt/day)
Conservative management		
0–2 yr	95–150 (400–630 kJ)	1.0–2.1
Children/adolescents	EAR for chronological age	1.0
Peritoneal dialysis		
0–2 yr	95–150 (400–630 kJ)	2.1–2.5**
Children/adolescents	EAR for chronological age	1.0–2.5
Haemodialysis		
0–2 yr	95–150 (400–630 kJ)	1.0–2.1
Children/adolescents	EAR for chronological age	1.0–1.8

EAR = Estimated average requirement (Dietary Reference Values, 1991 [9])

* These are guidelines which are rarely achieved in the acute stage because of fluid restriction

** If dialysis is prolonged, increased protein may be required

discussed with the medical and nursing staff so that the dietary prescription can be individualised for each child.

Nutritional assessment in ARF will include:

- Dietary history
  Should be obtained from the parents/carers.
- Growth parameters
  Height (if available) and weight plotted on a growth chart [7]. Weight recordings prior to the onset of ARF will help determine a more accurate estimation of dry weight.
- Fluid
  Allowances need to be determined (20 ml/kg or 400 ml/m²)
- Biochemical assessment
  Plasma levels of potassium, urea, creatinine, sodium, albumin, calcium and phosphate will be of particular relevance (Tables 11.2a and 11.2b).

Methods of feeding

Enteral feeding

The child with ARF may initially take oral fluids willingly because of thirst, but vomiting is commonplace.

Table 11.2a Reference range: guidelines for normal plasma values in childhood (as used at Nottingham City Hospital Trust)

Sodium (mmol/l)		132–142
Potassium* (mmol/l)	<1 mth	3.0–6.6
	>1 mth	3.0–5.6
Bicarbonate (mmol/l)		22–32
Urea (mmol/l)		2.5–6.5
Albumin (g/l)**		34–45
Calcium* (mmol/l)	<1 yr	2.4–2.8
	1–2 yr	2.3–2.7
	3–16 yr	2.2–2.6
Phosphate* (mmol/l)	<4 wks	1.2–3.1
	5 wks–6 mths	1.5–2.4
	6 mths–1 yr	1.5–2.1
	1–3 yr	1.2–2.0
	3–6 yr	1.0–1.8
	6–15	1.0–1.7
	Adult	0.8–1.4
PTH (ng/l)		12–72
Alkaline Phosphatase* (iu/l)	<10 days	180–740
	11 days–4 wks	183–945
	5 wks–6 mths	230–1197
	6 mths–2 yr	180–961
	3–9 yr	177–912
	9–11 yr	203–1069
	12–15 yr	216–1151
	>16 yr	80–280
Glucose (mmol/l)		3–5

* Age related

** Measured by bromocresol purple dye binding assay (those done by bromocresol green tend to be 5 g/l higher)

Table 11.2b Reference range guidelines for normal plasma creatinine values in childhood

Age (yrs)	Plasma creatinine (μmol/l)
<5	<44
5–6	<53
6–7	<62
7–8	<71
8–9	<80
9–10	<88
10+	<106

Ketones interfere positively
Bilirubin interferes negatively

The majority of children fail to meet the necessary nutritional goals via the oral route and as the duration of the acute illness is unknown, it is recommended that a fine bore nasogastric tube is placed. This can be done at the time of sedation or anaesthetic for other procedures such as insertion of a peritoneal dialysis catheter or arterial line [5]. This allows the provision of prompt nutritional support as anorexia, vomiting or refusal to take the nutritional prescription can complicate management and often cause anxiety for the parents.

A continuous 24 hour feed using an enteral feeding pump may be advantageous in the initial stages of treatment. As the oral intake improves the transition from continuous to overnight feeding provides the remaining nutritional prescription until appetite has returned sufficiently to allow tube feeding to be withdrawn.

Parenteral nutrition (PN)

The parenteral route is only considered if enteral nutrition is not tolerated. Established hospital PN regimens are usually not suitable for the child with ARF because of fluid restriction and electrolyte composition. A suitable daily nutritional prescription to meet individual requirements should be agreed by the dietitian and medical staff. The use of high nitrogen, electrolyte-free solutions can be considered to allow for the provision of increased energy from carbohydrate and fat solutions if fluid is limited. Electrolyte-free solutions allow flexibility in management based on blood biochemistry. The addition of water soluble vitamins and trace minerals should be included within the prescription when possible. For most children parenteral nutrition is temporary with re-establishment of the enteral route as soon as possible.

Nutritional considerations

Energy

Little is known about the energy requirements of infants and children with ARF [8]. The estimated average requirement (EAR) for energy (DRV 1991) [9] for healthy children of the same chronological age can provide an approximate guideline as shown in Table 11.1. Although such recommendations are unlikely to be achieved during acute treatment it is important to provide the maximum energy intake

tolerated within the fluid allowance. The prompt use of glucose polymers added to drinks of choice and flavoured according to preference is recommended. A concentration of 1 kcal (4 kJ)/ml (25% carbohydrate concentration) should be encouraged, but will depend on individual tolerance. Liquid glucose polymers may also be used but often require dilution to be acceptable to children. If fluid is severely restricted ice cubes and lollies can be prepared with an energy dense solution and offered at frequent intervals. Traditional bottled Lucozade (0.73 kcal/ml, 3 kJ/ml) may prove useful as an alternative for those children who refuse to drink prescribed energy supplements. Combined energy supplements of carbohydrate and fat or, alternatively, fat emulsions together with glucose polymers can also be considered (Table 11.3). These can be successfully added to infant formulas to increase the energy content. An energy density of 0.85–1 kcal/ml (3.6–4 kJ/ml) of formula can be achieved in infants up to 6 months of age. Infants of 8 to 12 months of age should tolerate concentrations of 1.0–1.5 kcal/ml (4–6 kJ/ml) without adverse effects. In children over 8 months of age or whose weight is greater than 8 kg it may be advantageous to consider prescribing a nutritionally complete feed which can be modified if necessary to meet individual requirements (Table 11.3).

Some children may have insulin resistance and hyperglycaemia can occur, exacerbated by the absorption of glucose from the peritoneal dialysis fluid and the intake of high carbohydrate supplements. Insulin infusions are rarely required but should be considered to control blood glucose levels along with dietary modification of carbohydrate.

Protein

Protein intake should be reduced when treatment is first initiated and then gradually increased on dialysis with increased solute removal and possible protein losses. The reference nutrient intake (RNI) values for protein (DRV 1991) [9] are not appropriate for the child with ARF and requirements should be individually determined. The age and weight of the child, the biochemistry and dialysis therapy if implemented will all need to be considered. Nutritional guidelines are shown in Table 11.1.

Nutritional supplements via the nasogastric route are frequently relied on to meet protein requirements in the initial stages of treatment. For infants, the commercially available whey-based formulas which

Table 11.3 Nutritional supplements

Supplement	Suggested use
Energy	
Glucose polymers	
(powder) e.g. Polycal, Polycose, Supersoluble Maxijul	Add to infant formula, baby juice, cow's milk, squash, fizzy drinks, tea, milk, ice cubes and lollies
(liquid) e.g. Polycal, Maxijul	Dilute with soda water, fizzy drinks of choice (unless fluid restricted); add to jelly
Fat emulsion	
e.g. Calogen, Liquigen	Add to infant formula, cow's milk, nutritionally complete supplements
Combined fat and carbohydrate	
e.g. Supersoluble Duocal Powder, Liquid Duocal	
Protein	
Protein powders	Add to infant formula, Liquid Duocal, modular feed components
e.g. Protifar, Supersoluble Maxipro HBV	
Renal Specific Infant Formula	
Kindergen PROD	For infants with CRF*
Powder/100 g (7.5 g protein, 507 kcal [2200 kJ], 93 mg phosphate, 3 mmol potassium, 10 mmol sodium)	
20 g powder made up to 100 ml with water (1.5 g protein, 101 kcal [422 kJ], 18.6 mg phosphate, 0.6 mmol potassium, 2 mmol sodium)	
Nutritionally complete	
Nutrini (2.8 g protein, 100 kcal [420 kJ], 39 mg phosphate, 2.6 mmol potassium, 2.3 mmol sodium/100 ml)	For oral or supplementary tube feed infants/children >8 months age and weight >8 kg
Nutrini Extra (3.4 g protein, 150 kcal [627 kJ], 50 mg phosphate, 4 mmol potassium, 3.5 mmol sodium/100 ml)	
Fortijuce (4 g protein, 125 kcal [523 kJ], 60 mg phosphate, 0.7 mmol potassium, 0.5 mmol sodium/100 ml)	
Fortisip (5 g protein, 150 kcal [627 kJ], 80 mg phosphate, 3.8 mmol potassium, 3.4 mmol sodium (sweet and neutral); 7.1 mmol (savoury)/100 ml)	
Suplena (3 g protein, 201 kcal [840 kJ], 79 mg phosphate, 2.9 mmol potassium, 3.5 mmol sodium/100 ml)	
Nepro (7 g protein, 200 kcal [836 kJ], 72 mg phosphate, 2.7 mmol potassium, 3.5 mmol sodium/100 ml)	
Low protein milk substitute	
Sno Pro (0.2 g protein, 67 kcal [280 kJ], <30 mg phosphate, <1.3 mmol potassium, <3.3 mmol sodium, <15 mg calcium/100 ml)	Use as a substitute for cow's milk to reduce protein and phosphate intakes.

* CRF chronic renal failure

are low in phosphate are recommended and can be modified as required. Kindergen PROD, a renal specific low phosphate, low potassium infant formula (Table 11.3) may prove to be beneficial if the infant is not receiving dialysis or is receiving intermittent haemodialysis when serum biochemistry levels are proving difficult to control. The nutritionally complete, high energy feeds for infants which are now available (Infatrini, SMA High Energy) may be considered if blood biochemistry allows. The phosphate content of these products is higher than in standard infant formulas and therefore their use may be limited. For the older child there are a number of nutritionally complete supplements available. Their composition of protein, phosphate and potassium should be assessed prior to use (Table 11.3).

If semi-elemental formulas or feeds are indicated they should be modified to meet individual requirements (pp. 74–6). Introduction should be gradual and delivery is usually by the nasogastric route. Once the child's appetite improves and protein intake is met by diet, energy supplemented drinks can then replace protein containing supplements. Prescribable low protein products can contribute to the energy content of the diet but are rarely necessary. Most children either refuse them or do not take sufficient quantity to be of any value in the diet.

Fluid

The volume of fluid prescribed during conservative treatment is based on insensible fluid requirements of 400 ml/m² body surface area/day or approximately 20 ml/kg body weight/day, with a 12% increase for each degree centigrade above normal body temperature, and a reduction if the child is ventilated. Insensible losses should be added to the previous day's urine output to give the total daily fluid allowance. If the child is being dialysed, the fluid prescription will be determined by monitoring the volume of fluid removed by ultrafiltration plus insensible losses. Ideally fluid removal on dialysis should be flexibly managed to allow for increased 'nutritional space'. Maximal nutrient intakes using supplements should be provided within the fluid allowance and divided as evenly as possible throughout the day. A written prescription plan should be provided for the ward nurses and families.

Electrolytes

Initially, intakes of electrolytes such as potassium, sodium and phosphate are likely to be restricted. Plasma levels and the use of dialysis will dictate requirements thereafter.

High potassium-containing foods which include citrus fruits and fruit juices, bananas, potato crisps and chocolate are among the foods commonly brought into hospital by relatives. All carers should be advised about potassium restriction so that rich food sources are withdrawn and lower potassium alternatives given (Table 11.4). Phosphate restriction can partly be achieved when protein intake, particularly that of dairy products, is reduced (Table 11.5).

Table 11.4 Potassium-rich foods and suggested alternatives

Potassium-rich foods*	Suggested alternatives
Bananas, apricots, kiwi fruit, cherries, avocado, citrus fruits, e.g. oranges, grapefruit; dried fruit, e.g. raisins; tinned fruit in fruit juice; melon, plums, rhubarb, blackcurrants	Apples, pears, tinned fruit in syrup
Fruit juices, e.g. orange, apple, tomato Instant coffee and coffee essence Malted drinks, e.g. Horlicks Cocoa, drinking chocolate	Squash, bottled Lucozade, lemonade and fizzy pop, tea
Potato crisps and potato type snacks, nuts, salt substitutes, Bovril, Marmite	Corn or rice snacks (take account of sodium content), sweetened popcorn, jam, honey, marmalade, syrup
Jacket potatoes, chips (oven and frozen), roast potatoes	Rice (boiled or fried), spaghetti, pasta, bread, chapatti, nan, crackers
Mushrooms, spinach, tomatoes, spaghetti in tomato sauce, baked beans, soups	Carrots, cauliflower, swede, broccoli, cabbage
Chocolate and all foods containing it, toffee, fudge, marzipan, liquorice	Boiled sweets, jellies, mints, marshmallows
Chocolate biscuits	Biscuits – plain, sandwich, jam filled, wafer
Chocolate cake, fruit cake	Cake – plain sponge filled with cream and/or jam Jam tarts, apple pie, doughnuts
Milk, yoghurt, evaporated and condensed milk	Low protein milk substitutes, e.g. double cream and water, Coffeemate, Coffee Compliment

* Allowance will depend on individual assessment

Table 11.5 Phosphate-rich foods and suggested alternatives

Phosphate-rich foods*	Suggested alternatives
Cow's milk (full cream, semi-skimmed, skimmed) Dried milk powder and other milk products	*Infants* Whey-based infant formula, e.g. Farleys First, Cow & Gate Premium for at least 1–2 yrs *Children* Reduce intake, consider low protein milk substitute
Yoghurt, fromage frais, mousse, ice cream, custard made with milk	Reduce intake Custard made with double cream and water or milk substitute
Evaporated milk, condensed milk, single cream	Double cream, imitation cream
Cheese, e.g. Cheddar, processed cheese, cheese spread, Edam	Limit intake and/or encourage use of cottage cheese (within protein allowance) or full fat cream cheese
Egg yolk	Meringues
Cocoa, chocolate and chocolate-containing foods, toffee, fudge	Boiled sweets, mints, dolly mixtures
Sardines, pilchards, tuna	
Baked beans	
Nuts, peanut butter, marzipan	Jam, honey, marmalade, syrup
Coca Cola, and other cola drinks, Dr Pepper and any others containing phosphoric acid	Squash, lemonade, Lucozade

* Allowance will depend on individual assessment

Cow's milk is generally restricted or eliminated from the diet during the acute phase because of its high protein, phosphate and potassium content. Avoidance of cow's milk also reduces the potential cow's milk protein or lactose intolerance which may follow the diarrhoeal prodrome in patients with HUS. If milk restriction proves difficult for some children, the use of a low protein milk substitute, e.g. Sno Pro, can be advantageous (Table 11.3). Reduction of sodium can be achieved by the avoidance of salted snacks and no added salt (Table 11.6). The level of the above restrictions will depend on each individual child and should be frequently monitored so as not to unnecessarily restrict and compromise the overall diet.

Micronutrients

Vitamin supplementation need only be considered if the dialysis treatment is prolonged. A general vitamin supplement should be adequate for the majority of children as appetite improves. Iron supplementation may be indicated in some children during the recovery phase, particularly in those who had a poor diet history prior to the onset of ARF.

Recovery phase

When the acute episode has subsided and the child is passing urine, dialysis can be suspended and dietary restrictions can be gradually reduced. Attention to serum electrolytes and dietary intakes is essential, as replacement therapy may be required if there are major losses of, for example, potassium during the diuretic phase.

Prior to discharge, advice should be given on the gradual reintroduction of foods previously restricted while renal function gradually improves, minimising the risk of vomiting on returning home when normal diet is reintroduced. The opportunity to educate the child and family about the principles of a well-balanced diet should also be taken. Some children may need to continue on energy and vitamin supplements for a short time, with monitoring of their progress in clinic.

Table 11.6 Sodium-rich foods and suggested alternatives

Sodium-rich foods	Suggested alternatives
Salted crisps, nuts and savoury snacks	Herbs and spices instead of salt
Tinned and packet soups	Salt 'n' Shake crisps (without salt)
Pot savouries	Sweet snacks instead of savoury
Other tinned foods with added salt	Unsmoked meats and fish
Smoked meats and fish	* Lower salt tinned products, e.g. reduced salt
Bacon, sausages and other processed meats	baked beans
Cheese	Fresh and home-made foods
Marmite, Bovril, pickles, sauces and chutneys	

* Many processed/manufactured foods contain high amounts of salt and even lower salt varieties can have a high salt content

Outcome of ARF

The prognosis for children with ARF is generally very good. A small percentage of children with HUS and other causes of ARF may be left with impaired renal function and may require ongoing dietary advice.

NEPHROTIC SYNDROME

Nephrotic syndrome (NS) is an uncommon condition and is characterised by heavy proteinuria (>40 mg/hr/m² body surface area or >200 mg/mmol creatinine in an early morning urine) leading to hypoalbuminaemia (<25 g/dl) and oedema. The syndrome can be subdivided into congenital, primary (idiopathic) and secondary types. It is more common in males (2:1) and in Asian children, and characteristically affects the pre-school child. The majority of cases found in childhood are in the primary category, so-called minimal change nephrotic syndrome (MCNS). Such children generally respond to corticosteroid treatment and are classified as having steroid sensitive nephrotic syndrome (SSNS) [10]. Their prognosis is generally good with the likelihood of few long term dietary problems. However, children who relapse frequently and are steroid dependent may require ongoing dietary intervention to monitor and maintain nutritional status and prevent obesity [6]. Growth failure remains an important issue in the long term management [6, 11]. Children who are classified as having steroid resistant nephrotic syndrome (SRNS) have rare disorders with varying responses to treatment and often have a poor prog-

nosis. They should be managed under the direction of a paediatric nephrologist and receive dietetic advice in the long term. The persistent hypoalbuminaemia and hyperlipidaemia could contribute to an increased risk of coronary artery disease which could hasten the progression of renal failure as well as the long term concerns regarding coronary vascular lesions. Such children may benefit from lipid lowering agents [12].

Nutritional issues

In past years, both high and low protein diets have been advised. Animal studies have shown that although albumin synthesis is increased with protein augmentation, there is no significant benefit on plasma albumin concentration or growth [13, 14]. Although a decrease in albuminuria has been shown with low protein diets in animal studies [15], there remains the risk of malnutrition and poor growth, particularly in childhood. Both high and low protein diets are often impractical, resulting in dietary imbalances and additional family anxieties.

Nutritional assessment

The dietitian should be involved following diagnosis and should obtain a detailed dietary history and chart growth parameters for both weight and height [7], including those available prior to diagnosis. These can both help in the prediction of the child's acceptable dry weight and approximate nutritional requirements. Attention to fluid balance and plasma electrolytes is also important.

Nutritional management

Energy and protein

A balanced diet, adequate in both energy (EAR for children of the same chronological age) [9] and protein (1–2 g/kg body weight/day) should be adequate for most children. Energy intake may need to be reduced if the child gains weight rapidly while on corticosteroid therapy.

Sodium

Sodium intake is a major contributor to thirst and weight gain in children with nephrotic syndrome [16]. A 'no added salt' diet (NAS), particularly avoiding salted snacks such as crisps with advice about the high sodium contents of manufactured foods such as tinned and packet soups (fluid and salt containing) and pot savouries, is recommended (Table 11.6). Very low sodium diets and the use of specialist products are rarely necessary. A NAS diet is encouraged for the long term, as part of healthy eating advice, and is preferable to the stop/starting of salt restriction with each relapse of NS.

Fluid

Restriction of fluid should be combined with the 'no added salt' diet in the initial oedematous phase.

Fats/oils

Diet is unlikely to significantly reduce the raised lipid levels commonly recognised in nephrotic patients. However, as part of the initial general healthy eating advice, the use of mono- and polyunsaturated margarines and oils with a reduction of saturated fat intake should be advocated. Such advice should be given with care so as not to compromise total energy intake [12].

Ongoing management

For most children the introduction of steroid therapy can stimulate appetite enormously and in practice the common dietary problem is the prevention of excessive weight gain. Dietary advice to reduce the child's energy intake must be initiated early if obesity is to be prevented. Children will often feel hungry while on steroids and a reduction of in-between meal snacks such as biscuits, crisps, sweets, chocolate and sugar-containing drinks should be encouraged, with the substitution of suitable low energy alternatives. Healthy eating advice for all the family should be reinforced and a leaflet/booklet on healthy eating may be helpful [17].

Nutritional support may be required in children who have prolonged anorexia or where there is evidence of malnutrition. Nutritional supplements taken orally or administered via a nasogastric tube should be considered.

Food allergy

Some reports have suggested that food hypersensitivity, particularly to milk and dairy products, may be involved in the aetiology of glomerular damage of both young and adult patients [18, 19]. Some parents may become very concerned about the possibility of allergies and a trial of a few foods diet may need to be considered, but only under close dietetic supervision. This situation does not tend to commonly arise. Some families also seek advice from alternative medicine practitioners.

Follow-up

It is recommended that the dietitian should see all nephrotic patients at least once in clinic following discharge, to monitor their clinical progress. Dietary guidelines should be reinforced to ensure that the diet is practical and not unnecessarily restrictive.

Psychosocial support

Naturally there is a great deal of concern and worry expressed by parents when they realise that their child may have a chronic illness. Information about the management and treatment of nephrotic syndrome by means of a booklet is recommended (p. 181). A parents' group may enable the sharing of experiences and be of great benefit to parents who feel they are struggling alone.

CONGENITAL NEPHROTIC SYNDROME

Congenital nephrotic syndrome is rare and can present at birth or in the first few months of life.

Proteinuria of up to 5 g/l is unresponsive to treatment and may be associated with a deterioration in renal function. Unilateral or bilateral nephrectomy, dialysis and transplantation may be necessary in infancy. Such patients are likely to require intensive dietetic support and intervention.

Nutritional and medical management

It is likely that fluid intake will be restricted, allowing an intake equivalent to the child's insensible losses (400 ml/m² body surface area/day) plus the previous day's urine output. Sodium intake should also be carefully monitored as some infants have a higher requirement for salt, but will still require a fluid restriction (an appropriate balance needs to be negotiated). Energy intake should be maximised (115–150 kcal [480–630 kJ]/kg body weight/day) within the fluid allowed and a minimum protein intake of 2–4 g/kg body weight/day may be indicated. Serum levels of calcium and phosphate are likely to be deranged and phosphate restriction is often required. The prescription of phosphate binders (Table 11.7) and Alfacalcidol is usually indicated.

Breast fed infants are unlikely to meet dietary requirements and fluid balance may be difficult. Although expressed breast milk can be supplemented with protein and energy supplements, the medical staff and dietitian need to discuss the importance of ensuring adequate nutrition and fluid balance with the parents and supporting them in the possible decision to stop breast feeding. Infant formula may then be modified as required and normal weaning practices should be encouraged between 4 and 6 months of age.

Additional medications that may be prescribed include thyroxine, Captopril, Indomethacin and in some cases erythropoietin and iron therapy. Complete nutritional supplements should be considered for infants over 8 months of age or those who weigh greater than 8 kg as shown in Table 11.3. Many infants are anorexic and require nutritional support via a nasogastric tube or by a gastrostomy button, which may be more appropriate when prolonged supplementary feeding is anticipated [20].

Renal function declines with time and dietary management will change to accommodate the metabolic consequences of chronic renal failure. If the child undergoes bilateral nephrectomy and dialysis is imposed dietary management will be modified accordingly.

CHRONIC RENAL FAILURE

Chronic renal failure (CRF) may be recognised shortly after birth or can present later in life with growth failure and anorexia. The pathophysiology of growth retardation in children is multifactorial and involves malnutrition, metabolic acidosis, renal osteodystrophy and hormonal disturbances. The progression of CRF can be divided into four stages:

(1) *Mild CRF* Glomerular filtration rate (GFR) 50–80 ml/min/1.73 m². Few clinical or biochemical abnormalities are evident when the GFR is above 60% of normal.
(2) *Moderate CRF* GFR 25–50 ml/min/1.73 m². Plasma urea, creatinine and parathyroid hormone (PTH) concentrations start to increase. Mild

Table 11.7 Phosphate binders

	Elemental calcium mg (mmol per tablet)	Dosage	Flavour
Calcium carbonate			
Titralac tablets (420 mg)	168 (4.2)	1–3 tds	Mint
Setler's Tums tablets (500 mg)	200 (5.0)	1–3 tds	Spearmint, peppermint, various fruit flavours
Calcium carbonate (10% solution)	200 (5.0) per 5 ml	5–15 ml tds	—
Rennie Tablets Digestif/Spearmint (680 mg)	272 (6.8)	1 tds	Peppermint/Spearmint
Remegel tablets (800 mg)	320 (8.0)	1–3 tds	Mint
Calcichew tablets (1250 mg)	500 (12.6)	1 tds	Orange
Calcium acetate			
Phosex Tablets (1000 mg)	250 (6.25)	1–3 tds	(swallow whole)

Table 11.8 Causes of chronic renal failure in childhood

Cause	%
Chronic glomerulonephritis, e.g. focal glomerulosclerosis	32
Reflux nephropathy and urinary tract malformation	22
Hereditary – familial, e.g. Alport's syndrome	16
Renal hypoplasia/dysplasia	12
Other diagnosis, e.g. Henoch Schönlein purpura	12
Uncertain	6

anaemia and the reduced renal regulation of water and electrolyte balance may be accompanied by acidosis.

(3) *Severe CRF* GFR $10–25 \, ml/min/1.73 \, m^2$. Marked anaemia, hyperphosphataemia, hypocalcaemia and renal osteodystrophy become evident. Uraemia, anorexia and growth retardation may occur.

(4) *End stage renal failure (ESRF)* GFR $<10 \, ml/min/1.73 \, m^2$. This stage implies the need for dialysis and transplantation [21].

An information booklet about chronic renal failure and its management is recommended (p. 181). The causes of chronic renal failure are shown in Table 11.8.

Management

Children with progressive CRF should be managed under the direction of a specialist centre where the dietitian is a key member of the multidisciplinary team. Since CRF can have a profound effect on growth and development, dietetic advice and support is required early in management and throughout the child's treatment. Dietary aims are to ensure optimal nutrition sufficient for growth and development and to maintain/improve nutritional status and acceptable blood biochemistry. Adequate energy and micronutrients should be ensured, with modification of protein, phosphate, sodium and dietary fats in an attempt to maximise growth and delay progression of renal dysfunction [22]. Individualised dietary prescriptions must be practical if goals are to be achieved and compliance maintained.

Once the child reaches ESRF, many families find nutrition to be one of the most stressful parts of treatment and an understanding of the psychosocial effects of feeding such children is as important as the nutritional advice [23]. Although families may have to travel long distances to the unit, continuity of the dietetic education is essential on the ward or at clinic visits. Regular telephone contact and visits to the home, nursery and school can be invaluable supportive measures. Good communication is essential with other team members to help develop practice, management strategies and shared team philosophies which ultimately lead to better patient and family care. Adequate dietetic time is crucial to provide the close and frequent supervision which is required to monitor and maintain qualitative standards of care for each child, due to the changing needs for growth and development. Attendance on ward rounds, outpatient clinics and psychosocial team meetings are essential. Infants with CRF present particular problems with anorexia and vomiting and nutritional support is now recognised to be crucial in management [20].

Most children with CRF pass through three stages of treatment:

- Pre-dialysis or conservative management
- Dialysis — peritoneal / haemodialysis
- Transplantation.

Dialysis is seen as a 'holding' measure before renal transplantation, although unfortunately some children may remain on dialysis for prolonged periods. There is an increasing trend to transplant children before dialysis is required (pre-emptive transplantation). Living related donor transplantation (LRD) is also being increasingly offered to families. Children with failing renal transplants will inevitably return to the pre-dialysis and dialysis programme and will need individual dietary support.

The stage of treatment and age of the child will influence the nutritional prescription. The overall principles of dietary management for dialysis are discussed.

Nutrition and chronic dialysis

Chronic peritoneal dialysis (CPD) is the preferred dialysis treatment in most centres [24], as it is technically easier than haemodialysis (HD) and the child can be managed at home. Generally, CPD allows a more liberal diet because of the continuous removal of wastes, electrolytes and fluid. Continuous ambulatory peritoneal dialysis (CAPD) involves three to four manual bag changes a day while continuous cycling peritoneal dialysis (CCPD) is performed automatically by a machine overnight. CCPD is now preferred in most units, as it enables the child and family to be free of dialysis bag changes by day. Optichoice allows flexibility in the older child to have a daytime exchange, enabling them to start on dialysis later in the evening. Compared with CAPD, this results in a smaller volume of dialysate in the abdomen during the day and hence reduces the feeling of fullness which may affect appetite.

Haemodialysis (HD) is an intermittent process lasting 3–6 hours, usually performed in hospital three times a week. Diet and fluid on HD is generally more restricted when compared with CPD to minimise the biochemical and fluid fluctuations between dialysis days.

A booklet is available on dietary advice for families (p. 181).

Nutritional assessment in CRF

Children who are commenced on chronic dialysis programmes require a dietary prescription together with the prescription of dialysis and medications. Such advice should meet individual requirements based on frequent nutritional assessment. The clinical and physical examination combined with the nutritional assessment and monitoring techniques all form part of the subjective global assessment in paediatric patients, where anthropometry is the most sensitive marker.

Anthropometry

The accurate measurement and recording of weight and height in older children, and weight, length and head circumference in children under 2 years should be regularly plotted on the appropriate chart to monitor growth [4]. Plotting growth for preterm infants should be corrected up to the age of 2 years. Height velocity should be calculated and recorded annually.

The growth chart may also assist in determining the child's nutritional requirements:

- If the child is within the normal percentile ranges for height (>2nd percentile), energy and micronu-

trient requirements can be based on the recommendations for children of the same chronological age (DRV 1991) [9].
- If the child falls below the normal percentile ranges for height (<2nd percentile), the child's height age may be used to determine acceptable baseline energy and micronutrient requirements when compared with recommended intakes (DRV 1991) [9] and adjusted accordingly thereafter.

Body mass index (BMI) can also form part of the nutritional assessment when calculated and plotted on a BMI chart [25]. Midarm circumference (MAC) may be measured 6 monthly and compared to norms for age, and X-rays of hands and wrists may be measured annually to determine bone age. Skinfold thicknesses (triceps and subscapular) may assist in assessing body protein and fat stores when compared with normal values. They should be carried out under a standard protocol, preferably by the same individual [26], but in practice children are reluctant to participate with the measurement and it tends to be used more for research purposes. Standard deviation scores relative to age, sex and height in the case of severe growth retardation, must always be used when calculating height, weight, height velocity, BMI, MAC and skinfold thicknesses.

Dietary assessment

A 24 hour dietary recall in clinic followed by the recording of a 3 day dietary diary (inclusive of one weekend day) are invaluable when estimating nutritional intakes and individual baseline requirements. The information on prescribed medications, presence or absence of nausea, vomiting, diarrhoea, constipation and energy levels can be helpful in the child's nutritional and medical assessment.

Nutrients should be computer analysed and a written report to the nephrologist and renal nurse, where appropriate, can reinforce discussions and recommendations made with the child and family.

Biochemical/haematological parameters

Comparing and discussing individual serum values with normal age specific reference ranges (Tables 11.2a and 11.2b) will identify abnormalities requiring adjustment in the dietary, medication(s) and/or dialysis prescriptions. The plasma values of particular relevance include:

- Urea, creatinine, sodium, potassium, bicarbonate, albumin, calcium, phosphate, alkaline phosphatase, parathyroid hormone (PTH), glucose, cholesterol and triglyceride.

  Serum albumin is a classical marker of nutritional status and has been shown to correlate with anthropometric indices of the nutritional state and subjective global assessment in adult patients [27]. However, it must be interpreted with care as rapid changes can be related to non-nutritional factors such as the PD loss of albumin, variations in states of hydration, the presence of systemic disease and acute phase response, liver function and a persistent nephrotic state [28].
- Haemoglobin (11–12 g/dl), ferritin (>100 ng/ml) and percent hypochromic cells (<10%) can be used to assess iron status in combination with serum iron and total iron binding capacity (TIBC) to calculate the percent transferrin saturation (TSAT; serum iron × 100 divided by TIBC) which should be maintained at greater than 20%.
- The glomerular filtration rate (GFR), if accurately measured, usually by Cr^{51} EDTA clearance can be used by the nephrologist to predict when dialysis is likely to be required. The nephrologist will often estimate GFR using the Schwartz formula: $40 \times$ ht (cm)/plasma creatinine (μmol/l).

Medications

Many of the prescribed medications are nutrition related (e.g. phosphate binders, oral iron, sodium supplements, vitamins) and should be periodically reviewed by the dietitian as part of the dietary assessment. Children and their families should be advised on the correct administration and timing of medications to ensure compliance, optimise absorption and minimise potential side effects. Ongoing discussion with education and information about each medication should be routine with each dietetic review. The practicalities of taking medications, e.g. at school, should be identified and regimens adjusted accordingly following medical and team discussion.

Fluid balance

This should be assessed as part of the clinical/physical examination as estimations of the child's pre-

dicted dry weight is relevant to the dietary prescription. Fluid allowance will depend upon the aetiology of renal disease, urine output and the fluid removed, if on dialysis.

Psychosocial assessment

As part of the overall nutritional assessment it is essential for the dietitian to become familiar with each child's psychosocial environment. Psychosocial team meetings are invaluable and ideally a home visit made with the renal nurse or social worker prior to, or at initiation of, chronic dialysis is recommended. Thereafter, a 6 monthly update visit made with the renal nurse for those receiving enteral feeding is ideal to reassess knowledge, prescriptions (dialysis, dietary, medications) and management [29].

Dialysis prescription and adequacy

The monitoring of dialysis prescriptions (dose of dialysis, cycles, solution(s), ultrafiltration) and urine output should be carried out in clinic by the nephrologist, renal nurse and dietitian. Dialysis adequacy is monitored by urea kinetic modelling, in particular by calculation of Kt/V (normalised whole body urea clearance) and PNA (protein nitrogen appearance). It is termed as the minimally acceptable dose of dialysis and refers to the dose of dialysis below which a significant increase in morbidity and mortality would occur. In contrast to adult patients, it is difficult to define in paediatrics and as a consequence, published data on delivered dialysis doses, peritoneal transport characteristics and correlations in clinical outcome is limited [28], although in a recent longitudinal analysis of 51 children both the peritoneal transport properties and the intensity of dialysis were shown to independently affect the physical development of children on PD [30].

Evidence based clinical practice guidelines for dialysis prescription that resulted from the National Kidney Foundation – Dialysis Outcomes Quality Initiative (NKF–DOQI) [31] can be used as a basis in paediatric patients, although it should be noted that practice guidelines vary amongst units and currently there is insufficient evidence to make recommendations. Measurements of adequacy should only be used in combination with the medical, clinical and nutritional assessment with each unit having their own protocol.

Dietary principles in CRF

The dietary aims in managing children with CRF require attention to:

- Adequacy of energy intake
- Regulation of protein
- Fluid balance and electrolytes
- Regulation of calcium and phosphate
- Adequacy of micronutrient and iron intakes.

Recommendations depend upon age, stage of management and nutritional assessment.

Energy

The provision of adequate energy is essential to promote growth in all children with CRF, but is particularly important during the pre-dialysis stage of treatment and for children undergoing haemodialysis, when protein intake may be restricted. The EAR for energy for either height age (if the child's height is <2nd percentile) or chronological age if the child falls within percentile ranges, can be used as baseline guidelines as shown in Table 11.9. Raised serum urea levels in combination with increased serum potassium may suggest catabolism and the need to increase energy intake.

High energy, low protein foods

These should be encouraged where possible, e.g. sugar, glucose, jam, marmalade, honey, syrup. The liberal use of poly- or monounsaturated oils in cooking or margarines spread on bread, toast or added to vegetables can also contribute significantly to the child's energy intake.

Energy supplements

These are relied upon to help achieve the child's requirements, because of anorexia, protein restriction and in some cases fluid restriction. There are a number of supplements available which enables a flexible approach with prescription (Table 11.3). They are most commonly used in children pre-dialysis when protein intake is moderated.

Combined fat and carbohydrate supplements, e.g. Duocal powder, or glucose polymer alone if additional fat is not tolerated, can be successfully added to infant formulas and supplementary tube feeds and

the concentrations should be increased gradually. Liquid glucose polymers are more popular if diluted with a fizzy drink or diluted squash but the volume allowed will depend upon fluid allowance. Powdered glucose polymers are useful for those children who drink plenty of water, squash or baby juice. The use of scoops to measure powders ensures better compliance at home and, should the child be admitted into hospital, the prescription can be continued by the nursing staff.

Peritoneal dialysis and energy

Glucose is absorbed from the dialysis fluid during peritoneal dialysis and Edefonti *et al.* reported a mean energy contribution of 9 kcal (38 kJ)/kg body weight/day [32]. For children who require an additional energy supplement while undergoing CPD, it may be of value to consider using a nutritionally complete supplement (Table 11.3) in preference to a high carbohydrate supplement, particularly as protein requirements are increased and because of recognised raised triglyceride levels in children on CPD. Where possible the use of complex carbohydrate foods such as bread, potatoes and cereals should continue to be encouraged. Extraneal PD solution, currently not licensed for children, containing Icodextrin (7.5%) as opposed to glucose as the osmotic agent may in the future be beneficial in paediatric patients to aid ultrafiltration and reduce carbohydrate load.

Protein

The RNI for protein is not generally appropriate for the child with CRF when undergoing dialysis as requirements vary according to the type of dialysis and clinical status and therefore the parameters of nutritional assessment will assist in the individual prescription of protein intake (Table 11.9).

Alterations to protein intake should always be made in conjunction with ensuring adequacy of energy intake. Particular attention to plasma urea, albumin and phosphate levels will help determine protein requirements.

Pre-dialysis

Protein intake is generally reduced and energy optimised during this stage of management to:

Table 11.9 Nutritional guidelines for the child with chronic renal failure (CRF)

	Energy (per kg body wt/day)		Protein (per kg body wt/day)
	(kcal)	(kJ)	(g)
Pre-dialysis			
Infants			
Preterm	120–180	500–750	2.5–3.0
0–0.5	115–150	480–630	1.5–2.1
0.5–1.0	95–150	400–630	1.5–1.8
1.0–2.0	95–120	400–500	1.0–1.8
Children/adolescents			
2.0–puberty	Minimum of EAR		1.0–1.5
pubertal	for chronological age (use height		1.0–1.5
post-pubertal	age if <2nd percentile for height)		1.0–1.5
Peritoneal dialysis (CCPD/CAPD)			
Infants			
Preterm	120–180	500–750	3.0–4.0
0–0.5	115–150	480–630	2.1–3.0
0.5–1.0	95–150	400–630	2.0–3.0
1.0–2.0	95–120	400–500	2.0–3.0
Children/adolescents			
2.0–puberty	Minimum of EAR		1.5–2.0
pubertal	for chronological age (use height age		1.4–1.8
post-pubertal	if <2nd percentile for height)		1.3–1.5
Haemodialysis			
Infants			
Preterm	120–180	500–750	3.0
0–0.5	115–150	480–630	2.1
0.5–1.0	95–150	400–630	1.5–2.0
1.0–2.0	95–120	400–500	1.5–1.8
Children/adolescents			
2.0–puberty	Minimum of EAR		1.0–1.5
pubertal	for chronological age (use height age		1.0–1.5
post-pubertal	if <2nd percentile for height)		1.0–1.5

These are guidelines which will require adjustments based on individual nutritional assessment.
EAR = estimated average requirement (Dietary Reference Values, 1991 [9])

- Minimise uraemia
- Preserve renal function by decreasing hyperfiltration, which may delay the progression to end stage renal disease (ESRD)
- Control hyperphosphataemia (phosphate intake is reduced when protein intake is restricted) [33].

Protein containing supplements are rarely required as most children usually receive sufficient protein from formula or diet.

Peritoneal dialysis

The protein requirements of children on CPD should be generally increased to allow for the reported peritoneal dialysate losses of protein and amino acids, with greatest losses being seen in the smaller, younger child [34]. However, the intake of cow's milk, dairy products and other high phosphate foods (Table 11.5) must be restricted if hyperphosphataemia is to be controlled. Most infants and children require complete nutritional supplements either as sip or tube feeds to meet recommended intakes (Table 11.3).

Peritonitis

The protein requirements of children during episodes of peritonitis or other intercurrent infections are increased. Serum albumin levels are likely to fall and increased intakes of nutritionally complete supplements should be prescribed and encouraged accordingly. Supplementary tube feeding should be considered for those children who fail to take sufficient nutrition by the oral route.

Nutrineal PD solution uses a mixture of amino acids instead of glucose as the osmotic agent. It was developed for use in adults with protein or protein-energy malnutrition and there is little experience of its use in children. However, it may have a place in the management of some children who are in need of nutritional support who are not receiving it, or in children whose protein requirements cannot be met from diet and/or supplements without providing additional dietary phosphate.

Haemodialysis

The protein intakes of children undergoing HD should be adequate for growth but be regulated to minimise fluctuations in pre-dialysis blood urea levels (Table 11.9).

Protein supplements

Infants   Protein powders which are relatively low in phosphate can be added to normal infant formulas, in combination with energy supplements (Table 11.3). Alternatively, infant formulas can be concentrated gradually to provide an increased balance of all nutrients. Frequent monitoring of biochemistry will be required, particularly with respect to potassium, phosphate and urea. Prior to dialysis, Kindergen PROD (a renal specific low phosphate and potassium infant formula) may be beneficial when serum phosphate levels and potassium prove difficult to control, however potassium and phosphate levels may drop too low. A combination of Kindergen PROD with a normal infant formula may be indicated with phosphate and potassium intakes determined by biochemistry. For infants older than 8 months of age, or whose weights are greater than 8 kg, nutritionally complete supplements can be considered (Table 11.3). Com-

bining supplements to achieve specific intakes is a common practice to achieve nutritional and biochemical goals.

Children/adolescents   It is recommended that a nutritionally complete low phosphate supplement is routinely prescribed on the commencement of peritoneal dialysis [35] (Table 11.3) as part of their overall nutritional and dialysis prescription. Such supplements may also be required for children undergoing haemodialysis who fail to achieve recommended intakes. Prescribed supplements should be treated as a medication and if taken orally they are best taken in divided amounts (preferably after food) during the day or as a drink before bed.

Fluid and electrolytes

Fluid

Individual fluid prescription can be devised by calculation of the insensible fluid losses (400 ml/m² body surface area/day) plus the volume of urine output from the previous day. On peritoneal dialysis the volume of fluid removed by ultrafiltration should also be included. Peritoneal dialysis will allow greater flexibility of fluid management as the strengths of glucose solution used in the dialysis fluid can be varied to increase fluid removal. Care must be taken to ensure an adequate fluid intake in those children who are polyuric.

Fluid balance in children on haemodialysis is generally difficult as weight gain between dialysis sessions can be problematic and ideally should not exceed 2–5% of the child's estimated dry weight. Accurate weighing of patients with careful interpretation of the intake and output of fluids is important. The volume of nutritional supplements (Table 11.3) needs to be accounted for and foods with high water content, e.g. jelly, gravy, sauces, custard, may need to be considered when fluid is severely restricted. Education with ongoing discussion and written guidelines may improve compliance.

Sodium

Requirements will be determined by the:

- Aetiology of the renal disease
- Presence of hypertension and oedema
- Stage of management and fluid restriction.

Prior to dialysis a 'no added salt diet' with avoidance of salted snacks should be recommended (Table 11.6). However, there are some diseases which are associated with loss of sodium into the urine and supplements of sodium chloride and/or sodium bicarbonate (if the child is acidotic) are indicated. These should be taken with formula feeds/food, 3–4 times daily to maintain plasma levels. Alternatively, they can be added to a 24 hour feed volume, provided the child is likely to receive the total amount.

The child undergoing CPD should be taught the principles of a 'no added salt diet'. If the child is hypertensive, oedematous or if fluid intake has to be regulated then careful attention to avoid increased sodium intake is important. Dietary assessment and regular discussions are required to remind children and families about salt in the diet.

Infants on chronic dialysis but particularly those on CPD, are at risk of becoming hyponatraemic (Na < 130 mmol/l) when increased strengths of dialysis glucose solutions (e.g. 2.27–3.86%) are required to increase the ultrafiltration of fluid. Sodium intakes of 4–7 mmol/kg body weight/day may be required to maintain sodium balance and medicinal salt supplements are needed.

On haemodialysis a 'no added salt' diet should be encouraged to reduce thirst and fluid intake. This may help in the control of interdialytic weight gain and hypertension. An intake of 1–3 mmol/kg body weight/day is usually acceptable.

Potassium

The dietary management of potassium is dependent on the:

- Aetiology of the renal disease
- Glomerular filtration rate (GFR)
- Stage of management and/or dialysis therapy.

The aim of management is to prevent:

Hyperkalaemia, which generally does not occur until the GFR is <10% of normal (however individual biochemical assessment will dictate requirements).

Possible causes of hyperkalaemia include:

- High dietary intake of potassium
- Catabolism, i.e. inadequate energy intake
- Anti-hypertensive and potassium sparing drugs, e.g. Captopril, Spironolactone
- Constipation.

A haemolysed blood sample will show a falsely high serum potassium level and serum bicarbonate levels must be maintained within the normal range.

Hypokalaemia, which can occur in some renal tubular disorders such as cystinosis where potassium supplements are usually necessary, but will be withdrawn as renal function deteriorates. Other causes of hypokalaemia include the use of diuretics (e.g. Frusemide) and anorexia.

Peritoneal dialysis, because of its more continuous removal of solutes, generally allows a moderate intake of potassium. A good urine output also helps to liberalise potassium restriction. However, care must still be taken against the child indulging in potassium rich drinks and foods, e.g. squash should be encouraged instead of fruit juice to drink; crisps may be taken occasionally but corn snacks are preferable. Particular care should always be taken with infants and children who are anuric or anephric. As haemodialysis is intermittent, more careful dietary control will be necessary to minimise problems with hyperkalaemia (Table 11.4). If treats such as chocolate and crisps are allowed they should be eaten within the first half an hour of dialysis and amounts need to be clearly specified. Hyperkalaemia can result in fatal cardiac arrhythmias; the dangers of hyperkalaemia must be explained and reinforced periodically during management. Ion exchange resins, e.g. calcium resonium, may be required if serum potassium levels are dangerously high, but should only be used at a time of crisis when diet and/or feed prescriptions can be modified no further.

Advice about potassium intake should be modified for each individual and discussed with the child and family. A photographic album of foods rich in potassium and the showing and discussion of potassium results may be helpful in management of the older child who needs to take responsibility for their own care. Intakes need to be reviewed at frequent intervals alongside blood biochemistry and dietary analysis.

Calcium and phosphate

The maintenance of normal serum calcium and phosphate biochemistry and parathyroid hormone (PTH) levels is crucial to achieve normal bone growth and to prevent renal osteodystrophy (combination of both rickets and hyperparathyroidism).

Abnormalities of bone mineral metabolism can be quite advanced before there are any significant changes in serum calcium, phosphate and alkaline phosphatase levels or evidence of changes on bone X-rays. PTH levels are a more sensitive marker and should be monitored regularly – ideally monthly in infants and no less than 3 monthly in older children. Careful management early on in the treatment of CRF includes:

- Dietary phosphate restriction (dairy produce in particular)
- Prescription of a Vitamin D analogue (1α hydroxycholecalciferol; 20–40 ng/kg body weight/day) with monitoring of PTH and plasma calcium values
- Phosphate binders.

Dietary phosphate restriction

Advice to reduce phosphate in the diet should apply throughout all stages of CRF management (Table 11.5) and is likely to be beneficial when the GFR is <75 ml/min/1.73 m² (Norman LJ *et al.*, unpubl. observ.). Normal whey-based infant formulas should be encouraged for infants for at least 1–2 years. Kindergen PROD, usually in combination with a normal infant formula, can be used. Thereafter, cow's milk may be introduced in a restricted amount for each individual child. Nutritional supplements should contain as little phosphate as possible and should be included within the dietary allowance. Guidelines for phosphate intake:

- <400 mg/day in infants
- 400–600 mg/day in children <20 kg body weight
- <800 mg/day in children >20 kg body weight.

During the pre-dialysis stage of treatment or for children undergoing haemodialysis, phosphate intake will be reduced because of protein restriction. However, dietary restriction of phosphate often proves difficult on peritoneal dialysis when protein intake is usually increased. Calcium intake is often compromised when phosphate restriction is adhered to and when there is no additional source of calcium from phosphate binders. Supplementation may need to be considered in some patients.

Vitamin D analogues

The prompt initiation of a Vitamin D analogue (Alfacalcidol, Calcitriol) will help to control hyperparathy-roidism by enhancing the absorption of calcium in the small intestine. Children with GFRs of 50 ml/min/ 1.73 m² or less should ideally be in receipt of such therapy. Prescription is based on serum calcium and PTH levels and is reduced or suspended if calcium levels are above the normal range (Table 11.2a).

Phosphate binders

Calcium carbonate is the first choice phosphate binder and is prescribed when dietary phosphate restriction can no longer control serum phosphate levels (Table 11.7). Tablets should be chewed and taken preferably just before meals/snacks as a lower pH improves binding capacity. Alternatively tablets can be crushed to a fine powder or used in solution which can be added to bottle feeds or overnight/daytime bolus feeds. Calcium carbonate impairs the absorption of iron so should not be taken at the same time as oral iron supplements. Approximately 20–30% of calcium contained in the phosphate binder will be absorbed so raising serum calcium to unacceptable levels in some patients.

Calcium acetate (Phosex) is a more potent phosphate binder and its smaller dosage delivers less elemental calcium to the patient. It must be taken during meals and swallowed whole, which is likely to limit its use in young children. However, it may prove beneficial in the older child who dislikes calcium carbonate preparations and where poor compliance and large doses of medicine are issues. Sevelamer hydrochloride (Renagel capsules) has most recently become available. It is calcium and aluminium-free and acts as a phosphate and cholesterol binder. Its potential to bind essential micronutrients may be of concern and it is not currently licensed for paediatric patients. Some patients with sustained hypercalcaemia and hyperphosphataemia may require a combination of the aforementioned phosphate binders to optimise management. Most PD patients require low calcium dialysate.

Micronutrients

Little is known about the essential micronutrient requirements of children with CRF. They vary with different age, appetite, growth and stage of renal disease. Individualised dietary assessment is therefore essential, taking into account the intakes from diet, micronutrient supplements, infant formulas and nutritionally complete supplements, the latter often being the sole source of nutrition for many patients. Only then can supplementation be individually and safely prescribed, if indicated. The RNIs [9] for healthy children of the same age and sex provide guidelines [36].

Adult renal studies have shown that there are potential dialysate losses of vitamins C, B_6 and folic acid [37]. Published adult recommendations for these vitamins are likely to be too high for the majority of paediatric patients. Recommended intakes based on the RNI and from the few paediatric studies available [38] would suggest intakes of:

- Vitamin C 15 mg (infants) – 60 mg/day
- Vitamin B_6 0.2 mg (infants) – 1.5 mg/day
- Folate 60 μg (infants) – 400 μg/day.

Caution regarding excessive intakes of vitamin C is advised to prevent elevated oxalate levels which could lead to the development of vascular complications [39]. Vitamin A supplementation should be avoided, since elevated levels have been associated with hypercalcaemia, anaemia and hyperlipidaemia [40]. Vitamin D-containing micronutrient supplements should also be avoided so as not to affect the management of renal bone disease. Further research on the links between vitamin B status and homocysteine, an amino acid intermediate, with cardiovascular disease [41] may affect recommendations in the future. Dietary intakes of zinc and copper are often found to be below recommended intakes, with some children requiring supplementation.

Children most at risk of possible micronutrient deficiencies include those who are anorexic and not under the direct care of a specialist unit and dietitian. Children who have prolonged periods on restricted diets (i.e. pre-dialysis) or who have prolonged time on dialysis complicated by peritonitis or other intercurrent infections are also of concern. Infants and children who are receiving nutritional support with the use of complete nutritional supplements, usually by an enteral tube feeding route, may not require supplementation in contrast to older children where diet may be poor and compliance with oral nutritional supplements is questionable.

There is no approved or specially formulated micronutrient supplement currently available for children with renal disease. However, a new supplement with a nutritional profile derived by the specialist interest paediatric renal dietitians group in the UK and Ireland has recently been piloted. Until this formulation is commercially available, prescribed supplements should be free of vitamins A, D, calcium, phosphate, sodium and potassium. To ensure compliance it is important that the taste and presentation of the supplement is acceptable to children. Ketovite tablets providing vitamins C, E and B complex (1–3/day) are currently the most appropriate choice.

Anaemia, iron and chronic renal failure

Most children will develop anaemia by the time their GFR has fallen below 40 ml/min/1.73 m^2, the primary cause being the insufficient production of erythropoietin by the kidneys. Other factors associated with this anaemia include nutrition (iron and/or folate, vitamin B_6 and B_{12} deficiency), blood loss during haemodialysis and gastrointestinal loss, a shortened red blood cell survival, hyperparathyroidism and circulatory inhibitors of erythropoiesis. Management should aim to prevent the development of iron deficiency anaemia and to maintain adequate iron stores with frequent monitoring and discussion of iron status. This requires close team collaboration between nephrologists, dietitians and renal nurses.

Nutritional/dietary assessment Attempts should always be made to encourage foods rich in iron, folic acid and vitamins C and B_{12}, and ensure children are achieving recommended intakes for age and sex (DRV) [9]. Advice to encourage haem iron and advice about non-haem iron and its potential inhibition by phytates in cereal grains and legumes, polyphenols such as tannin in tea, coffee and cocoa and calcium in milk and dairy products should also be given.

Oral iron supplements Oral iron supplements should be prescribed when dietary iron is insufficient to maintain adequate iron stores. Many children can be treated successfully with oral iron, unless their anaemia is severe and their tolerance poor, in which case intravenous iron can be given in addition or instead. Children managed on HD are most likely to require the latter two options, whereas children being conservatively managed or those undergoing peritoneal dialysis are likely to require only oral iron.

Type, dosage and administration The variety of iron preparations available allows a more individualised prescription of liquid, tablet or capsule format. Vitamin C is known to enhance the absorption of iron, but care must be taken not to oversupplement when a combined vitamin C and iron supplement is prescribed. Oral iron should be prescribed at a daily dose of 2–3 mg of elemental iron/kg body weight/day and given in two to three divided daily doses. It is best absorbed in the absence of medications (antacids/phosphate binders), food, infant formulas, milk or nutritional supplements. Ideally, it should be taken 1 hour before or 2 hours following a feed or meal and if possible taken with a micronutrient supplement if one is prescribed. It is not surprising that problems with compliance are common, particularly with the potential side effects such as nausea, vomiting and constipation. The ideal prescription often tends to be impractical and a flexible approach which is conducive to the child's feeds/diet, school and family should be advised. Intravenous iron therapy is increasingly being used for children on HD and in some children on CPD where iron status cannot be successfully improved following oral supplementation.

Information sheets are available designed for professionals to provide dietary advice for children with chronic renal failure on each of the mentioned dietary principles (p. 181).

Nutritional considerations for infants with CRF

Increasing numbers of infants are now receiving treatment for CRF due to improved clinical experience in dialysis techniques and renal transplantation. Although the ultimate goal is a renal transplant, this is a more difficult procedure in the very small child and many centres prefer to promote the growth of the child to a size (>10 kg) where the transplant operation will be easier and, hence, more successful. Optimal nutrition, with or without early dialysis, is therefore essential in the care of such infants and has been one of the most important factors responsible for the improved outcomes and improved growth seen in recent years [42, 43]. Data on growth (without the use of growth hormone) and the dietetic contact necessary to manage and support children and their families receiving chronic peritoneal dialysis and nutritional support was published in 1999 [44]. The data illustrates the essential role of paediatric renal dietitians in the management of such families. The provision of adequate nutrition for growth requires frequent adjustments of nutritional prescriptions in

accordance with blood biochemistry, particularly in children receiving nutritional support and in preschool children.

When diagnosis is first made, there may be a period of conservative management to determine if renal function improves or stabilises. However, supplementary tube feeding may be indicated early to achieve and maintain adequate nutrition for growth. For infants requiring dialysis, CCPD has become the preferred choice and supplementary tube feeding programmes should be commenced at the initiation of dialysis. Nasogastric tubes and percutaneous endoscopic gastrostomy (PEG) tubes are popular in many units; gastrostomy feeding using a gastrostomy button device is also a feeding route of choice (pp. 34–5) [20, 45]. Coleman *et al.* insert a gastrostomy button at the same time as insertion of a chronic dialysis catheter in children under 5 years of age and increasingly practise this in older children when it is anticipated that there will be a struggle to meet the nutritional prescription. Tube feeding reduces some of the parental pressures associated with oral feeding while assuring nutritional and medication prescriptions are met. It is preferable to force feeding, which frequently results in vomiting and/or refusal of formula or food which can have a detrimental effect on normal oral feeding behaviour in the long term [46].

Vomiting can be a persistent problem for some infants and feeding prescriptions should be closely monitored and altered appropriately. Fluid balance should always be enquired about in relation to vomiting as some infants are sensitive to changes in their fluid balance. It cannot be overemphasised how stressful and upsetting this vomiting is for families, particularly mothers, and close dietetic and team support is required in the long term [23]. Gastro-oesophageal reflux and disturbances in gastrointestinal motility may be evident in infants [47] and efforts to detect and treat appropriately are essential. Vomiting of a psychogenic nature may be responsible in some children, particularly those under stressful family circumstances [48]. Families, particularly those of infants, need to be frequently reminded that lack of interest in food and poor eating is very common.

Weaning should be encouraged from the normal age of 4–6 months to develop and maintain normal oral feeding experiences. Long term tube feeding does not preclude oral feeding and following successful renal transplantation normal feeding and drinking will be resumed in the majority of children [43].

Feeding regimens providing a balanced fat and carbohydrate profile to meet energy requirements do not enhance hyperlipidaemia [49].

Nutritional support

The initiation of enteral nutritional support should always be considered when the child's oral intake fails to meet recommended nutritional intakes and when growth velocity is not maintained. If oral supplementation is unsuccessful, then supplementary tube feeding should be instigated early and not after significant nutritional deficits and aversive feeding interactions have developed between the child and family. Discussion with the family and team members as to the most appropriate feeding route for each child should be implemented. Essentially, a shared team philosophy of early and sustained nutritional support is required [20]. Play preparation, with the use of videos, photograph albums, booklets and dolls can assist in teaching and some families find it helpful to talk to others with similar experiences.

Supplementary tube feeding should preferably be carried out overnight by means of an enteral feeding pump to allow oral feeding to be encouraged during the day. However, in practice the majority of infants will require intermittent bolus feeds by day to maintain adequate intakes. Continuous 24 hour feeds, ideally delivered by a portable feeding pump, should only be considered if the latter regimens are not tolerated.

DIET FOLLOWING RENAL TRANSPLANTATION

The ultimate goal for the child with end stage renal failure is a successful renal transplant to restore normal physiology and metabolic function without the aid of dialysis and dietary manipulation. Nutritional management remains an important aspect of treatment and the dietitian should continue to be involved with the ongoing management.

Initial management

Feeding can be commenced on the return of bowel sounds and if there are no complications the child will usually develop an appetite with improving renal function. Children who experience acute tubular necrosis following renal transplantation may require a period of conservative management or dialysis therapy, with dietary prescription, until adequate renal function is achieved. Chronic rejection will result in the child returning to a dialysis programme with appropriate dietary intervention as for chronic renal failure.

Despite successful transplantation with normal renal function there remain concerns that there may be a prolonged transition to exclusive oral nutrition in infants and children who commenced nutritional support via an enteral tube feeding route early in management [50]. Feeding dysfunction and impaired oral motor development appear to be more evident in infants who received nasogastric feeding than in those who had gastrostomy buttons for feeding [51]. It is recommended to cease gastrostomy feeding whenever possible at the time of renal transplantation, in order to stimulate appetite as renal function is restored and higher doses of corticosteroids are prescribed. To do this successfully the medical staff, dietitian and team members need to provide ongoing support to families. Most children do very well and resume normal eating and drinking post-transplant [43, 51]. There will always be exceptions to this approach with some children requiring short periods of nutritional support, particularly in the first few weeks post-transplantation. In such patients a planned and agreed strategy to wean off enteral tube feeding must be implemented. Common experience is that some young children take time to adapt to drinking more fluids. In such cases fluid boluses delivered via the enteral feeding tube may be useful.

Although a renewed appetite is favourable in the initial stages of management, care must be taken to prevent excessive weight gain, which may lead to obesity in the long term. Both the child and family should be reminded of this early in treatment and should follow appropriate dietary advice to prevent this from happening. The principles of a healthy eating, well balanced diet for all the family should be encouraged prior to discharge from hospital. It is advised by the chief medical officer that all patients on immunosuppressive therapy should take care with food hygiene and avoid foods which carry a high risk of food poisoning, e.g. listeria and salmonella, and this needs to be discussed with each child and family.

Hypertension may be present following transplantation and antihypertensive therapy may be required. Weight control and advice about a 'no added salt' diet as part of the healthy eating advice should be encouraged.

Hyperlipidaemia is evident in a large number of patients following transplantation and may put them at risk of developing premature cardiovascular disease [52]. The use of mono- and polyunsaturated fats and oils, with reduction of the total fat intake, should be advised where possible.

Ongoing management

Particular attention should be given to those children who are receiving nutritional support. A transition period to encourage the oral route should be agreed with families and reviewed at clinic appointments. Ideally, bolus feeds should be avoided during the day with minimal feed delivered overnight to stimulate appetite. Many children require a course of post-transplant oral iron despite an adequate intake from diet, which can be confirmed by monitoring iron status. Vitamin and/or trace mineral preparations may be required in those children whose micronutrient intakes are poor.

Adolescents

The prevention of rapid weight gain leading to obesity can be a difficult problem in this age group where body image is important. The patient who was anorexic prior to transplantation may object to advice to reduce food intake to control body weight. Adolescents who experience rapid weight gain and change of body image may be at risk of crash dieting and possible fasting to lose weight. Healthy eating and exercise should always be encouraged, including information on the health risks of alcohol and smoking.

An information booklet for families, on renal transplantation, is recommended (p. 181).

NEPHROGENIC DIABETES INSIPIDUS

Nephrogenic diabetes insipidus (NDI) is a rare inherited disorder where there is renal resistance to anti-diuretic hormone (ADH). The infant with NDI cannot concentrate its urine above 100 mOsm/kg H_2O and therefore presents in the first weeks of life with polyuria, polydipsia, dehydration and hypernatraemia. The excessive fluid intake needed to excrete a normal renal solute load leads to a preference for water intake with consequent failure to thrive, exacerbated by anorexia and vomiting. Diagnosis is made by finding a low urine osmolality which does not respond

to a water deprivation test or anti-diuretic hormone replacement therapy. Decreasing the renal solute load of the feed reduces the volume of urine required for its excretion. Drug treatment is also initiated: thiazides such as Chlorothiazide can reduce the polyuria by as much as 50%; a non-steroidal anti-inflammatory drug, Indomethacin, also reduces urinary output [53] but may cause deleterious side effects so is used with caution.

Nutritional managemen of NDI

A feed presenting a renal solute load of 15 mOsm/kg H_2O per kg body weight will require a fluid intake of greater than 200 ml/kg body weight for excretion. Fluid intakes above this are hard to achieve consistently in young infants and may cause vomiting. The nutritional management of NDI is to provide adequate fluid intake from a low solute feed while providing the EAR for energy and the RNI for protein for height age [9]. The renal solute load of the feed should therefore be reduced to 15 mOsm/kg H_2O per kg body weight or less to decrease obligatory urine excretion. An estimate of the renal solute load of a feed can be made using the following formula:

Ion/protein	Contributory solute load (mOsm/kg H_2O)
1 mmol Na	1
1 mmol K	1
anions	$2 \times (Na + K)$
1 g protein	4

Worked example

Six month old boy weighing 6.8 kg taking 700 ml feed with additional 700 ml water
Feed volume = 100 ml/kg
Water volume = 100 ml/kg
Total fluid volume = 200 ml/kg

	Energy kcal (kJ)	Protein g	Sodium mmol	Potassium mmol
90 g SMA Gold	472 (1973)	10.8	4.9	12.7
45 g Maxijul + water to 700 ml	171 (723)	0	0.4	0.1
Total	643 (2696)	10.8	5.3	12.8
Per kg	95 (396)	1.6	0.8	1.9
Req/kg	95 (396)	1.6		

Renal solute load $= Na + K + (2 \times [Na + K])$
$+ (4 \times protein)$
$= 5.3 + 12.8 + (2 \times [5.3 + 12.8])$
$+ (4 \times 10.8)$
$= 97.5 \text{ mOsm/kg H}_2\text{O}$
$= 14.3 \text{ mOsm/kg H}_2\text{O per kg}$
body weight

Energy supplements are routinely used to meet energy requirements as the amount of formula must be limited to control renal solute load. Weaning solids should be started at the usual age of 4–6 months and should be low in sodium. Some authors suggest a sodium restriction of 1 mmol/kg/day [54] to control the craving for fluids while others consider a 'no added salt' diet to be adequate [53] provided the child is on long term diuretics. If an increase in dietary salt leads to an increase in fluid intake that inhibits appetite for food, then salt intake must be decreased. Regular dietary assessment is necessary to ensure that the child is meeting recommended intakes for energy, protein and micronutrients (DRV) [9]. A high energy diet is to be encouraged using fats and sugars; glucose polymers added to the free water are a useful way to improve energy intake; most infants and children take adequate nutrition orally but if growth falters enteral feeding should be considered. The child must have free access to fluid day and night.

RENAL STONES

Renal stones are relatively uncommon in children within the UK. Presentation is generally between 6 and 15 years of age and boys are affected twice as frequently as girls. Hypercalciuria is present in 40–60% of children with stones. Calcium is the most frequent component of stones occurring in children (90%), although phosphate and oxalate are also present. Normal serum calcium with low to normal phosphate levels are characteristic [55]. Dietary management should include a diet history and 3 day food diary to accurately analyse dietary intake. In children with hypercalciuria, calcium intake should be limited to the recommended intake for chronological age (DRV) [9] and salt intake should be decreased to lessen calcium excretion. The level of calcium in the local water supply should be checked and if necessary deionised water may be indicated. Fluid intake should be encouraged to decrease the renal solute load and

advice about suitable reduced sugar drinks to prevent dental caries should be given. Milk and milk products will usually need to be restricted.

HYPERCALCAEMIA

There are a number of causes of hypercalcaemia [56] which can be defined if the serum calcium is sustained at a level above 2.5 mmol/l with a normal serum phosphate level.

Infants who present with hypercalcaemia, e.g. William's syndrome, are anorexic, irritable and are often constipated. Breast or formula milk is often refused in preference to water. A dietary assessment to determine the child's intake should be performed. Calcium intake should be reduced so as not to exceed recommended levels (DRV) [9]. The prescription of a low calcium formula, e.g. Locasol (0.2 mmol calcium per 100 ml) may be indicated and modified with energy supplements in the infant failing to thrive. It is also advisable to check the level of calcium in the local water supply and to use deionised water if necessary. Other rich sources of dietary calcium, e.g. dairy produce, should be limited.

REFERENCES

1 Siegel NJ, Van Why SK, Boydstun II *et al.* Acute renal failure. In: Holliday MA, Barratt TM, Avner ED (eds) *Paediatric Nephrology*, 3rd edn. Baltimore: Williams & Wilkins, 1994, pp. 1176–81.
2 Brocklebank JT Renal failure in the newly born. *Arch Dis Childh*, 1988, **63** 991–4.
3 Milford DV, Taylor CM New insights into haemolytic uraemic syndrome. *Arch Dis Childh*, 1990, **65** 713–15.
4 Watson AR The management of acute renal failure. *Current Paediatr*, 1991, **1** 103–7.
5 Coleman JE, Watson AR Nutritional support for the child with acute renal failure. *J Hum Nut Diet*, 1992, **5** 99–105.
6 Haycock GB Renal disease. In: McLaren DS, Burman D, Belton NR, Williams AF (eds) *Textbook of Paediatric Nutrition*, 3rd edn. Edinburgh: Churchill Livingstone, 1991, pp. 240–42.
7 Freeman JV *et al.* Cross sectional and weight reference curves for the UK 1990. *Arch Dis Childh*, 1995, **73** 17–24.
8 Grupe WE Nutritional issues in acute renal insufficiency. In: Grand RJ, Sutphen JL, Dietz WH (eds) *Paediatric Nutrition, Theory and Practice*, London: Butterworths, 1987, pp. 582–4.

9 Department of Health Report on Health and Social Subjects No 41. *Dietary Reference Values for Food, Energy and Nutrients for the United Kingdom*, London: The Stationery Office 1991.

10 Report of workshop by British Association for Paediatric Nephrology and Research Unit, Royal College of Physicians. Consensus statement on management and audit potential for steroid responsive nephrotic syndrome. *Arch Dis Childh*, 1994, **70** 151–7.

11 Rees L, Greene SA, Adlord P *et al.* Growth and endocrine function in steroid sensitive nephrotic syndrome. *Arch Dis Childh*, 1988, **63** 484–90.

12 Coleman JE, Watson AR Hyperlipidaemia, diet and simvastatin therapy in steroid resistant nephrotic syndrome of childhood. *Pediatr Nephrol*, 1996, **10** 171–4.

13 Blainey JD High protein diets in the treatment of the nephrotic syndrome. *Clin Sci*, 1954, **13** 567–81.

14 Al-Bander H, Kaysen GA Ineffectiveness of dietary protein augmentation in the management of nephrotic syndrome. *Paediatr Nephrol*, 1991, **5** 482–6.

15 Feehally J, Baker F, Walls J Dietary manipulation in experimental nephrotic syndrome. *Nephron*, 1988, **50** 247–52.

16 Grupe WE Nutritional issues in glomerular damage. In: Grand RJ, Sutphen JL, Dietz WH (eds) *Paediatric Nutrition, Theory and Practice*, London: Butterworths, 1987, pp. 579–81.

17 Watson AR, Coleman JE Dietary management in nephrotic syndrome. *Arch Dis Childh*, 1993, **69** 179–80.

18 Genova R *et al.* Food allergy in steroid resistant nephrotic syndrome. *Lancet*, 1987, 1315–16.

19 Lagrue G, Laurent J, Rostoker G, Lang D Food allergy in idiopathic nephrotic syndrome. *Lancet*, 1987, 277.

20 Watson AR, Coleman JE, Warady BA When and how to use nasogastric and gastrostomy feeding for nutritional support. In: Fine RN, Alexander SR, Warady BA (eds) *CAPD/CCPD in Children*, 2nd edn. Boston: Kluwer Academic Publishers, 1998, 281–301.

21 Watson AR Disorders of the urinary system. In: Campbell AGM, McIntosh N (eds) *Forfar and Arneils Textbook of Paediatrics*, 5th edn. New York: Churchill Livingstone, 1998, 978–84.

22 Wingen A-M, Fabian-Bach C, Schaefer F, Mehls O Randomised multicentre study of a low protein diet on the progression of chronic renal failure in children. *Lancet*, 1997, **349** 1117–23.

23 Norman LJ, Coleman JE, Watson AR Nutritional management in a child on chronic peritoneal dialysis: a team approach. *J Hum Nutr Diet*, 1995, **8** 209–13.

24 Balfe JW, Vigneux A, Williamson J *et al.* The use of CAPD in the treatment of children with end stage renal disease. *Perit Dial Bull*, 1981, **1** 35.

25 Cole TJ *et al.* BMI reference curves. *Arch Dis Childh*, 1995, **73** 25–9.

26 Nelson P, Stover J Principles of nutritional assessment and management of the child with ESRD. In: Fine RN,

Gruskin AB (eds) *End Stage Renal Disease in Children*. Philadelphia: WB Saunders, 1984, pp. 209–26.

27 Churchill DN, Wayne Taylor D, Keshaviah PR *et al.* Adequacy of dialysis and nutrition in continuous peritoneal dialysis: association with clinical outcomes. *J Am Soc Nephrol*, 1996, **7** 198–207.

28 Shaefer F Adequacy of peritoneal dialysis in children. In: Fine RN, Alexander SR, Warady BA (Eds) *CAPD/CCPD in Children*, 2nd edn. Boston: Kluwer Academic Publishers, 1998, pp. 99–118.

29 Wright E, Gartland CE, Watson AR An update programme for children on home peritoneal dialysis. *EDTNA/ERCA*, 1995, **3** 25–7.

30 Shaefer F, Klaus G, Mehls O and the Mid-European Paediatric Dialysis Study Group Peritoneal transport properties and dialysis dose affect growth and nutritional status in children on chronic peritoneal dialysis. *J Am Soc Nephrol*, 1999, **10** 1786–92.

31 National Kidney Foundation Dialysis Outcome Quality Initiative Clinical practice guidelines; peritoneal dialysis adequacy. *Am J Kid Dis*, 1997, **30**(Suppl 2) S67–136.

32 Edefonti A, Picca M, Damiani B *et al.* Dietary prescription based on estimated nitrogen balance during peritoneal dialysis. *Pediatr Nephrol*, 1999, **13** 253–8.

33 Jureidini KF, Hogg RJ, van Renen MJ *et al.* Evaluation of long term aggressive dietary management of chronic renal failure in children. *Pediatr Nephrol*, 1990, **4** 1–10.

34 Quan A, Baum M Protein losses in children on continuous cyclic peritoneal dialysis. *Pediatr Nephrol*, 1996, **10** 728–31.

35 Coleman JE, Watson AR Vitamin, mineral and trace element supplementation of children on chronic peritoneal dialysis. *J Hum Nutr Diet*, 1991, **4** 13–17.

36 Coleman JE Micronutrient supplements for children. *Br J Ren Med*, 1998, **3** 21–3.

37 Kopple JD, Blumenkrantz M Nutritional requirements for patients undergoing continuous ambulatory peritoneal dialysis. *Kidney Int*, 1989, **24** (Suppl 16) 295–302.

38 Warady BA, Kriley M, Uri SA *et al.* Vitamin status of infants receiving long-term peritoneal dialysis. *Paediatr Nephrol*, 1994, **8** 354–6.

39 Shah GM, Ross EA, Sabo A *et al.* Effects of ascorbic acid and pyridoxine supplementation on oxalate metabolism in peritoneal dialysis patients. *Am J Kid Dis*, 1992, **20** 42–9.

40 Norman LJ, Coleman JE, Watson AR *et al.* Nutritional supplements and elevated serum vitamin A levels in children on chronic dialysis. *J Hum Nutr Diet*, 1996, **9** 257–62.

41 Makoff RM, Dwyer J, Rocco MV Folic acid, pyridoxine, cobalamin and homocysteine and their relationship to cardiovascular disease in end stage renal disease. *J Ren Nutr*, 1996, **6** 2–11.

42 Neu AM, Warady BA Special considerations in the care of the infant CAPD/CCPD patient. In: *CAPD/CCPD*

in Children, 2nd edn. Boston: Kluwer Academic Publishers, 1998, pp. 281–301.

43 Ledermann SE, Shaw V, Trompeter, RS Long-term enteral nutrition in infants and young children with chronic renal failure. *Pediatr Nephrol*, 1999, **13** 870–75.

44 Coleman JE, Norman LJ, Watson AR Provision of dietetic care in children on chronic peritoneal dialysis. *J Ren Nutr*, 1999, **9** 145–8.

45 Coleman JE, Watson AR, Rance CH *et al*. Gastrostomy buttons for nutritional support on chronic renal dialysis. *Nephrol Dial Transpl*, 1998, **13** 2041–6.

46 Warady BA, Kriley M, Belden B *et al*. Nutritional and behavioural aspects of nasogastric tube feeding in infants receiving chronic peritoneal dialysis. In: Khanna R (ed) *Advances in Peritoneal Dialysis*. Toronto: University of Toronto Press, 1990, **6** 265–8.

47 Ravelli AM Gastrointestinal function in chronic renal failure. *Pediatr Nephrol*, 1995, **9** 756–62.

48 Gonzalez-Heydrich J, Kerner JA, Steiner H Testing the psychogenic vomiting diagnosis: four paediatric patients. *Am J Dis Childh*, 1991, **145** 913–16.

49 Kari JA, Shaw V, Valance DT *et al*. Effect of enteral feeding on lipid subfractions in children with chronic renal failure. *Pediatr Nephrol*, 1998, **12** 401–404.

50 Strologo LD, Principato F, Sinibaldi D *et al*. Feeding dysfunction in infants with severe chronic renal failure after long-term nasogastric tube feeding. *Pediatr Nephrol*, 1997, **11** 84–6.

51 Coleman JE, Watson AR Growth post-transplantation in children previously treated with chronic dialysis and gastrostomy feeding. In: Khanna R (ed) *Advances in Peritoneal Dialysis*. Toronto: University of Toronto Press, 1990, **14**, 271–3.

52 Drukker A, Turner C, Start K *et al*. Hyperlipidaemia after renal transplantation in children on alternate day corticosteroid therapy. *Clin Nephrol*, 1986, **26** 140–45.

53 Stern P Nephrogenic defects of urinary concentration. In: Edelman CM (ed) *Pediatric Kidney Disease*, 2nd edn. London: Little Brown, 1992.

54 Knoers N, Monnens L Nephrogenic diabetes insipidus. In: Holliday MA, Barratt TM, Avner ED (eds) *Pediatric Nephrology*, 3rd edn. Baltimore: Williams & Wilkins, 1994.

55 Teotia M, Teotia SPS Paediatric nephrolithiasis renal tract stone. In: Wickham JEA, Buck AC (eds) *Metabolic Basis and Clinical Practice*. Edinburgh: Churchill Livingstone, 1990, 439–49.

56 Levene M Metabolic disorders. In: Levene MI (ed) *Jolly's Diseases of Childhood*, 6th edn. Oxford: Blackwell Science, 1991, p. 22.

INFORMATION RESOURCE

All the following are available from: Research Secretary, c/o Children and Young People's Kidney Unit, Nottingham City Hospital NHS Trust, Hucknall Road, Nottingham NG5 1PB

Childhood Nephrotic Syndrome, 2nd edn, 1997.

Your Child and Chronic Renal Failure, 2nd edn, 1998.

Dietary Advice for Children on Dialysis: A guide for families, 1997.

Information sheets designed for professionals to provide dietary advice for children with chronic renal failure, 1998.

Bertie Button. A children's story about gastrostomy button feeding.

Kidney Transplantation in Childhood: A guide for families, 2nd edn, 1999.

CHAPTER 12

The Cardiothoracic System

CONGENITAL HEART DISEASE

The incidence of congenital heart disease (CHD) is approximately 8 in every 1000 live births. It is the largest single group of congenital abnormalities and accounts for approximately 30% of the total. Eight lesions make up 80% of cases, the most common of which are ventricular septal defect, patent ductus arteriosis, atrial septal defect and tetralogy of Fallot.

Congestive heart failure (CHF) describes a set of symptoms and clinical signs which show myocardial dysfunction and cardiac output inadequate to meet the metabolic demands of the body. In infants and children it may be caused by increased cardiac workload. Congenital heart disease is the cause of most congestive heart failure during infancy and childhood. Severe anaemia may also produce congestive heart failure at any age.

Malnutrition and growth retardation are both commonly associated with congenital heart disease and congestive heart failure during infancy [1–9]. Wynn Cameron et al. [10] found that acute and chronic malnutrition occurred in 33% and 64% respectively of hospitalised infants and children with CHD. Although early total surgical correction of the congenital heart lesion may be the optimal treatment for affected infants, in practice not all complex defects are correctable during the neonatal period, with infants being managed on supportive therapy or undergoing palliative surgery. The prolonged nutritional deficits and secondary growth disturbances related to heart defects in infants not undergoing early operative correction may ultimately result in increased surgical risks. It is therefore important that wherever possible nutritional deficits are corrected [11]. Many factors may contribute to reduced growth and poor weight gain in infants and children with congenital heart disease.

Reasons for poor growth in infants with CHD

Many studies have tried to determine the reason for the poor growth seen in many infants and children with CHD. Leitch et al. looked at resting energy expenditure (REE), total energy expenditure (TEE), and energy intake in infants with cyanotic congenital heart disease (CCHD) compared with normal controls. They found that at 2 weeks and 3 months of age infants with CCHD weighed significantly less than infants in the control group. In this study no significant difference was seen in energy intake or REE between the two groups during either period. TEE was slightly increased in the CCHD group at 2 weeks, but a significant increase was seen at 3 months. They concluded that increased TEE but not REE is a primary factor in the reduced growth in infants with CCHD [12, 13]. Other studies have concluded that poor intake was the primary cause of the failure to thrive seen in infants with CHD [14].

Lundell et al. looked at lipid metabolism in two groups of infants with CHD. One group had ventricular septal defects, the other group had cyanotic CHD. The cyanotic group all had transposition of the great arteries and the mean oxygen saturation was 68%. Both groups were given an intravenous (IV) lipid load. Severe growth retardation in infants in both groups was correlated to higher peak levels (after IV lipid load) of linoleic acid in the plasma free fatty acids. The peak levels of linoleic acid in the triglyceride fraction were positively correlated to weight standard deviation score. Peak glycerol levels were higher in the most growth retarded infants, indicating faster intravascular lipolysis. They concluded that their results supported the hypothesis that lipid metabolism is disturbed in infants with CHD [15].

Some or all of the following factors may be involved in the poor growth seen in infants with CHD:

- Fatigue on feeding leading to low total intake
- Fluid restriction
- Poor absorption
- Increased metabolic expenditure
- Early satiety
- Anorexia
- Frequent infections
- Frequent use of antibiotics affecting gut flora.

All these factors will compromise the nutritional adequacy of the child's dietary intake. It is often necessary therefore to manipulate the diet so that a higher concentration of nutrients is obtained from the amount of feed being tolerated.

Intestinal functional in children with CHD

The intestinal function of children with CHD and CHF has been assessed by a number of studies [16–18]. The main findings in these studies were that some of the cardiac infants exhibited mild absorptive abnormalities, mild steatorrhoea, bile salt loss, delayed gastric emptying and excessive enteric protein loss.

The studies concluded that no consistent pattern of gastrointestinal abnormalities was detectable. The mild gastrointestinal defects found were felt to be unrelated to the type or severity of the cardiac lesion, but were thought to be severe enough to be of potential nutritional significance. All the studies concluded that if sufficient energy was provided, weight gain and linear growth could be achieved. Yahov *et al.* [19] found a good correlation between energy intake and weight gain in all their study patients; however a constant weight gain was observed in all patients only when energy intake exceeded 170 kcal (710 kJ)/ kg/day. Below this the most severely nutritionally depleted infants continued to lose weight.

Feeding the infant with cardiac abnormalities

Breastfeeding or expressed breast milk (EBM) is the optimum feed for infants with CHD. In cases of severe fluid restriction, i.e. less than 100 ml/kg, fortification of the breast milk would be necessary. This may be done by the addition 3–5% of an infant formula powder, or by using one of the commercially available breast milk fortifiers (pp. 13, 61). If breast milk is not available it will be necessary to use an infant formula. To meet the nutrient requirements for infants with CHD it is necessary to use a formula with a higher nutrient density than a standard infant formula. Two such formulas are available:

| SMA High Energy | providing 91 kcal (380 kJ)/100 ml 2.0 g protein per 100 ml |
| Infatrini | providing 100 kcal (420 kJ)/100 ml 2.6 g protein per 100 ml |

Table 12.1 shows a comparison of the energy and protein obtained from standard infant formula and fortified infant formula fed at increasing volumes, illustrating the volumes and concentration of feed necessary to facilitate growth in infants with CHD.

A high to very high energy feed may be needed to achieve adequate weight gain and appropriate catch-up growth in infants with CHD. The strength and volume of feed given can be increased as shown in Table 12.2.

If no weight gain is being achieved on full strength Infatrini fed at 150 ml/kg and it is not possible to increase the volume of feed given, then a further gradual increase in energy density of the feed should be undertaken with the addition of Duocal in 0.5% daily increments up to a maximum of 3.5% until weight gain is achieved. The final feed provides an energy density of 1.2 kcal (5kJ)/ml. It may be necessary to reduce the energy density of the feed if it is not being absorbed, significant aspirates are being obtained or the infant develops diarrhoea. When the infant is once more absorbing the feed or diarrhoea has settled, then energy density should be gradually increased again.

Methods of feed administration

The cardiac infant will commonly fail to complete feeds offered orally. This may be due to fatigue brought on by the effort of sucking, anorexia or experiencing a feeling of early satiety. If an infant is regularly failing to complete feeds one of the following strategies should be employed:

- Offer smaller more frequent feeds orally
- Complete feeds via nasogastric tube if necessary
- Give small frequent bolus feeds via nasogastric tube
- Top up small frequent daytime feeds with continuous feeds overnight via an enteral feeding pump
- Give feeds continuously over 24 hrs via an enteral pump.

Table 12.1 A 3 month old infant with a congenital cardiac defect, weight 3.5 kg. Comparison of energy and protein intake from standard infant formula and Infatrini when fed at 100, 120 and 150 ml/kg.

			Energy		Protein
			(kcal)	(kJ)	(g)
Feeding 100 ml/kg					
Total fluid intake 360 ml					
Feeding 45 ml × 3 hourly × 8 feeds					
(a) 360 ml standard infant formula		=	233	974	5.3
	per kg	=	66	276	1.5
(b) 360 ml Infatrini		=	360	1512	9.3
	per kg	=	100	420	2.6
DRV	per kg	=	100 (EAR)*	418	2.1 (RNI)**
Suggested requirements	per kg	=	140+	585	3–4.5
Feeding 120 ml/kg					
Total fluid intake 440 ml					
Feeding 55 ml × 3 hourly × 8 feeds					
(a) 440 ml standard infant formula		=	286	1195	6.6
	per kg	=	81	339	1.8
(b) 440 ml Infatrini		=	440	1848	11.4
	per kg	=	120	505	3.1
DRV	per kg	=	100	418	2.1
Suggested requirements	per kg	=	140+	585	3–4.5
Feeding 150 ml/kg					
Total fluid intake 520 ml					
Feeding 65 ml × 3 hourly × 8 feeds					
(a) 520 ml standard infant formula		=	341	1432	7.8
	per kg	=	97	405	2.2
(b) 520 ml Infatrini		=	520	2184	13.5
	per kg	=	150	630	3.5
DRV	per kg	=	100	418	2.1
Suggested requirements	per kg	=	140+	585	3–4.5

*   Estimated average requirement (Dietary Reference Values) [22]
** Reference nutrient intake (Dietary Reference Values) [22]

Table 12.2 Increasing feed strength and fluid volume using Infatrini

	Fluid ml/kg	Feed	kcal/kg	kJ/kg
Day 1	120 ml	80% Infatrini	96	405
Day 2	120 ml	90% Infatrini	108	455
Day 3	120 ml	100% Infatrini	120	505
Day 4	140 ml	100% Infatrini	140	590
Day 5	150 ml	100% Infatrini	150	630

There have been a number of studies looking at the efficacy of methods of feed administration in infants with CHD. Schwarz *et al.* [20] compared oral feeding, oral daytime feeds plus 12 hours continuous nasogastric feeding overnight, and 24 hours continuous nasogastric feeding in a small group of infants with CHD and CHF. For all patients the feed used was fortified to an energy density of 1 kcal (4 kJ)/ml. During the 5 months of the study only the group of infants receiving 24 hour continuous nasogastric feeds achieved intakes in excess of 140 kcal (585 kJ)/kg/day.

Vanderhoof *et al.* [11] studied a small group of children with complex congenital heart lesions who were all given feeds continuously via a nasogastric tube. These children had all failed to achieve adequate weight gain despite the use of orally administered fortified feeds. Continuous feeding was instigated using the same fortified feeds as had been offered orally. Energy intake and weight measurements were obtained at weekly or monthly intervals. Both mean daily energy intake and mean daily weight gain were greater after initiation of continuous nasogastric feeding. Heymsfield *et al.* [21] suggested that continuous feeding caused a smaller rise in basal metabolic rate and heart rate than occurs after bolus feeds.

Sodium supplementation of infant feeds

Some infants with CHD may be failing to gain weight on an energy intake in excess of 140 kcal (585 kJ)/kg. These infants may need to have to their feeds supplemented with sodium. A 24 hour urine sodium balance should be done to establish urinary sodium losses. Once the level of sodium loss is known, sodium supplementation should be discussed with the medical staff. It should be remembered that an infant feeding 150 ml/kg of a standard infant formula would be receiving 0.9 mmols Na^+/kg (the reference nutrient intake for sodium for an infant aged 0–3 months is 1.5 mmol Na^+/kg [22]).

CHYLOTHORAX

Chylothorax is the accumulation of chyle in a pleural cavity from an internal lymphatic fistula. The origin of the fistula can be congenital, obstructive or traumatic [23]. It is usually right–sided as most of the duct is within the right hemithorax; with damage at the level of the aorta, chyle will appear on the left side.

Figure 12.1 shows the anatomy of the thoracic duct.

Constituents of chyle

Chyle contains fat from the intestinal lacteal system which gives it a characteristically milky appearance and allows an initial bedside test for thoracic duct damage. Sixty to seventy per cent of absorbed dietary fat passes through this system at a concentration of 5–30 g/l. Chyle contains lymphocytes, immunoglobulins, enzymes, triglycerides, cholesterol and fat soluble vitamins. The loss of these nutrients if unchecked would invariably lead to serious metabolic deficit. The concentration of triglycerides in chyle is higher than that of plasma, which can aid differentiation of chylous pleural effusions from those of other origin [24].

This condition can be treated conservatively using a minimal long chain triglyceride (LCT) diet [25, 26],

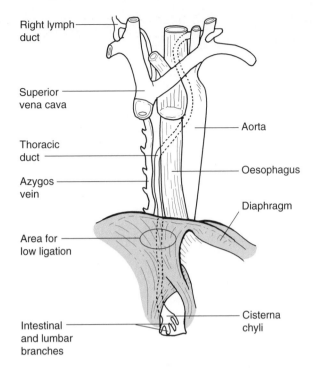

Fig. 12.1 Anatomy of the thoracic duct (Source: Merrigan *et al.* [24])

or a surgical repair of the fistula can be performed [26, 27].

The aim of conservative treatment is to reduce the lymph flow and so allow the fistula to heal. The transport of ingested fats is the principal function of thoracic duct lymph. A minimal LCT diet greatly reduces the lymph flow. After hydrolysis in the intestinal lumen, dietary fats are absorbed as glycerol and fatty acids. In the mucosal cell, long chain fatty acids (12 or more carbon atoms) are re-esterified to triglyceride and pass into the lymph as chylomicra. The medium chain fatty acids (6–10 carbon atoms), however, do not undergo resynthesis and pass directly into the portal vein, where they are transported in the form of 'free fatty acids' bound to albumin (Fig. 12.2).

In humans dietary fat is mainly composed of long chain triglyceride (LCT). Medium chain triglyceride (MCT) containing fatty acids 6–10 carbon atoms in length does not constitute more than a minor proportion of normal dietary fats.

The flow of lymph in the thoracic duct can be increased by up to ten times its resting volume following a high fat meal. A lesser but definite increase

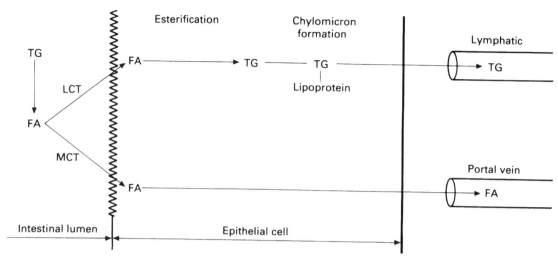

FA = Fatty acid
TG = Triglyceride

Fig. 12.2 Scheme of the pathways of absorbtion of LCT and MCT

is seen after ingestion of a balanced meal containing protein, carbohydrate and fat [28].

Dietary treatment of chylothorax

Minimal LCT diet   A general guide is to give not more than 1g of LCT per year of life up to a maximum of 4 to 5 g LCT per day.

Addition of MCT   The addition of MCT to the diet increases the energy value and palatability.

Vitamin and mineral supplementation   Since a wide range of foods must be either excluded from the diet or taken in reduced quantities, it is essential to check the vitamin and mineral content of the diet, giving supplements as necessary.

Minimal fat feed for the infant with chylothorax

- Monogen
- MCT Pepdite 0–2
- Minimal LCT modular feed based on Peptide Module 767.

Table 12.3 Nutritional content of standard dilution Monogen per 100 ml

Energy	74 kcal/311 kJ
Protein equivalent	2 g
Carbohydrate	12 g
Fat	
MCT	1.86 g
LCT	0.14 g

Monogen

Monogen is a minimal LCT, whole whey protein infant formula. The fat sources are fractionated coconut oil and walnut oil. Table 12.3 shows the nutritional composition of standard dilution Monogen (17.5%).

Monogen should be introduced at half strength, i.e. 8.5% dilution for a minimum of 12 hours. Standard dilution provides 70 kcal (293 kJ)/100 ml. It may therefore be necessary to slowly increase both concentration and energy density of the feed further, particularly in cases of severe fluid restriction. Feed concentration should be increased in 1% increments up to a maximum of 19.5% and then by 0.5% increments up to a maximum of 20.5%. The carbohydrate concentration in Monogen is 12% at standard

Table 12.4 Plan for introduction and increased concentration of Monogen

Monogen dilution	Energy kcal/kJ per 100 ml	Protein g/100 ml	% CHO	% Fat	g LCT
8.5% (half strength)	35/146	1	6	1	0.07
17.5% (full strength)	74/310	2	12	2	0.14
18.5%	78/329	2.1	12.6	2.1	0.15
19.5%	82/346	2.2	13.3	2.2	0.15
20%	84/355	2.25	13.6	2.25	0.16
20.5%	87/364	2.3	13.9	2.3	0.16

CHO = carbohydrate
LCT = long chain triglyceride

dilution and therefore additional carbohydrate should not be added to the feed until after all the preceding stages have been achieved. Monogen is a complete infant formula and does not need to be supplemented with essential fatty acids (EFAs).

Table 12.4 gives the nutritional values of varying concentrations of Monogen used during its introduction and increases in concentration.

If whole cow's milk protein is contraindicated, e.g. in the infant who has had necrotising enterocolitis or where the infant has a proven cow's milk protein intolerance, Monogen would also be contraindicated. In this situation the choice of feed would be MCT Pepdite 0–2.

MCT Pepdite 0–2

MCT Pepdite 0–2 is a low LCT infant formula where the protein source is hydrolysed non-milk protein and amino acids. The LCT content of MCT Pepdite 0–2 is 17% of total fat (0.45 g/100 ml) compared with 7% (0.14 g/100 ml) in Monogen. This level of LCT may not be low enough to adequately reduce chyle flow in some infants with chylothorax.

If MCT Pepdite 0–2 is used, EFA supplements must be given; this will increase the total LCT content of the feed. If chyle flow continues after 48 hours of feeding MCT Pepdite 0–2, a change to a modular minimal LCT feed should be considered.

Minimal LCT modular feed

This is a modular feed using Peptide Module 767 as a minimal fat protein source. To produce a nutritionally adequate infant feed carbohydrate, a suitable fat source, electrolytes, minerals and vitamins must be added. An example of this feed is shown in Table 12.5.

Once the full strength feed is tolerated, weight gain should be reviewed. It may be necessary to increase the energy density of the feed to facilitate weight gain. This should be done by gradual increments of glucose polymer (1% daily) and MCT emulsion, e.g. Liquigen (0.5% daily). A total of 12% carbohydrate as glucose polymer and 4% fat as MCT emulsion should be tolerated.

Points to note:

- The feed may be low in vitamin D and supplementation with Mothers' and Children's Vitamin Drops A,D,C may be necessary
- This feed when taken as the sole source of nutrition does not provide sufficient folate and supplementation will be necessary. 0.1 ml Lexpec should be given daily.

Essential fatty acids

Essential fatty acids (EFAs) in phospholipids are important for maintaining the function and integrity of cellular and subcellular membranes. They also participate in the regulation of cholesterol metabolism, being involved in its transport, breakdown and ultimate excretion. It has been postulated that in infants there may be a specific dietary requirement for these longer chain fatty acids during rapid brain development [29]. A deficiency state arising from an inadequate intake of linoleic acid has been demonstrated in children [30]. Although a specific deficiency state arising from inadequate dietary alpha-linolenic acid has not been demonstrated in healthy humans, it is

Table 12.5 A modular feed for a 3 month old infant who presents with or develops a chylothorax post-surgery and where whole cow's milk protein is contraindicated. Weight = 4 kg Fluid volume = 150 ml/kg

	Na$^+$ (mmol)	K$^+$ (mmol)	Energy (kcal/kJ)	CHO (g)	Prot (g)	MCT (g)
16 g Peptide Module 767			55/231		13.8	
60 g Glucose polymer	0.5	neg	230/965	57		
28 ml Liquigen	0.3		126/530			14
10 g Paediatric Seravit	0.1		30/125	7.5		
5 ml KCl (2 mmol/ml)		10				
4 ml NaCl (1 mmol/ml)	4					
+ water to 600 ml						
Totals	4.9	10	441/1850	64.5	13.8	14
per 100 ml	0.8	1.6	73/308	10.7	2.3	2.3
per kg	1.2	2.5	110/462		3.4	

Day 1	Day 2	Day 3
4 g Peptide Module 767	8 g Peptide Module 767	12 g Peptide Module 767
15 g Glucose polymer	30 g Glucose polymer	45 g Glucose polymer
7 ml Liquigen	14 ml Liquigen	28 ml Liquigen
2.5 g Paediatric Seravit	5 g Paediatric Seravit	7.5 g Paediatric Seravit

Aims in constructing feed: 3 g protein per kg; 70 kcal (239 kJ) per 100 ml; 10% carbohydrate concentration.
The feed concentration should be gradually increased daily as shown to achieve the full strength.

Table 12.6 Comparison of the % energy derived from linoleic and alpha-linolenic acids in current minimal LCT feeds.

	% Energy from C18:2	% Energy from C18:3
Monogen	1.1	0.25
MCT Pepdite 0–2	3.9	0.02
Minimal LCT modular feed	0	0

regarded as a dietary essential [30]. It has been recommended that the neonate requires at least 1% of energy intake from linoleic acid (C18:2) and at least 0.2% of energy from alpha-linolenic acid (C18:3) [22]. Table 12.6 gives a comparison of EFA content of feeds used in the treatment of infants with chylothorax.

If using any of the feeds shown in Table 12.6 other than Monogen, supplementation with a source of EFA is necessary. This should be done using walnut oil. The fatty acid content of this oil will provide linoleic and alpha-linolenic in an acceptable quantity and ratio with a minimum of LCT. Walnut oil contains 55 g linoleic and 12 g alpha-linolenic acids per 100 ml.

EFA supplementation of feeds

The addition of:

- 0.07 ml of walnut oil per 100 ml feed to MCT Pepdite 0–2
- 0.15 ml of walnut oil per 100 ml feed to the minimal LCT Peptide Module 767 based feed

will provide EFA (and at the same time contribute a minimum amount of LCT) to a minimum of:

- 1% energy from linoleic acid
- 0.2% energy from alpha-linolenic acid.

As the energy content of the feed is increased it will be necessary to increase the EFA supplementation proportionately.

Minimal LCT weaning diet

The following foods contain minimal LCT and can be introduced as weaning solids:

- Puréed vegetables, e.g. potato, carrots, swede, green beans
- Puréed fruit, e.g. pears, apples, banana, peaches
- Puréed boiled rice mixed with minimal fat milk
- Baby rice reconstituted with minimal fat milk
- Tins and jars of baby foods containing less than 0.2 g of LCT per 100 g may be included in the diet. These are mainly the fruit based tins and jars. Other dried packet baby foods, tins and jars contain too much LCT and should be avoided.

Even when solids are introduced into the diet of the infant, a minimal LCT milk formula will continue to form a major part of his nutritional intake providing energy, protein, vitamins and minerals. A sample day's menu for the toddler on a minimal LCT diet is given in Table 12.7. The mimimal fat milk can be flavoured with Nesquik powder, fruit Crusha syrups or low fat chocolate flavour topping. It can also be used on breakfast cereals, to make custard or in cereal puddings. Extra energy can be added to the diet by increasing the concentration of glucose polymer in the milk or by using 10–15% solution of glucose polymer to make up fruit squash. Increased energy intake can be achieved by the addition of Liquigen to suitable foods such as mashed potatoes or other root vegetables.

Feeding the older child and adolescent with chylothorax

Keeping the LCT intake to a minimum necessitates the exclusion of many foods including animal and vegetable fats such as butter, lard, margarine and vegetable oils. It also makes it necessary to strictly limit or exclude the protein foods which also have a high fat content such as meat, fatty fish, full fat milk, cheese and eggs. All cakes, pastry and biscuits made with LCT fats must also be avoided. The diet relies on skimmed milk fortified with carbohydrate and MCT as a source of energy, protein, minerals and vitamins. MCT can be added to the diet in the form of MCT oil or MCT emulsion. The use of MCT oil allows fried foods to be included in the diet, such as fried fish, chips and crisps. MCT oil and MCT emulsion can both be used in baking, cakes, biscuits, pastry; all these foods are valuable sources of energy and can greatly enhance the acceptability of the diet to the patient. Table 12.8 lists foods containing minimal LCT which can be used freely in the diet.

Table 12.7 Sample day's menu for a toddler on a minimal LCT diet

Minimal fat milk (MFM)

60 g skimmed milk powder	Provides 500 kcal (2090 kJ)
35 ml Liquigen	22 g protein
30 g glucose polymer	0.8 g LCT
8 g Paediatric Seravit	
+ water to 600 ml	
Use throughout the day as drinks and mixed with appropriate foods	

Breakfast	10 g Rice Krispies + 60 ml MFM Glass MFM (100 ml)
Mid AM	Glass MFM (100 ml) 2 MCT biscuits
Lunch	80 g baked beans + 50 g MCT chips 50 g very low fat fromage frais Glass fruit squash + glucose polymer
Mid PM	Glass MFM (100 ml) Meringue or Rice Krispie cake
Supper	40 g white fish steak fried in MCT oil Fat free mashed potatoes plus 2 teaspoons Liquigen 40 g carrots 50 g very low fat ice cream Jelly
Bedtime	Glass MFM (100 ml)

Total LCT intake for the day = 2 g

Table 12.8 Free foods for minimal LCT diet

All fruits fresh, tinned or frozen (except olives and avocado pear)
All vegetables, fresh, tinned or frozen
Sugar, honey, golden syrup, treacle, jam, marmalade
Jelly and jellied sweets such as Jelly Tots, Jelly Babies, wine gums or fruit pastilles
Boiled sweets, mints (not butter mints)
Fruit sorbets, water ices, ice lollies
Meringue, egg white, Rite Diet egg replacer
Spices and essences
Salt, pepper, vinegar, herbs, tomato ketchup, most chutneys, Marmite, Oxo, Bovril
Fruit juices, fruit squashes, Crusha fruit flavouring syrups, Nesquik fruit flavouring powder, chocolate flavour topping, bottled fruit sauces.
Fizzy drinks, lemonade, cola, Lucozade

The weights and fat contents of foods which can be used to construct a day's meals containing minimal fat for the child or adolescent with chylothorax are given in Table 12.9.

Table 12.9 LCT content of foods suitable for use in LCT diet

Food	LCT per 100 g	Average portion size (g)	LCT per portion (g)
Breakfast cereals			
Cornflakes	0.85	25	0.2
Frosties	0.55	20	0.1
Sugar Puffs	0.85	25	0.2
Special K	1.0	20	0.2
Cocopops	1.0	20	0.2
Rice Krispies	0.8	25	0.2
Ricicles	0.5	20	0.1
Weetabix	2.5	35 (1)	0.9
Puffed Wheat	2.6	15	0.4
Bread			
White, large thin slice	1.6	35	0.4
Matzos	1.0	20	0.2
Crumpets, toasted	1.0	40 (1)	0.4
Dairy foods			
Reduced fat cottage cheese	1.4	50	0.7
Very low fat fromage frais	0.4	50	0.2
Condensed milk, skimmed sweetened	1.0	50	0.5
Very low fat ice cream	0.4	50	0.2
Fish			
White cod fillet, raw	0.7	100	0.7
White cod steak, raw	0.6	100	0.6
Grilled white haddock fillet	0.6	100	0.6
Steamed whiting	0.9	100	0.9
Steamed smoked haddock	0.9	100	0.9
Fish finger	7.2	25 (1)	1.8
Tuna	0.5	100	0.5
Shell fish			
Prawns – peeled	1.7	80	1.4
Crabsticks	0.1	50	neg
Crab (canned)	0.9	50	0.4
Shrimps (canned)	1.2	50	0.6
Cockles, boiled	0.3	50	0.1
Mussels	2.0	50	1.0
Meat and poultry			
Roast turkey, light meat	1.4	70	1.0
Roast chicken, light meat	4.0	25	1.0
Roast lamb, lean	8.0	25	2.0
Roast beef, lean only topside	4.4	45	2.0
Silverside, lean only	4.9	40	2.0
Tinned ham	5.0	40	2.0
Legumes, pasta, rice			
Baked beans in tomato sauce	0.5	200	1.0
Tinned spaghetti in tomato sauce	0.4	125	0.5
White rice, boiled	0.3	150	0.4
White pasta, boiled	0.8	130	1.0

Table 12.10 Day's meals for a 14 year boy with chylothorax (Aim: 4–5 g LCT per day)

Daily milk allowance

Fortified skimmed milk (FSM)
100 g skimmed milk powder
100 g glucose polymer
50 ml Liquigen
+ water to 1000 ml

20% Glucose polymer solution
40 g glucose polymer
+ water to 200 ml

1000 ml FSM provides: 950 kcal (3971 kJ), 36 g protein, 1.3 g LCT

Breakfast	25 g cornflakes + FSM 120 ml orange juice and glucose polymer Apple
Mid AM	Glass of FSM + meringue + 2 MCT biscuits
Lunch	70 g roast turkey (light meat only) 150 g mashed potatoes + 15 ml Liquigen 60 g carrots 120 g tinned fruit + 120 ml custard made with FSM Glass fruit squash made with glucose polymer solution
Mid PM	250 ml FSM + 1 sachet strawberry Build-up + banana + 2 MCT biscuits
Supper	200 g baked beans + 100 g MCT chips Apple pie made with MCT pastry + 100 g very low fat fromage frais
Bedtime	Glass of FSM

Table 12.11 Nutritional analysis of minimal LCT diet for a 14 year old boy showing comparison with current dietary reference values

			DRV*
Energy	(kcal)	2700 (11.3 MJ)	2200 (9.2 MJ)
Protein	(g)	87	42
LCT	(g)	5	
Na	(mmol)	100	70
K	(mmol)	130	80
Ca	(mmol)	42	25
Fe	(μmol)	330	200
Vitamin D	(μg)	13	10
Vitamin A	(RE**μg)	1200	600
Vitamin C	(mg)	165	35

*   Dietary Reference Values [22]
** Retinol equivalent

The final diet may contain 40–70 g MCT, depending on the age and energy requirement of the patient. This would be gradually introduced over a period of 7–10 days in order to avoid abdominal discomfort.

A day's meals for a 14 year old boy with chylothorax is shown in Table 12.10. Table 12.11 gives a nutritional analysis of the diet.

REFERENCES

1 Webb JG, Kiess MC, Chan Yan CC Malnutrition and the heart. *Canad Med Ass J*, 1986, **135** 753–9.
2 Bougle D *et al.* Nutritional treatment of congenital heart disease. *Arch Dis Childh*, 1961, 799–801.
3 Naeye RL Organ and cellular development in congenital heart disease and in alimentary malnutrition. *J Pediatr*, 1965, Sept, 447–8.
4 Krieger I Growth failure and congenital heart disease: energy and nitrogen balance in infants. *Am J Dis Childh*, 1970, **120** 497–504.
5 Pittman JG, Cohen P The pathogenesis of cardiac cachexia. *N England J Med*, 1964, **271** 403–409.
6 Varan B, Tokel K, Yilmaz G Malnutrition and growth failure in cyanotic acyanotic heart disease with and without pulmonary hypertension. *Arch Dis Childh*, 1999, **81** 49–52.
7 Mehrizi A, Drash A Growth disturbance in congenital heart disease. *J Pediatr*, 1962, **61** 418–22.
8 Feldt R, Strictler G, Weidman W Growth of children with congenital heart disease. *Am J Dis Childh*, 1969, **117** 573–9.
9 Huse D, Feldt RH, Nelson RA, Novak LP Infants with congenital heart disease food intake, body weight and energy metabolism. *Am J Dis Childh*, 1975, **129** 65–9.
10 Wynn Cameron J, Rosenthal MD, Olson AD Malnutrition in hospitalized children with congenital heart disease. *Arch Pediatr Adolesc Med*, 1995, **149** 1098–102.
11 Vanderhoof JA, Hofsschire PJ, Baluff M *et al.* Continuous enteral feedings: an important adjunct to the management of complex heart disease. *Am J Dis Childh*, 1982, **136** 825–7.
12 Leitch CA, Karn CA, Peppard RJ *et al.* Increased energy expenditure in infants with cyanotic congenital heart disease. *J Pediatr*, 1998, **133** 755–60.
13 Ackerman IL, Karn CA, Denne SC *et al.* Total but not resting energy expenditure is increased in infants with ventricular septal defects. *Pediatrics*, 1998, **102** 1172–7.
14 Thommessen M, Heiberg A, Kase B Feeding problems in children with congenital heart disease: the impact on energy intake and growth outcome. *Eur J Clin Nutr*, 1992, **46** 457–64.
15 Lundell KH, Sabel KG, Eriksson BO Plasma metabolites after lipid load in infants with congenital heart disease. *Acta Paediatr*, 1999, **88** 718–23.
16 Sonheimer JM, Hamilton JR Intestinal function in infants with severe congenital heart disease. *J Pediatr*, 1978, **92** 572–8.
17 Cavell B Gastric emptying in infants with congenital heart disease. *Acta Paediatr Scand*, 1981, **70** 517–20.
18 Davidson JD *et al.* Protein-losing gastroenteropathy in congestive heart failure. *Lancet*, 1961, **1** 899.
19 Yahov J *et al.* Assessment of intestinal and cardiorespiratory function in children with congenital heart disease on high calorie formulas. *J Pediatr Gastroenterol Nutr*, 1985, **4** 778–85.
20 Schwarz SM *et al.* Enteral nutrition in infants with congenital heart disease and growth failure. *Pediatr*, 1990, **86** 368–73.
21 Heymsfield SB, Hill JO, Evert M Energy expenditure during continuous intragastric infusion of fuel. *Am J Clin Nutr*, 1987, **45** 526–33.
22 Department of Health Report on Health and Social Subjects No. 14 *Dietary Reference Values for food. Energy and Nutrients for the United Kingdom.* London: The Stationery Office, 1991.
23 Bessone LN, Ferguson TB, Burford TH Chylothorax collective review. *Annals Thorac Surg*, Nov 1971, **12** 527–45.
24 Merrigan BA, Winter DC, O'Sullivan GC Chylothorax. *Brit J Surg*, 1997, **84** 15–20.
25 Cooper P, Paes ML Bilateral chylothorax. *Brit J Anaes*, 1991, **66** 387–90.
26 Puntis JWL, Roberts KD, Handy D How should chylothorax be managed? *Arch Dis Childh*, 1987, **62** 593–6.
27 Stringer G, Mercer S, Bass J Surgical management of persistent postoperative chylothorax in children. *Canad J Surg*, 1984, **27** 543–6.
28 Issalbacher KJ, Senior ED Mechanisms of absorption of long and medium chain triglycerides. In: *Medium Chain Triglyceride*. Philadelphia: University of Pensylvania, 1968.
29 Crawford MA, Sinclair AJ Nutritional influences in the evolution of mammalian brain. In: Elliot T, Knight J (eds) *Lipids, Malnutrition and the Developing Brain.* Amsterdam: Elsevier, 1972.
30 Hanson AE *et al.* Eczema and essential fatty acids. *Am J Dis Childh*, 1947, **73** 1–18.

FURTHER READING

Congenital heart disease

Krauss A, Auld A. Metabolic rate of neonates with congenital heart disease. *Arch Dis Childh*, 1975, **50** 539–41.

Mitchell I, Davies P, Day J, Pollock J, Jamieson M, Wheatley D Energy expenditure in congenital heart disease before and after cardiac surgery. *J Thorac Cardiovasc Surg*, 1994, **107** 374–80.

Chylothorax

Hopkins, RL, Akingbola OA, Frieberg EM Chylothorax: Key References. *Ann Thorac Surg*, 1998, **66** 1845–6.
Gracey M, Burke V, Anderson CM Medium chain triglyc-erides in paediatric practice. *Arch Dis Childh*, 1970, **45** 445–52.
Ramos W, Faintuch J Nutritional management of thoracic duct fistula. A comparative study of parenteral verus enteral nutrition. *J Parent Ent Nutr*, 1986, **10** 519–21.
Bond SJ, Guzzetta PC, Snyder ML, Randolph JG Management of paediatric postoperative chylothorax. *Ann Thorac Surg*, 1993, **56** 469–72.
Kosloke AM, Martin LW, Schubert WK Management of chylothorax in children and medium chain triglyceride feedings. *J Ped Surg*, 1974, **9** 365–71.

CHAPTER 13

The Immune System

FOOD ALLERGY AND INTOLERANCE

Food allergy and intolerance is a controversial area to which many symptoms have been attributed. Some of the controversy has come about as a result of problems with definition. Food intolerance has been defined as a reproducible adverse reaction to food or to any of its components which can occur even when the food is eaten unknowingly (blind) [1]. This includes allergy (or hypersensitivity). Food aversion on the other hand is a psychological avoidance caused by emotions associated with food and which does not occur when the food is given blind.

MECHANISMS RESPONSIBLE FOR FOOD INTOLERANCE

A variety of mechanisms are responsible for food intolerance and are listed below, but much controversy exists:

- Some food intolerance occurs as a result of enzyme deficiency such as lactase deficiency or disorders of amino acid or intermediary metabolism, e.g. phenylketonuria. Such intolerances are well documented and are discussed elsewhere in this book.
- Alternatively, some foods may have an unpleasant pharmacological effect, e.g. caffeine in coffee and cola; vasoactive amines in cheese and wine; phenylethylamine in chocolate.
- Some food such as shellfish and strawberries contain histamine-releasing agents which cause adverse reactions.
- An important cause of food intolerance is food allergic disease which may be defined as an adverse clinical reaction to food(s) due to any type of abnormal immune response [1].

- Some symptoms have been reported as being related to food allergy or intolerance but there is much difference of opinion and controversy and aetiology is unknown. These include severe migraine, attention deficit hyperactivity disorder (ADHD), enuresis, arthritis and autism.

The latter two points are discussed in this chapter and the pros and cons of dietary management are reviewed.

FOOD ALLERGY OR INTOLERANCE

Food allergy/intolerance is a large subject and this chapter can only provide an introduction. An effort has been made to concentrate on dietetic principles. The interested reader is directed to the references and particularly to the Further Reading section for information on immunological mechanisms related to food allergy.

Symptoms of food allergy or intolerance may come on quickly or slowly. An immediate reaction can occur when the subject has been exposed to a very small amount of the provoking food and is often (but not always) associated with antibodies of the immunoglobulin E (IgE) class. There is usually little doubt about which food(s) has caused this. Reactions may, however, occur slowly over hours or days and only after a considerable amount of the food has been consumed. This means that it is difficult if not impossible to identify the provoking foods especially if they are foods eaten at every meal, e.g. milk or wheat. Some of the slow onset food intolerance is allergic in nature and probably T cell mediated.

The many symptoms which have been attributed to food allergy are listed in Table 13.1. Some are more

Table 13.1 Symptoms of food allergy/intolerance

	IgE mediated Immediate onset* Within 2 hours	Non-IgE mediated Delayed onset** Within a few hours to 3 days
Gastrointestinal	Swelling of lips, tongue, mouth Oral allergy syndrome Vomiting Colic	Reflux Abdominal pain, bloating Enteropathy Failure to thrive Allergic colitis, rectal bleeding Diarrhoea Constipation
Cutaneous	Urticaria Angio-oedema Erythema, pruritis	Eczema Urticaria (rarely)
Respiratory	Cough/wheeze/sneeze Laryngeal oedema Bronchospasm	Asthma
Systemic	Cardiac arrhythmia Hypotension Anaphylaxis	
Controversial		Migraine Migraine with epilepsy ADHD Enuresis Rheumatoid arthritis Autism

* Occasionally immediate symptoms are not IgE mediated
** 'Late phase' IgE mediated reactions may occur after 4–48 hours

firmly established than others as food related or having an immunological basis.

DEVELOPMENT OF ALLERGIC DISEASE

Allergic disease seems to be on the increase [2]. Although the tendency to develop allergies is inherited it is thought that environmental factors in modern society predispose to allergic disease in susceptible individuals. Hanson and Telemo have reviewed the evidence [3]. They cite several studies showing that children living in clean affluent areas have a greater risk of developing allergies that those in poorer more industrialised areas. There is also some evidence that lack of infectious exposure early in life (including immunisation as opposed to contracting the disease) may predispose to the development of allergic disease. It is also suggested that a normal intestinal flora, e.g. lactobacilli, bifidobacteria, play a major role in the development of the immune system in early life. Babies born in hospital, by caesarian section or fed with formula are colonised by different bacteria, e.g. clostridia, from those traditionally born at home and breast fed and there are suggestions that this change due to modern life may predispose to allergic disease.

Although children tend to grow out of their food allergies it is becoming evident that allergic disorders change and progress from eczema and food allergy to asthma and rhinitis. This phenomenon is referred to as the 'allergic march'. Allergen sensitisation is predominantly against foods in infancy but is largely replaced by inhalants such as house dust mite and pollen in later childhood [4, 5].

TESTS FOR DIAGNOSIS OF FOOD ALLERGY OR INTOLERANCE

IgE mediated allergy

Skin prick tests (SPT)

The skin prick test indicates the presence of allergen specific IgE. Drops of food extract and positive (histamine) control and negative (saline) control are applied using skin pricks. Antihistamine treatment should be discontinued prior to the test. Food allergens eliciting wheals at least 3 mm larger than those induced by the negative control are considered positive; all others are considered negative. However, the positive predictive accuracy of SPTs is less than 50% (when compared with results from double-blind placebo-controlled food challenge studies (DBPCFC)). Negative predictive accuracy is 95% [6]. This means that negative SPT responses are a worthwhile means of excluding IgE mediated allergies, but positive SPT responses only indicate the atopic individual and exclusion diets should not be based on these results.

Radio allergo sorbent test (RAST)

RAST is an *in vitro* assay for identifying food specific IgE antibodies from serum but is considered less sensitive than SPTs. It is also more expensive. This test may be preferred when patients have dermatographism, patients have severe skin disease and limited surface area for testing, patients have difficulty discontinuing antihistamines, or patients have suspected exquisite sensitivity to certain foods [6]. Interpretation of results is as difficult as with SPTs. However SPTs and RAST tests provide useful contributory information when interpreted by clinicians who are familiar with them and taking into account the clinical picture.

Intradermal test

A report of the British Society for Allergy and Environmental Medicine (BSAEM) with the British Society for Nutritional Medicine (BSNM), entitled *Effective Allergy Practice*, does not recommend the use of intradermal tests and states that the significance of positive tests with foods is a matter of controversy [7]. Other medical authorities do not recommend it either and fatalities have been reported after intradermal testing [6].

Non-IgE mediated allergy

Results of non-specific laboratory tests may be abnormal in non-IgE mediated food allergy and for gastrointestinal allergies biopsies may provide much information. However, there are no tests which can identify foods responsible for the symptoms [6]. 'Diagnosis' can only be made by dietary manipulation, i.e. exclusion followed by challenge.

Commercial allergy testing services

Advertised diagnostic methods such as applied kinesiology, hair tests or electrodermal tests were evaluated in a Consumer Association report [8]. The verdict was that known allergies in individuals were not picked up, the services exaggerated the number of allergies and this could result in unnecessarily restricted and inadequate diets. The report suggests that people should not waste their money on these tests.

INFANT FORMULAS FOR COW'S MILK ALLERGIC INFANTS

Protein hydrolysate formulas

The hypoallergenic or semi-elemental infant formula is often the choice for an infant with immediate or delayed adverse reactions to cow's milk. There are a

Table 13.2 Molecular weight range of some hydrolysed infant formulas. (Adapted from Bindels & Boerma 1994 [12] with permission)

Formula	ESPACI classification	<1.5 kDa(%)	1.5–3.5 kDa(%)	3.5–6.0 kDa(%)	>6.0 kDa(%)
Hydrolysed casein					
Alimentum	eHF	96.5	2.5	0.5	0.5
Nutramigen	eHF	95.5	3.5	0.5	0.5
Pregestimil	eHF	97.0	2.0	0.5	0.5
Hydrolysed whey					
Alfare	eHF	88.0	8.0	1.5	2.5
Nan HA	pHF	54.0	20.5	7.5	18.0
Nutrilon Pepti	pHF	84.0	12.0	2.0	2.0
Pepti-Junior	eHF	85.0	11.5	1.5	2.0
Profylac	eHF	83.5	11.5	2.5	2.5

ESPACI = European Society for Paediatric Allergology and Clinical Immunology
eHF = extensively hydrolysed formula
pHF = partially hydrolysed formula

variety of such formulas where the protein has been extensively hydrolysed (Table 6.6). Casein hydrolysates have been in use for over 50 years, whey hydrolysates for rather less time and hydrolysates of pork/soya have been more recently introduced. All these products are regarded as extensively hydrolysed and are in regular use in the UK. However, there is some variation in the degree of hydrolysis, casein products being the most highly hydrolysed with peptide size mostly below 1200 daltons. The slight difference between extensively hydrolysed casein and whey products, which may be clinically insignificant, is illustrated in Table 13.2.

A major problem with these products is palatability: the infant will take them quite readily; the child over 1 year or so will not. Sweetening and flavouring improve the taste. Whey, soya and meat hydrolysates taste marginally better than casein hydrolysates.

Much of the literature on the subject of the use of these formulas relates to IgE mediated allergy. As far as cow's milk sensitive enteropathy is concerned both casein and whey extensively hydrolysed formulas (eHF) have been shown to be satisfactory [9].

It should not be assumed that these formulas will always be tolerated. Anaphylactic reactions have been described with both casein and whey hydrolysates and this has been reviewed by Sampson [10]. Also, late onset adverse reactions to eHF have been reported by Hill *et al.* [11]. Bindels and Boerma suggest that the small amount of peptides larger than 6000 Da present accounts for the rare occurrence of adverse reactions to these products [12]. In fact, the majority of cow's milk allergic infants will tolerate any of the eHF. The highly allergic infant may tolerate one and not another. It is possible that in such a case, casein hydrolysate (being the most highly hydrolysed) will be most successful. On the other hand, a formula based on hydrolysed soy may be preferable for the very highly cow's milk-allergic infant. There is a case for introducing eHF slowly under supervision for such an infant.

There are partially hydrolysed whey based formulas (pHF) available in some European countries, Canada and the USA, but they are not yet available in the UK. They are much more palatable than eHF and much cheaper but have a much larger proportion of peptides larger than 4000 Da, e.g. Nan HA (Table 13.2). They are intended for prophylactic use and are not considered suitable for the treatment of cow's milk allergy/intolerance; there have been many reports of adverse reactions to these products.

Many health workers are troubled by the confusion of names under which these products are marketed worldwide [13]. Classification of molecular weight range is not standard and there is confusion between eHF and pHF. Bindels and Boerma have critcised the classification of eHF and pHF in the European Society for Paediatric Allergology and Clinical Immunology (ESPACI) position paper on hydrolysates published in 1993, as they feel that Nutrilon Pepti should be regarded as eHF not pHF [12].

A study by Rugo *et al.* illustrates the great differences in allergenic activities (using *in vivo* and *in vitro* methods) between the eHF and pHF when looking at children with IgE mediated allergy. There were also some differences between the various eHF studied, casein hydrolysates having the least residual antigenic activity [14].

A joint statement by ESPACI and the European Society for Paediatric Gastroenterology, Hepatology and Nutrition (ESPGHAN) was published in 1999, where current developments and unresolved issues are discussed regarding products used in infants for treatment and prevention of food allergy [15]. They state that 'attempts have been made to classify products according to degree of protein hydrolysis but there is no unanimous agreement on which to base such a classifiation'. It has been recommended by the American Academy of Pediatrics Nutritional Committee that dietary formulas for the treatment of cow's milk protein allergy in infants should be tolerated by at least 90% (with 95% confidence) of groups of infants with documented cow's milk allergy [16].

Amino acid-based formulas

For those few cow's milk allergic children who cannot tolerate eHF an alternative must be found. Neocate (Chapter 6, Table 6.9), a formula where the protein source is pure synthetic amino acids, has been shown to be tolerated by infants and children with both slow onset and quick onset food allergy/intolerance [10, 11, 17, 18, 19]. There are very few reports of adverse reactions to Neocate [20]. McLeish *et al.* compared feed tolerance, palatability and growth in children randomised to receive a whey hydrolysate formula or an amino acid based formula, and there was little difference between the two [21].

Formulas based on whole soy protein isolate

Infant formulas based on whole soy isolate have been available without prescription for many years and no doubt have been used inappropriately, without medical supervision for vague symptoms on a large scale (Chapter 6, Table 6.4). There is a difference of opinion among clinicians as to their usefulness.

Cantini *et al.* feel that the allergenicity/antigenicity of soy formulas has been overemphasised in the literature [22]. Businco *et al.* critically reviewed the literature on the safety of feeding soy formulas to babies with cow's milk allergy. They state that soy formulas are the preferred formulas for children with IgE mediated cow's milk allergy unless there is evidence that the child is allergic to soy [23]. Zeiger *et al.* recently studied the prevalence of soy allergy in children with IgE associated cow's milk allergy. Only 14% of 99 children were allergic to soy and the authors concluded that soy formula is safe for the majority of such children [24].

However, there are frequent reports of adverse reactions to soy formula in cow's milk-intolerant children with slow onset enteropathy or enterocolitis. The American Academy of Pediatrics published recommendations on the use of soy-based formulas for infants in 1998 [25]. Their recommendations are described, with comments in italics:

- Soy based formulas have *no* advantage over cow's milk based formulas for normal infants as a supplement for breast milk. *The report states clearly that breast is best.*

- Soy based formulas are suitable for lactose intolerance.
- The routine use of soy based formula has no proven value in the prevention or management of infant colic. *A systematic review of trials looking at the effectiveness of treatments for infantile colic [26] shows that removing cow's milk protein from the diet (one week trial initially) may be beneficial. The effectiveness of soy was unclear when only trials of good methodological quality were considered. The authors comment that the use of soy formula is debatable and that more research on dietary treatment is necessary.*
- The routine use of soy based formula has no proven value in the prevention of atopic disease in healthy or high risk infants (p. 210).
- Infants with documented cow's milk protein enteropathy or enterocolitis frequently are sensitive to soy and should not be given soy based formula routinely.
- Most infants with documented IgE mediated allergy do well on soy based formula.
- Soy based formulas are not designed or recommended for preterm infants who weigh <1800 g.

Soy formulas are known to be high in aluminium. The American report states that 'term infants with normal renal function do not seem to be at substantial risk of aluminium toxicity from soy based formulas'.

Soy formulas are also high in phytoestrogens of the isoflavone class. The report says that limited human data suggests that soy phytoestrogens have a low affinity for human post-natal oestrogen receptors and low potency in bioassays. *Indeed, Setchell argues that exposure to these phytoestrogens early in life may have long term benefits for hormone dependent diseases such as cancer, osteoporosis and cardiovascular disease [27]. However, phytoestrogens have been implicated as a possible cause of disease in some animal species and in view of the high intake of phytoestrogens by soy fed infants it is suggested that further investigation into the biological effects of long term consumption is needed [28]. Dietitians must be aware that some parents will not wish to use soy formulas for this reason.*

There are practical reasons for including soy in the diet when possible. The formulas taste better and are cheaper than hydrolysates. Soya-containing products such as desserts enhance the variability of a cow's milk-free diet.

Sheep and goat milk

Sheep and goat milk are not suitable for infants with cow's milk protein allergy as their nutritional composition is unsuitable for infant feeding, there is sometimes concern about microbial content and their proteins can be as sensitising as cow's milk protein. Dean *et al.* have shown that there is strong cross reactivity *in vitro* between allergens in all mammalian milks (except human milk) [29]. An infant formula based on goat milk (Nanny) is nutritionally suitable for infants but many cow's milk-allergic infants are likely to be allergic to this also.

Human milk

Breast milk should be encouraged for all infants. Occasionally infants exhibit allergic symptoms while exclusively breast fed. It is known that allergens from the mother's diet can appear in breast milk [30]. Breast fed infants with multiple allergies have been described [31]. The mother should be encouraged to avoid milk and egg and any other food which appears to upset the infant when she eats it. If symptoms cannot be controlled by maternal allergen avoidance breast feeding may very occasionally have to be stopped as a last resort. Isolauri says this particularly applies to infants with atopic dermatitis who have impaired growth [32]. Breast feeding mothers on exclusion diets should be reviewed by a dietitian to check adequacy of their diets as they may need supplements, especially of calcium.

IgE MEDIATED FOOD ALLERGY (USUALLY IMMEDIATE ONSET)

Some symptoms appear within minutes after a very small amount of food has been consumed. Immediate symptoms may affect the gut, the skin and/or the lungs. They include vomiting, abdominal pain, urticaria, angio-oedema (swelling of the face/throat), erythema, pruritis, wheeze and cough.

Symptoms of upper airway obstruction (larygeal oedema), lower airway obstruction (bronchoconstriction), hypotension, cardiac arrhythmias and even heart failure constitute the most severe and sometimes life-threatening reactions. This is known as anaphylactic shock and first symptoms may include sneezing and a tingling sensation on the lips, tongue and throat followed by pallor and feeling unwell, fearful, warm and lightheaded. Generalised erythema, urticaria and angio-oedema are common features but do not always occur. Severe symptoms may recur up to 6 hours after apparent resolution. The presentation of anaphylaxis is varied but the major causes of death are obstruction to the upper airway or shock, hypotension and cardiac arrhythmia [33].

The results of DBPCFC from several studies in the USA have shown that the most common foods to provoke immediate reactions are peanuts, tree nuts, milk, egg, soy and wheat, fish and shellfish [34]. Seeds (e.g. sesame) have also been implicated.

When adverse reactions to foods are immediate the culprit food is usually obvious. Problem food(s) should be avoided and the dietitian has an important role to play. Alternatives to staple foods need to be found, e.g. milk substitute for an infant or wheat substitute for an older child. Since adverse reactions can occur with minute amounts of food and since some sufferers have life-threatening symptoms on exposure to these foods, families must be taught how to avoid foods completely. Some foods, particularly milk or its derivatives, wheat and soy are present in many manufactured foods and parents and children must be taught to read and understand food labelling. However, there are loopholes in the food labelling system and people need to be aware of this too:

- *The 25% rule*. If a manufactured food contains a compound ingredient which comprises less than 25% of the whole, its ingredients do not have to be declared. Many food manufacturers are now voluntarily declaring the presence of peanuts and disregarding the 25% rule. It is hoped that this will, in future, apply to other common allergens such as milk, wheat and soya. In fact some food manufacturers are already doing this.
- *Factory contamination*. Tiny amounts of foods may be present as factory contamination from other food items packaged on the same production lines. For example, most chocolate manufacturers cannot rule out contamination with traces of nuts. This means that many manufactured foods have 'may contain' labels, usually for nuts.
- Goods sold loose or unwrapped, e.g. in bakeries, are generally unlabelled and pose a particular problem for people with severe allergies.

Eating out is also a real problem. Many people working in the catering industry do not understand the severity of the situation and do not take the sufferer's questions seriously. There may be confusion with naming of foods, e.g. peanuts are also known as ground nuts. There is always the danger that a meal may be contaminated from a serving spoon or a knife which has been used for the previous meal that was served.

Peanut allergy

Peanut allergy is of particular importance as it presents early in life, is often severe and does not resolve. It is increasing and 1.3% of under four year olds in Britain are sensitised to peanut. Peanut accounts for the majority of food-related anaphylactic fatalities and about 30% of all cases of anaphylaxis in the community. The status of peanut allergy has been reviewed by Hourihane [35]. Refined peanut oil (as found in most manufactured foods) is safe for most individuals allergic to peanuts but crude oil is sometimes a problem. Although arachis (peanut) oil present in topically applied medications is refined, there is a concern that peanut protein below the limits of detection using current bioassays may sensitise the peanut allergic with damaged skin (e.g. eczema). In fact, many pharmaceutical manufacturers no longer use arachis oil in their preparations. Individuals who are allergic to peanuts are frequently also allergic to tree nuts. However, other legumes do not pose significant problems (even though SPTs to legumes may be positive).

Anaphylaxis

Anaphylaxis is the most severe form of food allergy and may be life threatening. Although peanuts and other nuts are the most common cause of severe allergic reactions, any food is capable of triggering this, particularly milk and egg in young children. Patel *et al.* [33] say that risk factors for especially severe reactions have been poorly documented but may include: history of a previous severe reaction or of increasingly severe reactions; history of asthma; reintroduction of foods following elimination diets for eczema [36]; certain foods are especially noted for their ability to provoke severe reactions (nuts, cow's milk, egg, fish) but any food can be implicated. Such people need to carry injectable adrenaline in case of inadvertant ingestion of the trigger food. Mild allergic reactions may be greatly enhanced in people receiving β blockers.

The dietitian must be aware of the possible severity of adverse reactions and must help the clinician support children and their families to avoid their occurrence. Sampson reported on 6 fatal and 7 near fatal cases of anaphylaxis in children and adolescents. All had asthma. They or their parents were unaware that they had eaten an allergen and nearly all had had previous anaphylactic reactions to the same food. Five of the six fatal cases occurred in public places (four at school) and all the non-fatal cases occurred in private homes (only two in the patient's own home). A delay in administration of adrenaline may have contributed to the fatal or near fatal outcome [37]. There are several reports of anaphylactic reactions to food occurring only after exercise [38].

Food reintroductions

Children tend to grow out of specific food allergies (e.g. milk, egg, wheat, soy) but are less likely to grow out of others (peanuts, tree nuts, fish, shellfish) and so food reintroductions will need to be considered from time to time. As the potential exists for a severe reaction, challenges with foods which have been suspected of provoking immediate severe symptoms should be performed under professional supervision in experienced hospital units. The gold standard for confirming or refuting food allergy is the DBPCFC [34]. Although the DBPCFC is necessary for research, in practice open challenges are more common. However, many children are very reluctant to eat a food which they do not remember having eaten before, or which they have previously been told to avoid. Indeed it is not uncommon for children who have had previous severe reactions to foods to exhibit some degree of food avoidance. It is therefore often advisable to provide the challenge in a single blind form simply to ensure that the child consumes it.

Bock and Sampson have suggested that challenges for suspected immediate allergies should be done in a graded fashion. The starting quantity should be less than that estimated to be required to provoke symptoms in that patient. The dose is then doubled every 15 to 60 minutes until 8–10 g of the dried food (or the equivalent amount of 'wet' food) has been given in a single dose. By this time the subject may have consumed 15–20 g of dried food [34]. In fact, a reasonable serving is probably a good guideline and this of course will vary with age: 8 g of dried food (equivalent to 90 ml fresh milk, or half a large egg) should contain plenty of protein to challenge a small child. Indeed, those who relapse on challenge usually do so on far less than the full dose. The challenge process should be slowed down if there is the slightest sign of a reaction and may take between 2 and 5 hours. If no reaction has occurred, the child can go home with instructions to incorporate that food gradually into the diet.

LATE PHASE OR NON-IgE MEDIATED FOOD ALLERGY (DELAYED ONSET)

Reactions to foods may develop slowly after hours or days and only when a considerable amount of food has been consumed [39]. As with immediate symptoms, adverse reactions can affect the skin, gut or lungs. Symptoms include chronic diarrhoea, abdominal pain, failure to thrive, enteropathy, allergic colitis, constipation, eczema and asthma. The gastrointestinal symptoms are discussed in Chapter 6. More controversial problems which may be related to food allergy/intolerance are migraine, migraine with epilepsy, enuresis, attention deficit hyperactivity disorder (ADHD) and rheumatoid arthritis. Dietary manipulation (elimination and challenge) is the mainstay for diagnosis and treatment of possible delayed food intolerance.

The dietary manipulations involved

The dietary manipulations used for diagnosis are broadly similar whatever the symptoms may be. They may help not only to establish a diagnosis but also to exclude a diagnosis that has been wrongly made. Since restricted diets require a considerable effort on the part of the family a number of points must be considered before a diet is embarked upon.

- Are the clinical symptoms severe enough to warrant a diet? For example, a child with eczema should not be put on a diet unless he has failed to respond to optimum topical treatment.
- Is the child/parent motivated and able to adhere to the diet? Non-compliance renders the diet trial a waste of time.
- Unless a relationship with food seems likely from diet history, other disease should be excluded before embarking on a diet trial, particularly if symptoms are severe (e.g. diarrhoea).

The diagnosis and treatment of food allergy/ intolerance by diet involves three phases of dietary manipulation. The first comprises an appropriate 'diagnostic' elimination diet which should be used for 3 to 6 weeks. The length of time will depend on frequency of symptoms, degree of restriction of diet and type of symptoms involved (improvement in gastrointestinal symptoms may occur within a day or two whereas improvement in eczema may take several weeks). If successful, the diet will result in significant relief of symptoms. The second phase involves a sequential open reintroduction of foods in an effort to identify provoking foods. The third phase is the adherence to a nutritionally adequate maintenance diet excluding the foods which have caused problems.

Attention must always be paid to nutritional adequacy during these dietary manipulations. The initial diagnostic diet may not be nutritionally adequate and supplements of vitamins and calcium may be used (Table 13.5). However, this initial diet is used for only a short time and it can be argued that supplements are unnecessary at this stage. Indeed, highly food intolerant children may be adversely affected by the supplements themselves. Close attention must be paid to nutritional adequacy during the reintroduction phase so that the final diet is adequate and supplements incorporated if necessary.

Throughout the period of dietary manipulations and for at least a week before any diet starts it is extremely useful for the parent (or patient) to keep a symptom score diary. It is then possible to be reasonably objective about change in severity of symptoms. Physical symptoms can be listed at the end of each day and a numerical score can be given for each one (e.g. 0 for no symptoms, 1 to 3 for symptoms which are mild, moderate or severe). Where attention deficit and hyperactivity are concerned it is useful to use a shortened form of the Conners' scale (Table 13.3) [40].

Phase 1: initial diagnostic diet

A full diet history is mandatory before embarking on a diet and may indicate possible provoking foods. It is often stated that parents' histories are notoriously unreliable. This may be true but they are a useful starting point. It is not uncommon for parents to be mistaken as to which foods affect their child and intolerance to staple foods eaten several times a day, such as milk and wheat, often go unnoticed. Keeping a food

Table 13.3 Short form of Conners' Scale for hyperactivity

Observation date . . .	Degree of activity			
	Not at all	Just a little	Pretty much	Very much
Restless or overactive				
Excitable, impulsive				
Disturbs other children				
Short attention span				
Constantly fidgeting				
Inattentive, easily distracted				
Demands must be met immediately				
Cries often and easily				
Mood changes quickly and drastically				
Temper outbursts, explosive and unpredictable behaviour				

diary for some weeks before starting a diet may provide a baseline but seldom adds any useful information about suspect foods which has not been revealed by diet history. A diagnostic elimination diet should avoid disliked foods and foods which are craved or eaten in large amounts. The initial diet may exclude one or a large number of foods. The choice of diet is a matter of clinical judgement taking into account age, severity of symptoms and whether diets have already been tried. There are broadly three levels of dietary restriction – an empirical diet, a few foods diet or an elemental diet.

Empirical diet

An empirical diet is used where food allergy/intolerance is suspected and causative agents are not known. One or several of the most commonly provoking foods are avoided. Studies with children who have delayed reactions to food indicate anecdotally that the most common provoking foods are similar to those listed for immediate reactions to foods except that intolerance to some food additives and chocolate appears more common and intolerance to fish and nuts less common. In infants the most frequent offender is cow's milk based infant formula so a cow's milk-free diet is often used. A diet avoiding egg and milk, together with any known problem foods, is sometimes used for eczema (p. 205). It is not unusual for paediatric gastroenterologists to use a diet free of milk, egg, wheat, rye and possibly soya for children with gastrointestinal symptoms. Several adult centres use a diet free of all grains (some include rice), egg, milk, chocolate and additives. This is sometimes known as a 'hunter gatherer' diet. A very similar diet was described by Rowe and Rowe in 1959 for the diagnosis and treatment of food induced asthma [41].

Additives that are most commonly cited as being potential problems are artificial colours (azo, coal tar and erythrosine dyes; E102–E219), benzoate preservatives (E210–E219), sulphur dioxide preservatives (E220–E224) and nitrite preservatives (E249–E252). However, there are reports of intolerance to some natural colours [42]. Foods containing the above additives usually also contain flavours which do not have E numbers and these cannot be assumed to be inert. Since most manufactured foods containing additives usually include several additives it is difficult to get a picture of which ones give the most problems. An empirical additive-free diet could be considered to avoid artificial colours, benzoate, sulphur dioxide, nitrite preservatives and food flavours where possible. This will automatically exclude major sources of natural colours.

There is some evidence that urticaria may sometimes be provoked by aspirin and this has been used as an argument for removing fruits and vegetables containing natural salicylates from the diet. A self-help group also suggests hyperactive children may be affected by these fruits and vegetables. The only available analysis of salicylate content of fruits and vegetables has been carried out by Swain and Truswell [43] and it is not clearcut which foods should be avoided on such a diet. Intolerance to fruits should not be assumed to be due to salicylate content. Many food intolerant children are affected adversely by some fruits but can tolerate others which contain salicylates.

Problems occur with empirical diets when excluded foods are inadvertently replaced by others which are equally capable of causing adverse reactions, e.g. a child on a milk-free diet may drink soya milk or orange juice instead and it is possible to be equally intolerant of these foods. Failure to respond to an empirical diet does not rule out the possibility of food intolerance. More restricted diets therefore have a role to play.

Few foods diet

There are considerable difficulties in teaching people how to avoid a large number of foods. For very restricted diets it is easier to decide on which foods the child can eat and teach the diet in terms of which foods are allowed rather that concentrating on those that are forbidden. This is the basis for the few foods diet. Three to four weeks is the longest time one should consider using a very restricted diet, although improvement may occur in a shorter time.

The simplest few foods diet to have been described consists of lamb, pears and spring water only. Diets using one meat, one carbohydrate source, one fruit and one vegetable have been used [44]. If no improvement occurs a second diet containing a different set of foods can be used (Table 13.4) [45, 46]. In extreme circumstances one could include rarely eaten foods such as rabbit, venison and sweet potatoes [47].

Since the above diets are extremely rigorous, slightly less restricted diets have been used which make adherence less of a problem (Table 13.5) [48, 49, 50, 51]. It is much more difficult to find a completely different set of foods for a second attempt if the first is not helpful. However, it is possible to monitor progress closely and change or further restrict the diet during the third or fourth week in an

Table 13.4 Two examples of few foods diets

Under two year olds require a nutritionally adequate milk substitute. This diet should not be used for longer than 4 weeks

A	B
Turkey	Lamb
Cabbage, sprouts, broccoli, cauliflower	Carrots, parsnips
Potato, potato flour	Rice, rice flour
Banana	Pear
Soya oil	Sunflower oil
Calcium and vitamins (see Table 13.5)	Calcium and vitamins
Tap water	Tap water

Possible additions: whey-free margarine, sugar for baking
Possible variations: bottled water; rabbit instead of above meats; peaches and apricots, melon, pineapple instead of above fruits

Table 13.5 Less restricted few foods diet

This diet should be used for no more than 4 weeks. Under two year olds require a nutritionally adequate substitute for milk

Choose two foods from each food group

Meat	Lamb, rabbit, turkey, pork
Starchy food	Rice, potato, sweet potato
Vegetables	Broccoli, cauliflower, cabbage, sprouts (brassicas)
	Carrots, parsnips, celery
	Cucumber, marrow, courgettes, melon
	Leeks, onions, asparagus
Fruit	Pears, bananas, peaches and apricots, pineapple

Also included: Sunflower oil, whey-free margarine
　　　　　　　Plain potato crisps
　　　　　　　Small amount of sugar for baking
　　　　　　　Tap or bottled water
　　　　　　　Juice and jam from allowed fruits
　　　　　　　Salt, pepper and herbs in cooking

A calcium (300–400 mg/d) and vitamin supplement is advisable: calcium gluconate effervescent 1 g × 3 daily; or calcium lactate 300 mg × 6 daily; or Sandocal 400 g × 1 tablet daily. Abidec 0.6 ml daily

attempt to achieve eventual success. A diet rather similar to that in Table 13.5 has been described by Bock and Sampson [34].

The acceptability of the few foods diet depends greatly on the dietitian's advice as regards planning menus, giving ideas for meals and recipes for cooking with the foods allowed. Ideas for packed lunches should be given as school canteens cannot be expected to cope adequately with such a restricted diet. For vegetarians one would have to allow a larger range of vegetables, including pulses. The dietitian should keep in touch with the family and be available by telephone. Cost of the diet may be a problem and should be discussed with the family. The few foods diet is most difficult to carry out in the toddler age group. Such children may still be very reliant on milk or formula. Ideally they should take a hydrolysate formula but it may be refused. The diet can be altered to suit the individual. In some circumstances one can make it less restricted by including a larger range of meats, fruits and vegetables.

Few foods diets are generally carried out in the home environment. It is important that the child's lifestyle is not altered, otherwise changes in symp-

toms could be attributed to factors other than change in diet. Regular medication should not be altered preceding or during the diet trial for the same reason. Children on regular medication such as anticonvulsants should remain on these but be switched to a colour/preservative-free version if possible. Attention should be paid to non-food items which may be consumed by small children such as toothpaste (a white toothpaste should be used), chalks and paints.

Hypoallergenic formula only

Hypoallergenic (semi-elemental or amino acid based) formulas can occasionally be justified for children who have not responded to a restricted diet, but this treatment should be very much a last resort as suitable products do not have good taste and tube feeding may be necessary to achieve adequate nutrition. This will involve a hospital admission. Suitable products for older children are listed in Table 6.10. These formulas have been used mainly for children with severe eczema and for gastrointestinal problems [52]. The hypoallergenic formula for the infant is an obvious choice, as discussed earlier in this chapter.

Phase 2: reintroduction of foods

The sufferer or the parent of a child who has experienced significant relief of symptoms on a diet will usually want to continue with it. Ineffective diets must be abandoned. Young infants who have done well on a cow's milk-free formula should not be challenged with cow's milk too soon. Between 9 and 12 months may elapse before a trial of cow's milk. In the meantime the infant should be weaned on to milk-free weaning foods or should follow a careful weaning plan as described (p. 211).

In an older child, if the initial diet avoids several foods, these should be reintroduced singly in order to try and identify trigger foods. Each new food may be tried in a small test quantity, then given in normal amount every day for a week and then incorporated into the diet as desired. A guide to reintroduction of foods is given in Table 13.6. The order of reintroduction should depend on the person's preferences and the need for nutritional adequacy.

Sometimes one sees children whose parents have already put them on diets and they come for advice because the diet is only partially successful or they are worried about nutritional adequacy. A full diet history

Table 13.6 Open reintroduction of foods

Each food should be given in normal quantities daily for a week before being allowed freely in the diet. A test dose may be recommended initially. The order of reintroduction depends on the patient's preference and on which foods were avoided initially

Oats	Porridge oats, Scottish oatcakes, home-made flapjacks (if sugar is already allowed)	Orange	Pure orange juice, oranges, satsumas. If oranges are tolerated all citrus fruit probably are too
Corn	Sweetcorn, home-made popcorn, cornflour, maize flour, cornflakes if malt is tolerated	Sugar	Use ordinary sugar on cereal, in drinks and baking. Some parents comment that small amounts are tolerated whereas larger amounts are not
Meats	Try meats (including offal) singly, e.g. chicken, beef, pork	Chocolate	Try only if sugar is tolerated. If diet is milk-free, use milk-free chocolate
Wheat	Wholemeal or unbleached white flour for baking, egg-free pasta, Shredded Wheat, Puffed Wheat		Cocoa powder in drinks and cooking
Yeast	Pitta bread; ordinary bread (this usually also contains soya)	Carob	Carob confectionery can be tried if chocolate is not tolerated. Check other ingredients – it may contain milk or soya
Rye	Worth trying if wheat is not tolerated; pure rye crisbread; pumpernickel	Tea/coffee	Add milk if this is already in the diet
Cow's milk	Fresh cow's milk, cream, butter, plain yoghurt, milk containing foods with tolerated ingredients, e.g. rice pudding. Try cheese separately later	Peanuts	Plain or salted peanuts (not for under four year olds) Peanut butter
Cow's milk substitute	If cow's milk is not tolerated try substitutes one by one. Infant soya formula or infant hydrolysate formula. Ewe's milk, goat milk for over one year olds (boiled or pasteurised). Supermarket liquid soya milk with additional calcium	Other nuts	Try singly or mixed
		Malt	Malt/malt flavouring is present in most breakfast cereals. Try Rice Krispies if rice is tolerated etc.
		Nitrite/nitrate	Corned beef if beef is tolerated, ham and bacon if pork is tolerated
Egg	Use one whole fresh egg per day for test period. It may be preferred to begin with small amounts of egg in baking	Sodium benzoate	Supermarket lemonade provided other ingredients are tolerated
Fish	Fresh or frozen (not smoked, battered etc.), e.g. cod, herring etc. If one type is not tolerated others may be. Try shellfish separately later	Sodium glutamate	Stock cubes, gravy mixes, flavoured crisps, provided the other ingredients are tolerated
Tomatoes	Fresh tomatoes, canned and pureed tomatoes, ketchup	Sodium metabisulphite	Some squashes, sausages provided the other ingredients are tolerated, dried fruit
Peas/beans	These include peas, green beans, kidney beans, lentils, baked beans in tomato sauce if tomato is tolerated	Vitamins Minerals	These may be given if needed to enhance nutritional adequacy and introduced singly to test tolerance

Other foods, e.g. fruit and vegetables, can be introduced gradually as desired. Manufactured foods such as ice cream, biscuits can be introduced taking into account known sensitivities. Many additives, e.g. colours, flavours, will be introduced as mixtures in manufactured foods such as sweets and canned/bottled drinks. For children with multiple cereal intolerances, flours such as buckwheat, soya, gram (chickpea), wheatstarch may be tried. Some of the special dietary products for gluten-free and low protein diets may be suitable but other ingredients must be checked (they are not strictly prescribable for food allergy)

is essential. The dietitian has an important role to play in ensuring provoking foods are completely avoided and in reintroducing foods in a sequential way to arrive at the broadest possible diet which is nutritionally adequate.

It is not unusual to find that children with multiple symptoms and multiple food allergies/intolerances react differently to different foods. Immediate and delayed reactions can occur in the same individual [53]. It is possible to have immediate reactions to one or more foods and slow onset reactions to others. Where there is a perceived risk of a severe reaction to a food reintroduction, that food should either be avoided or challenged in hospital as previously described. Alternatives must be found for avoided foods especially if they are staples such as milk and wheat. Some older children who cannot manage cow's milk may wish to try sheep or goat milk to see if they tolerate it.

Phase 3: maintenance diet

The maintenance diet has been achieved when the introduction of all foods has been attempted and the child is having the widest possible variety of foods. Nutritional adequacy is paramount and supplements are sometimes necessary. Children without milk will need a calcium supplement [54, 55]. The dietitian plays a vital role in ensuring that people know how to avoid the necessary foods, suggesting alternatives to avoided foods, giving recipes and meal plans where necessary and ensuring adequacy.

Since children often lose their intolerances over time, attempts should be made every 6–12 months to introduce the avoided foods (particularly if they are staples such as milk or wheat). This may happen in an unsupervised way as the result of an accidental or deliberate break in the diet. It is extremely important that introductions of food are performed at home only if there is no danger of a severe immediate reaction.

PRACTICAL TIPS FOR DIETITIANS SUPERVISING EXCLUSION DIETS

A small child who has to avoid cow's milk or formula and has been prescribed Neocate or a hydrolysed protein formula may find it more acceptable if the milk to be discontinued is gradually phased out by mixing with increasing quantities of the new formula. A covered mug may be preferred to an open cup. Flavouring, e.g. with Nesquick if allowed, improves the taste considerably. A different carer other than the main carer may persuade the child to take the new milk. Some older children who have a long history of milk allergy come to dislike milk substitutes (and even dislike milk itself after the intolerance has been outgrown). Drinks which look like milk, based on oats, pea protein and rice as well as soy, are quite popular as vehicles for cereal but children who have these will need a calcium supplement as will any child who does not have milk.

Parents find recipes very useful. Some examples are cakes without egg, biscuits and cakes without wheat, and gravy and sauces without wheat. A general discussion about menu planning is helpful. Advice

may include ideas for packed lunches and weaning foods. Other carers may need to be contacted, e.g. school caterers.

Parents also find lists of manufactured foods useful, e.g. biscuits without milk or soya, margarine without whey, bread without soya, and chocolate without milk. Parents still need to be taught to interpret ingredients lists on manufactured foods and to check that the lists they have are not out of date.

Although children with wheat allergy cannot strictly have gluten-free foods prescribed for them, some general practitioners will prescribe bread, pasta etc. if requested. It is very helpful for parents to have lists of gluten-free/wheatstarch-free foods which are also egg, milk and soya-free if necessary. They may choose to buy some of the items as well as obtain some on prescription (many are not prescribable anyway). It is also useful to tell parents about wheat-free items readily available in supermarkets, e.g. puffed rice cakes, Thai rice noodles. Most supermarkets have a customer helpline and these telephone numbers can be given to parents so they can get information themselves.

CONFIRMATION OF FOOD ALLERGY/INTOLERANCE WITH SPECIAL REFERENCE TO DELAYED FOOD ALLERGY/INTOLERANCE

Double-blind placebo-controlled food challenges (DBPCFC) are regarded as the 'gold standard' for the confirmation of food allergy or intolerance and are essential for some research designs. Bock and Sampson *et al.* have produced a manual recommending DBPCFCs as an office procedure [34]. It states that before a DBPCFC can be designed for an individual, one needs the following information:

- The suspected food(s)
- The timing between ingestion of food and onset of symptoms
- The smallest quantity of food that is suspected to produce symptoms
- The frequency and reproducibility of the reaction
- Whether exercise was associated with the reaction
- The most recent occurrence of food reaction
- A description of signs such as urticaria, asthma, diarrhoea.

This document mainly deals with rapid adverse reactions where the procedure can be performed on a day-care basis. It does briefly discuss delayed reactions but in practice it is much more difficult to perform DBPCFCs for perceived delayed reactions to food [56].

In a series of studies designed to look into a possible relationship between diet and migraine and also hyperactivity [46, 47, 48, 49, 50, 51] children had foods introduced openly after an initial few foods diet in order to target foods for DBPCFC. Where foods appeared to result in a relapse it was very common for parents to report this after up to 3 days or even longer after eating normal amounts of food. It was necessary for the design of the DBPCFC to take these open findings into account. This involved giving challenge and placebo phases each for a week with a 1–2 week washout period in between. During these studies there were many open reports of foods causing problems in the raw but not the cooked state (e.g. raw apple or tomato as opposed to the cooked version). Such phenomena have been described anecdotally by others [57]. It was felt, therefore, that the DBPCFC should involve challenge foods in their native state or at least in the state in which they appeared to cause problems openly. An additional problem was sometimes the amount of food which seemed to be needed to provoke a reaction openly. It was often impossible (e.g. with wheat) to disguise the necessary amount for DBPCFC. This meant that DBPCFCs could only be performed on a subgroup of the patients who relapsed during open reintroductions of foods. Those designing research protocols for perceived slow onset food intolerance must be aware of these potential problems.

Before embarking on DBPCFCs for delayed onset food intolerance, attention should be given to the following points:

- The required amount of provoking food must first be established. It is extremely important to ensure that enough of the food is given. This is just as important as ensuring that only a tiny dose is given initially for suspected severe immediate reactions.
- The provoking food must be hidden in other food and this (placebo and excipient) must be food which is known to be tolerated in the amount to be used.
- A challenge performed during a quiescent phase of the disease may give a different result from a challenge performed at another time.
- The placebo must be indistinguishable from the challenge.

- The provoking food should be given in the same form as that which caused a relapse on open reintroduction, e.g. dried milk cannot be assumed to affect the individual in the same way as fresh milk.
- When dealing with children the material must be palatable or the child will refuse it. Amounts must be small enough for a child to manage.
- The child must not break the diet during the DBPCFC. Those who are subject to adverse reactions to food may also be intolerant of inhaled substances or skin contact. Such a reaction during DBPCFC may remain undetected and give spurious results.
- Owing to the subjective nature of some delayed symptoms (e.g. headaches) it has been suggested that more than one challenge and placebo period should be performed. If each period lasts 1 week the time span is more than most parents would tolerate.

DISCUSSION OF SPECIFIC SYMPTOMS

Eczema

The majority of children with eczema respond well to emollients and intermittent topical steroids. Diet may be considered in those whose eczema remains troublesome. The role of diet is controversial and environmental allergens (e.g. house dust mite, smoke and pollen), heat, infected skin (often *Staphylococcus aureus*) and stress as well as food may cause exacerbation of eczema. These multiple triggers can make the role of diet difficult to ascertain.

There are differences in approach between people working in this field [58]. In several studies in the USA the initial approach has been to perform skin prick and RAST tests, followed by DBPCFCs for foods which gave positive tests; 8–10 g dried food was given which may provoke an erythematous rash (and gastrointestinal and/or respiratory symptoms) after 2 hours or so [59, 60]. Elimination diets were based on these DBPCFC results. This study design seems to make the assumption that the immediate rashes result in worsening of eczema and also precludes the possibility of looking for delayed adverse reactions to larger amounts of food. However, significant improvement in eczema has been reported on the above diets. Sampson has described a 'late phase' IgE response to food which continues to have effect 24–48 hours later and establishes the more chronic inflammatory picture [61]. It has been estimated that approximately 40% of infants and young children with moderate/severe atopic dermatitis have food allergy but that this is not a common cause in older children and adults [62].

Others have used different study designs, getting improvement by open diet manipulation and then confirming the diagnosis with DBPCFC. Hill and Hosking identified three groups of children with cow's milk allergy [39]. The first, an IgE sensitised group, shows features of immediate cutaneous eruptions and anaphylaxis. The second, non-IgE sensitised group develops gastrointestinal symptoms within hours of ingesting moderate amounts of milk and the third, non-IgE sensitised group shows gastrointestinal symptoms with or without eczematous and/or bronchitic symptoms after ingesting milk over hours or days. Also, Sloper *et al.* reported exacerbation of eczema after 1–3 days in a study comprising a food elimination diet followed by DBPCFC. They commented that eczema improved in 74% of patients and response was not affected by age. Immediate skin changes in this study were unusual [63]. Sloper *et al.* also report that the clinical outcome of food elimination could not be predicted by the initial SPT, serum immunoglobulins, or total or specific IgE [64].

A popular view in the UK is that children with eczema can be affected by food in several ways:

● Immediate allergic symptoms
This can happen within minutes to 2 hours or so and after small (sometimes minute) amounts of food have been eaten. Skin symptoms may include erythema, urticaria and angio-oedema, but gastrointestinal symptoms, wheeze etc. may also occur. Anaphylaxis is an occasional occurrence.

● Delayed food allergy/intolerance
This can happen up to 3 days or so after starting a food which is then given regularly. This may cause eczema to worsen. Diarrhoea and abdominal pain may also occur. Caffarelli *et al.* looked specifically at the prevalence of gastrointestinal symptoms in children with eczema and concluded that diarrhoea, regurgitation and vomiting are significantly more common in children with eczema (especially those with diffuse distribution) than in control children [65].

● Scratching
Itching may occur after certain foods. If children then rub and scratch their skin this will cause inflam-

mation and bleeding and will make infection more likely.

Possible criteria for selecting children for a diet trial include [58]:

● Positive SPTs and RASTs
This indicates an allergic child but as already discussed, children frequently are clinically tolerant of foods which give positive test results. If successful diets have been based on these results it must be borne in mind that the child may be avoiding more foods than is necessary. Negative results invariably preclude IgE mediated food allergy but not food allergy mediated by other immune mechanisms.

● Parental reports of food intolerance
These reports can be very inaccurate but a detailed diet history is essential as the dietitian may be able to obtain useful information. Also, reports of severe immediate reactions to foods must be taken seriously.

● Clinical criteria
Although there is no strong data to back this up it is common to offer diet trial to those with the most extensive eczema, those with multiple symptoms and those under 3 years old (and particularly those under 1 year).

● Parental wishes to try dietary approach

DBPCFCs are rarely performed in the UK outside research studies. The most usual procedure for children who have not responded to optimum topical treatment is to try a milk and egg-free diet, also avoiding known triggers [58, 63]. If an empirical diet has failed one may be tempted to try a few foods approach. Results of studies using this approach have been disappointing. Pike *et al.* found that a few foods approach appeared to benefit some children but DBPCFCs did not confirm this [47]. Mabin *et al.* found that children given a few foods diet failed to show any benefit when compared with a control group [66].

Several UK reports describe the results of dietary manipulation for eczema as disappointing [58, 67]. Perhaps this is particularly so where older children are investigated and in tertiary referral centres which see the patients who have already failed to respond to diet.

A link between food allergy and eczema is a popular conception. If the child fits some of the possible criteria above and the parents wish to try this approach they should have the opportunity to explore the diet approach with professional help. Otherwise they are likely to try it alone with all the nutritional hazards that this might involve. Parents must be encouraged to carry on with prophylactic topical treatment even if diet is successful.

Asthma

Asthma can be induced by food but the prevalence is low [68]. People who have food-induced asthma almost always have cutaneous and/or gastrointestinal symptoms as well as asthma [68, 69] and tend to be young [68]. Asthma, especially poorly controlled asthma, is a risk factor for anaphylactic reactions to food. Food-induced asthma reactions are said to be usually immediate [70] but there are anecdotal reports of delayed reactions in adults [71]. There is a view that 'late phase' IgE mechanisms as well as immediate ones may be involved [72]. It is possible that food-induced asthma may manifest itself only in the presence of another trigger, e.g. inhaled allergens such as birch pollen, oral allergy syndrome to fruits, cross reacting foods, or exercise, all of which may also increase bronchial reactivity [69].

Migraine and epilepsy

Cheese, chocolate and red wine sometimes provoke migraine, allegedly owing to the presence of a pharmacologically active ingredient, tyramine.

However, children with severe migraine who have failed to benefit from avoidance of cheese and chocolate have been shown to respond to a few foods diet and the most common provoking foods on food re-introduction were those which are implicated in food allergy/intolerance generally [46]. When migraine attacks are fewer than one per week it is difficult to use a diet approach. If symptoms are infrequent, 3 weeks of few foods diet would not be long enough to assess change in rate of attacks and the reintroduction phase would be very muddled. However, for children with severe frequent migraine who have not responded to medication, a diet trial is a worthwhile procedure.

Sometimes children with severe migraine have other symptoms and epilepsy may be one of these. A minority of children with epilepsy who also have migraine respond to diet whereas children with epilepsy alone do not [49]. As with migraine, the diet approach cannot be tried unless seizures are frequent. A trial of diet for such children who have not responded to conventional treatment is worth considering.

Attention deficit hyperactivity disorder (ADHD)

The question of diet and ADHD is very controversial. In 1975 Ben Feingold, an American allergist, claimed that hyperactive children would benefit from avoiding food containing salicylates together with artificial flavours and colours. Later, food preservatives were also excluded. The results of studies aimed at testing Feingold's hypothesis indicate that only a few hyperactive children respond to the elimination of food additives from their diets. Problems with methodology and interpretation of these studies have been discussed by Taylor [73]. Five studies by Egger *et al.* [48], Kaplan *et al.* [74], Boris *et al.* [75], Carter *et al.* [51] and Schmidt *et al.* [76] have looked at the relationship between food (not just additives) and behaviour. There are indications from this work that the idea that food can affect behaviour should be taken seriously, although the proportion of children who might benefit is not known. Although food additives may adversely affect hyperactive children, foods can do so also and the most common provoking foods are the same as those which cause food allergy/intolerance generally. Unfortunately, it is not always possible to carry out a diet trial as many children (especially those over 7 or 8 years) may be completely out of control and non-compliant.

Many hyperactive children have cravings and bizarre eating habits and the first line of approach may be to enforce a more 'normal' diet. Any improvement may be due to firmer parental control than anything else. An 'additive'-free diet may serve the same purpose. However, to look into the possibility of food intolerance properly one must use an empirical diet or few foods diet as described. This should only be attempted where the problems are severe as the difficulties of adhering to a diet can easily be worse than the behaviour problem it is supposed to treat. It must be stressed to parents that this is a little researched area and that dietary management might not be the answer for their child. Other treatments such as behaviour modification or stimulant medication may be more effective although some children may end up on a combination of these treatments. Parents of children with severe ADHD who wish to explore the dietary approach should be given the opportunity to do so, otherwise they will be tempted to experiment with diet unsupervised.

Rheumatoid arthritis (RA)

Darlington and Ramsey published the results of a placebo-controlled blind study of dietary manipulation in rheumatoid arthritis in adults and there was significant objective improvement during periods of diet therapy compared with periods of placebo treatment [77]. The literature was reviewed in 1993 and it was concluded that there was sufficient evidence to suggest that in some adults with RA, dietary therapy may influence at least the symptoms and possibly the progression of the disease. The most common provoking foods were said to be corn, wheat, bacon/pork, oranges, milk, oats, rye, eggs and many others to a lesser extent. The review concluded that more research was needed to further confirm the role of food intolerance with DBPCFCs, to test the idea that essential fatty acid supplements are useful and to look into the possibility of abnormal gut flora playing a role in RA [78]. Brostoff and Gamlin, in another review, felt that food intolerance may play a role in as many as 30% of adults with RA [79]. The above work involved adults only.

Autistic spectrum disorder (ASD)

ASD is a collection of behavioural, perceptual and psychological abnormalities characterised in particular by poor verbal language development, poor socialisation and ritualistic behaviour. There are indications that a subgroup of autistic children have family backgrounds of allergy, attention deficit disorder, hyperactivity and autoimmune dysfunction [80].

Panskepp noted the similarity between autistic symptoms and those of long-term chronic exposure to opioid substances [81]. Reichelt took seriously parental reports that their autistic children reacted unfavourably to some foods and suggested that the breakdown products of proteins from gluten and casein could be a problem. He reported on the presence of urinary peptides in autistic children not normally present [82].

Shattock *et al.* at the Autism Research Unit, University of Sunderland, have continued to research this area and have looked at the raised urinary peptides of many autistic children using high performance liquid chromatography (HPLC). They believe that autistic people have elevated levels of opioid peptides in the central nervous system and that these may come from the incomplete breakdown of foods in particular gluten and casein. Their theory is that these peptides (exorphins) may have direct opioid activity or, alternatively, they may bind to and inhibit the peptidase enzymes which would break down the opioid peptides (endorphins) which occur naturally in the central nervous system. Peptidase enzymes in the gut may be underfunctioning and/or the gut/blood barrier or the blood/brain barrier may be 'leaky'.

In the absence of published research in this area the medical profession is likely to find these ideas unacceptable. Parents have therefore been experimenting either on their own or with the help of interested professionals with gluten and/or casein-free diets. There are many anecdotal reports of success but very little published research. Lucarelli *et al.* studied 36 autistic children and noted a marked improvement in behaviour after an 8 week period on a milk-free diet [83]. They found high levels of IgA antigen specific antibodies for casein, lactalbumin and β-lactoglobulin and IgG and IgM for casein compared to a control group of healthy children. Shattock's group put 22 autistic children on a gluten-free diet for 5 months and noted improvement on a number of behavioural measures but there was no reduction in urinary peptides [84]. Knivsberg and Reichelt found a decrease in autisitic behaviour in 15 subjects after 1 year on a gluten and casein-free diet and normalisation of urine patterns was noticed [85]. These were all open studies.

Another strand to the story relates to the work of Rosemary Waring [80]. Her view is that children with ASD may have a deficiency in the phenol-sulphurtransferase enzyme system. This involves the oxidation of sulphur-containing compounds to produce sulphate. Autistic children tend to have low plasma sulphate levels. The mucin layer which lines the gut needs to be sulphated and with inadequate sulphate may become discontinuous and so render the gut wall more 'leaky'. Sulphate is also needed for inactivation of neurotransmitters. Dietary neurotransmitters (such as serotonin in bananas, phenylethylamine in chocolate and tyramine in cheese) may not be metabolised efficiently. Flavenoids (present in foods such as red wine, citrus fruit) may possibly also be problem foods for similar reasons.

A number of dietary measures are being used in the UK in different centres:

- Gluten and/or casein-free diet based on urinary HPLC results from Paul Shattock's department. Many people feel it is premature to base diets on these results.
- Gluten and casein-free diet.
- Gluten and casein-free diet and also avoiding bananas, citrus fruit, chocolate and sometimes also artificial colours and preservatives.
- Low sugar, yeast-free diet with antifungal medication. No work has been published on this but there are anecdotal reports of success.
- 'Hunter gatherer' diet.

Recommended length of time to try a diet varies from 3 to 12 months but the more restricted the diet the more difficult it is to follow for an extended period.

Many dietitians will wonder if they should be involved in this under-researched field. There is not enough evidence for dietitians to advocate diet treatment. Indeed, which diet should be recommended? However, if parents wish to try a diet for their child the dietitian could help to implement the diet properly, to ensure nutritional adequacy, to ensure that there is an end point so that unhelpful diets are abandoned and most importantly to have some kind of outcome measure. This could be, for example, some form of diary describing behaviours which might be expected to improve in the short term. Motivated parents who wish to try diet treatment will do it with or without professional help. It is important to point out to parents that diet treatment is experimental at this time. Also the problem of expense of the diet must be discussed in view of the fact that special gluten and milk-free products (e.g. bread, pasta and biscuits) are not prescribable for this condition.

It is important that the referring doctor supports a diet trial and shows some interest. The ideal format would be a team consisting of dietitian, doctor and a specialist in psychological medicine. There is a subgroup of autistic children who have physical symptoms, particularly gastrointestinal problems. The dietitian may have an important role here working alongside a paediatrician to find out if the physical symptoms at least may be responsive to an exclusion diet.

Many ASD children are hyperactive and children with ADHD who are food intolerant can be adversely affected by a large range of foods and additives. Perhaps some autistic children are adversely affected by foods other than or as well as casein and gluten. The problems of putting autistic children on diets are probably as great as attempting diets on children with ADHD. They may have bizarre eating habits and refuse to eat a restricted diet. Further research is needed in this field and controlled diet studies will be hard to achieve because of the difficulties of carrying out blind food provocations as previously described in this chapter.

NOVEL APPROACHES

Probiotics

Probiotics are live bacteria which, if taken orally, are said to improve intestinal microbial balance and exert beneficial effects on health. The most important are lactic acid bacteria and they must be capable of surviving passage through the stomach and small intestine. The intestinal microflora is an important constituent of the gut mucosal barrier [86]. Majamas and Isolauri studied two groups of infants with eczema [87]. One group took a hydrolysed formula and the other took the same formula and a probiotic – lactobacillus GG. The group with lactobacillus showed significant skin improvement after 1 month whereas the other group did not. There were also some changes in markers of intestinal inflammation. The results suggest that probiotic bacteria may act as a useful tool in the treatment of eczema and food allergy by promoting endogenous barrier mechanisms and by alleviating intestinal inflammation.

Prebiotics

Prebiotics are growth substrates intended to stimulate the growth of beneficial bacteria already in the colon. They are oligosaccharides which are not digested in the small intestine such as fructo oligosaccharides and inulin. They are intended as an additional (or alternative) approach to probiotics.

It is to be hoped that further research will elucidate the role of both pre- and probiotics in the treatment of food allergy.

PROBLEMS WITH DIETARY TREATMENT

In this controversial area of medicine it is important to avoid giving inappropriate emphasis to dietary treatment. However, people who feel that diet plays a role in their child's illness should have the opportunity to discuss in an unbiased fashion the possibilities of dietary treatment and, where appropriate, have the opportunity to try a diet. A lack of sympathetic approach may lead to self-imposed diets (likely to be inadequate) or self-referral to an unqualified practitioner. Whatever the prejudices of the professionals involved, the question of diet must be discussed as the child may be on an inadequate and inappropriate diet. Although some children may be on unhelpful diets, others benefit dramatically from the correct exclusion diet. The role of the dietitian is to assist in maintaining helpful diets and broaden the diet as much as possible. It is equally important to encourage people to abandon unhelpful diets. An open-minded approach is necessary. Occasionally parents will not take advice and in exceptional cases the restrictions imposed by the parent on the child may be regarded as a form of child abuse [88].

PREVENTION OF FOOD ALLERGY

There is considerable interest in the idea of preventing the onset of food allergy in babies born into allergic families (affected parent or sibling). It is presumed that breast feeding has a preventative effect compared with cow's milk formula feeding but the effect remains controversial. In a study from Finland nonselected infants were followed up to age 17 years. Breast feeding was associated with lower rates of eczema and food allergy at 1 and 3 years and also a lower score of respiratory allergy at 17 years compared with cow's milk formula fed infants [89].

Several prospective studies looking at the effect of allergen avoidance in high risk infants have been published. The studies cannot be compared as the study designs were different. Hide *et al.* followed a prophylactic group where infants were breast fed (with mothers on an exclusion diet) or fed an extensively hydrolysed formula, were weaned carefully and were living in a house where house dust mite was strenuously reduced; they compared them with a control group at age 4. At this age a significant advantage remained in the prophylactic group [90]. Chandra followed up infants for 5 years and concluded that exclusive breast feeding or feeding with a partial whey hydrolysate is associated with lower incidence of atopic disease and food allergy as compared with conventional cow's milk formula or soy feeding [91]. Zeiger followed a prophylactic and control group for 7 years. The mothers were on exclusion diets during the last trimester of pregnancy and during lactation. The infants were breast fed or given a casein hydrolysate and weaned carefully. Although there was significant reduction in food allergy before 2 years, there was little difference between the two groups at age 7 [92]. Oldaeus *et al.* studied 155 at-risk infants for 18 months. Breast feeding mothers were on a diet, solids were carefully introduced and at weaning they were randomised to receive either an extensively hydrolysed formula (eHF) or a partially hydrolysed formula (pHF) or a regular formula. The findings supported an allergy preventative effect of eHF but not pHF during the first 18 months of life [93]. These studies involved several interventions and their possible individual benefits need to be unravelled.

Maternal diet during pregnancy

Although work is in progress looking at the possibility of allergic priming *in utero* [94], there is no conclusive evidence for a protective effect of a maternal exclusion diet during pregnancy [15, 95]. However, the report on peanut allergy by the Committee on Toxicity of Chemicals in Food, Consumer Products and the Environment (COT) advises that pregnant women from atopic families may wish to avoid peanuts in pregnancy [96]. The report stresses that the advice is precautionary because of the potential seriousness of peanut allergy.

Maternal diet during lactation

Some studies indicate that the preventative effect of breast feeding may be enhanced by maternal avoidance whereas other studies do not confirm this finding [15]. Zeiger feels that maternal avoidance diets must be considered experimental at this time [95]. A recent study by Hattvig *et al.* looked at the effects of maternal dietary avoidance during lactation in children at 10 years of age and concluded that the results did not support general recommendations to implement prophylactic maternal dietary avoidance during lactation in allergy-prone families [97]. The authors comment that in their study there was a lower rate of atopic dermatitis at 6 months and one year and in Zeiger's study [92] a lower rate in infancy, indicating some early beneficial effect. They go on to say that individual recommendations to families with pronounced heredity might thus be considered, providing adequate dietetic follow-up can be given and the parents are informed that there is no real evidence of a long term benefit. The COT report on peanut allergy advises against the intake of peanuts for breast feeding women for the same reason as during pregnancy [96].

Careful weaning

Exclusive breast feeding should be encouraged for at least the first 4 months of life. An extensively hydrolysed formula appears to be the best alternative to breast milk. Controversial views exist on the use of whole soy formulas and further studies are needed to clarify this [15].

It is not clear what best advice is as regards weaning but it would appear prudent to begin with a limited number of foods of low allergenicity [15]. The dietitian will be asked to advise on feeding and weaning of at-risk infants. A prevention programme can be tried which should also involve avoidance as far as possible of aeroallergens such as house dust mite and cigarette smoke. This may at least delay the onset of symptoms even if it does not prevent them.

The relationship between weaning and the development of food allergic disease has been little studied but Cant and Bailes suggested a system of introducing one food group at a time and leaving the most common provoking foods until last [98]. They suggested breast feeding until 6 months if possible or at least until 4 months. At 6 months a supplement of 0.3 ml Abidec and 2.0 ml Niferex iron supplement should be given if weaning is not well in progress. Foods should then be introduced in the following order:

- Milk-free baby rice
- Puréed root vegetables: potatoes, carrot, parsnip, swede, turnip
- Puréed fruit: apple, pear, banana (not citrus fruit until 8 months)
- Other vegetables: peas, beans, lentils
- Other cereals (not wheat until 8 months)
- Lamb, turkey and then other meats
- Fish (not until 10–12 months)
- Cow's milk products, ordinary infant formula (not until 10–12 months). If breast milk has diminished before that a supplementary feed will be needed as infant soya formula or preferably a hydrolysate
- Eggs: not until 1 year.

The COT report suggests that children from allergic families should not have peanuts until at least 3 years of age [96].

A joint statement from ESPACI (European Society for Paediatric Allergology and Clinical Immunology) and ESPGHAN (European Society of Paediatric Gastroenterology, Hepatology and Nutrition) discusses current developments and unresolved issues in the dietary prevention of food allergy [15]. The summary of the report is as follows:

- Exclusive breast feeding during the first 4–6 months of life might greatly reduce the incidence of allergic manifestations and is strongly recommended.
- Supplementary foods should not be introduced before the fifth month of life.
- In bottle fed infants with a documented hereditary atopy risk (affected parent or sibling), the exclusive feeding of a formula with a confirmed reduced allergenicity is recommended.
- More studies comparing the preventative effects of formulas that have highly reduced allergenicity (eHF) with formulas that have moderately reduced allergenicity (pHF) are needed.
- Dietary products used for preventive purposes in infancy need to be evaluated carefully with respect to their preventative and nutritional effects in appropriate clinical trials. (There is no evidence for or against the use of formulas based on soy protein isolate.)
- There is no conclusive evidence to support the use of formulas with reduced allergenicity for preventative purposes in healthy infants without a family history of allergic disease.

REFERENCES

1 Walker Smith J (chair) Report of a BSACI working party. Food allergy and intolerance. *Clin Exp Allergy*, 1995, **25** suppl 1.
2 Shamssain M, Shamsian N Prevalence and severity of asthma, rhinitis and atopic eczema: the north east study. *Arch Dis Childh*, 1999, **81** 313–17.
3 Hanson L, Telemo E The growing allergy problem (invited commentary). *Acta Paediatr*, 1997, **86** 916–18.
4 Kjellman NIM, Nilsson L From food allergy and atopic dermatitis to respiratory allergy. *Pediatr Allergy Immunol*, 1998, **9** (suppl 1) 13–17.
5 Kulig M, Bergmann R *et al.* Natural course of sensitization to food and inhalant allergens during the first 6 years of life. *J Allergy Clin Immunol*, 1999, **103** 1173–9.
6 Sampson H Food allergy. Part 2: Diagnosis and management. *J Allergy Clin Immunol*, 1999, **103** 981–9.
7 The first report of the BSAEM/BSNM. *Effective*

allergy practice, 1994. The British Society for Allergy and Environmental Medicine with the British Society for Nutritional Medicine, PO Box 28, Totton, Southampton SO40 2ZA.

8 Food allergy testing. *Health Which*, Dec 1998, 12–15.

9 Walker Smith J, Digeon B *et al*. Evaluation of a casein and a whey hydrolysate for treatment of cow's-milk-sensitive enteropathy. *Eur J Pediatr*, 1989, **149** 68–71.

10 Sampson HA, James JM *et al*. Safety of an amino acid-derived infant formula in children allergic to cow milk. *Pediatr*, 1992, **90** 463–5.

11 Hill DJ, Cameron DJS *et al*. Challenge confirmation of late-onset reactions to extensively hydrolysed formulas in infants with multiple food protein intolerance. *J Allergy Clin Immunol*, 1995, **96** 386–94.

12 Bindels JG, Boerma JA Hydrolysed cow's milk formulae. (Letter to the editor.) *Pediatr Allergy Immunol*, 1994, **5** 189–90.

13 Hide D, Wharton B Hydrolysed protein formulas: thoughts from the Isle of Wight meeting. *Eur J Clin Nutrit*, 1995, **49** (1) S100–S106.

14 Rugo E, Wahl R *et al*. How allergenic are hypoallergenic infant formulae? *Clin Exp Allergy*, 1991, **22** 635–9.

15 Høst A, Koletzko B *et al*. Dietary products used in infants for treatment and prevention of food allergy. A joint statement of the European Society for Paediatric Allergology and Clinical Immunology (ESPACI) and the European Society for Paediatric Gastroenterology, Hepatology and Nutrition (ESPGHAN). *Arch Dis Childh*, 1999, **81** 80–84.

16 Kleinman RE, Bahna S *et al*. Use of infant formulas in infants with cow milk allergy. A review and recommendation. *Paediatr Allergy Immunol*, 1991, **4** 146–55.

17 Vanderhoof JA, Murray ND *et al*. Intolerance to protein hydrolysate infant formulas: an under-recognized cause of gastrointestinal symptoms in infants. *J Pediatr*, 1997, **131** 741–4.

18 De Boissieu D, Matarazzo P *et al*. Allergy to extensively hydrolysed cow milk proteins in infants: identification and treatment with an amino acid-based formula. *J Pediatr*, 1997, **131** 744–7.

19 Isolauri E, Sutas Y *et al*. Efficacy and safety of hydrolysed cow milk and amino acid-derived formulas in infants with cow milk allergy. *J Pediatr*, 1995, **127** 550–57.

20 Strauss RS, Koniaris S Allergic colitis in two infants fed with an amino acid formula (short communication). *J Pediatr Gastoenterol Nutr*, 1998, **27** 362–5.

21 McLeish CM, Macdonald A *et al*. Comparison of an elemental with a hydrolysed whey formula in intolerance to cow's milk. *Arch Dis Childh*, 1995, **73** 211–15.

22 Cantani A, Lucenti P *et al*. Natural history of soy allergy and/or intolerance in children and clinical use of soy-protein formulas. *Pediatr Allergy Immunol*, 1997, **8** 59–74.

23 Businco L, Bruno G *et al*. Soy protein for the prevention and treatment of children with cow-milk allergy. *Am J Clin Nutr*, 1998, **68** (suppl) 1447S–52S.

24 Zeiger RS, Sampson HA *et al*. Soy allergy in infants and children with IgE-associated cow's milk allergy. *J Pediatr*, 1999, **134** 614–22.

25 American Academy of Pediatrics. Committee on Nutrition. Soy protein-based formulas: recommendations for use in infant feeding. *Pediatr*, 1998, **101** 148–53.

26 Lucassen PLB, Assendelft WJJ *et al*. Effectiveness of treatments for infantile colic: systematic review. *Brit Med J*, 1998, **316** 1563–9.

27 Setchell KDR, Zimmer-Nechemias L *et al*. Isoflavone content of infant formulas and the metabolic fate of these phytoestrogens in early life. *Am J Cin Nutr*, 1998, **68** (suppl) 1453S–61S.

28 Essex C Soy based infant formula and phytoestrogens (comment). *Paediatr Today*, 1996, **4** 39–40.

29 Dean TP, Adler BR *et al*. In vitro allergenicity of cow's milk substitutes. *Clin Exp Allergy*, 1992, **23** 205–10.

30 Barau E, Dupont C Allergy to milk proteins in mother's milk or in hydrolysed cow's milk infant formulas as assessed by intestinal permeability measurements. *Allergy*, 1994, **49** 295–8.

31 De Boissieu D, Matarazzo P *et al*. Multiple food allergy: a possible diagnosis in breastfed infants. *Acta Paediatr*, 1997, **86** 1042–6.

32 Isolauri E, Tahvanainen A *et al*. Breast feeding in allergic infants. *J Pediatr*, 1999, **134** 27–32.

33 Patel L, Radivan FS *et al*. Management of anaphylactic reactions to food. *Arch Dis Childh*, 1994, **71** 370–75.

34 Bock SA, Sampson HA *et al*. Double-blind, placebo-controlled food challenge (DBPCFC) as an office procedure: a manual. *J Allergy Clin Immunol*, 1986, **82** 986–97.

35 Hourihane JO'B Peanut allergy – current status and future challenges. *Clin Exp Allergy*, 1997, **27** 1240–46.

36 David TJ Anaphylactic shock during elimination diets for severe atopic eczema. *Arch Dis Childh*, 1984, **59** 983–6.

37 Sampson HA, Mendelson L *et al*. Fatal and near-fatal anaphylactic reactions to food in children and adolescents. *N Engl J Med*, 1992, **327** 380–84.

38 Tilles S, Schoket A *et al*. Exercise induced anaphylaxis related to specific foods. *J Pediatr*, 1995, **127** 587–9.

39 Hill DJ, Hosking CS The cow milk allergy complex: overlapping disease profiles in infancy. *Eur J Clin Nutr*, 1995, **49** (suppl 1) S1–S12.

40 Conners CK Rating scales for use in drug studies with children. *Psychopharmacol Bull* (Special issue pharmacotherapy with children), 1973, **9** 24–8.

41 Rowe AH, Rowe A Bronchial asthma due to food allergy alone in ninety-five patients. *JAMA*, 1958, **169** 104–8.

42 Young E, Stoneham MD *et al*. The prevalence of reaction to food additives in a survey population. *J Royal Coll Physicians*, 1987, **21** 241–7.

43 Swain AR, Dutton S *et al.* Salicylates in foods. *J American Dietetic Assoc*, 1985, **85** 950–60.

44 Minford AMB *et al.* Food intolerance and food allergy in children: a review of 68 cases. *Arch Dis Childh*, 1983, **57** 742–7.

45 Atherton DJ Dietary treatment in childhood atopic eczema. *Proceedings of the second food allergy workshop*, 1983, Oxford: The Medicine Publ Foundation, 109–110.

46 Egger J, Carter C *et al.* Is migraine food allergy? *Lancet*, 1983, ii 865–9.

47 Pike MG, Carter CM *et al.* Few foods diet in the treatment of atopic eczema. *Arch Dis Childh*, 1989, **64** 1691–8.

48 Egger J, Carter C *et al.* Controlled trial of oligoantigenic diet in the hyperkinetic syndrome. *Lancet*, 1985, i 540–45.

49 Egger J, Carter CM *et al.* Oligoantigenic diet treatment of children with epilepsy and migraine. *J Pediatr*, 1989, **114** 51–8.

50 Egger J, Carter CM *et al.* Effect of diet treatment on enuresis in children with migraine or hyperkinetic behaviour. *Clin Pediatr*, 1992, **31** 302–307.

51 Carter CM, Urbanowicz M *et al.* Effects of a few foods diet on attention deficit disorder. *Arch Dis Childh*, 1993, **69** 564–8.

52 Devlin J, David TJ *et al.* Elemental diet for refractory atopic eczema. *Arch Dis Childh*, 1991, **66** 92–9.

53 Bishop JM, Hill DJ *et al.* Natural history of cow milk allergy: clinical outcome. *J Pediatr*, 1990, **116** 862–7.

54 David TJ, Waddington W *et al.* Nutritional hazards of elimination diets in children with atopic eczema. *Arch Dis Childh*, 1984, **59** 323–5.

55 Devlin J, Stanton RHJ *et al.* Calcium intake and cow's milk free diets. *Arch Dis Childh*, 1989, **64** 1183–93.

56 Carter C Double-blind food challenges in children: a dietitian's perspective (comment). *Current Medical Literature – Allergy*, 1995, **3** 95–9.

57 Morrow Brown H Milk allergy and intolerance (clinical aspects). In: DLJ Freed (ed.) *Health Hazards of Milk*. London: Bailliere Tindall, 1984.

58 David TJ, Patel L *et al.* Dietary regimens for atopic dermatitis in childhood. *J R Soc Med*, 1997, **90** 9–14.

59 Sampson HA, McCaskill CC Food hypersensitivity and atopic dermatitis: evaluation of 113 patients. *J Pediatr*, 1985, **107** 669–75.

60 Burks AW, James JM *et al.* Atopic dermatitis and food hypersensitivity reactions. *J Pediatr*, 1998, **132** 132–6.

61 Sampson HA Food sensitivity and the pathogenesis of atopic dermatitis. *J R Soc Med*, 1997, **90** (suppl 30) 2–8.

62 Sicherer SH, Sampson HA Food hypersensitivity and atopic dermatitis: pathophysiology, epidemiology, diagnosis and management. *J Allergy Clin Immunol*, 1999, **104** S114–22.

63 Sloper KS, Wadsworth J *et al.* Children with atopic eczema. I: Clinical response to food elimination and subsequent double-blind food challenge. *Quarterly J Med*, 1991, **New Series 80** (292) 677–93.

64 Sloper KS, Wadsworth J *et al.* Children with atopic eczema. II: Immunological findings associated with dietary manipulations. *Quarterly J Med*, 1991, **New Series 80** (292) 695–705.

65 Caffarelli C, Cavagni G *et al.* Gastrointestinal symptoms in atopic eczema. *Arch Dis Childh*, 1998, **78** 230–34.

66 Mabin DC, Sykles AE *et al.* Controlled trial of a few foods diet in severe atopic dermatitis. *Arch Dis Childh*, 1995, **73** 202–207.

67 Atherton DJ Diet and atopic eczema. *Clin Allergy*, 1988, **18** 215–28.

68 Onorato J, Merland N *et al.* Placebo-controlled double-blind food challenge in asthma. *J Allergy Clin Immunol*, 1986, **78** 1139–46.

69 Novembre E, de Martino M *et al.* Foods and respiratory allergy. *J Allergy Clin Immunol*, 1988, **81** 1059–65.

70 James JM, Eigenmann PA *et al.* Airway reactivity changes in food allergic, asthmatic children undergoing double-blind placebo-controlled food challenges. *Am J Respir Crit Care Med*, 1996, **153** 597–603.

71 Wraith D Food allergy. *Respiratory Disease in Practice*, March 1983, 8–13.

72 Sampson HA Food allergy, Part 1: Immunopathogenesis and clinical disorders. *J Allergy Clin Immunol*, 1999, **103** 717–28.

73 Taylor E Toxins and allergens. In: Rutter M, Casaer P (eds) *Biological Risk Factors for Psychosocial Disorders*. New York: Academic Press, 1992.

74 Kaplan BJ, McNichol J *et al.* Dietary replacement in preschool-aged hyperactive boys. *Pediatr*, 1989, **83** 7–17.

75 Boris M, Mandel FS Foods and additives are common causes of the attention deficit disorder in children. *Annals of Allergy*, 1994, **72** 462–7.

76 Schmidt MH, Mocks P *et al.* Does oligoantigenic diet influence hyperactive/conduct disordered children – a controlled trial. *Eur Child Adol Psych*, 1997, **6** 88–95.

77 Darlington LG, Ramsey NW *et al.* Placebo-controlled, blind study of dietary manipulation in rheumatoid arthritis. *Lancet*, 1986, i 236–8.

78 Darlington LG, Ramsey NW Review of dietary therapy for rheumatoid arthritis. *Br J Rheumatol*, 1993, **32** 507–14.

79 Gamlin L, Brostoff J Food sensitivity and rheumatoid arthritis. *Environ Toxicol Pharmacol*, 1997, **4** 43–9.

80 Waring RH, Klovrza LV Sulphur metabolism in autism. *J Nutr Environ Med*, 2000, **10** 25–32.

81 Panskepp J A neurochemical theory of autism. *Trends in Neuroscience*, 1979, **2** 174–7.

82 Reichelt KL, Hole K *et al.* Biologically active peptide-containing fractions in schizophrenia and childhood autism. *Adv Biochem Psychopharmacol*, 1981, **28** 627–43.

83 Lucarelli S, Frediani T *et al.* Food allergy and infantile autism. *Panminerva Medica*, 1995, **37** 137–41.

84 Whiteley P, Rodgers J *et al.* A gluten-free diet as an intervention for autism and associated spectrum disorders: preliminary findings. *Autism*, 1999, 3 45–65.

85 Knivsberg AM, Reichelt KL *et al.* Autistic syndromes and diet: a follow-up study. *Scandin J Educat Res*, 1995, 39 223–36.

86 Fuller R Probiotics in human medicine. *Gut*, 1991, 32 439–42.

87 Majamas H, Isolauri E Probiotics: a novel approach in the management of food allergy. *J Allergy Clin Immunol*, 1997, 99 179–85.

88 Warner JO, Hathaway MJ Allergic form of Meadow's syndrome (Munchausen by proxy). *Arch Dis Childh*, 1984, 59 151–6.

89 Saarinen *et al.* Breast feeding as prophylaxis against atopic disease – prospective follow up until 17 years old. *Lancet*, 1995, 346 1065–9.

90 Hide DW, Matthews S *et al.* Allergen avoidance in infancy and allergy at 4 years of age. *Allergy*, 1996, 51 89–93.

91 Chandra RK Five-year follow-up of at-risk infants with family history of allergy who were exclusively breast-fed or fed partial whey hydrolysate, soy, and conventional cow's milk formulas. *J Pediatr Gastroenterol Nutr*, 1997, 24 380–88.

92 Zeiger RS, Heller S The development and prediction of atopy in high risk children: follow-up at age seven years in a prospective randomized study of combined maternal and infant food allergen avoidance. *J Allergy Clin Immunol*, 1995, 95 1789–90.

93 Oldaeus G, Anjou K *et al.* Extensively and partially hydrolysed infant formulas for allergy prophylaxis. *Arch Dis Childh*, 1997, 77 4–10.

94 Jones AC, Miles EA *et al.* IFN gamma and proliferative responses from fetal leucocytes during 2nd and 3rd trimesters of pregnancy. *J Allergy Clin Immunol*, 1995, 9 380.

95 Zeiger RS Prevention of food allergy and atopic disease. *J R Soc Med*, 1997, 90 (suppl 30) 21–33.

96 Committee on Toxicity of Chemicals in Food, Consumer Products and the Environment (COT) Peanut Allergy, 1998, Dept of Health.

97 Hattvig G, Sigurs N *et al.* Effects of maternal dietary avoidance during lactation on allergy in children at 10 years of age. *Acta Paediatr*, 1999, 88 7–12.

98 Cant AJ, Bailes JA How should we feed the potentially allergic infant? *Hum Nutr: Applied Nutr*, 1984, 38A 474–6.

FURTHER READING

Sampson HA Food allergy, Part 1: Immunopathogenesis and clinical disorders. *J Allergy Clin Immunol*, 1999, 103 717–28.

Sampson HA Food allergy, Part 2: Diagnosis and management. *J Allergy Clin Immunol*, 1999, 103 981–9.

Playfair JHL *Immunology at a Glance*, 6th edn. Oxford: Blackwells, 1996.

Joneja JV *Dietary Management of Food Allergies and Intolerances. A comprehensive guide*, 2nd edn. Vancouver: JA Hall, 1998.

Sicherer SH Food allergy: when and how to perform oral food challenges. *Pediatr Allergy Immunol*, 1999, 10 226–34.

Ortolani C, Bruijnzeel-Koomen C *et al.* Controversial aspects of adverse reactions to food. Position Paper. *Allergy*, 1999, 54 27–45.

Committee on Toxicity of Chemicals in Food, Consumer Products and the Environment (COT) Adverse Reactions to Food and Food Ingredients, 2000, Dept of Health.

Food allergy – getting move out of your skin prick tests. Editorial, *Clin Exper Allergy*, 2000, 30 1495–8.

USEFUL ADDRESSES

Anaphylaxis Campaign
PO Box 149, Fleet, Hampshire, GU13 9XU Tel. 01252 542029 www.anaphylaxis.org.uk

British Allergy Foundation
Deepdene House, 30 Bellgrove Rd, Welling DA16 3PY Tel. 020 8303 8525 www.allergyfoundation.com

Food Allergy Network
www.foodallergy.org

American Academy of Allergy Asthma and Immunology
www.aaaai.org

IMMUNODEFICIENCY SYNDROMES

These are a heterogeneous group of disorders characterised by defects of B-lymphocytes, T-lymphocytes or neutrophils. The most common disorders and the associated gastrointestinal complications are summarised in Table 13.7.

The dietetic treatment of children with these disorders depends on the type of immune deficiency, the nature and severity of the gastrointestinal complications and whether they also present with failure to thrive.

Table 13.7 Immunodeficiency syndromes (Adapted from Walker-Smith and Murch [10])

Immunodeficiency	Gastrointestinal complications
B-lymphocyte defects	
IgA deficiency	Malabsorption, coeliac disease, gut infection
Transient IgA/IgG subclass deficiency of infancy	Malabsorption, food allergy
Hypogammaglobulinaemia (X-linked)	Malabsorption, steatorrhoea; disaccharidase deficiencies [9]
Common variable immunodeficiency	Gut infection
T-lymphocyte defects	
T-cell activation defects	Autoimmune enteropathy
Di George's syndrome	Diarrhoea and intestinal infection
Class II MHC deficiency	Chronic diarrhoea
Wiskott-Aldrich syndrome	Malabsorption, food allergy
CD40 ligand deficiency	Gut infection, lymphoma of the small intestine, liver disease
Severe combined immunodeficiency: Autosomal recessive X-linked Sporadic ADA, PNP deficiency	Infectious diarrhoea
HIV	Enteropathy, malabsorption
Neutrophil immunodeficiencies	
Chronic granulomatous disease	Diarrhoea, protein-losing enteropathy, pancolitis, small bowel obstruction [18]
Leucocyte adhesion deficiency	Mucosal infection and inflammation, appendicitis, perirectal abscesses [18]

B-LYMPHOCYTE DEFECTS

Immunoglobulins are secreted by plasma cells which are terminally differentiated B-lymphocytes. Therefore immunodeficiencies affecting the B-cell system are linked to abnormal synthesis of immunoglobulins. The B-lymphocyte defects that require the most dietetic input are discussed below.

IgA and IgG/IgG subclass deficiency

Immunoglobulin A (IgA) accounts for about 20% of the total serum immunoglobulins. It is synthesised mainly in the lamina propriae underlying the respiratory tract, the gut and other mucosae. It helps to protect the mucosal surface of the small intestine and regulates antigen entry. Deficiency of IgA is over-represented in children with food allergy. It is estimated that 7% of atopic individuals have transient IgA deficiency [1]. Protection of such infants from excessive antigen stimulation during the susceptible time when IgA is low is recommended in order to prevent the development of atopic disease later [2, 3]. If patients with IgA deficiency develop symptoms in early life, it may be appropriate to follow the careful weaning guidelines developed by Cant and Bailes [4], in an effort to prevent atopic symptoms later in life. This system was developed for weaning infants with a family history of food allergy and involves introducing one food group at a time, leaving the most commonly provoking foods (e.g. cow's milk, fish, eggs) until last. These guidelines are discussed in detail earlier (p. 211).

Children with low immunoglobulin G (IgG) or low IgG subclasses (commonly IgG2 and IgG4) also commonly have food allergy estimated at 32% of patients with an IgG subclass deficiency [5]. The dietetic management of children with food allergy or intolerance is discussed earlier (p. 195).

Selective IgA deficiency is associated with coeliac disease. The incidence of selective IgA deficiency in coeliac patients is 10–16 fold higher than in the general population [6]. The only difference between these and other children with coeliac disease is that IgA deficiency persists when on a gluten-free diet despite the return of normal mucosa. A gluten-free diet is always indicated [7, 8] (p. 77).

Hypogammaglobulinaemia

Disaccharidase deficiencies, most commonly lactase, have been reported in children with congenital X-linked and idiopathic acquired hypogammaglobulinaemias [9]. The authors observed that symptoms of milk intolerance can be ameliorated by withdrawal of lactose from the diet. However, it is not clear whether the disaccharidase deficiencies were the result of the primary immunodeficiency or of coincidental infection. Furthermore, in the above study, lactose as well as milk protein was withdrawn from the diet and it is therefore possible that the improvement of symptoms was at least partly due to the withdrawal of milk protein. Although villous atrophy has been described, this rarely responds to a gluten-free diet [10].

Children with any of the above immunodeficiencies frequently present with failure to thrive which further complicates the dietetic treatment. The nutritional requirements for children with the above immunodeficiencies are not well established. One should aim for at least the dietary reference values for energy, protein and other nutrients, depending on the age of the child, increasing further if growth is compromised particularly in children with frequent periods of inflammation and infection. Nutritional support in the form of nasogastric or gastrostomy feeding can be very useful, enabling adequate nutritional intake. Extensively hydrolysed protein feeds may be better tolerated and a diet free of milk, wheat, egg and soya is also often used empirically. Details of suitable feeds are given in Chapter 6, Tables 6.6, 6.9 and 6.10.

T-LYMPHOCYTE AND COMBINED DEFECTS

Impairment of T-lymphocyte function leads to defective cell-mediated immunity and increased susceptibility to a wide range of pathogens including viruses, parasites and intracellular bacteria. The commonest T-cell defects are summarised in Table 13.7. The dietetic management of these conditions is empirical. However, a common approach can generally be applied.

Susceptibility to infections

These patients suffer not only from severe and persistent infections due to common pathogens, but are also vulnerable to a range of opportunistic organisms. Care should be taken to avoid the risk of infection by food-borne organisms. Patients are advised to follow general food hygiene precautions, to boil water before use and to avoid the use of products which contain unpasteurised milk, uncooked eggs/fish and live yoghurt. In our institution, these patients do not follow the very strict 'clean diet' precautions that are applied to those undergoing allogeneic bone marrow transplantation (p. 26).

Autoimmune enteropathy

The mucosal changes in T-cell-mediated immunodeficiencies have a complex aetiology. They are probably associated commonly with infection but less frequently with autoimmune enteropathy [11]. In autoimmune enteropathy, enterocyte autoantibodies are found in association with crypt hyperplastic villous atrophy. Such infants present with chronic diarrhoea and failure to thrive. They are often maintained for extended periods on intravenous fluids to maintain hydration but nutrition is inadequate, particularly in the presence of recurrent infections which result in increased nutrient requirements [10]. Malnutrition itself leads to a worsening of mucosal and pancreatic function [12–15] thus inducing a vicious cycle of further malnutrition. A period of parenteral nutrition may initially be necessary although it is important to continue some oral/enteral feeding to the maximum tolerated level in order to exert a trophic effect on gut mucosa. Parenteral nutrition should continue until successful enteral nutrition is established.

Once an oral rehydration solution (e.g. Dioralyte) is tolerated, enteral feeding should commence. Extensively hydrolysed protein or amino acid-based feeds can be used. Both, particularly amino acid formulations, have a higher osmolality than normal infant formulas and therefore care should be taken to avoid osmotic diarrhoea. Feed concentration should be increased slowly. If these feeds are not tolerated, a modular feed (e.g. using comminuted chicken meat) could be tried (p. 84).

Introduction of foods should be done carefully. Empirically, the weaning programme suggested by Cant and Bailes [4] could be used for the infant who has not previously been exposed to significant amounts of solid food (p. 211).

For the older child food reintroduction could follow a procedure similar to that described in the 'few foods diet' section (p. 201), starting with one type of food unlikely to cause problems (e.g. rice or chicken) and thereafter introducing slowly one additional food at a time. Empirically, the order of food reintroduction described in Table 13.6 could be followed. The progression of feeding depends on the severity of the disease. For some patients excluding milk, egg, wheat and soya from the diet is sufficient to control symptoms.

Combined immunodeficiency

Combined immunodeficiency, including severe combined immunodeficiency (SCID), comprises a group of congenital deficiencies of both T-cell and B-cell function. SCID is fatal in early childhood if untreated. Infants usually present with intractable diarrhoea due to chronic gastrointestinal infection and autoimmune enteropathy [10] and vomiting due to gastro-oesophageal reflux [16]. All of these factors contribute to failure to thrive. Nutritional support in the form of tube feeding may be necessary. Infants who are breast fed appear to have more resistance to infections so a delay in the introduction of infant formula seems prudent. For infants or children with persistent diarrhoea, extensively hydrolysed protein feeds (Chapter 6, Tables 6.6 and 6.10) or amino acid-based feeds (Chapter 6, Tables 6.9 and 6.10) may be more efficiently absorbed and so promote weight gain. Intake of solids should be monitored to avoid diarrhoea, as described above, in children with autoimmune enteropathy. The energy and protein requirements of children with SCID are probably higher than healthy children of the same age, particularly during periods of infection.

Bone marrow transplantation

Bone marrow transplantation is used to treat certain severe immunodeficiencies. In patients with SCID, bone marrow transplant from a histocompatible sibling can result in 76% probability of disease-free survival [17]. The outcome could be positively influenced by the nutritional state and absence of infection at the time of transplant.

During the procedure, patients are nursed in isolation with a filtered air system to protect against environmental pathogens. 'Clean diet' precautions are imposed to reduce the risk of infection with food borne organisms. Empirically, most units will feed infants with a pasteurised extensively hydrolysed protein or amino acid feed or with breast milk. In most units, expressed breast milk is no longer tested for microbial contamination nor is it pasteurised before use. Food for the older child is produced under a filtered laminar airflow system and food utensils are sterilised by γ-irradiation. The provision of 'clean' meals is discussed on p. 26. Clean precautions are lifted once bacterial resistance has increased. This may take between 3 weeks and 6 months as indicated by the blood neutrophil count.

Children receiving allogeneic bone marrow transplantation need intensive immunosuppressive conditioning treatment for about 10 days before the transplant, to ablate recipient haemopoietic and lymphoid stem cells. This disrupts the rapidly dividing mucosal cells of the gut and mouth leading to poor tolerance of oral feeds and diet. Local anaesthetic sprays are sometimes helpful. Where possible, some oral feeding should continue, even if most of the nutrition is provided parenterally. This will preclude the loss of the sucking reflex and also minimise gut atrophy. To protect against oral infections such as cytomegalovirus, candida or herpes, antifungal and antiviral agents are usually given pre- and post-transplant. In addition, in neutropenic patients, prophylactic antibacterial mouth washes are used.

After the transplant, during immunological reconstitution, food 'intolerance' due to the gut healing and immune disregulation may appear, but will usually subside over 12 months. For this reason, a diet avoiding milk, egg and sometimes wheat is sometimes recommended. The timing of reintroduction of these potential antigens is usually dictated by immune function and foods are introduced one by one. Usually wheat is introduced first, followed by milk and finally egg. If the transplant is successful, dietetic intervention will no longer be needed.

REFERENCES

1 Kaufman HS, Hobbs JR Immunoglobulin deficiencies in an atopic population. *Lancet*, 1970, 2 (7682) 1061–3.
2 Taylor B, Norman AP, Orgel HA, Stokes CR, Turner MW, Soothhill JF Transient IgA deficiency and pathogenesis of infantile atopy. *Lancet*, 1973, 2 (7821) 111–13.
3 Ludviksson BR, Eiriksson TH, Ardal B, Sigfusson A, Valdimarsson H Correlation between serum immunoglobulin A concentrations and allergic manifestations in infants. *J Pediatr*, 1992, 121 23–7.
4 Cant AJ, Bailes JA How should we feed the potentially allergic infant? *Hum Nutr: Appl Nutr*, 1984, 38A 474–6.
5 Goldblatt D, Morgan G, Seymour ND, Strobel S, Turner MW, Levinsky RJ The clinical manifestations of IgG subclass deficiency. In: Levinsky RJ (ed.) *IgG Subclass Deficiencies*. London: Royal Society of Medicine Services, 1989.
6 Cataldo F, Marino V, Ventura A, Bottaro G, Corazza GR Prevalence and clinical features of selective immunoglobulin A deficiency in coeliac disease: an Italian multicentre study. Italian Society of Paediatric Gastroenterology and Hepatology (SIGEP) and 'Club del Tenue' Working Groups on Coeliac Disease. *Gut*, 1998, 42 362–5.
7 Klemola T, Savilahti E, Arato A, Ormala T, Partanen J, Eland C, Koskimies S Immunohistochemical findings in jejunal specimens from patients with IgA deficiency. *Gut*, 1995, 37 519–23.

8　Crabbe PA, Heremans JF Selective IgA deficiency with steatorrhea. *Amer J Med*, 1967, **42** 319–26.

9　Dubois RS, Roy CC, Fulginiti VA, Merrill DA, Murray RL Disaccharidase deficiency in children with immunologic deficits. *J Pediatr*, 1970, **3** 377–85.

10　Walker-Smith JA, Murch SH The immune system of the small intestine. In: *Diseases of the Small Intestine in Childhood*, 4th edn. Oxford: Isis Medical Media Ltd, 1999, 45–61.

11　Murch SH, Fertleman CR, Rodrigues C, Morgan G, Klein N, Meadows N, Savidge TC, Philips AD, Walker-Smith JA Autoimmune enteropathy with distinct mucosal features in T-cell activation deficiency: the contribution of T cells to the mucosal lesion. *J Pediatr Gastroenterol Nutr*, 1999, **28** 393–9.

12　Chandra RK Nutrition, immunity and infection: present knowledge and future directions. *Lancet*, 1983, **1** (8326) 688–91.

13　Chandra RK Nutrition and the immune system. *Proc Nutr Soc*, 1993, **52** 77–84.

14　Good RA, Fernandes G, West A Nutrition, immunity and cancer – a review. *Clin Bull*, 1979, **9** 3–12.

15　Morgan G What, if any, is the effect of malnutrition on immunological competence? *Lancet*, 1997, **349** (9066) 1693–5.

16　Boeck A, Buckley RH, Schiff RI Gastroesophageal reflux and severe combined immunodeficiency. *J Allergy Clin Immunol*, 1997, **99** 420–23.

17　Fischer A, Landais P, Friedrich W, Morgan G, Gerritsen B, Fasth A, Porta F, Griscelli C, Goldman SF, Levinsky R, Vossen J European experience of bone marrow transplantation for severe combined immunodeficiency. *Lancet*, 1990, **336** (8719) 850–54.

18　Klein N, Jack D Immunodeficiency and the gut: clues to the role of the immune system in gastrointestinal disease. *Ital J Gastroenterol Hepatol*, 1999, **31** 802–6.

HIV AND AIDS

Human immunodeficiency virus (HIV) is the virus that causes acquired immune deficiency syndrome (AIDS). The infection may be transmitted vertically from an infected mother to child, via blood or blood products or by sexual intercourse. In 1994 the Center for Disease Control (CDC), USA, revised the clinical classification system for HIV infection in children less than 13 years of age (Table 13.8) [1]. HIV infection can be diagnosed in non-breast-feeding infants as early as 1 month of age, using a molecular amplification technique such as PCR (polymerase chain reaction). Children over the age of 18 months can be tested for HIV antibody [2]. A total of 882 HIV-infected children have been reported in the UK; 269 (30%) are known to have died [3].

Paediatric HIV infection differs from the adult infection in a number of ways. The incubation period is shorter with a higher mortality rate. Bacterial infections and lymphocytic pneumonia are more common and Kaposi's sarcoma, malignancies and some opportunistic infections, e.g. toxoplasmosis, are rare. Chronic growth and developmental problems are a complication of the disease itself. Frequent infections, fevers, diarrhoea, neurological and social problems result in malnutrition and can affect both adults and children alike.

COMPLICATIONS ASSOCIATED WITH AIDS

Common infections

Pneumocystis carinii pneumonia (PCP) is the most common and often the first opportunistic infection to appear in the paediatric patient. PCP is characterised by a dry cough, shortness of breath and increased respiratory rate. Severe coughing causes fatigue and limits oral intake. Lesions in the mouth and oesophagus caused by recurrent or long episodes of candidiasis make sucking, chewing and swallowing painful. Bottle and food refusal is common.

Diarrhoea

Fat, protein and carbohydrate malabsorption is a feature of paediatric HIV infection, not always asso-

Table 13.8 CDC classification of paediatric HIV infection

Category	
N	No symptoms
A	Mildly symptomatic
B	Moderately symptomatic
C	Severely symptomatic:
	(1) Serious bacterial infections, multiple or recurrent
	(2) Opportunistic infections
	(3) Severe failure to thrive/wasting syndrome
	(4) HIV encephalopathy
	(5) Malignancy

ciated with diarrhoea [4]. Decreased oral intake and enteric infections with malabsorption will contribute to growth faltering in HIV infected infants and children. *Cryptosporidium Parvum, Giardia lamblia, Mycobacterium avium-intracellulare* (MAI), *Clostridium difficile, Salmonella, Shigella, Campylobacter*, cytomegalovirus, adenovirus, rotavirus and herpes simplex virus have been found as enteric pathogens [5]. Diarrhoea occurs less frequently with use of anti-retroviral treatment, although it may be present in new cases. Lactose intolerance may occur, in which case a lactose-free formula/diet may be used for 4–6 weeks. A semi-elemental or elemental formula may be required.

HIV encephalopathy

HIV-associated progressive encephalopathy can affect up to 30–60% of children and adolescents [6], characterised by impaired brain growth, motor dysfunction and neurodevelopmental decline. Regular developmental assessment involving physiotherapy, occupational therapy and psychology specialities can help to identify the developmental issues affecting each child. Little is known about the relationship between nutrient deficiencies and the central nervous system in paediatric HIV infection. A dietary assessment to exclude any nutritional deficiencies would be valuable.

Social problems

Many HIV infected children in the UK are born to mothers from high prevalence countries, particularly sub-Saharan Africa, and to a lesser extent intravenous drug using families. Associated poor/temporary housing facilities, isolation, physical and mental health of other family members may contribute to poor nutrition.

Confidentiality and fears of disclosing the diagnosis of HIV can be a hindrance to liaising with appropriate health and social support providers.

DRUG TREATMENT

Highly active anti-retroviral treatment (HAART) has been used to great effect in the last few years. At present, HAART is mainly available in developed countries. In developing countries it is rarely available in sufficient quantity or regularity to carry out an effective treatment programme. Treatment is usually initiated when clinical symptoms develop or on the basis of deteriorating immune function (rising viral load, decreasing CD4 count). HAART cannot eradicate the virus but it can slow the spread of HIV and reverse some of the deleterious effects. Taking HAART will be life-long and therefore requires careful planning with each child and their carer(s). A combination of three or four drugs may be used, many of which are now available in liquid/suspension formulation. The drugs currently in use, with details of food interactions, side effects and drug interactions, are shown in Table 13.9.

DIET THERAPY

With HAART treatment, children now experience fewer intercurrent infections with improvements in nutritional status, intestinal function [7] and growth. Some children are now even presenting with obesity. Additional dietary challenges include hyperlipidaemia and possibly lipodystrophy (signs in adults include fat redistribution and metabolic abnormalities).

Although the nature of nutrition and paediatric disease is changing with HAART, the aims of nutritional management remain the same:

- Providing the greatest opportunity for normal growth and development
- Supporting the optimal functioning of the immune system [8].

The energy requirements of children with HIV are likely to be 100% of the estimated average requirement for age, with adjustments for mobility, infections and catch-up growth. To maintain nitrogen balance the protein requirement has been estimated to be 150–200% of recommended dietary allowances (American guidelines) [8]. Vitamin and mineral supplements are not routinely given to infants and children (to minimise the quantity of medicines taken) unless intakes are shown to be less than the reference nutrient intake. Diet therapies used in the treatment of some common problems arising in HIV disease are shown in Table 13.10.

Food safety advice should be given where necessary in order to reduce the prevalence of food-borne disease. During periods of acute illness, enteral or parenteral feeding may be necessary.

Table 13.9 HAART: food restrictions, drug interactions and side effects

Drug	Food restrictions	Side effects[1]	Drug interactions	Possible long term side effects[2]
Non-nucleoside reverse transcriptase inhibitors (NNRTIs)				
Efavirenz Sustiva™ liquid	None	Dizziness/light-headedness	In adults – caution with other drugs, e.g. rifabutin and rifampicin	Continuing CNS symptoms
Nevirapine Viramune™ liquid and tablets	None	Rash, fever, nausea, headache	As above	Liver problems
Protease inhibitors (PI)				
Amprenavir Agenerase™ liquid and capsules	None, although eating before a dose can help prevent nausea	Diarrhoea, rash, tiredness, unusual feelings around the mouth	None known	Lipodystrophy
Nelfinavir Viracept™ tablets and powder	With or after food (helps absorption and reduces nausea)	Diarrhoea (can be controlled with loperamide), nausea	In adults – not to be recommended in conjunction with rifampicin	Persistent diarrhoea
Ritonavir Norvir™ liquid and capsules	Best with or after food	Headache, nausea or vomiting, diarrhoea, tingling/numbness in mouth, tiredness	Ritonavir and ddl should be taken 1 hour apart from each other	Lipodystrophy, diabetes, kidney problems, hypertriglyceridaemia
Nucleoside reverse transcriptase inhibitors (NRTIs)				
Lamivudine (3TC) Epivir™ liquid and tablets	None, although eating just before can help prevent nausea	Nausea or vomiting, abdominal pain, diarrhoea or constipation, headache, tiredness	None known	Neutropenia, link with body fat loss, hair loss
Zidovudine (AZT) Retrovir™ liquid	None	Nausea, vomiting, headache, sore muscles, trouble sleeping	Not to be prescribed with stavudine	Neutropenia if also on Septrin
Stavudine (D4T) Zerit™ liquid and capsules	None, although eating just before a dose can help prevent nausea	Peripheral neuropathy, headache, nausea or vomiting, diarrhoea or constipation	Not to be prescribed with AZT	Lipodystrophy, pancreatitis
Abacavir Ziagen™ liquid or tablets	None, although eating before a dose can stop feelings of nausea	Nausea, vomiting, dizziness, diarrhoea, abdominal pain, headache, trouble sleeping	None known	
Didanosine (ddl) Videx™ liquid	Taken at least 1 hour before or 2 hours after food	Diarrhoea, nausea, peripheral neuropathy, stomach cramps, vomiting, rash	Food. H$_2$ antagonists	Peripheral neuropathy, pancreatitis, (in children, eyes need to be checked every 4–6 weeks)

[1] In general, children do not suffer from side effects as much as adults
[2] Reported in adults, although some have been observed in infants and children

Table 13.10 Dietary intervention in paediatric HIV patients

Problem	Interventions
Poor appetite/oral intake	High energy/nutrient dense food
	Age appropriate supplements
	Small frequent meals
	Limit mealtimes to half an hour at most
	Involve child in food choices
Sore mouth	Oral hygiene
	Appropriate medical treatment
	Soft, non-acidic or spicy food and drink
	Use straw to bypass any lesions
Neurodevelopmental deficit	Assess feeding techniques and mealtime behaviour
	Modify consistency of food
	Finger foods
	Establish daily routines
	Involve speech and language therapy
	Consider gastrostomy feeding

Breast feeding

Breast feeding approximately doubles the risk of vertical HIV transmission [9]. In developed countries, mothers generally use infant formula feeds, while in rural settings in developing countries the negative impact on overall infant morbidity and mortality of not breast feeding may outweigh the benefit of avoiding HIV transmission from breast milk [10].

WHO and UNICEF, working with UNAIDS, support several developing countries to reduce mother-to-child transmission. Programmes include HIV testing, with pre- and post-test counselling, advice on infant feeding choices, short course antiretroviral treatment, obstetric services that include best practices for minimising transmission, maternal nutrition support and support to ensure access to adequate breast milk substitutes where women decide not to breast feed [11].

REFERENCES

1 *Morbidity and Mortality Report*: 1994. Revised classification system for Human Immunodeficiency Virus Infection codes and official guidelines for coding and reporting. ICD-9-CM.
2 Gibb D *Guidelines for management of children with HIV infection*, 3rd edn. Horsham: AVERT, 1998.
3 Communicable disease report. *CDR Weekly*, 1999, **9** 18.
4 The Italian Paediatric Intestinal/HIV Study Group, Intestinal malabsorption of HIV-infected children: relationship to diarrhoea, failure to thrive, enteric microorganisms and immune impairment. *AIDS*, 1993, **7** 1435–40.
5 Winter H Gastrointestinal tract function and malnutrition in HIV-infected children. *J Nutr*, 1996, **126** 2620S–2622S.
6 Mintz M Neurological and developmental problems in pediatric HIV infection. *J Nutr*, 1996, **126** 2663S–73S.
7 Berni R Ritonavir combination therapy restores intestinal function in children with advanced HIV disease. *J Acq Imm Defic Syndr*, 1999, **21** 307–12.
8 Heller L Nutrition support for children with HIV/AIDS. *J Amer Diet Assoc*, 1997, **5** 473–5.
9 Dunn DT, Newell ML, Ades AE, Peckham CS Estimates of the risk of HIV-1 transmission through breastfeeding. *Lancet*, 1992, **340** 585–8.
10 Mofenson L Update on prevention of perinatal HIV transmission. *J HIV Ther*, 1999, **4** 57–63.
11 Csete J HIV and Infant Feeding: a Programme Challenge. Field Exchange, 1999, **6**. Emergency Nutrition Network www.tcd.ie/ENN.

USEFUL ADDRESS

AVERT
11–13 Denne Parade, Horsham, West Sussex RH12 1JD. Tel. 01403 210202. e-mail: avert@dial.pipex.com

CHAPTER 14

Ketogenic Diet for Epilepsy

Epilepsy is a common disorder that is a symptom of cerebral dysfunction; it is classified according to the type of manifestations produced, but these categories should not be regarded as separate disease entities. A convulsion or other epileptic manifestation is thought to occur when there is a sudden disorganised discharge of electrical activity from a group of neurones producing symptoms ranging from sensory abnormalities to convulsive movements and unconsciousness. In children it presents typically as myoclonic epilepsy (massive violent muscular contractions) that can co-exist with other types of fits.

The ketogenic diet is a high fat, low carbohydrate and protein diet that was first used as a treatment in 1921, at a time when the only anti-epileptic drugs available were phenobarbitol and bromides [1]. It was noted that fasting decreased the frequency of epileptic seizures and this effect was thought to be due to a combination of acidosis, ketosis and dehydration. The ketogenic diet was designed to mimic these physiological effects of starvation. Usage of the diet decreased when new anti-epileptic drugs were introduced from the 1950s onwards. The diet has regained popularity in recent years, since the side effects and potential toxicity of drugs became apparent.

MODE OF ACTION

A number of hypotheses have emerged about the mode of action of the ketogenic diet and these have been summarised by Schwartzkroin [2].

(1) Energy metabolism

Absence of glucose as a fuel induces non-glycolytic pathways. A high ATP:ADP ratio and increased creatine levels have been shown in the ketotic brain but no abnormality in mitochondrial function has been described in most types of epilepsy.

(2) Cell membrane changes

The ketogenic diet may lead to changes in the properties of the cell membrane, which cause decreased excitability. These changes could be due to the results of altered ATP or other metabolites. A change in the composition of the cell membrane may occur due to the insertion of fatty acid molecules resulting from the high fat intake.

(3) Neurotransmitter function

Higher levels of betahydroxybutyrate in the brain (because of the production of ketones) cause interaction with gamma amino butyric acid (GABA), a brain neurotransmitter, and with glutamate. This may alter neurotransmitter function, which in turn may alter synaptic transmission.

(4) Changes in circulating neuromodulatory substances

A change in secretion of substances such as insulin and other hormones, neurosteroids and peptides, which is a feature of ketosis, exerts direct action on the excitability of neurones via specific receptors. CNS neurones are also sensitive to glucose levels directly, and this may have an effect.

(5) Changes in the extracellular milieu of the brain

Dehydration or altered distribution in the brain may result from fluid restriction or by enhanced metabolism of lipid. pH changes occur as a result of altered metabolic processes. The ketogenic diet may affect blood flow or the properties of the blood-brain barrier and may alter the movement of other molecules into or out of the brain.

There is some evidence to support all the hypotheses listed, but it is still not clear whether the efficacy of the diet is due to ketosis itself, dietary energy restriction, high levels of fatty acids, lack of glucose or altered hormonal levels. Other unanswered questions are why age appears to be important – children are more sensitive than adults – why the diet appears to work on a number of seizure types which have different causes, and why the diet is efficacious in only 50% of children.

TYPES OF DIET

A number of different forms of the diet exist and are used in the USA and the UK; there is currently no standardisation of different regimens, and variations on the main types of diets also exist. There has been only one controlled study examining differences in outcome between the classical ketogenic diet, the MCT ketogenic diet and the Radcliffe diet (which incorporated both MCT and LCT), and this found no difference in outcome between the three [3]. The three diets in most common use in the UK, the classical diet, the Johns Hopkins diet and the MCT diet, are described below.

EFFICACY

The ketogenic diet appears to be most effective for myoclonic, absence and atonic or drop seizures. However, it has been shown to be useful for other forms of epilepsy. A large prospective study at Johns Hopkins showed that approximately 30% of children achieved >90% seizure reduction and 50% achieved >50% reduction. Children aged 8 years and over were less likely to show significant improvement; those with more frequent seizures did as well as those entering the study with fewer seizures; there was no significant difference in terms of efficacy according to seizure type [4]. A smaller multicentre study in the USA using the Johns Hopkins protocol found similar results [5]. In the UK a retrospective study using three different ketogenic diets found that 40% had >90% reduction in seizure frequency and a total of 80% had >50% reduction. There was no difference in outcome between the three different dietary regi-

mens [3]. A 50% reduction in seizure frequency has become the benchmark for the efficacy of drugs, and the ketogenic diet offers this to about 50% of children with refractory epilepsy. There is normally a significant decrease in the number of medications prescribed and cost of medication was estimated to be reduced by 70% in one study after the initiation of a ketogenic diet [6]. The effects of the diet are long-lasting and discontinuation of the diet after a period of 1–2 years should not result in resumption of seizure activity.

IMPLEMENTATION OF THE DIET

Implementation of the diet is difficult: the diet is complicated and unpalatable and compliance may be poor. It is estimated that about 20 hours of dietetic time is needed for one admission, including pre-admission work-up, plus at least 1 hour per week for each outpatient – although some parents who need a good deal of support will take more time than this. In order to be successful a number of core staff are needed: a skilled paediatric dietitian is central to the team; a paediatrician who is preferably also a neurologist and a specialist nurse are needed. Ideally regular home visits should be carried out and close liaison with the school and other carers is essential [7]. It is essential to have access to a paediatrician at all times, as often medical decisions need to be made in emergencies by a clinician who understands the dietary regimen. The diet needs careful and regular monitoring, and the paediatrician must be prepared to carry out the necessary tests. This is a difficult and complicated regimen and a protocol should be drawn up and agreed by the team before a child is taken onto a ketogenic diet programme, so that the carers and ward, community and other hospital staff know what to expect. The protocol should include initiation of diet, timing and type of monitoring and a planned length of the trial; it should also include clear instructions for illness (see later section).

Selection of patients should be according to agreed criteria and some of the following points need to be borne in mind. The epilepsy should be refractory and control should have failed to be achieved on at least two drugs previously. The diet appears to work best in young children under the age of 8 years [3]; infants under the age of 1 year have difficulty in becoming ketotic and are prone to hypoglycaemia. The diet must be rigidly controlled and under close medical and dietetic supervision – there is very little flexibility or room for manoeuvre – and some families may not accept this degree of discipline or may not be able to change their food habits sufficiently. Cost may be an issue as although some preparations are prescribable, butter and cream must be purchased as well as other foods not normally included in the family diet. The implications of the diet must be explained to parents and there must be considerable commitment from them and other carers. Children who are very selective in their eating are unlikely to tolerate the restricted and prescriptive nature of the diet. Children who lead an independent social life without direct carer supervision will find the diet very difficult to manage outside the confines of the home and school.

PRACTICAL MANAGEMENT

(1) A full diet history should be taken prior to accepting the child onto a ketogenic diet programme, in order to obtain meal patterns, food preferences and current energy intake. This is used as a basis for calculating the diet.

(2) A diary should be kept by the parents and other carers, starting approximately 1 month prior to commencing the diet. It should record number, frequency and type of seizures and dose and frequency of medication. General well-being, mood, communication, concentration etc. should be assessed and recorded. The ability and motivation of the carers to keep such a diary will predict likely compliance as well as providing baseline data on which to make objective judgements about response to the diet.

(3) The practice in many centres is to fast the child prior to starting the diet – up to as much as 48 hours [8]. A number of centres in the UK do not fast children prior to the diet, or do not fast them for as long as the Johns Hopkins regimen. A full classical diet should induce ketosis within 48 hours without the need for prior fasting.

(4) A hospital admission for 3–5 days is usual in the UK, although it may be possible to initiate the diet as an outpatient if the regimen does not include a period of fasting.

(5) Drugs should be energy-free and a change to energy-free drugs should be made well in advance of starting the diet. Some children find it difficult to take tablets if they have been accustomed to liquid medication and the action of a drug may be different for different types of preparations [9]. Any carbohydrate contained in medication should be calculated as part of the carbohydrate allowance. In addition, care should be taken to ensure that toothpaste is also energy-free if the child is likely to swallow it.

(6) A fluid restriction is recommended in some protocols, but there is no evidence that this is necessary and many centres allow unrestricted fluids or normal requirements. Better control may be achieved by giving small amounts of liquid spaced throughout the day rather than a few large volume drinks.

(7) A supplement of vitamins, minerals, trace elements and calcium should be taken daily.

(8) A meal plan of three main meals per day plus a bedtime snack is successful at maintaining ketosis as it reduces the time of the overnight fast, which tends to decrease urinary ketones. Eating in between meals should be discouraged as it reduces ketosis.

(9) No foods other than those on the diet sheet are allowed. No sweet foods or sugar are allowed.

(10) Restricted foods both in the hospital and at home should be weighed.

(11) Foods which are generally unrestricted in the classical and MCT diets appear in Table 14.1. Foods marked with a * contain some carbohydrate and/or protein and may need to be calculated into the diet if ketosis is difficult to achieve. It is important to try to make some foods unrestricted to provide bulk and alleviate hunger. Children with low energy requirements may only be allowed a very small amount of carbohydrate and 'free foods' may need to be calculated if they make a significant contribution to the carbohydrate and protein content of the diet.

(12) The fat intake should be spread fairly evenly throughout the day; this is particularly important if a special milk is used.

(13) The ratio of fat:carbohydrate + protein should be correct for each eating occasion (meal or snack). It is not sufficient to achieve the ratio for the day overall.

(14) A recipe for a meal replacement in the form of a milk shake should be calculated and given to parents in case of food refusal or emergency situations. The milk shake can be kept frozen so that it is always available.

Table 14.1 Free foods for ketogenic diet*

Drinks	Tea and coffee – no milk or sugar Sugar-free squash and fizzy drinks Mineral water
Salad vegetables	Celery, chicory, cucumber, lettuce, spring onion, watercress, mustard and cress, radishes, tomatoes
Vegetables	Asparagus, French and runner* beans, beansprouts, broccoli*, Brussels sprouts*, cabbage*, cauliflower*, courgettes, marrow, mushrooms, peppers, spinach*, turnips
Fruits	Rhubarb, stewed without sugar, gooseberries raw or cooked without sugar*, lemons and pure lemon juice, olives*
Flavourings	Vinegar, salt, pepper, garlic, beef extract, yeast extract, Worcester sauce, Tabasco, curry powder, food essences and colourings, gelatine
Sweeteners	Aspartame can be used in moderation. The aspartame contained in sugar-free drinks can contribute to the non-fat calories if consumed in large quantities. Saccharin can be used without restriction. *Do not* use sweeteners containing sorbitol, glucose, lactose or fructose

Items marked * contain >0.5 g protein + carbohydrate per average portion and may need to be calculated into the diet.

(15) The use of bulk sweeteners such as sorbitol, mannitol, polydextrose or maltodextrin is contraindicated.

Nutritional requirements

The ketogenic diet may be followed for lengthy periods of time and it is important that it provides adequate nutrients for optimum growth and development. Normal growth and biochemical parameters were found in one study after 6 months on the classical diet [10].

The diet is generally restricted in energy. If excess energy is taken in the diet it will be stored as fat and will not be used as fuel. This will upset the ratio of fat : carbohydrate and protein being metabolised by the body and will compromise ketosis. The degree of energy restriction depends on the type of regimen followed. Weight gain will be slower than it was prior to the diet, particularly during the first 6 months, and the weight centile will gradually drop. The energy prescriptions given for the three types of diet are very general and the level of activity of the child must be taken into account when deciding energy requirements. The energy content of the diet can be adjusted in the light of weight gain – if weight is being gained too quickly, decrease energy intake in increments of 100 kcal (420 kJ) per day. If weight gain is judged to be too slow, increase the energy intake by 100 kcal (420 kJ) per day initially. It may be necessary to increase the ratio of the diet to compensate for a higher energy intake.

A protein intake of 1 g/kg body weight is suggested for most regimens. However there is no reason in older children why protein intake should not be reduced to the minimum WHO recommendations when using the classical diet (p. 274), providing that the majority of protein is of high biological value. This will allow more carbohydrate and may improve the palatability of the diet.

The diet is deficient in water soluble vitamins and calcium. A complete vitamin, mineral and trace element such as Forceval Junior capsules for children is recommended, plus a sugar-free source of calcium. The diet may be high in vitamin A, depending on the fat source used. There is no supplement that is low in or free of vitamin A and parents should be advised to reduce the quantities of foods high in vitamin A such as cream, margarine, butter and vegetable oil and to use a proprietary product such as Calogen instead.

In order to minimise hyperlipidaemia, polyunsaturated fats are recommended, in a ratio 3 : 1 to saturated fats. This recommendation may be difficult because of compliance [10]. The ketogenic diet is low in sources of carnitine. The additional metabolism of fatty acids may increase carnitine requirements and the anti-epileptic drug valproate also reduces blood carnitine levels and may result in hyperammonaemia [11]. Serum carnitine levels should be monitored. Both free carnitine and total carnitine are measured. Normal values for free carnitine are 30–90 μmol/l and a blood level of <20 μmol/l suggests deficiency. The ratio of acylcarnitine : free carnitine is a more precise marker of status and a ratio of <0.4 indicates deficiency. A supplement of 50–100 mg/kg/day should be given to children [12]. Carnitine sources in the UK are likely to contain sorbitol or other potential sources of carbohydrate. Children most at risk of carnitine deficiency are those in the younger age groups and those receiving valproate medication.

Illness

If the child is dehydrated then the diet must take second place to necessary treatment. Low carbohydrate oral rehydration solutions such as Dioralyte may not upset ketosis. If intravenous fluids are used, saline should be used initially unless the child is hypoglycaemic. Intravenous dextrose-saline will usually eliminate ketosis so it is important that it is not given unnecessarily as it can provoke convulsions. A low blood sugar in itself is not an indication for intravenous dextrose.

Where intravenous fluids are not indicated frequent drinks of carbohydrate-free liquids (e.g. sugar-free lemonade) can be given for 24–48 hours. If the child is unwell for more than 24 hours then medical advice should be sought. It is usually necessary to stop the fat and/or the MCT for a short time, particularly if the child is vomiting. If the child is able to eat, then use exchanges with smaller bulk. If the child is unable to eat, give drinks such as milk or unsweetened fruit juice but avoid concentrated sugary drinks, while remaining within exchanges.

If ketosis is lost for a few days the diet should be restarted slowly using smaller quantities for a few days. If the child is on a high fat:carbohydrate + protein ratio (e.g. 4:1 or 5:1) the ratio can be dropped to 3:1 for a day or two. Slowly restart protein and carbohydrate or calorie exchanges if used, beginning with one quarter of the normal allowances. At the same time reintroduce fat or MCT. If a special milk is used a half strength dilution should be given initially, building up to full strength over 2–3 days. Where diarrhoea is a problem it may be necessary to begin with one quarter strength and build up over 4–5 days.

Special occasions

There is very little flexibility in the diet and any deviation from the diet prescription is likely to lead to break-through seizures. Diabetic foods are generally contraindicated as they are likely to contain sorbitol or other bulk sweeteners. Sugar-free fruit gums and mints can be used occasionally. Some foods can be kept as 'special' – cheesecake made from cottage cheese and cream, and eclairs filled with cream with a small amount of plain chocolate brushed on top, are popular. However, it is important that the family tries to make occasions such as birthdays, Christmas and Easter less food-focused and the child is given other treats such as comics, games, videos etc. or is taken on outings.

The classical diet

The diet provides 90% energy from fat, 10% energy from protein + carbohydrate and contains a ratio of 4 g fat to each 1 g protein and carbohydrate combined; in children under 18 months a ratio of 3:1 may be used (87% energy from fat). The dietary energy content is normally 75 kcal/kg (314 kJ/kg). However, this can be adjusted according to age and size – older children may not require as much as 75 kcal/kg and the EAR for age should be considered when calculating the energy prescription. The protein intake should be about 1 g/kg or sufficient to meet the WHO protein requirements for age or size (p. 274). Many centres in the UK do not restrict fluids and allow a normal fluid intake.

A calculation of a classical 4:1 diet is shown in Table 14.2. The diet is divided into three meals or three main meals plus a bedtime snack. Whole meals or half meals (snacks) are calculated and carers or children select the appropriate number of meals or snacks each day. Most meals include a quantity of Calogen to be used at the mealtime. This must be diluted with at least an equal quantity of water and can be flavoured with vanilla essence, instant coffee or sugar-free fruit squash. It can be coloured with food colourings to improve its appearance. Drinks are best served chilled and may be taken more readily through a straw. Alternatively the Calogen and water can be frozen and served as an ice lolly on a stick or as a 'slush'.

The Johns Hopkins diet

For fuller details of the practical management and calculation of this diet see the book produced by the Johns Hopkins team [13]. A computer software

Table 14.2 Calculation of a 4:1 classical diet, boy aged 5 years, weight 18.5 kg

Nutrient	Allowance		Daily prescription
Energy	75 kcal/kg (EAR* = 88 kcal/kg)	75 × 18.5	1385 kcal
Protein	0.88 g/kg	0.88 × 18.5	16.3 g
Fat	90% energy	1385 × 0.9 = 1246 kcal	138.5 g
Protein + carbohydrate	10% energy	1385 × 0.1 = 138.5 kcal	34.6 g
Carbohydrate	By difference	34.6–16.3	18.3 g

Nutrient	Daily	Breakfast	Lunch	Tea	Bedtime
Protein	16.3 g	4.65 g	4.65 g	4.65 g	2.35 g
Fat	138.5 g	39.6 g	39.6 g	39.6 g	19.8 g
Carbohydrate	18.3 g	5.2 g	5.2 g	5.2 g	2.6 g

<table>
<tr><td colspan="4" align="center">Examples of meals</td></tr>
<tr><td>Food</td><td>protein (g)</td><td>carbohydrate (g)</td><td>fat (g)</td></tr>
<tr><td>Half Weetabix (7.5 g)</td><td>0.9</td><td>5.3</td><td>0.2</td></tr>
<tr><td>30 g raw egg</td><td>3.7</td><td>—</td><td>4.0</td></tr>
<tr><td>70 ml Calogen</td><td>—</td><td>—</td><td>35.0</td></tr>
<tr><td>Total</td><td>4.6</td><td>5.3</td><td>39.2</td></tr>
<tr><td>10 g crisps</td><td>0.6</td><td>4.9</td><td>3.6</td></tr>
<tr><td>20 g cheese triangle</td><td>3.7</td><td>—</td><td>4.6</td></tr>
<tr><td>15 g mayonnaise</td><td>0.3</td><td>—</td><td>11.8</td></tr>
<tr><td>Free salad vegetables</td><td>—</td><td>—</td><td>—</td></tr>
<tr><td>40 ml Calogen</td><td>—</td><td>—</td><td>20.0</td></tr>
<tr><td>Total</td><td>4.6</td><td>4.9</td><td>40.0</td></tr>
<tr><td>15 g roast chicken</td><td>3.7</td><td>—</td><td>0.8</td></tr>
<tr><td>20 g roast potato</td><td>0.6</td><td>5.5</td><td>1.0</td></tr>
<tr><td>Free vegetables</td><td>—</td><td>—</td><td>—</td></tr>
<tr><td>10 g butter</td><td>—</td><td>—</td><td>8.0</td></tr>
<tr><td>60 ml Calogen</td><td>—</td><td>—</td><td>30.0</td></tr>
<tr><td>Total</td><td>4.3</td><td>5.5</td><td>39.8</td></tr>
</table>

<table>
<tr><td colspan="4" align="center">Examples of snacks</td></tr>
<tr><td>Food</td><td>protein (g)</td><td>carbohydrate (g)</td><td>fat (g)</td></tr>
<tr><td>50 g avocado pear</td><td>2.1</td><td>0.9</td><td>11.1</td></tr>
<tr><td>8 ml oil + vinegar (free)</td><td>—</td><td>—</td><td>8.0</td></tr>
<tr><td>15 g cherries</td><td>0.1</td><td>1.6</td><td>—</td></tr>
<tr><td>Total</td><td>2.2</td><td>2.5</td><td>19.1</td></tr>
<tr><td>90 g single cream – flavoured as drink or frozen as ice cream</td><td>2.2</td><td>2.9</td><td>19.1</td></tr>
</table>

* EAR Estimated Average Requirement (Dietary Reference Values, 1991) 1 kcal = 4.18 kJ

Table 14.3 Dietary units in the Johns Hopkins diet (Adapted from Freeman *et al.* 1996 [13])

Diet ratio	Energy value per unit	Fat component per unit	CHO + protein per unit
2:1	22	2g	1g
3:1	31	3g	1g
4:1	40	4g	1g
5:1	45	5g	1g

CHO carbohydrate

Table 14.4 Calculation of the Johns Hopkins diet (Adapted from Freeman *et al.* 1996 [13])

Girl aged 6 years, weight 20 kg (50th centile)
Ketogenic ratio = 4:1
EAR for energy = 82 kcal/kg = 1640 kcal
Energy prescription = 80% of EAR = 1310 kcal
Number of dietary units = 1310/40 = 33 units
Quantity of fat = 4 × 33 = 132 g/day
Quantity of carbohydrate + protein = 1 × 33 = 33 g/day
Quantity of protein = 1 g/kg = 20 g
Quantity of carbohydrate = 13 g/day
One unit = 4 g fat + 0.6 g protein + 0.4 g carbohydrate

Meal plan	Fat (g)	Protein (g)	Carbohydrate (g)
Breakfast 11 units	44	6.6	4.4
Lunch 11 units	44	6.6	4.4
Evening meal 11 units	44	6.6	4.4

program has been developed to simplify dietary calculations for the Johns Hopkins regimen and details are available in the Johns Hopkins book. However, this is of little practical use in the UK as it is based on American foods.

Energy prescription is 75% of the USA RDA; it should be remembered that USA recommendations are slightly higher than the UK EAR for energy, particularly for girls and a prescription of 80–85% of the EAR may be more appropriate. The calculation is based on the child's ideal weight and is dependent on age and height. For overweight children the prescription is based on a lower weight than the current one; for underweight children, however, the current weight rather than the ideal weight is used to prevent rapid weight gain. Energy intake can be gradually increased once seizure control is achieved. The Johns Hopkins regimen only allows for a weight gain of approximately 1 kg per year – any additional weight gain is considered to be excessive and the energy content of the diet is decreased.

The protein intake is a minimum of 1 g/kg ideal body weight on a 4:1 ratio. More protein can be included on 3:1 or 2:1 ratios. Fluid is restricted to 65 ml/kg body weight or 1 ml per dietary kilocalorie. The amount of liquid contained in the cream used is counted into the fluid allowance. Additional fluid can be given to very active children or during very hot weather. The diet is supplemented with an energy-free multivitamin preparation and a calcium supplement of approximately 600 mg daily. The initial ketogenic ratio is usually 4:1 fat:carbohydrate + protein and may increase to 4.5:1 or 5:1. For children under the age of 15 months a 3:1 ratio is started.

The diet is based on 'dietary units' which have a different composition according to the ketogenic ratio used (see Table 14.3). The initial stage of diet calculation after estimating energy requirements is to calculate the number of dietary units to be included. The fat allowance is determined by multiplying the number of dietary units by the fat component in the diet. Protein should be a minimum of 1 g/kg and the quantity of carbohydrate is calculated by difference. An example of a calculated prescription is given in Table 14.4. The prescription is divided into three equal meals. Meal plans are calculated using food tables and a system of exchange lists. These consist of fruits containing 10% and 15% carbohydrate, vegetables with very low quantities of carbohydrate (such as cabbage and green pepper) and those with a higher content (such as carrots or mushrooms). There are very few 'free' foods; most are calculated into the diet prescription.

The MCT ketogenic diet

A diet based on medium chain triglycerides (MCT) induces a greater degree of ketosis than a diet containing an equivalent amount of long chain fat [14]. This means that the diet can be more generous in the amount of energy and protein + carbohydrate that it contains. The appropriate EAR for energy can be prescribed and a wider variety of foods included in the diet. The diet comprises 60% energy from MCT, 10% energy from protein, 12% from long chain fat and 18% from carbohydrate; an alternative

Table 14.5 Calculation of MCT diet

8 year old boy, weight 26 kg
Estimated energy intake (from diet history) = 1800 kcal
60% energy = 1080 kcal = 130 ml MCT oil or 260 ml Liquigen
40% energy intake = 720 kcal = 7 × 100 kcal exchanges

Table 14.6 100 kcal exchanges for ketogenic diets

High protein	Lower protein
150 ml whole cow's milk	45 g bread
300 ml skimmed milk	30 g unsweetened breakfast cereal
25 g Cheddar-type hard cheese	85 g cooked pasta
20 g Stilton or cream cheese	80 g boiled rice
200 g natural low-fat yoghurt (1% fat)	125 g boiled potato
70 g raw egg	115 g jacket potato with skin
60 g ham or gammon	65 g roast potato
50 g cooked chicken or turkey	40 g chips
40 g cooked beef, lamb, pork	20 g crisps
20 g salami-type sausage	155 g baked beans
30 g English sausage	200 g eating apple
30 g beefburger	125 g banana
100 g steamed/baked white fish	160 g grapes
50 g fatty fish	280 g orange
40 g fried fish finger	270 g pear

approach is to provide 60% of energy from MCT and 40% from normal foods [15]. An example of a calculation for an MCT diet is given in Table 14.5. MCT oil or emulsion (Liquigen) is used either as a drink or mixed with foods. In the UK a system of 50 kcal (209 kJ) and 100 kcal energy exchanges is used, and examples of 100 kcal (418 kJ) exchanges are given in Table 14.6. In order to ensure an adequate protein intake it is important that carers are instructed to include 2–3 high protein exchanges. Fluid is not normally restricted in the MCT diet.

There are some advantages to the MCT diet compared with regimens that use long chain fat. The high levels of cholesterol and triglycerides seen in the classical and Johns Hopkins regimens are reduced in the MCT diet [14]. The diet itself is more varied and contains more protein. However, the diet is said to be less palatable and more inclined to cause vomiting because of the MCT. MCT needs to be introduced much more slowly (over about 5–10 days) than long chain fat as it is likely to cause abdominal cramps,

diarrhoea and vomiting if introduced rapidly. During the introduction period only half the prescribed allowance of ordinary food is given.

ENTERAL FEEDS

Enteral feeds delivered by nasogastric tube or gastrostomy should be based on the same total and percentage nutrient content as the oral diet. On the classical diet double cream or Calogen will form the basis of the feed; on regimens containing MCT, Liquigen will be used. Protein and carbohydrate modules such as Maxipro and a glucose polymer or whole milk can provide the protein and carbohydrate. It is important that a complete vitamin, mineral and trace element supplement (e.g. Paediatric Seravit) is included in the feed.

MONITORING

The diet is monitored by regular testing of urinary ketone levels, the aim being to produce a ketone level in the region of 3.9–7.8 mmol/l. If an initial starvation period is not instigated prior to the commencement of the diet, then testing for ketones should not be expected until the diet has been followed for about 48 hours.

Testings should be undertaken twice daily initially, but can be reduced to once daily in the morning once the diet is well established. Variations in levels occur throught the day, with lowest levels in the morning (around 1.5 mmol/l) and highest in the afternoon. In babies, or children who are not dry, urine can be collected by placing a cotton wool ball in the napkin. A record of ketone levels should be kept as this can be correlated with seizure patterns. A sudden fall in urinary ketones is often an indication of illness or the initial stages of an infection; ketones will reappear on recovery.

If ketone levels are low or absent, the following points need to be checked:

(1) Is the diet being strictly adhered to, are the prescribed foods being exceeded, are free foods being consumed in excess, are forbidden foods being given (perhaps by relatives) and have sugar containing drugs been prescribed?
(2) The last intake of fat and/or MCT should not be consumed too early in the day. Fat/MCT should be spread out during the day. A redivision of the

foods may be necessary and a bedtime snack in the correct ratio will help maintain morning ketosis.

(3) Excess fluids are not being consumed – it may be necessary to restrict fluids to 1000 ml daily.
(4) The child is not gaining weight rapidly. This would indicate a need to reduce the energy content of the diet.

If ketosis and/or seizure control is not regained, then it may be necessary to further decrease the energy content or increase the ketogenic ratio of the diet.

An EEG examination should be carried out at least every 6 months. A regular 24 hour EEG is more useful than a short one, but may not be practical. EEG results may not show a correlation with seizure reduction. A diary of seizure time, frequency and type should be kept for the whole duration of the diet. Carers at school should also maintain this diary. As well as seizure occurrence other factors such as behaviour, concentration, communication and mood should be described.

Weight, height, mid arm circumference and head circumference (if appropriate) should be measured every 3 months and centiles plotted in order to monitor growth. A diet history should be taken every 3 months, although this will be more frequent intitially.

Biochemical measurements should include haemoglobin and folate status if compliance with supplements is suspected to be poor; these can be measured after 6 months and then at least annually. Vitamin A status needs to be measured if there are concerns that intake is high. Carnitine should be measured every 6 months in patients considered to be at risk of developing deficiency.

ADVERSE EFFECTS AND GROWTH

Short term complications occurring during the first few days of diet initiation include dehydration, drowsiness, hypoglycaemia, nausea, vomiting and diarrhoea [9]. These symptoms ususaly resolve after a few days on the diet, but it is important to initiate the diet slowly over a few days in order to minimise these early side effects. Hypoglycaemia is particularly common and blood sugar levels should be checked every 4 hours during this period. If symptoms of hypoglycaemia occur (pallor, sweating, dizziness etc.)

and the blood sugar is <2.4 mmol/l (40 mg/100 ml), then a small amount of carbohydrate (3–5 g) should be given in a rapidly absorbed form and blood sugars repeated hourly. If the blood sugar falls below 1.5 mmol/l (25 mg/100 ml) without symptoms the same action should be taken. If hypoglycaemia causes severe symptoms such as a change in consciousness, a 5% dextrose infusion should be started immediately.

A number of other adverse effects have been noted after the initiation of the diet. In one study 10% of children reported adverse symptoms. Most of the complications occurred within 1 month of initiation of diet. Later adverse events may be precipitated by an intercurrent illness. Adverse events include oedema secondary to protein depletion, haemolytic anaemia, thrombocytopenia and abnormal liver function tests. Complications were more common in patients who were receiving valproate as part of their therapy, and an interaction between the diet and valproate is postulated [12].

Both a ketogenic diet and valproate medication are risk factors for carnitine deficiency and carnitine deficiency may precipitate the hepatotoxic effects of valproate [16]. One case of pellagra has been noted, emphasising the importance of vitamin supplements for this diet [17]. Elevated serum lipids, mainly cholesterol and LDL [18] and very long chain fatty acids [19], have been described, but the long term effects of these are not known.

Constipation is a common complication [4]. This is probably due to a number of factors including fluid restriction, a low food intake and a low intake of fibre from fruits, cereals and vegetables. If the diet restricts fluid, an increase of 100–150 ml/day may improve the problem. A small amount of MCT oil to replace long chain fat may also be useful. It may be necessary to prescribe a sugar-free laxative if emptying the bowels is difficult and causes distress.

Renal stones have been described in 5–8% of patients receiving a ketogenic diet [18] and raised values of plasma uric acid have been described [3]. A reduction in bone density occurs if the diet is continued long term without adequate calcium supplementation [19].

Infants under the age of 1 year may not grow well initially and most children will show a reduction in growth velocity [9]. However, growth does not appear to be adversely affected in the long term and catch-up growth occurs in pre-pubertal children when the diet is discontinued [10].

DURATION AND DISCONTINUATION OF THE DIET

Generally a trial of between 1 and 3 months is advocated to see whether the diet does result in a decrease in seizure activity. If there is little or no improvement after this time it is reasonable to discontinue if the parents or carers so wish. Some late improvements have been shown to occur as long as 6 months after diet initiation. In a large trial in the USA it was found that 50% of patients experienced sufficient benefit to continue on the diet for one year. Numbers remaining on the diet at 3 months and 6 months after initiation were 83% and 71% respectively [4]. The Johns Hopkins regimen recommends that after one year with no seizures the ratio of the diet can be reduced in order to allow greater portions of restricted or free foods. After 2–3 years normal diet may be resumed without return of seizures [4]. In the UK the diet is followed for between 1 and 4 years. If the diet is to be continued for more than a few months it is necessary to re-evaluate energy and nutrient requirements at least six-monthly.

When the decision is made to discontinue the diet it is imperative that the dietary restrictions are released slowly over a 5 day period; the length of time taken should be determined by the length of time that the child has been on the diet. A sudden increase in dietary carbohydrate or a drop in ketone levels can precipitate seizures and this is potentially dangerous. The following steps to relax the diet are suggested:

- Reduce fat by 5 g (10 ml emulsion) each day until a normal fat intake is achieved
- Increase protein until normal size protein portions are reached
- Introduce unrestricted cow's milk after 7 days
- Introduce increased quantities of carbohydrate foods after 7 days, avoiding concentrated sugars

The Johns Hopkins regimen decreases the ratio gradually over the course of a year from 4:1 to 3:1 for 6 months and 2:1 for a further 6 months. Once the child has been free of ketones for a few months, a normal diet can be gradually introduced, leaving very sweet, sugary foods until the last. If at any stage the seizures reappear or become more severe, food consumption should revert to a stage where control was acceptable. Once the child is stable the relaxation of the diet should be resumed at a slower rate.

REFERENCES

1 Wilder RM The effects of ketonuria on the course of epilepsy. *Mayo Clin Bull*, 1921, **2** 307.

2 Schwartzkroin PA Mechanisms underlying the anti-epileptic efficacy of the ketogenic diet. *Epilepsy Res*, 1999, **37** 171–80.

3 Schwartz RH, Boyes S, Aynesley Green A Metabolic effects of three ketogenic diets in the treatment of severe epilepsy. *Dev Med Child Neurol*, 1989, **31** 152–60.

4 Freeman JM, Vining EP, Pilas DJ, Pyzik PL, Casey JC, Kelly MT The efficacy of the ketogenic diet: a prospective evaluation of intervention in 150 children. *Pediatr*, 1998, **102** 1358–63.

5 Vining EP, Freeman JM Multi-Center Ketogenic Diet Study Group. Multi-center study of the efficacy of the ketogenic diet. *Arch Neurol*, 1998, **55** 1433–7.

6 Gilbert DL, Pyzik PL, Vining EP, Freeman JM Medication cost reduction in children on the ketogenic diet: datas from a prospective study. *J Child Neurol*, 1999, **14** 469–71.

7 Casey JC, McGrogan J, Pillas D, Pyzik P, Freeman J, Vining EP The implementation and maintenance of the ketogenic diet in children. *J Neurosci Nurse*, 1999, **31** 294–302.

8 Freeman JM, Vining EP Seizures decrease rapidly after fasting: preliminary studies of the ketogenic diet. *Arch Pediatr Adolesc Med*, 1999, **153** 946–9.

9 Schwartz RH, Eaton J, Bowyer BD, Aynesley Green A Ketogenic diets in the treatment of epilepsy: short-term clinical effects. *Dev Med Child Neurol*, 1989, **31** 145–51.

10 Couch SC, Schwarzman F, Carroll J, Koenigsberger D, Nordli DR, Deckelbaum RJ, DeFelic AR Growth and nutritional outcomes of children treated with the ketogenic diet. *J Am Dietet Assoc*, 1999, **99** 1573–5.

11 Gidal BE, Inglese CM, Meyers JF, Pitterle ME, Antonopolous J, Rust RS Diet and valproated induced transient hyperammonaemia. *Pediatr Neurol*, 1997, **16** 301–305.

12 DeVivo DC, Bohan TP, Coulter DL, Dreifuss FE, Greenwood RS, Nordli DR, Shields WD, Stafstrom CE, Tein I L-carnitine supplementation in childhood epilepsy: current perspectives. *Epilepsia*, 1998, **39** 1216–25.

13 Freeman JM, Kelly MT, Freeman JB *The Epilepsy Diet Treatment: An Introduction to the Ketogenic Diet*, 2nd edn. New York: Demos Vermade, 1996.

14 Huttenlocher P Ketonemia and seizures: metabolic and anticonvulsant effects of two ketogenic diets in childhood epilepsy. *Pediatr Res*, 1976, **10** 536–40.

15 Clarke BJ, House FM Medium chain triglyceride oil

ketogenic diets in the treatment of childhood epilepsy. *J Hum Nutr*, 1978, **32** 111–16.

16 Ballaban-Gill K, Callahan C, O'Dell C, Pappa M, Moshe S, Shimmar S Complications of the ketogenic diet. *Epilepsia*, 1998, **7** 744–8.

17 Swink TD, Vining EP, Freeman JM The ketogenic diet: 1997. *Adv Pediatr*, 1997, **44** 227–329.

18 Theda C, Woody RC, Naidu S, Moser AB, Moser HW Increased very long chain fatty acids in patients on a ketogenic diet: a cause of diagnostic confusion. *J Pediatr*, 1993, **122** 724–6.

19 Hahn TJ, Halstead LR, De Vivo DC Disordered mineral metabolism produced by ketogenic diet therapy. *Calcif Tissue Int*, 1979, **28** 17–22.

SECTION 5

Inborn Errors of Metabolism

CHAPTER 15

Disorders of Amino Acid Metabolism, Organic Acidaemias and Urea Cycle Defects

DISORDERS OF AMINO ACID METABOLISM

PHENYLKETONURIA

Phenylketonuria (PKU) is an autosomal, recessive, genetic disorder [1] usually caused by a deficiency of the hepatic enzyme phenylalanine hydroxylase (phenylalanine 4-mono-oxygenase, EC 1.14.16.1). This is a mixed function oxidase which catalyses the hydroxylation of phenylalanine to tyrosine, the rate limiting step in phenylalanine catabolism [2]. Deficiency of this enzyme leads to an accumulation of phenylalanine, resulting in hyperphenylalaninaemia and abnormalities in the metabolism of many compounds derived from aromatic amino acids. The enzyme deficiency varies from complete absence of detectable activity to a residual activity up to 25% or more [3]. Treatment is by a strict low phenylalanine diet.

PKU is particularly common in Turkey, Ireland, Poland, the Czech Republic and Yemenite Jews. Overall, the frequency among Caucasians is approximately 1 in 10000, corresponding to a carrier frequency of about 1 in 50. In Asian populations PKU is rare and incidence figures range from approximately 1 in 16500 in China to 1 in 120000 in Japan [4]. An autosomal recessive gene transmits PKU. There is a one in four incidence of PKU in siblings of index cases and there is an equal sex ratio.

Fölling first recognised classical PKU in 1934. In 1947, Jervis [5] observed that the administration of phenylalanine to normal humans led to prompt elevation in serum tyrosine but this response was absent in patients with PKU. In 1952, the enzyme system that converts phenylalanine to tyrosine was identified [6]. Woolf and Vulliamy [7] first suggested a low phenylalanine diet for the treatment of PKU and this was given to a 2 year old child with PKU in 1953. The child

had severe developmental problems, unable to stand, walk, or talk and spent her time groaning, crying and head banging. During treatment with a low phenylalanine diet there was a gradual improvement in the child's mental state. She learnt to walk, crawl, stand, climb on chairs, ceased head banging and her hair grew darker. A blind challenge with 5 g L-phenylalanine led to the child becoming distressed and a recurrence of the head banging within 6 hours. Within 20 hours, she could no longer stand and could hardly crawl [8].

CLASSIFICATION OF PKU

Phenylalanine hydroxylase deficient hyperphenylalaninaemia can be divided into two main types depending on residual enzyme activity:

- *Classical or severe PKU* Usually characterised by plasma phenylalanine concentrations over 1000 μmol/l (an arbitrary threshold) at presentation [9], but sometimes in excess of 3000 μmol/l. There is almost a complete loss of enzyme activity [10] and in the liver phenylalanine hydroxylase activity is 0.3% or less of normal [11]. Historically, the condition is called 'classical' and in the UK almost 80% of all patients fall into this category of hyperphenylalaninaemia [1].
- *Persistent hyperphenylalaninaemia* A milder form of the disorder where there is only a partial reduction in the activity of the phenylalanine hydroxylase enzyme from 2 to 5% of normal [10]. On a normal diet plasma phenylalanine concentrations will range from 120 to 1000 μmol/l. In the UK, 21% of all patients who have elevated phenylalanine have mild hyperphenylalaninaemia [1]. It is recommended that all children who have phenyl-

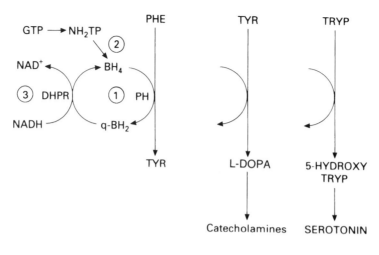

DHPR = Dihydropteridine reductase
PH = Phenylalanine hydroxylase
GTP = Guanosine triphosphate
NH_2TP = Dihydroneopterin triphosphate
BH_4 = Tetrahydrobiopterin
$q\text{-}BH_2$ = Quinoid-dihydrobiopterin
NAD = Nicotinamide adenine dinucleotide

1 Classical PKU
2 }Defects in tetrahydrobiopterin
3 }metabolism

From McLaren DS *et al.* (eds) *Textbook of Paediatric Nutrition*, 3rd edn. Edinburgh: Churchill Livingstone, 1991. By kind permission.

Fig. 15.1 Hydroxylation of phenylalanine (phe), tyrosine (tyr) and tryptophan (tryp)

alanine concentrations of 400 µmol/l or above should follow a low phenylalanine diet [12] at least in early childhood.

There are also rarer forms of hyperphenylalaninaemia due to a deficiency of reductase or other enzymes involved in the biosynthesis of tetrahydrobiopterin [13, 14, 15]. These tetrahydrobiopterin deficiency disorders are sometimes referred to collectively as malignant hyperphenylalaninaemias, but the clinical picture is variable and some patients are only moderately affected, presenting late with mental retardation. A low phenylalanine diet is not effective. In Caucasian populations only 1–2% of cases of hyperphenylalaninaemias have tetrahydrobiopterin deficiency defects [16].

BIOCHEMISTRY

The hydroxylation of phenylalanine to tyrosine is a complex biochemical reaction involving three reactions, each catalysed by a separate enzyme. Phenyl-

alanine hydroxylase catalyses the hydroxylation of phenylalanine to tyrosine in the presence of the co-factor tetrahydrobiopterin (BH_4). During this reaction the co-factor is oxidised to quinoid dihydrobiopterin, which is subsequently reduced to the tetrahydro form by dihydropteridine reductase (DHPR) (Fig. 15.1).

Normally, hydroxylation of phenylalanine contributes up to 50% of the tyrosine that is incorporated into tissue protein [3]. Tyrosine is essential for the synthesis of the catecholamine neurotransmitters such as dopamine and norepinephrine. In classical PKU, there is an inability to convert phenylalanine into tyrosine, subsequently patients with PKU tend to have low–normal or reduced concentrations of tyrosine unless they are given specific supplementation.

DIAGNOSIS

PKU is detected by routine neonatal screening between 6 and 14 days. Whole blood is obtained by heel prick and may be analysed by the Guthrie bacterial inhibition test, fluorimetry, thin layer or paper chromatography [17], or high pressure liquid chromatography. The Medical Research Council (MRC) Working Group on PKU recommends that diagnosis and treatment should begin by 20 days [12].

CLINICAL OUTCOME

Untreated PKU leads to mental retardation, hyperactive behaviour with autistic features and seizures [18]. If treatment is started within the first 3 weeks of life, irreversible mental retardation is prevented [19]. Although patients with PKU treated continuously and carefully, following neonatal diagnosis, have demonstrated that a low phenylalanine diet prevents mental retardation, there is still some anxiety about the intellectual and neurological outcome of early treated children. Most early treated children who have started diet by 4 weeks of age fall within the broad normal range of general ability and attend mainstream schools [20, 21]. However, studies have indicated that the IQ of children with PKU is still about 0.5 standard deviations below population norms and below unaffected siblings [22, 23, 24]. There is strong evidence to indicate that outcome is closely related to the quality of blood phenylalanine control, particularly during pre-school and early school years [21]. A persistently raised concentration of blood phenylalanine over 400 μmol/l correlates quantitatively with a reduction in intelligence quotient (IQ) [22, 23]. However, the risk of intellectual deterioration declines dramatically in adolescence. Neurological signs, e.g. excessively brisk tendon jerks, ankle clonus and intention tremor, have been noted in children with early treated PKU with high blood phenylalanine concentrations and in young adults returned to a normal diet [3, 25].

TREATMENT

The aim of treatment is to prevent excessive phenylalanine accumulation in the blood. Over the years the duration of the diet has been the subject of much discussion and policy change. In the 1960s and 1970s, many PKU centres stopped diet as early as 4 or 8 years, when it was argued brain development would be substantially complete. However, a series of studies showing deterioration in IQ in children under 12 years of age [26, 27] and neurological signs and neuropsychological deficits in problem-solving in young adults has led to the recommendation of diet for life.

PRINCIPLES OF DIETARY MANAGEMENT

The goals of dietary management in children are threefold:

● To prevent excessive phenylalanine accumulation by strict control of natural protein intake in combination with the administration of a phenylalanine-free protein substitute
● To achieve normal growth and micronutrient biochemical status
● To ensure the diet is palatable, flexible and compatible with a modern day lifestyle.

There are five key elements to dietary management:

● Restriction of dietary phenylalanine to maintain blood phenylalanine concentrations within desirable PKU reference ranges in children. As phenylalanine comprises 4–6% of all dietary protein, high protein foods such as meat, fish, eggs, cheese, nuts and soya, e.g. tofu, are not generally included in the diet as portion sizes are small and contribute so little energy to the diet.
● Daily allocation of dietary phenylalanine from measured quantities of lower protein containing foods to provide phenylalanine requirements. These are given in the form of an exchange system, whereby one food can be exchanged or substituted for another of equivalent phenylalanine content.
● Provision of a phenylalanine-free protein substitute, with added tyrosine in order to meet nitrogen and tyrosine requirements.
● Maintenance of a normal energy intake by encouraging liberal use of foods naturally low in phenylalanine, and specially manufactured low protein foods such as bread, pasta and biscuits.
● Provision of all vitamins and minerals to meet dietary requirements. These can either be given together in the phenylalanine-free protein substitute or as modules.

Phenylalanine exchanges

Phenylalanine tolerance is variable and is dependent on the genotype and residual enzyme activity [28]. For

Table 15.1 Theoretical phenylalanine requirements (Adapted from: Acosta [29] and Francis [58])

Age	Approximate theoretical phenylalanine requirements (mg/kg/day)
0–3 months	50–60
4–6 months	40–50
7–12 months	30–40
1–2 years	25–30
2–3 years	20–25
4–6 years	15–25
7–8 years	15

Table 15.2 Protein and phenylalanine content of fruit and vegetables containing phenylalanine between 50 and 100 mg/100 g

Fruit and vegetables	Phenylalanine (mg/100 g) [59]	Protein (g/100 g) [60]	Current status
Phenylalanine 50–75 mg/100 g			
Raisins	51	2.1	free
Banana	53	1.2	100 g/exchange
Leeks	53	0.7	free
Sultanas	58	2.7	free
Mushrooms	65	1.8	free
Mange tout	66	3.2	30 g/exchange
Avocado	71	1.9	55 g/exchange
Mushrooms, fried	75	2.4	free
Phenylalanine 76-100 mg/100 g			
Broccoli	76	3.1	30 g/exchange
Asparagus	84	3.4	1 serving/day
Cauliflower	89	2.9	free
Brussels sprouts	92	2.9	35 g/exchange
Beansprouts	93	2.9	1 serving day
Yam	97	1.7	60 g/exchange

children with classical PKU to maintain a blood phenylalanine within the target range of 120–360 µmol/l, an intake of 200–500 mg of phenylalanine daily is usually tolerated. Phenylalanine requirements are highest in early infancy. Acosta *et al*. [29] reported that to maintain blood phenylalanine concentrations between 60–324 µmol/l in infants, mean phenylalanine requirements per day were: at 0–3 months 55 mg/kg; 4–6 months 36 mg/kg; 7–9 months 31 mg/kg; 9–12 months 27 mg/kg. After the age of one year, there is a small continuous decline in phenylalanine requirements per kg body weight in both males and females with PKU (Table 15.1). This parallels decreasing growth rate and protein requirements. However, total daily phenylalanine requirements remain mainly unchanged on a strict diet [30].

In the UK, phenylalanine is given in the form of a 50 mg exchange system, whereby one food can be exchanged or substituted for another of equivalent phenylalanine content. This is quite different from systems used in other countries, e.g. in the USA and Australia, where a 15 mg phenylalanine exchange system is used and they calculate the phenylalanine content of all foods given in the diet [31, 32].

A 50 mg phenylalanine exchange is equivalent to about 1 g protein and for most foods, when phenylalanine data analysis for specific foods is not available, it is acceptable to estimate phenylalanine content from protein analysis. However, this does not apply to fruit and vegetables and most only yield 30–40 mg phenylalanine per 1 g of protein. It is better to estimate phenylalanine exchanges for fruit and vegetables from phenylalanine rather than protein analysis.

The allocation of fruits and vegetables in the 50 mg phenylalanine exchange system has caused controversy and debate. Some which contain phenylalanine

between 50 and 100 mg/100 g (e.g. leeks, mushrooms, cauliflower) are allowed freely, whereas others (broccoli, sprouts, yam) are counted as part of the phenylalanine exchange system [33] (Table 15.2). There is evidence that all fruits and vegetables containing phenylalanine less than 75 mg per 100 g do not elevate plasma phenylalanine concentrations [34]. In addition, vegetables containing phenylalanine between 76 and 100 mg do not increase plasma phenylalanine concentrations when eaten in small portions. However, the Medical Advisory Committee for the NSPKU does not yet advise that fruits and vegetables containing phenylalanine between 51 and 100 mg/100 g be allowed as part of the free food system.

It is probably better to use basic foods such as potatoes, breakfast cereal, rice, baked beans and sweetcorn for phenylalanine exchanges for a child on a strict diet. Theoretically, any foods can be eaten for exchanges. However, high protein foods can only be permitted in small amounts. Some children may have difficulty in accepting that they are unable to have more of these foods and this may lead to cheating. In addition, if a child eats ordinary bread, biscuits or chocolate for their phenylalanine allowance it may make low protein equivalent foods less acceptable. A

Table 15.3 50 mg food exchanges [33]

Milk	30 ml	**Cereals**	
Single cream	40 ml	Kellogg's Cornflakes	15 g
Double cream	60 ml	Kellogg's Frosties	20 g
Soured cream	35 ml	Kellogg's Rice Krispies	15 g
		Sugar Puffs	15 g
Vegetables		Weetabix, Weetaflakes	10 g
Potatoes		Shredded Wheat	10 g
Boiled, boiled and mashed	80 g	Ready Brek (Weetabix)	10 g
milk-free, jacket		Original	
(all these ways of cooking)		Puffed Wheat	5 g
Roast	55 g	Bran Flakes	10 g
Chips – frozen, fresh, oven,	45 g	Oatmeal (raw) and rolled oats	10 g
crinkle		Rice (raw) white or brown	15 g
Canned, new (drained	100 g	Rice (boiled) white or brown	45 g
weight)			
Croquette	30 g	**Fruits**	
Instant mashed potato – dry	10 g	Avocado pear, flesh only	55 g
powder		Passion fruit	35 g
Baked beans – ordinary, barbecue,	20 g		
curried			
Bamboo shoots, raw	60 g		
Peas – fresh, frozen and petit	25 g		
pois			
Spinach, boiled	25 g		
Sweetcorn kernels and baby	35 g		
corn – canned drained			
Corn on the cob, raw or	55 g		
cooked weight			
Length of cob	4 cm		

list of basic 50 mg phenylalanine exchanges is given in Table 15.3. Figures for the weight of food are rounded off to the nearest 5 g. All phenylalanine exchanges should be weighed unless the weight is stated on the packaging. Parents/carers should be issued with or encouraged to purchase scales to measure in 2 g or 5 g increments.

Ideally phenylalanine exchanges should be spread evenly throughout the day so that a load of dietary phenylalanine is not given at any one time. However van Spronsen *et al.* [35] showed that plasma phenylalanine concentrations only increased above baseline by 10–18% when 50% of the total daily phenylalanine allowance was given at once and 8–26% when 75% of the total daily phenylalanine allowance was given at once. This is in contrast to normal individuals and may be because patients with PKU have a lower ratio of phenylalanine intake relative to plasma pool size [36].

Protein substitutes

These can be categorised into six groups:

- Protein hydrolysate powders – rarely used in the UK
- Amino acid powders ± carbohydrate and without vitamins and minerals
- Amino acid powders with added vitamins and minerals but minimal carbohydrate
- Amino acid powders with added carbohydrate, ± fat, vitamins and minerals
- Amino acid capsules and tablets without added carbohydrate, vitamins and minerals
- Amino acid bars without vitamins and minerals.

The main types and features of protein substitutes designed for children over the age of 1 year are given in Table 15.4.

Table 15.4 Protein substitutes: presentation and composition

Type	Amino acid g/100 g	Protein Equiv. g/100 g	Energy kcal/ 100 g	Energy kJ/ 100 g	Added CHO g/100 g	Added fat g/100 g	Added vitamins/ minerals	Advantages	Disadvantages	Presentation	Supporting research studies
L-amino acids											
PK Aid 4 (SHS)	93.2	77.8	326	1387	Nil	Nil	Nil	• Flexible • Low bulk • Easy to prepare	• No carbohydrate • Poor palatability	Powder (400 g tub)	Associated with selenium deficiency (Lipson *et al.* [44], Wilke *et al.* [45])
Aminogran Food Supplement (UCB)	97.2	—	400	1675	Nil	Nil	Nil			Powder (500 g tub)	
Phlexy-10 Drink Mix (SHS)	50	41.7	343	1456	44	Nil	Nil	• Flavoured • Palatable • Convenient • Moderate bulk • Flexible	• No added vitamins/ minerals • Available in only one flavour	20 g sachets (powder)	Shown to result in better compliance and improved phenylalanine control when compared with other protein substitutes (Clark *et al.* [61])
L-amino acids with added vitamins/minerals but minimal carbohydrate											
Milupa PKU 2 (Milupa)	80.1	66.8	300	1275	8.2	Nil	Some	• Low bulk • Age specific • Easy to prepare	• Inflexible • Does not contain all vitamins/ minerals • Minimal carbohydrate • Poor palatability • Poor compliance • Unsuitable for all age groups	Powder (500 g)	
Milupa PKU 3 (Milupa)	81.6	68	288	1222	3.9	Nil	Some			Powder (500 g)	
L-amino acids with added CHO/ vitamins/minerals											
P Maxamaid (SHS) X	30	25	300	1260	51	Nil	Yes	• Age specific • Easy to prepare • Contains all added vitamins/ minerals	• Inflexible • Bulky • Poor palatability • Poor compliance • Unsuitable for all age groups	Powder (500 g)	Growth normal (Acosta *et al.* [29], Wardley *et al.* [62]) XP Maxamaid associated with low ferritin concentrations (Bodley *et al.* [47])
XP Maxamum (SHS)	47	39	290	1226	34	Nil	Yes			Powder (500 g)	

Table 15.4 *Continued*

| Type | Amino acid g/100 g | Protein Equiv. g/100 g | Energy | | Added CHO g/100 g | Added fat g/100 g | Added vitamins/ minerals | Advantages | Disadvantages | Presentation | Supporting research studies |
			kcal/ 100 g	kJ/ 100 g							
Novel presentations											
Phlexy-10 bar (SHS)	23.8	19.8	371	1562	48.8	10.7	Nil	• Palatable • Convenient	• Bulky • No vitamins/ minerals • High calorie • Product fatigue	Bar (42 g)	Bars been shown to score highly on acceptability rating but did not improve compliance (Prince *et al.* [40])
Phlexy-10 capsules (SHS)	100	83.3	350	1470	4.5	Nil	Nil	• Convenient • No mixing	• Need large numbers • No vitamins/ minerals • Suitable for older patients only	Capsules (0.5 g amino acid per capsule)	In a single case, compliance better than with conventional supplement (Keckskemethy *et al.* [63]). Two out of 19 patients preferred capsules to conventional products (Clark *et al.* [74])
Aminogran Food Supplement tablets (UCB)	97.2	—	400	1675	Nil	Nil	Nil			Tablets (1.0 g amino acid per tablet)	

Requirements

In the child with PKU, protein substitute requirements appear high. Insufficient protein substitute may affect plasma phenylalanine and growth. Although there is debate regarding protein substitute requirement, generous quantities of protein substitute should:

• Lead to increased nitrogen retention
• Improve phenylalanine tolerance
• Help prevent an imbalance of amino acid transport across the blood–brain barrier.

Guidelines for the total protein requirements per kg body weight (i.e. protein from phenylalanine exchanges and protein substitute) are given in Table 15.5.

Timing of protein substitute intake

It has been traditionally recommended that protein substitute should be taken three times daily with meals. The effect of timing of protein substitute has

Table 15.5 Guidelines for total protein requirements in PKU and other amino acid disorders

Age (Years)	Amino acids* g/kg body weight/day	Total protein** g/kg body weight/day
0–2	3.0	3.0
3–5	2.0	2.5
6–10	2.0	2.0
11–14		1.5
>14		1.0

* MRC guidelines on PKU [12]. No recommendation was made for teenagers

** Total protein = protein equivalent from protein substitute/amino acid supplement and phenylalanine exchanges (natural protein)

been extensively studied and it is better to give protein substitute in small frequent doses, three to four times daily spread evenly throughout the day, than once or twice daily [34]. Theoretically it is better given with some of the phenylalanine allowance; protein substitute with added carbohydrate may reduce leucine oxidation and increase net protein synthesis [37]. There is evidence that infrequent administration of large doses of protein substitute increases nitrogen excretion as well as oxidative utilisation of amino acids so this practice is not advocated. In nine patients with PKU and one with hyperphenylalaninaemia, protein substitute was taken in one or two doses on day one, and on day two in three equal doses with meals [38]. In eight patients, excretion of nitrogen decreased from between 6.3 and 12.4 g/day to between 4.7 and 10.8 g/day when the total amount of amino acid mixture was given in smaller and more frequent doses.

Administration of protein substitute

The traditional method of administering protein substitute is in the form of a drink. When dissolved in water it is bitter tasting and produces a hyperosmolar solution (e.g. XP Maxamaid osmolality [1:5 dilution] 968 mOsmol/kgH$_2$O). If diluted with less water, it may cause abdominal pain, diarrhoea or constipation. Communication from parents in PKU newsletters and the Internet constantly reports major difficulties in persuading children to take protein substitute in this format. It was reported from a study on feeding problems in young children that it took on average an hour to drink the protein substitute, with one child taking as long as 7 hours each day [39].

Ideally, if protein substitute is given as a drink, it should be prepared just prior to use, mixed with cold water and taken from a covered beaker to disguise the smell. If it is diluted with less water than recommended by the manufacturers, an additional drink of water should be taken at the same time.

Reports of mixing protein substitute with food are few. Prince *et al.* [40] tried adding a new amino acid blend, containing lower quantities of unpalatable sulphurous and dicarboxylic amino acids, to foods such as tomato sauce and lemon pudding. Compliance did not appear to be any better and it is quite messy and time consuming to mix amino acid products in this way.

Protein substitute (e.g. Aminogran Food Supplement, XP Maxamaid) can be given as a paste. A small amount of water and flavouring, such as concentrated fruit juice, Crusha syrup or Nesquik, is added to each dose of protein substitute to make a thick paste. A teaspoon of fruit purée helps to take away the gritty texture of the paste. An additional drink of water should be given with each dose to dilute this hyperosmolar mixture. It is important the paste receives minimal handling, as excessive mixing may release sulphur containing amino acids. At Great Ormond Street Hospital for Children protein substitute (Aminogran Food Supplement plus vitamins and minerals) has been introduced as a paste from 4 months of age, starting with 1 teaspoon once daily, when additional protein substitute supplementation is necessary. This practice has been adopted by others in the UK and surprisingly is well accepted by most young infants.

Hints for giving protein substitute

- Always treat protein substitute as a medicine
- Establish a time routine – always give at the same time each day
- Always supervise
- Be firm, but give positive encouragement
- Do not allow excuses
- Be consistent
- If taken with meals, try and give before food to ensure it is taken.

TYROSINE

In PKU, the inability to convert phenylalanine into tyrosine makes tyrosine an essential amino acid. Consequently, patients are dependent on a dietary source of tyrosine. To ensure an adequate intake, the PKU MRC Working Group [11] suggested that protein substitutes should supply 100–120 mg/kg/day tyrosine. All prescribable protein substitutes are supplemented with tyrosine and should supply this intake of tyrosine providing adequate protein substitute is given to meet protein requirements. Extra tyrosine may need to be given during pregnancy.

LOW PHENYLALANINE FREE FOODS

Energy requirements are normal in children with PKU [41]. The majority of energy is provided in the form of carbohydrate, with only 20–25% energy from fat [42]. Many patients have low cholesterol levels and a poor long chain polyunsaturated fatty acid (LCPUFA) status [43]. Endogenous synthesis should compensate for the physiological need for cholesterol, but the need for supplementary LCPUFAs in PKU and infancy is being considered.

There are a number of foods naturally low in phenylalanine which can be eaten without restriction:

- *Fruits and vegetables*: phenylalanine content less than 50 mg/100 g (Table 15.6).
- *Fats*: butter, ghee, margarine, lard, dripping and solid vegetable oils, vegetable oils.
- *Sugars and starches*: cornflour, custard powder, sago, tapioca, arrowroot, sugar, glucose, jam, honey, marmalade, golden syrup, treacle and sweets <0.3 g protein/100 g.
- *Miscellaneous*: vegetarian jelly, agar-agar, salt, pepper, herbs, spices and vinegar. Tomato and brown sauce, pickles, chutneys and sandwich spreads <1.5 g protein/100 g. Baking powder, bicarbonate of soda and cream of tartar. Food essences and colouring. Gravy browning <0.3 g protein/100 g. 'Cook in sauces' <1.0 g protein/100 g.
- *Drinks*: aspartame-free squash, lemonade, cola and fruit juice. Tea, coffee, tonic water, soda water and mineral water.
- *Low protein special foods*: a selection of low protein breads, flour mixes, pizza bases, pasta, biscuits, crackers, breakfast cereals, egg replacers. Low protein milks, cheese, cheese sauces (the protein content of these products needs to be counted in the diet) and chocolate are available (Table 15.7). The Advisory Committee on Borderline Substances (ACBS) approves the vast majority for prescription on FP10.

It is important to introduce a variety of low phenylalanine foods into the diet as early as possible to give variety and adequate energy to meet estimated average requirements. Families need lots of simple ideas on how to incorporate free foods into the diet effectively. They need help in interpreting food labels so they can fully utilise all free foods on the market. PKU recipe books, cookery workshops and cookery demonstrations can all help parents prepare free foods. Unfortunately, however, low protein flour mixes are very difficult to handle and as a consequence, low protein cooking failure rate is high. Home cooking was not rated as highly by children with PKU as by control children, particularly home-made cakes and pastry [34]. This in turn can lead to disillusionment and abandoning of low protein special cooking except in the most dedicated of parents. Boredom, hunger and poor compliance may be the inevitable consequence.

Table 15.6 Fruits and vegetables allowed freely (phenylalanine content less than 50 mg/100 g)

Fruits	Vegetables
Most types (fresh, tinned,	artichoke (globe and Jerusalem)
raw or cooked in sugar) including:	aubergine
apples	butternut squash
apricots fresh and dried	beans (French)
bilberries	beetroot
blackberries	cabbage
cherries	capers
clementines	carrots
cranberries,	celeriac
currants (black, red and dried)	celery
damsons	chicory
figs (fresh *not* dried)	courgettes
fruit pie filling	cucumber
fruit salad	endive
gooseberries	fennel
grapes	gherkin
grapefruit	kohl rabi
greengages	lady's finger (okra)
guavas	leek
lemons	lettuce
limes	marrow
loganberries	mooli
lychees	mustard and cress
kiwi fruit	onion, pickled onion
kumquats	parsley and all herbs
mandarins	parsnip
mango	peppers (red, green, yellow, orange)
melon, water melon	pumpkin
medlars	radish
mulberries	swede
nectarines	sweet potato
olives	tomato
oranges	turnip
paw paw	watercress
peaches (*not* dried)	
pears	
pineapple	
plums	
pomegranate	
prunes	
quince	
raspberries	
rhubarb	
satsumas	
strawberries	
tangerines	
mixed peel, angelica, glace cherries and ginger	

Table 15.7 Manufactured low protein/low phenylalanine foods (ACBS approved, available on FP10 prescription in the UK)

	Weight (g)		Weight (g)
Biscuits		Promin Low Protein Tricolour Pasta (four shapes)	
General Dietary Limited		Shells	250
Valpiform Low Protein Shortbread Biscuits	120	Spirals	250
Valpiform Low Protein Cookies with	150	Alphabets	250
Chocolate Nuggets and Hazelnut Flavour		Elbows	250
		Promin Low Protein Pastameal	500
Gluten Free Foods Limited		Promin Low Protein Imitation Rice	500
Aminex Low Protein Rusk	200		
Aminex Low Protein Biscuits	200	*Ultrapharm Limited*	
Aminex Low Protein Cookies	150	Aproten Pastas	
		Macaroni (Rigatini)	500
SHS International Limited		Flat Noodles (Tagliatelle)	250
Loprofin Low Protein Sweet Biscuits	150	Short Macaroni (Ditalini)	500
Loprofin Low Protein Orange Cream Wafers	100	Spaghetti Rings (Anellini)	500
Loprofin Low Protein Vanilla Cream Wafers	100	Spaghetti	500
Loprofin Low Protein Chocolate Cream	100	Aglutella Rice	500
Wafers			
Loprofin Low Protein Crackers (Savoury)	150	**Bread, flour and mixes**	
Loprofin Low Protein Cinnamon Cookies	100	*SHS International Limited*	
Loprofin Low Protein Chocolate Chip Cookies	100	Loprofin Low Protein Loaf – sliced and	400
Loprofin Low Protein Chocolate Flavour	100	unsliced	
Cream Biscuits		Loprofin Low Protein Mix	500
Juvela Low Protein Cinnamon Cookies	150	Rite-Diet Low Protein Flour Mix	500
Juvela Low Protein Orange Flavour Cookies	150	Rite-Diet Low Protein Baking Mix	500
Juvela Low Protein Chocolate Chip Cookies	130	Loprofin Low Protein White Bread with no	
		added salt (canned)	
Ultrapharm Limited		Loprofin Bread Rolls	6 × 4 rolls
Aproten Low Protein Biscuits	180	Loprofin Low Protein – Part Baked Bread	6 × 4 rolls
Aproten Crispbread	260	Rolls	
Ultra PKU Savoy Biscuits	150	Rite-Diet Low Protein White Bread with	400
Ultra PKU Cookies – Aniseed Flavour	250	Added Fibre	
Ultra PKU Biscuits	200	Juvela Low Protein Mix	500
		Juvela Low Protein Loaf (vacuum packed,	400
Pasta		whole and sliced)	
SHS International Limited		Juvela Low Protein Bread Rolls	5 × 70 g
Loprofin Low Protein Pasta Spirals	500		
Loprofin Low Protein Macaroni Penne	500	*Ultrapharm Limited*	
Loprofin Low Protein Vermicelli	250	Aproten Low Protein Flour	300
Loprofin Low Protein Short Cut Spaghetti	500	Aproten Low Protein Bread Mix	250
		Aproten Low Protein Cake Mix	300
Orgran		Ultra PKU Flour Mix	500
Low Protein Pasta – spiral tubes	500	Ultra PKU Fresh Bread	400
		Ultra PKU Fresh Pizza Base	5 × 80 g
First Play Dietary Foods Limited			
Promin Low Protein Pasta (six shapes)		**Cereals**	
Macaroni	250	*SHS International Limited*	
Short Cut Spaghetti	250	Loprofin Low Protein Breakfast Cereal	4 × 375 g
Shells	250	Loops	
Spirals	250		
Alphabets	250		
Elbows	250		

Table 15.7 *Continued*

	Weight (g)		Weight (g)
Fat and carbohydrate products		**Low protein drinks** (These products	
SHS International Limited		contain some phenylalanine)	
Calogen LCT Emulsion – plain and butterscotch	250 ml and 1 litre bottles		
Duocal – liquid	250 ml and 1 litre bottles	*Milupa*	
Duocal – super soluble	400 g can	Milupa lpd	400
		250 ml = half an exchange when made as instructions	
Egg replacers			
SHS International Limited		*SHS International Limited*	
Loprofin Egg Replacer	250	Loprofin PKU Long Life Milk Drink	200 ml cartons
		Contains approximately half an exchange per carton	
General Dietary			
Ener-G Egg Replacer	454	Sno Pro Drink	200 ml cartons
Tel: 0208-336-2323		Contains half an exchange per carton	
Protein-free high energy bar		**Low protein cheeses**	
SHS International Limited		*General Dietary Ltd*	
Duobar available in Natural and Strawberry	8 × 45 g bars	Ener-G Low protein imitation cheeses	
		Ener-G Cheddar (30 g = one exchange)	
		Ener-G Mozzarella (45 g = one exchange)	

VITAMIN AND MINERAL SUPPLEMENTATION

Comprehensive vitamin and mineral supplementation is added to some protein substitutes (e.g. XP Maxamaid and XP Maxamum) and providing adequate quantities of protein substitute are taken no additional supplementation is necessary. Other protein substitutes (e.g. PK Aid 4, Aminogran Food Supplement and Phlexy 10) contain no vitamins and minerals so complete supplementation is necessary, whereas others contain only partial supplementation with vitamins and minerals (e.g. Milupa PKU 2 and Milupa PKU 3).

Reports of vitamin and mineral deficiency are common. This is due to three main reasons:

- Failure of a protein substitute or vitamin and mineral supplement to contain a specific micronutrient, e.g. selenium deficiency has been commonly associated with lack of added selenium to the supplement [44, 45]. The only clinical symptom that has been reported is a dysrhythmic ventricular tachycardia in a 9 month old infant [46].
- Low bioavailability of micronutrients added to supplements. Low ferritin concentrations have

been reported in a high percentage of children aged 1–12 years despite normal haemoglobin and mean corpuscular concentrations [47] and adequate dietary iron supplementation. Similar results were reported by Bohles *et al.* [48].

- Non-compliance with the protein substitute with added vitamin and mineral supplement or separate vitamin and mineral supplement. Vitamin B_{12} deficiency is commonly reported in older teenagers and young adults and is attributed to failure to take prescribed supplements. An 18 year old female with PKU who had avoided all animal products and irregularly consumed her protein substitute presented with paraparesis, tremor, disorientation, slurred speech, distractibility and megaloblastic anaemia. She had low serum vitamin B_{12} and her symptoms gradually responded to oral vitamin B_{12}. In the same clinic a further 12 out of 37 adult patients had low or borderline vitamin B_{12} concentrations [49].

Complete vitamin and mineral supplementation is difficult as there are no ideal supplements available. The most useful products providing micronutrients are as follows.

Paediatric Seravit

The recommended daily dosage is dependent on the age, body weight and dietary vitamin and mineral intake:

0–6 months	14 g
6–12 months	17 g
1–7 years	17–25 g
7–14 years	25–35 g

Paediatric Seravit can be given as a drink (flavoured with suitable squashes or milk shake syrups) or given as a paste with extra drinks given at the same time. It is better to give in 2–3 dosages throughout the day. It is unpalatable.

Forceval Junior vitamin and mineral capsules with additional calcium

Forceval Junior does not contain calcium, sodium, potassium or chloride and contains only small quantities of magnesium. Although it is relatively easy to give an aspartame-free calcium supplement with Forceval Junior, it is difficult to supplement specifically with extra magnesium and phosphorus. No extra sodium and potassium supplement should be necessary for older children, but intake of all nutrients should be carefully monitored. Forceval Junior vitamin and mineral capsules are not recommended for children under 5 years of age because of difficulty in swallowing the hard capsules. It is recommended children over 5 years of age take two capsules per day. They should not be taken on an empty stomach. In older patients, one adult Forceval vitamin and mineral capsule daily can replace two Forceval Junior vitamin and mineral capsules.

Ketovite tablets and liquid and Aminogran Mineral Mixture or Metabolic Mineral Mixture

This combination is one of the original commercial vitamin and mineral supplements used in PKU. However, the composition of these supplements has remained unchanged since they were evaluated in the late 1970s.

Aminogran Mineral Mixture

This product does not contain selenium or chromium and unspecified trace quantities of molybdenum and iodine. Recommended daily dosage:

Infants	<5.5 kg	1.5 g/kg
	>5.5 kg	8 g
Children >1 year		8 g

For children >1 year, Aminogran Mineral Mixture can be given as a concentrated drink or paste; water or diluted drinks should be offered at the same time. If preferred, the unflavoured drink or paste may be given with suitable flavouring such as milk shake syrup. It is better to give in three doses with meals throughout the day. It is unpalatable.

Metabolic Mineral Mixture

This product does not contain selenium or chromium. Recommended daily dosage:

Infants <5.5 kg	1.5 g/kg
>5.5 kg until 3 years of age	8 g
>3 years of age	12 g

For children over 1 year, Metabolic Mineral Mixture can be given as a concentrated drink or paste; water or diluted drinks should be offered at the same time. If preferred, the unflavoured drink or paste may be given with suitable flavouring such as milk shake syrup. It is better to give in three doses with meals throughout the day. It is unpalatable.

Ketovite tablets and liquid

Recommended daily dosage:

Ketovite tablets	3
Ketovite liquid	5 ml

It is essential that these are given with Metabolic Mineral Mixture.

Monitoring of vitamin and mineral status

Annual testing of biochemical, haematological, vitamin and mineral status (e.g. haemoglobin, ferritin, selenium, zinc, copper and vitamin A), together with a dietary assessment is recommended. In particular, vitamin B_{12} concentrations should be monitored in non-compliant teenagers and adults [50].

ASPARTAME

Aspartame is an artificial sweetener which is derived from a dipeptide composed of phenylalanine and the methyl ester of aspartic acid. It is commonly added to squashes, fizzy drinks, chewing gums, sweets, desserts, tabletop sweeteners and even flavoured crisps. It should be avoided in PKU.

MONITORING THE DIET

Guidelines for desirable blood phenylalanine concentrations in PKU

Since the early 1960s it has been policy to maintain blood phenylalanine concentrations slightly above the normal concentrations of 30–70 μmol/l [51, 52, 53] to avoid the risk of phenylalanine deficiency as there is evidence that this is harmful to intellectual, neurological and nutritional status [22, 54].

A recent UK MRC Working Group [12] published a set of guidelines that included monitoring of blood phenylalanine concentrations in PKU. Recommendations include:

- Reference blood phenylalanine concentrations in PKU:
  - children 0–4 years   120–360 μmol/l
  - children 5–10 years   120–480 μmol/l
  - over 11 years   120–700 μmol/l
- Frequency of blood phenylalanine monitoring:
  - children 0–4 years   weekly
  - children 5–10 years   fortnightly
  - over 11 years   monthly
- Blood phenylalanine concentrations should be taken at a standard time each day, preferably before the first dose of protein substitute in the morning when blood phenylalanine concentrations are usually at their highest [39].

Parents should be taught how to collect heel or thumb prick blood samples at home by a specialist nurse. If blood samples are not taken before the first protein substitute dose in the morning, timing should be noted as blood levels may vary by as much as 150 μmol/l per day. Blood samples are then posted to the hospital. Analysis of blood samples by fluorimetry or high pressure liquid chromatography is preferable because of its greater accuracy, although some centres still use the Guthrie bacterial inhibition technique.

The dietitian should contact the parents with the results to discuss their interpretation and instruct on any dietary changes as soon as possible.

Possible explanation for high phenylalanine levels

- Inadequate intake of protein substitute either due to poor compliance or inadequate quantity prescribed

- Catabolism caused by infection, trauma or surgery
- Too much dietary phenylalanine: too much prescribed, excess eaten inadvertently or poor dietary compliance.

A high blood phenylalanine concentration should always be discussed with the parents or patient before any reduction of phenylalanine intake, as high phenylalanine concentrations are due to many reasons. Phenylalanine intake should be decreased by 25 to 50 mg ($\frac{1}{2}$–1 exchange) daily if blood phenylalanine concentrations are consistently high and there appears no other explanation for this (Table 15.8). Phenylalanine intake should not be decreased below a total of three phenylalanine exchanges (150 mg) daily.

Possible explanation for low phenylalanine levels

- Inadequate prescription of dietary phenylalanine
- Failure to eat all phenylalanine exchanges
- Vomiting
- Anabolic phase, following an intercurrent infection.

Prolonged inadequate intake of phenylalanine, especially in infants, may result in a skin rash (commonly seen around the nappy area) and growth failure. If the early morning blood concentration is below 120 μmol/l, dietary phenylalanine should be increased by 25–50 mg ($\frac{1}{2}$–1 exchange) daily (Table 15.8).

FEEDING DIFFERENT AGE GROUPS WITH PKU

Infants

All infants with blood phenylalanine concentrations consistently above 400 μmol/l are treated for PKU. However, the initial treatment will depend upon the diagnostic phenylalanine concentration.

Phenylalanine concentration >1000 μmol/l

A protein substitute is given only. The phenylalanine source (breast or infant formula) is temporarily stopped. This is to achieve a rapid fall in plasma phenylalanine concentrations; a decrease of between 300 and 600 μmol/l per day is normal during this period. The protein substitute should be given on demand and a minimal intake of 150 ml/kg/day should be encouraged. When concentrations are

Table 15.8 Adjustment of dietary phenylalanine against plasma levels

Plasma phenylalanine level (µmol/l)	50 mg phenylalanine exchanges
<60	Increase by 1
60–120	Increase by $\frac{1}{2}$–1
120–360	No change
360–600	Decrease $\frac{1}{2}$–1
>600	Decrease by 1

below 1000 µmol/l, breast milk or 50 mg/kg/day phenylalanine from formula feeds is reintroduced. It is important that the breast-feeding mother is encouraged to express breast milk when breast feeding is temporarily stopped. She should be supplied with a breast feeding pump and also given good support by her midwife during this time. Ideally, plasma phenylalanine concentrations should be measured daily to monitor the rate of decrease and prevent possible phenylalanine deficiency.

Phenylalanine concentrations 600–1000 µmol/l

It is not necessary to completely stop the phenylalanine source. From the time of diagnosis, either breast feeds in combination with a protein substitute or approximately 50 mg/kg/day phenylalanine from infant formula and a protein substitute is given.

Phenylalanine concentrations 400–600 µmol/l

Phenylalanine concentrations should be monitored weekly to ensure they are consistently over 400 µmol/l before dietary treatment is started. Minimal restriction of phenylalanine may be all that is necessary. Dietary restriction of phenylalanine should always be given in combination with a protein substitute.

Breast feeding

Breast feeding is easy to maintain in the infant with PKU and it should always be encouraged. It has several advantages:

- It is low in phenylalanine (46 mg/100 ml of breast milk compared with approximately 60 mg/100 ml in whey based formula)

- It contains LCPUFAs
- It is convenient and reduces the number of bottles which need to be given
- It helps establish good mother-infant bonding
- It helps the mother maintain some control over the feeding process.

The quantity of breast milk produced is suppressed by giving a measured quantity of protein substitute before breast feeds. The baby can breast feed on demand, varying the quantity of feeds from day to day providing a protein substitute is always given first. The quantity of protein substitute given at each feed will vary according to plasma phenylalanine concentrations, but is usually between 40 and 60 ml for infants presenting with plasma phenylalanine concentrations over 1000 µmol/l. Once stabilised, if plasma phenylalanine concentrations are greater than 360 µmol/l, the protein substitute is increased by 10 ml at each feed to decrease the volume of breast milk taken, e.g. if six breast feeds are taken in a day an additional 60 ml protein substitute will be given. If phenylalanine concentrations are below 120 µmol/l, the protein substitute is decreased by 10 ml per feed to increase the quantity of breast milk taken.

Initially, the mother may need much reassurance and support as she may feel the baby is taking little breast milk and the baby may be slow to recommence sucking. Plasma phenylalanine concentrations should be checked twice weekly until they have stabilised and the baby weighed weekly. Breast feeding can continue as long as mother and infant desire.

Bottle feeding

Once phenylalanine concentrations are below 1000 µmol/l, 50 mg/kg/day of phenylalanine from normal infant formula should be introduced (Table 15.9). The total daily amount of calculated infant formula is divided between 6 and 7 feeds and given first to ensure the entire phenylalanine source is given. Infant protein substitute is usually given second in a separate bottle to make up the rest of the feed. The infant is given a total feed volume of 150–200 ml/kg/day (Table 15.10).

It is possible to mix the infant formula and protein substitute in the same bottle, providing all the feed is taken. However, when phenylalanine from food exchanges is introduced and the quantity of normal formula is reduced, the remaining protein substitute may taste less acceptable.

The quantity of infant formula is adjusted by 25–50 mg/day of phenylalanine according to plasma phenylalanine concentrations. If plasma phenylalanine concentrations are less than 120 μmol/l, the infant formula is increased. If the plasma phenylalanine is greater than 360 μmol/l, the daily dietary phenylalanine is decreased by 25–50 mg, providing the infant is well and drinking adequate quantities of protein substitute. Initially phenylalanine concentrations should be checked twice weekly until they have stabilised.

Infant protein substitutes

Analog LCP   This is a phenylalanine-free, otherwise nutritionally complete infant protein substitute, which contains the LCPUFAs arachidonic (AA) and docosahexaenoic acids (DHA). Analog LCP maintains DHA and AA concentrations in red blood cell membrane phospholipids closer to that of breast-fed infants compared to non-supplemented formula [55]. This formula provides 72 kcal (300 kJ)/100 ml and 1.95 g/100 ml of protein which is in the form of L-amino acids. It is made up in the standard way, i.e. 1 scoop + 30 ml water.

XP Analog   This is a phenylalanine-free, otherwise nutritionally complete infant protein substitute. This formula provides 72 kcal (300 kJ)/100 ml and 1.95 g/100 ml of protein which is in the form of L-amino acids. It is made up in the standard way, i.e. 1 scoop + 30 ml water.

Lofenalac   This is a protein hydrolysate, which contains 122 mg/l phenylalanine that should be included in all calculations. It does not contain added chromium, molybdenum or selenium. It provides 2.3 g protein/100 ml as a casein hydrolysate plus amino acids. It is made up 1 scoop + 60 ml water.

Introduction of solids

Solids should be introduced at the normal recommended age of 4–6 months. Usually infants start with one to two teaspoons of low phenylalanine foods such as homemade or commercially puréed fruits or vegetables (less than 50 mg phenylalanine/100 g (Table 15.6)). Useful first weaning foods include

Table 15.9 Phenylalanine content of whey-based infant formula

Type	Amount equivalent to 50 mg phenylalanine exchange	Protein content per 100 ml	Phenylalanine content per 100 ml
Premium (Cow & Gate)	90 ml	1.4 g	60 mg
Aptamil First (Milupa)	90 ml	1.9 g	60 mg
Farleys First (H J Heinz)	80 ml	1.45 g	63 mg
SMA Gold (SMA Nutrition)	90 ml	1.5 g	*

* data available from manufacturer

Table 15.10 Calculation of daily feeding plan for 4 kg infant on infant formula having 50 mg phe/kg

- Total fluid intake 150 ml/kg/day (i.e. 600 ml daily)
- 90 ml Cow & Gate Premium = 50 mg phenylalanine
- Total number of feeds 6 daily

Phenylalanine requirement 50 mg/kg = 4 × 50 mg = 200 mg phenylalanine daily
- Daily formula intake from Cow & Gate Premium = 360 ml = (approximately 200 mg phenylalanine)

Protein substitute
- Total fluid requirement = 600 ml
- Fluid from normal formula = 360 ml. Deficit = 240 ml
Therefore feed deficit made up with phenylalanine-free protein substitute, e.g. Analog LCP (i.e. 240 ml daily)

Feeding plan
1st feed   60 ml × 6 feeds of Cow & Gate Premium
2nd feed   40 ml × 6 feeds of Analog LCP

apple, pear, carrot or low protein rusk made from low protein flour mix, or Aminex rusk mixed with cooled boiled water to a smooth paste. Alternatives are low protein custard made with Sno Pro or Calogen, custard powder and sugar. Low phenylalanine weaning foods are usually offered after the breast or formula feeds so as not to inhibit appetite for the phenylalanine source and protein substitute. The quantity of weaning foods is gradually increased to three times daily. Once the infant is taking 6–10 teaspoons at a time, a 50 mg phenylalanine exchange from food is given instead of the equivalent quantity of infant formula or a breast feed. Gradually all breast or formula feeds are replaced with equivalent phenylalanine from solid food.

Finger foods such as low protein fingers of toast, soft fruits such as bananas, strawberries and peaches, fingers of low protein cheese (as phenylalanine exchanges), low protein rusks and biscuits can be given from 7 months of age. The infant protein substitute or low protein milk substitute can be given from a teacher beaker at 6 months of age.

Introduction of second stage protein substitute

As solids are introduced, the infant is usually unable to drink more protein substitute and from the age of 5–6 months will struggle to meet total protein requirements from infant protein substitute and phenylalanine exchanges alone. It therefore becomes necessary to introduce in small quantities a more concentrated protein substitute. This can be in the form of a non-supplemented L-amino acid mixture, e.g. PK Aid 4 or Aminogran Food Supplement powder mixed in a ratio of two scoops of food supplement to one scoop of minerals, e.g. Paediatric Seravit; or the vitamin and mineral supplemented unflavoured XP Maxamaid. These can both be mixed with a small quantity of water and given as paste pre-meals or added to the infant protein substitute. These products are hyperosmolar and should be given with extra fluid. They should be cautiously introduced and the effect on stools closely monitored.

Additional minerals and vitamins may need to be given with the unsupplemented amino acid mixtures when the volume of infant protein substitute is less than 500 ml daily. The intake of vitamins and minerals from XP Maxamaid should be carefully monitored: 10 g of XP Maxamaid provides 2.5 g protein equivalent, 2.5 mmol of sodium, 2.1 mmol of potassium and a vitamin and mineral profile which is slightly more concentrated than 100 ml of Analog LCP or XP Analog. Infants should not completely replace the infant protein substitute with the second stage protein substitute until they are 1 year old. The infant protein substitute can be stopped at 1 year; if it is continued after this stage it is usually as a late evening drink. A sample menu for a 9 month old infant is given in Table 15.11.

Table 15.11 Sample menu for infant aged 9 months with classical PKU

Weight 8.4 kg
On waking: phenylalanine-free formula, e.g. XP Analog

Breakfast	Exchanges
15 g XP Maxamaid or 1 scoop (5 g) Aminogran Food Supplement as paste	
1 × 50 mg phe exchange e.g. 10 g Weetabix plus protein-free milk or Sno Pro or Loprofin PKU drink	1
Low protein toast and butter	
Infant protein substitute, e.g. XP Analog	

Midday	
15 g XP Maxamaid or 1 scoop (5 g) Aminogran Food Supplement	
2 × 50 mg phe exchanges	
40 g mashed potato	1/2
10 g puree peas	1/2
purée free vegetables	
1 exchange yoghurt	1
Banana or soft fruit	
Fruit juice	

Evening meal	
15 g XP Maxamaid or 1 scoop (5 g) Aminogran Food Supplement	
50–60 g tinned spaghetti	1
Low protein toast and butter	
Low protein custard and fruit	
XP Analog	
	4

Bedtime
XP Analog

Expected daily intake	Protein intake (g)
500 ml XP Analog	9.8
45 g XP Maxamaid (or 15 g Aminogran Food Supplement + 7.5 g Paediatric Seravit)	11.3 (12.1)
4 phe exchanges	4
	25.1 g/day = 3 g/kg/day

Toddlers

Feeding problems are common in young children with PKU. MacDonald *et al.* [56] reported that 47% of mothers perceived their children to have at least three feeding difficulties. Principal problems were slowness to feed, a poor appetite, a dislike of sweet foods and a limited variety of foods consumed. Parents also perceived their children to have more gastrointestinal symptoms such as diarrhoea or constipation. Parents resorted to more mealtime coercive strategies to persuade children to eat, used less verbal encouragement at mealtimes and were more likely to feed their children in isolation. Particular difficulties were experienced with the administration of the protein substitute.

There are a number of reasons for feeding difficulties in PKU:

- *Energy content of protein substitutes.* Some of the common protein substitutes used with young children contain a significant amount of energy. XP Maxamaid contains 309 kcal (1.3 MJ)/100 g, providing 30% of a 1–3 year old's energy requirements. Parents may be unaware of the energy contribution from protein substitutes and so may have unrealistic expectations of how much food their children should eat and may try to coerce their children to eat when they are not hungry.
- *Refusal to eat phenylalanine exchanges.* Parents may become preoccupied in ensuring their children eat all phenylalanine exchanges. Repeated exchange refusal may lead parents to force feed their children and this usually results in an unpleasant mealtime situation.
- *Lack of verbal encouragement at mealtime.* Parents may have to prepare two family meals at mealtime. As a result, children with PKU may be fed first and given their meals alone. However, lack of pleasant conversation and eating in isolation can only have a negative effect on appetite and feeding.
- *Difficulty in giving the protein substitute.* Crying, screaming, gagging, vomiting and deliberately spilling the protein substitute are common in this age group and may lead to some of the feeding difficulties seen.

Overcoming feeding difficulties in toddlers

Some feeding problems may be quite difficult to overcome, but if consistently applied the following tips may be helpful:

- Children with PKU should eat at the same time as everyone else in the family, even though the food offered may be different.
- Small portions of food should be offered at mealtimes.
- Parents should be encouraged to make mealtime a positive experience so the child and family enjoy it. If a child is refusing to eat, negative communication such as 'hurry up' or 'you are a naughty child' should be minimised. Phenylalanine exchanges should be made up later in the day with yoghurt or milk. Bribery should not be used.
- Parents should offer a wide variety of low protein foods as early as possible and preferably during the weaning period. If a food is initially refused, parents should be persuaded to try it again and again.
- Children should start to cook with their foods as soon as possible: icing may be put onto low protein biscuits and decorated with suitable low protein sweets; they can help to choose low protein pizza toppings for their low protein pizza; they can crush low protein biscuits to use as a biscuit base for a dessert. Young children may be encouraged to grow their own low protein vegetables in the family garden. All of this helps to create an interest in food and eating.
- At mealtimes parents should be encouraged to prepare a similar dish for the child with PKU equivalent to that which the rest of the family is eating. For example, instead of spaghetti bolognaise, a low protein pasta dish with tomatoes and mushroom sauce could be given; low protein burgers or vegefingers could be given instead of beefburgers or fish fingers.
- Low protein dishes should be made as colourful and interesting as possible. For example, adding ingredients such as tomato purée, custard powder and brown sugar improves the colour of low protein flour dishes.
- The child's friends can be invited to low protein birthday parties, teas and picnics. If low protein food is eaten and enjoyed by peers, it will make the diet more acceptable.
- Parents should be persuaded not to become angry or frustrated if the protein substitute is refused. They should continue with positive encouragement, but should not allow the child to do anything else (e.g. watching television or playing) until the entire protein substitute is taken. Plenty of praise should be given immediately afterwards. If the

same routine is followed every day, a child will quickly learn this is the way it has to be, even though there may be a few protests from time to time.

Eating in nurseries or other childcare centres

It is increasingly common for young children to spend part of their day in nurseries, other childcare centres or with childminders. Nursery teachers and other childcare workers should understand the basic principles of the PKU diet, foods permitted and forbidden, necessity for protein substitute and phenylalanine exchanges. Ideally they should receive one-to-one verbal explanation from the dietitian or a specialist nurse working in PKU, but at the very least should receive written information about the diet. Parents should be encouraged to supply aspartame-free drinks or the cartoned low protein milk substitute drinks (Sno Pro or Loprofin PKU drink – each carton contains 25 mg phenylalanine) for breaktime drinks, low protein biscuits, a small tin of suitable sweets for treats and a packed lunch. Parents should be encouraged to liaise closely with the nursery about cookery sessions or parties so alternative, suitable PKU food can be provided.

An example of a meal plan for a 4 year old child is given in Table 15.12.

Schoolchildren

By the time a child is starting school, it is important that they have some basic understanding of their diet. Most parents give their children a packed lunch as the majority of school dinner systems are only able to offer a limited choice of foods and are not usually able to prepare special dishes from low protein mixes. The NSPKU produce a useful booklet on packed lunch ideas; a typical lunch box usually consists of low protein sandwiches (e.g. low protein cheese, salad and jam), crisps, salad vegetables, fruit, low protein biscuits or cakes and fruit juice.

Although the protein substitute should be given three times daily it is probably better not to give this at school as it may be a source of teasing for the child and result in the protein substitute becoming even less desirable. Instead, protein substitute can be given at breakfast, immediately after school and at bedtime providing that a source of phenylalanine is given with each dose.

Table 15.12 Menu plan for a 4 year old girl on 5×50 mg phenylalanine exchanges

Weight 18 kg

Breakfast	Exchanges
Protein substitute, e.g. 40 g XP Maxamaid	
1×50 mg phenylalanine exchange, e.g. 15 g	1
Cornflakes + protein free-milk substitute + sugar	
Low protein toast + fried mushrooms	
Fruit juice – aspartame-free	

Midday	
Protein substitute, e.g. 40 g XP Maxamaid	
Low protein bread + butter	
45 g Mozzarella low protein cheese	1
1 small banana	
Fruit juice – aspartame-free	

Mid-afternoon	
1 packet crisps	1

Evening Meal	
Protein substitute, e.g. 40 g XP Maxamaid	
45 g chips	1
20 g baked beans	1
Salad vegetables	
Low protein crumble + low protein custard	
Fruit juice – aspartame-free	

Bedtime	
Protein-free milk substitute	

Expected daily intake	Protein intake (g)
5×50 mg phenylalanine exchanges	5
120 g XP Maxamaid	30 (36 amino acids)
(or 40 g Aminogran Food Supplement + 20 g Paediatric Seravit)	35 g/day = 2 g/kg/day

Schoolchildren will gradually spend more time eating away from home, e.g. at friends' homes, parties, McDonalds and at other events. It is important that having PKU does not constrict social activities, but equally parents and children need to be sensible in their approach to the PKU diet. Children have to be trusted to eat the right things. They also need with them a good supply of appetising low phenylalanine free foods so they are less tempted to cheat if there are few suitable foods available.

Teenagers

This is perhaps the most difficult of age groups in which to maintain acceptable blood phenylalanine control. Teenagers regard PKU as a burden and the diet can be a major cause of friction within households. Although the aim of treatment is to maintain strict phenylalanine control as long as possible, even the MRC Working Group on PKU [21] accepted that it is a problem to maintain strict phenylalanine control in older children. They suggest for this age group that blood phenylalanine concentrations could be maintained as high as 700 μmol/l. However, at this concentration they acknowledge that there is evidence that performance on specific decision-making tasks may be sub-optimal. The MRC Working Group [20] suggest that adolescents and young adults should make their own choices about their phenylalanine intake, having been appraised of the risks of high phenylalanine concentrations.

If it is agreed that the diet will be relaxed from a strict regimen to one aiming to maintain phenylalanine concentration just below 700 μmol/l, the phenylalanine exchanges are gradually increased by one at a time. Plasma phenylalanine concentrations are monitored weekly or fortnightly until the new phenylalanine concentrations are achieved and levels have stabilised.

Compliance with protein substitute and phenylalanine exchanges may deteriorate substantially in teenage years. Schulz and Bremer [57] studied the dietary intake of 93 adolescents and young adults with PKU. Twenty per cent had stopped taking their protein substitute, phenylalanine intake varied between 521 and 936 mg daily, and intake of the following nutrients was low in most patients: thiamin, riboflavin, folate, calcium and iron. Generally non-complying teenagers tend to eat extra exchange foods, eat ordinary bread, biscuits and chocolate, but still avoid the higher protein foods such as meat and fish. If compliance with the protein substitute or separate vitamin and mineral mixture is poor, nutritional quality of the diet is a major concern. Some practitioners would recommend that if the teenager is not taking the protein substitute then they must be allowed free protein in the diet.

Even though compliance and blood phenylalanine control may be poor during teenage years, it is important to maintain contact and communication with the teenager. Health professionals should remain as helpful and supportive as possible.

Teenage pregnancy

This is a particular concern in PKU. It is important that teenage girls and their families are educated and reminded about the potential risks of high maternal phenylalanine concentrations to the fetus, including microcephaly, impaired fetal growth and congenital heart malformations. Head size, birth weight and intelligence of offspring have been shown to be associated with maternal phenylalanine concentrations [20]. They need to understand about the need to be on a strict low phenylalanine diet pre-conception aiming at a blood phenylalanine concentration of 60–250 μmol/l.

Illness management

High blood phenylalanine concentrations are common during illness due to catabolism. Appetite may be poor and management can be quite difficult. There is little work defining the best management during illness in PKU, but the following guidelines may be helpful:

- Continuation, if possible, of protein substitute intake. This will support anabolism and help suppress phenylalanine concentrations. It may be better for this to be given in smaller, frequent dosages throughout the day. Phenylalanine concentrations will quickly rise without protein substitute.
- Encouragement of frequent intake of high carbohydrate drinks, e.g. Lucozade, Ribena or glucose polymer solution.
- It is sometimes recommended that phenylalanine exchanges should be omitted for one or two days. However, catabolism will probably make a greater contribution to plasma phenylalanine than dietary phenylalanine. Some children suffer from frequent intercurrent infections and run the risk of phenylalanine deficiency if exchanges are stopped during each illness episode. It is probably unnecessary to specifically omit dietary phenylalanine, but a sick child should not be forced to eat every phenylalanine exchange.
- Other low phenylalanine foods should be offered to appetite.
- Aspartame-free medications should be used.

MAPLE SYRUP URINE DISEASE

Maple syrup urine disease (MSUD) is caused by a deficiency of branched-chain 2-ketoacid dehydro-

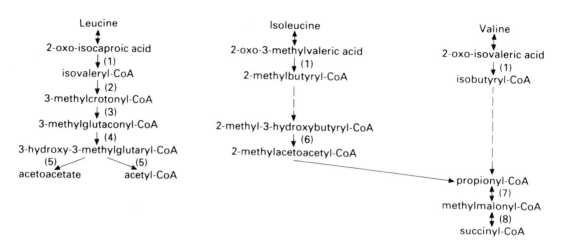

(1) Maple syrup urine disease

(2) Isovaleric acidaemia

(3) 3-methylcrotonyl-CoA carboxylase deficiency

(4) 3-methylglutaconyl-CoA hydratase deficiency

(5) 3-hydroxy-3-methylglutaryl-CoA lyase deficiency

(6) 2-methylacetoacetyl-CoA thiolase deficiency

(7) Propionic acidaemia

(8) Methylmalonic acidaemia

Fig. 15.2 Selected inborn errors of the catabolic pathways of branch chain amino acids

genase enzyme complex (Fig. 15.2). This results in accumulation of the three essential branch chain amino acids leucine, isoleucine and valine and their respective ketoacids in plasma and urine. Leucine and 2-oxo-isocaproate are thought to be the main toxic metabolites and responsible for irreversible neurological impairment.

MSUD can be classified clinically into three types [64].

Classical MSUD

Patients usually present within the first 1–2 weeks of life with a progressive and overwhelming illness with poor feeding, lethargy and seizures leading to coma. The main problem is toxic encephalopathy with varied signs including irritability, changes in tone and full fontanelle. Patients may have a marked metabolic acidosis. The characteristic smell of maple syrup in the urine may be present. Plasma leucine levels are grossly elevated, ranging from 1000–5000 µmol/l (normal reference range 65–220 µmol/l). Untreated, patients may die and survivors are severely mentally and physically retarded. Patients may also present later in infancy with developmental delay and neuro-

logical problems such as fits, but no acute metabolic decompensation in the neonatal period.

Intermittent MSUD

In this variant disorder patients are normally well between acute episodes which are usually precipitated by metabolic stress such as intercurrent infections or high dietary protein intake. Plasma branch chain amino acid levels are near normal between episodes with only a modest or no restriction of dietary leucine intake.

Thiamin responsive MSUD

Thiamin is a co-factor in the branched-chain 2-ketoacid dehydrogenase reaction and occasionally patients may respond to the pharmacological doses of the vitamin. In general presentation is less severe than in non-thiamin responders. Although dietary treatment is required in addition to thiamin supplementation, the degree of dietary restriction is much less severe than in the child with classical MSUD. A restricted protein intake may be sufficient, although it may be beneficial or necessary for some patients to

Table 15.13 Recommendations for plasma branch chain amino acid levels in MSUD

	Aim (μmol/l)	Normal reference range (μmol/l)
Leucine	200–500	65–220
Isoleucine	100–200	26–100
Valine	100–300	90–300

have supplements of branch chain-free amino acids (discussed later).

Dietary management of classical MSUD

Early diagnosis, combined with good long term metabolic control, is essential in minimising neurological impairment and poor intellectual outcome in MSUD [65, 66, 67, 68]. The aim of dietary treatment is to maintain branch chain amino acids (BCAA) close to the upper limit of the normal ranges to ensure an adequate rate of protein synthesis and prevention of protein deficiency. Recommendations for these are given in Table 15.13. Plasma leucine levels should, if possible, be maintained at the lower end of the recommended reference range as higher levels are associated with poorer intellectual outcome.

Plasma leucine is generally elevated much more than isoleucine and valine. The diet is therefore related to leucine intake. The quantity given is adjusted according to plasma leucine levels. Leucine requirements per kg body weight decrease with increasing age.

Considerable interindividual variations of BCAA requirements are reported during the first few months of life [69]. Personal experience has shown leucine requirements to be around 100–110 mg/kg body weight/day in 2–3 month old infants, decreasing towards the age of 1 year to around 40–50 mg/kg body weight/day. Most children with MSUD have leucine intakes between 400 and 600 mg per day.

Once stabilised, there is little variation in the total leucine intake irrespective of age – except during growth spurts or occasionally after prolonged infections when there has been a reduced intake of leucine.

Leucine intake is measured by an exchange system, i.e. the quantity of food providing 50 mg leucine is termed one leucine exchange. Leucine is usually provided by a variety of low biological value protein foods such as potato, vegetables, rice and cereals.

Foods of high biological value protein are invariably avoided because their leucine content is high and energy contribution is low. The leucine allowance is spread throughout the day, ideally evenly distributed, between three and four meals, to reduce fluctuations in plasma BCAA levels. Table 15.14 provides a list of leucine exchange foods for use in MSUD.

The dietary requirements for isoleucine and valine are lower than for leucine. The isoleucine and valine content of foods are always lower than that of leucine content (Table 15.14). Often the leucine exchanges will provide sufficient isoleucine and valine. If plasma concentrations of isoleucine and/or valine fall too low, a supplement of these amino acids is essential to prevent them becoming rate limiting for protein synthesis. An initial daily dose of 50–100 mg of amino acid, divided into two to three doses, is given with the amino acid supplement and leucine exchanges. If plasma isoleucine or valine levels remain low, the dose is increased until concentrations fall within the recommended reference range (Table 15.13). Isoleucine and valine are added to the diet as a solution of the pure L-amino acid. In practice, parents make this solution at home: 50 ml of water is added to 500 mg of amino acid in a medicine bottle (the amino acid is weighed accurately in pharmacy). The solution is refrigerated and kept for 7 days maximum. The medicine bottles are colour coded for the different amino acids, to avoid confusion.

Due to the severe restriction of leucine in the diet, the intake of natural protein is much less than that required for normal growth. It is therefore essential to give a supplement of amino acids free from BCAAs. Generous amounts of BCAA-free amino acids are required because of their synthetic nature and lower bioavailability. This will also help minimise disturbance of flux of amino acids across the blood–brain barrier [70]. No specific recommendations for intakes of amino acid supplements have been set for MSUD, so these are extrapolated from the PKU guidelines [11]. Table 15.5 gives guidelines for total protein intake expressed as protein equivalent from amino acid supplement (protein substitute) plus exchanges as natural protein. A number of BCAA-free amino acid supplements (protein substitutes) of differing composition are available (Table 15.15). The supplement is given as an evenly divided dose ideally with natural protein (leucine), three times per day in children, and more often in infants while they are still being demand fed.

To ensure adequate protein synthesis and normal

Table 15.14 Leucine exchanges for use in MSUD

Food	Weight (g)	Energy (kcal)	Energy (kJ)	Protein (g)*	Leucine (mg)**	Isoleucine (mg)**	Valine (mg)**
Milk							
SMA Gold	35 ml	23	96	0.5	***	***	***
Cow & Gate Premium	35 ml	23	98	0.5	54	31	33
Cow's milk	15 ml	10	42	0.5	50	27	36
Single cream	20 ml	40	167	0.5	48	26	36
Double cream	35 ml	157	656	0.6	52	30	38
Yoghurt (natural/flavoured)	10	10	42	0.4	57	31	34
Custard	15 ml	18	75	0.5	57	31	42
Ice cream	15	25	105	0.4	53	28	36
Milk chocolate	5	26	109	0.4	46	27	30
Plain chocolate	15	79	330	0.7	45	27	40
Cereals							
Rice – raw	10	36	150	0.7	56	26	39
Rice – boiled	25	35	146	0.6	47	22	32
Pasta – raw	5	17	73	0.6	53	28	32
Pasta – cooked	15	16	66	0.5	50	27	30
Vegetables (boiled)							
Asparagus	35	9	36	1.2	50		
Baked beans (canned)	15	13	53	0.8	51		
Broccoli	45	10	45	1.4	51		
Brussels sprouts	35	12	54	1.0	53		
Cauliflower	40	11	47	1.2	53		
Mushrooms (fresh)	50	7	27	0.9	53		
Okra (fried in oil)	35	94	392	1.5	52		
Peas	15	12	50	1.0	45		
Petit pois	15	7	31	0.8	51		
Spinach	20	4	16	0.4	54		
Spring greeens	25	5	20	0.5	51		
Sweetcorn (canned)	15	18	78	1.3	50		
Yams	45	60	255	0.8	49		
Potato†							
boiled, jacket	60	44	188	1.0	55		
roast	45	67	283	1.3	53		
chips	35	66	279	1.3	46		
Fruit (edible portion)							
Avocado	45	85	353	0.9	52		
Bananas	55	34	146	0.7	53		
Figs (green, raw)	90	39	166	1.2	51		
Kiwi fruit	90	44	186	1.0	51		
Dried fruits‡	60	162	693	1.4	56		

Sources:

*   *McCance and Widdowson's 'The Composition of Foods*, 5th edn. Royal Society of Chemistry, Ministry of Agriculture, Fisheries and Food. London: HMSO, 1991.

**   Paul AA, Southgate DAT, Russell J *First supplement to McCance and Widdowson's 'The Composition of Foods'*. London: HMSO, 1979, for milk and cereals; Leatherhead Food RA, Randalls Road, Leatherhead, Surrey, England, 1994, for fruits and vegetables. No data available for isoleucine and valine. Manufacturers' data for Premium.

*** Data available from manufacturer.

†   Potatoes – the leucine content of potato varies between old, new and different varieties: an average figure has been used.

‡   Dried fruits – the leucine content of different dried fruits is not too dissimilar, so an average figure has been used.

Table 15.15 Branch chain free amino acid products used in MSUD

Product*	Amino acids g/100 g	Protein equiv. g/100 g	Energy kcal/100 g	Energy kJ/100 g	Carbohydrate g/100 g	Fat g/100 g	Vitamins and minerals	Dilution	Osmolality mOsm/kg H₂O	Comment
MSUD Analog	15.5	13	475	1990	54	23	full range	15%	353	Infant formula. Reconstituted 1 scoop to 30 ml
MSUD Maxamaid	30	25	309	1311	51	<0.5	full range	1 to 5	782	Suitable from 1 year of age, can be given as a paste or drink
MSUD Maxamum	47	39	297	1260	34	<0.5	full range	1 to 5	1181	Suitable from 8 years of age, can be given as a paste or drink
MSUD Aid III**	93	77	326	1386	4.5	nil	calcium phosphorus only		332	Usually given as a paste

* All products are free from leucine, isoleucine and valine but otherwise contain all essential and non-essential amino acids
** Requires complete vitamin and mineral supplementation
All products are manufactured by Scientific Hospital Supplies and approved by the Advisory Committee Borderline Substances for prescription on FP10. Other MSUD products are manufactured by Milupa, Mead Johnson Nutritionals and Ross Laboratories, but are not currently available in the United Kingdom.

growth, an adequate energy intake must be provided. Plasma BCAA levels will rise if insufficient energy precipitates catabolism. Most infants if diagnosed early and not severely neurologically impaired will eat well orally. If however oral intake is inadequate, tube feeding is vital to prevent metabolic decompensation; both nasogastric and gastrostomy feeding have been successfully used. Long periods of fasting are avoided, especially in infants, as plasma BCAAs increase on fasting. Dietary energy is provided mainly by the following groups of foods which are allowed freely in the diet, although some is provided by exchanges and the amino acid supplement:

- Foods naturally very low in or free from leucine – most fruits and vegetables (Table 15.16); sugar and fats (Table 15.17)
- Specially manufactured low protein (low leucine) foods, e.g. bread, pasta, biscuits (Table 15.7)
- Energy supplements – glucose polymers, fat emulsions.

Supplements of all vitamins and minerals are necessary because of the limited range of foods that can be taken. Free fruits and vegetables may provide sufficient amounts of vitamin A and C. The source of the vitamins and minerals varies: they may be a constituent of the BCAA-free amino acid supplement (Analog, Maxamaid or Maxamum); or a separate supplement will be needed if using pure amino acids (MSUD Aid III). Paediatric Seravit is a comprehensive vitamin, mineral, trace element powder with a carbohydrate base but contains only trace amounts of sodium, potassium and chloride. It can be used for children of all ages, but palatability and quantity required may become a problem in older children. There is no ideal alternative vitamin and mineral supplement for older children. Forceval Junior Capsules or Forceval Capsules are usually given but these contain no sodium, potassium, calcium, phosphate, chloride, inositol or choline and only a small amount of magnesium. A separate calcium supplement will be needed, but the diet may provide sufficient phosphate and magnesium from fruits and vegetables. The diet and supplement together should provide the reference nutrient intake [71] for age for all vitamins and minerals. Alternative vitamin and mineral supplements have been reviewed in the PKU section (p. 246).

Table 15.16 Fruits and vegetables with low leucine content

Fruits

(less than 30 mg leucine/100 g (0.3–1.0 g protein/100 g))

Apple juice	Lemons	Passion fruit
Apples	Limes*	Peaches
Apricots	Lychees*	Pears
Blackberries*	Mandarins	Pineapples
Blackcurrants*	Mangoes*	Pineapple juice
Cherries	Melons	Plums
Cranberries	Mulberries*	Raspberries
Clementines	Nectarines	Rhubarb
Damsons	Olives	Satsumas
Gooseberries*	Orange juice	Strawberrries
Grapefruits	Oranges	Tangerines
Grapes	Paw paw*	Tomato juice
Guavas		

Commercial baby fruit jars/tins which contain ≤0.5 g protein/100 g

* No leucine data is available for these fruits. They are included on the free list because they contain less than 1 g protein/100 g and are consumed in small amounts, infrequently.

Vegetables

(less than 100 mg of leucine/100 g)

Aubergines	Fennel†	Parsley†
Artichokes†	Garlic†	Peppers
Beans (runner)**	Gherkins†	Plantains**
Beans (French)**	Gourd†	Pumpkins
Beansprouts**	Leeks**	Radishes
Beetroot	Lettuces**	Swedes
Cabbages**	Mange tout**	Sweet potatoes
Carrots	Marrows†	Tomatoes
Celery	Onions	Tomato puree
Chicory	Onions (spring)	Turnips
Courgettes	Onions (pickled)	Watercress†
Cucumbers	Parsnips**	

** These vegetables contain 50 to 100 mg of leucine/100 g and could contibute significantly to leucine intake if eaten regularly in large quantities.

† No leucine data is available for these vegetables. They are included on the free list because they are usually consumed in small amounts, infrequently.

Source: Leatherhead Food RA, Randalls Road, Leatherhead, Surrey, England, 1994.

Leucine content of foods

The only published UK data on amino acid content of foods is in the First Supplement to McCance and Widdowson's *The Composition of Foods*, The Sta-

Table 15.17 Foods with low protein (leucine) content

Fats	Butter, ghee, margarine, lard, dripping, solid vegetable fat, vegetable oils
Sugar and starches	Cornflour, custard powder (not instant), sago, tapioca, arrowroot Vegetarian jelly, agar agar Sugar, icing sugar, glucose Jam, marmalade, honey, golden syrup, maple syrup, treacle
Sweets Desserts	Sweets with ≤0.3 g protein/100 g Sorbet, ice-lollies, ice-cream wafers with ≤0.3 g protein/100 g Dessert sauces with ≤1.5 g protein/100 g
Drinks	Flavoured fizzy drinks, e.g. lemonade, cola, Lucozade Squash, cordials, Ribena Fruit juice Milk shake flavourings, e.g. Crusha syrup, Nesquik (not chocolate) Tonic water, soda water, mineral water Tea, fruit teas, coffee
Baking products	Baking powder, bicarbonate of soda, cream of tartar, food essences and colourings
Condiments and sauces	Salt, pepper, herbs, spices, pure mustard powder, vinegar Savoury sauces, vegetable spreads, chutney and pickles with ≤1.5 g protein/100 g Cook-in and pour-over sauces with ≤0.5 g protein /100 g Gravies (reconstituted) with ≤0.3 g protein /100 ml

tionery Office, London, 1979. As there were no plans to update or expand this very limited data, in 1994 the National Society for Phenylketonuria commissioned Leatherhead Food RA to analyse a range of fruits and vegetables for phenylalanine content. In conjunction these were also analysed for leucine content. The analyses were done at the Laboratory of the Goverment Chemist. At present the leucine data is unpublished and the author holds a copy of the leucine analyses. The leucine-free and 50 mg leucine exchange lists for fruits and vegetables in the text are derived from this data (Tables 15.14 and 15.16).

Traditionally manufactured foods have been omitted from the MSUD diet because of lack of detail of their leucine content. The protein content of food alone is perceived to be a poor indicator of leucine content because it is too variable, e.g. a 50 mg leucine exchange of cereal, flour and milk all provide about 0.5 g protein whereas a 50 mg exchange of vegetables and fruit provides 1 g of protein or more. The exclusion of manufactured foods in the diet has made it extremely limited and boring for children with MSUD. Therefore, in 1999 a group of UK metabolic dietitians addressed this issue and decided that 0.5 g protein from manufactured foods could be taken to be equivalent to a 50 mg leucine exchange. Some specialist centres had already been using this value and maintaining good metabolic control. It was also reasoned that more manufactured foods were likely to have flour, milk or cereal as their main ingredient so there would be approximately 50 mg leucine per 0.5 g protein in a food. A 50 mg leucine exchange from a manufactured food is calculated as 50 ÷ (g protein per 100 g of food).

Management of the newly diagnosed infant

On presentation the newly diagnosed baby with MSUD is acutely unwell, often encephalopathic and requiring intensive care. Plasma leucine level is usually greatly elevated and may be rapidly reduced with haemodialysis or haemofiltration [72], although this is not necessary in all cases. Dietary treatment is also started as soon as possible, usually as nasogastric feeding. As the plasma leucine level falls and the infant's clinical status improves, oral feeding can usually be established.

During the acute phase no dietary leucine is given until plasma leucine falls to around 800 μmol/l. Apart from dialysis, the major route of removal of leucine from the plasma pool in MSUD is into protein synthesis [73] and this is best achieved by aggressive supplementation with branch chain free amino acids, a high energy intake and frequent 2–3 hourly feeding. Continuous feeding may be necessary in those patients who have problems with vomiting or hypoglycaemia. The infant is fed the branch chain-free amino acid infant formula MSUD Analog, aiming to provide 3 g branch chain-free amino acids/kg body weight/day and at least the normal energy requirement for age. This may take a few days to achieve in the very sick infant, commencing with a more dilute MSUD Analog solution supplemented with glucose polymer to a final concentration of 10% carbohydrate.

Plasma BCAA levels should be measured frequently, ideally daily. If either the plasma isoleucine or valine levels fall below 100–150 μmol/l, a supplement (50–300 mg per day) is given to maintain plasma levels within the recommended reference range (Table 15.13). Leucine is usually introduced as normal infant formula beginning with 50–100 mg per day (35–70 ml infant formula) divided between several feeds. The leucine intake is then increased according to plasma levels, aiming to maintain plasma leucine between 200 and 500 μmol/l.

Feeding the infant and child with classical MSUD

The diet for the infant is provided by a combination of normal infant formula as the source of leucine and MSUD Analog. The leucine-containing formula is given in evenly divided doses. The frequency of feeding will to an extent be dictated by how often the infant demands feeds. Initially this may be up to eight times per day, but with age will decrease to five to six times per day. This is followed by a feed of MSUD Analog to appetite (Table 15.18). Weaning is commenced at the usual time between 4 and 6 months, starting with low leucine foods such as puréed apple, carrot or crushed low protein rusk or commercial baby desserts which contain ≤0.5 g protein per 100 g. The low leucine food is given after the leucine containing formula and during or after the MSUD Analog feed. It does not matter therefore if solids are not completed as they do not affect total leucine intake. As the infant takes more solids, the amount of infant formula offered is reduced by one leucine exchange and replaced with one exchange of food, e.g. 40 g cauliflower. The food exchange is given before the MSUD Analog. This process is continued throughout the first year until all the leucine is provided by solids and is given divided between three main meals.

MSUD Aid III (an amino acid supplement free from BCAA) is gradually introduced from around 4 to 6 months of age to condition the infant to its flavour and texture and, in some, to maintain an adequate supply of branch chain-free amino acids. The MSUD Aid III and vitamin and mineral supplement are mixed with water and milk shake flavouring, such as Nesquik or Crusha syrup, to form a paste. A teaspoon of fruit purée added to this mixture will make it less gritty and more palatable. A strong flavouring agent is essential to improve the taste of the product: in practice 10 g MSUD Aid III is mixed with 5 g Paediatric Seravit (a ratio of 2:1) plus 2–3 teaspoons water and Nesquik powder. Initially one

Table 15.18 Example of a feeding regimen for infant with MSUD aged 2 months, weight 4.5 kg

	Energy		Protein (g)	Amino acids (g)	Leucine (mg)	Isoleucine (mg)	Valine (mg)
	(kcal)	(kJ)					
300 ml Cow & Gate Premium 60 ml × 5 feeds	201	840	4.2		450	256	273
420 ml MSUD Analog 70 ml × 6 feeds	345	1442	9.4*	11.1	—	—	—
Totals	546	2282	13.6		450	256	273
Per kg	121	507	3.0		100	57	61
DRV per kg for 0–3 months [71]	115–100	480–420	2.1				
Aim per kg (Table 15.5)			3.0				

* Protein equivatent

teaspoon of this paste is given at one meal per day before the measured leucine exchange. The MSUD Aid III mixture is gradually increased in quantity and given at three meals per day and will eventually replace the MSUD Analog. The infant's acceptance of the MSUD Aid III will determine how quickly the quantity offered can be increased; force feeding must be avoided. As the amount of paste taken increases it is important to give a drink of water after it because of its high osmolality. Flexibility is necessary when introducing the MSUD Aid III paste; a combination of both Analog and MSUD Aid III may be more acceptable throughout the toddler years. If MSUD Aid III is not taken well as a paste, it may need to be added to the Analog feed to maintain an adequate intake of branch chain-free amino acids. Care must be taken as the feed will be hyperosmolar; 5 g of MSUD Aid III can be safely added to 150 ml MSUD Analog.

An alternative to MSUD Aid III paste is MSUD Maxamaid (branch chain-free amino acid supplement with added carbohydrate and full range of vitamins and minerals) which is given as a drink. This product is not recommended for children under the age of 1 year because of its high osmolality (Table 15.15). However, it can be introduced before 1 year of age as a diluted drink initially once per day, so the child can get used to the taste. The concentration is then gradually increased as tolerated to the recommended 1 in 5 dilution and the frequency to three times per day. These Maxamaid drinks are often taken in a greater concentration than 1 in 5 without a problem.

Maxamaid can also be given as a paste with a drink to follow. Compared to MSUD Aid paste mixture this is much more bulky because of its carbohydrate (CHO) content. A strong flavouring agent needs to be added to Maxamaid. An orange flavoured version of MSUD Maxamaid is available.

From around 1 year the diet should have progressed so that all leucine exchanges come from food, MSUD Aid III paste is taken and low leucine foods are taken to appetite. Table 15.19 provides a typical example of a child's daily diet. During childhood the branch chain-free amino acid supplement is increased to ensure an adequate intake of total protein (Table 15.5). MSUD Maxamum (Table 15.15) is a useful alternative branch chain-free amino acid supplement which provides more amino acids in a smaller dose. It is recommended for use from 8 years of age.

Monitoring branch chain amino acids

Plasma BCAAs should be measured once a week in infants because growth is rapid, and every 2 weeks in 1–3 year olds. Thereafter, frequency varies between 2–8 weeks depending on the stability of the child.

Leucine intake is altered according to plasma BCAA levels. There are several reasons for high leucine levels, apart from intercurrent infections. These include inadequate energy intake with poor growth, insufficient branch chain-free amino acid supplement, or dietary indiscretion. If the plasma leucine level is around 600–700 μmol/l leucine intake

Table 15.19 Sample menu for child with MSUD age 4 years, weight 15 kg providing 450 mg leucine (nine exchanges per day)

Branch chain-free amino acid supplement
35 g MSUD Aid III (2 g amino acids/kg)
20 g Paediatric Seravit
Flavouring e.g. Strawberry Nesquik
Add water to a paste ÷ 3
or
100 g MSUD Maxamaid (2 g amino acids/kg)
Flavouring e.g. blackcurrant juice
Add water to 450 ml
÷ 150 ml × 3 drinks

		Leucine Exchanges
Breakfast	⅓ amino acid supplement	
	3 × 50 mg leucine exchange	
	18 g Weetabix	3
	protein-free milk* + sugar	
	low protein bread + margarine + honey or jam	
Lunch	⅓ amino acid supplement	
	3 × 50 mg leucine exchange	
	120 g potato	2
	45 g broccoli tops	1
	low leucine vegetables and margarine	
	low protein apple crumble	
	low protein custard	
Supper	⅓ amino acid supplement	
	3 × 50 mg leucine exchange	
	30 g peas	2
	low protein pasta + margarine + tomato ketchup	
	15 g ice cream	1
	fruit, fresh or tinned in syrup	
Snacks	low protein biscuits, cake or cereal	
	Duobar high energy supplement or fruit	
	squash, fizzy drinks, protein-free milkshake*	

---

* Protein-free milks (Tables 15.7, 15.29)

is decreased by 50 mg to 100 mg daily (one to two leucine exchanges). If the plasma leucine level is less than 100–200 µmol/l, leucine intake is increased by 50–100 mg (one to two exchanges). If either plasma isoleucine or valine level is less than 100 µmol/l, while the concentrations of the other amino acids are normal, a supplement of 50–100 mg of the relevant amino acid is given. Any dietary alteration is reviewed with a follow-up blood test within 1–2 weeks. Diurnal changes in amino acids have been reported in MSUD, BCAA levels always being higher after an overnight

fast than post-prandially [75]. These factors need to be considered when interpreting plasma BCAA concentrations.

Monitoring the diet

Clinical, biochemical and nutritional status is monitored specifically looking for signs of protein deficiency such as skin rashes. Protein, zinc and isoleucine [74] deficiency have been seen in children with MSUD (pers. observ.). Periodic analysis of trace element status is important (Table 1.6). The diet is assessed regularly to ensure all nutrients, particularly trace elements and minerals, provide the RNI for age [71].

Dietary management during illness

During intercurrent infections plasma BCAA concentrations may rise rapidly, particularly that of leucine. This increase in leucine appears to be more attributable to inadequate energy intake than to the direct catabolic effect of the infection [76]. At the first sign of illness the emergency regimen (ER) is started to reduce the accumulation of leucine which could cause rapid neurological deterioration. If oral intake is poor, tube feeding should be commenced without delay. The usual leucine intake is stopped or substantially decreased. The standard ER (p. 287) of a high CHO intake from glucose polymer and frequent two to three hourly feeding or even 24 hour continuous feeding are instituted. Furthermore, supplements of branch chain-free amino acids are given to promote protein synthesis. As this is the major route of removal of leucine from the plasma pool, other losses are minimal. If branch chain-free amino acids are not given, other amino acids will become rate-limiting for protein synthesis and plasma leucine concentrations will remain high. The aim is to provide the child's usual intake of branch chain-free amino acids and at least the normal energy requirement for age, although this can be difficult to achieve. The infant is given MSUD Analog with additional glucose polymer to a total concentration of 10–12% carbohydrate, and the child either MSUD Maxamaid or Maxamum with glucose polymer added to 15–20% carbohydrate. If the child is on MSUD Aid III this should continue to be given, but it may be more acceptable and better tolerated as smaller more frequent doses. This is combined with high CHO drinks according to the standard ER (p. 287).

If the child normally has isoleucine and valine supplements and plasma levels are not high, it may be prudent to continue these, as plasma concentrations can fall to low levels during the recovery phase, particularly if plasma leucine levels have been high.

Plasma BCAA levels should be measured frequently throughout illness, to monitor progress and determine when leucine can be reintroduced. Once the plasma leucine has fallen to around 600–700 μmol/l or the child is improving, dietary leucine can be gradually reintroduced, increasing to the usual intake over a few days according to plasma levels. In milder illnesses plasma leucine may not necessarily increase above 600–700 μmol/l if the ER has been instituted at an early stage.

If the child does not tolerate the ER feeds then intravenous (IV) fluids (10% dextrose) are given. There are no branch chain-free parenteral amino acid solutions available in the UK. If needed, the best option is to combine IV fluids (dextrose and lipid) with a continuous nasogastric feed of branch chain-

free amino acids such as MSUD Aid III, beginning with a small amount such as 0.5 g amino acids/kg and increasing as tolerated. Illness in intermittent and thiamin responsive MSUD also necessitates use of an ER similar to classical MSUD. If the child is not on branch chain-free amino acids then the standard ER of high CHO feeds is used (p. 287).

TYROSINAEMIA TYPE I

Tyrosinaemia type I is caused by reduced activity of fumarylacetoacetate hydrolyase which catalyses the final step of tyrosine degradation (Fig. 15.3). Fumarylacetoacetate and maleylacetoacetate accumulate and are further metabolised to succinylacetone which is found in greatly increased quantities in plasma and urine. These metabolites are considered toxic and responsible for the clinical features of progressive liver failure with increased risk for hepatocellular carcinoma (HCC), renal tubular dysfunction

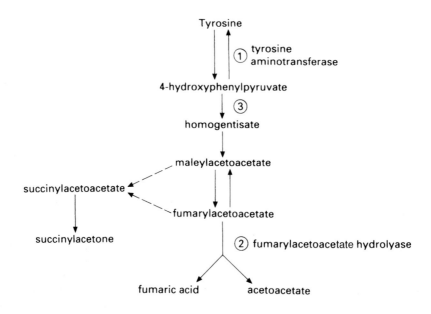

Fig. 15.3 Pathway of tyrosine degradation

with hypophosphataemic rickets and a porphyria-like syndrome [77, 78]. Tyrosinaemia type I can present at different ages with varying degrees of severity. In 1994 a new classification was proposed according to survival rate; this did not include data of patients treated with NTBC (discussed later) [79].

Age of onset	symptoms	1 and 2 year survival rates
Very early onset	<2 months	38%, 29%
Early onset	2 to 6 months	74%, 74%
Late onset	>6 months	96%, 96%

At presentation plasma tyrosine concentration is usually moderately increased (two to four times upper normal limit). Plasma methionine concentration can also be markedly increased. This is due to secondary inhibition of s-adenosylmethionine synthetase [77]. High plasma methionine may affect normal liver function [80].

In the past, tyrosinaemia type I was treated with a low tyrosine, low phenylalanine diet to minimise formation of toxic succinylacetone. Initially, a reduced methionine intake was also used. Dietary treatment was shown to improve renal tubular dysfunction and growth. Liver function (in particular pro-thrombin time) sometimes improved a little but diet could not prevent the development of hepatoma and some patients developed progressive liver failure or had lethal porphyric crises. Until recently liver transplantation was the only really effective treatment for tyrosinaemia type I. However, in 1992 Lindstet *et al.* described the use of 2-(2-nitro-4-trifluoromethylbenzoyl)-1, 3-cyclohexanedione (NTBC) as an alternative treatment [81]. NTBC inhibits the enzyme 4-hydroxyphenylpyruvate dioxygenase and blocks the tyrosine degradation pathway at this level (Fig. 15.3). This prevents the formation of the hepatotoxic and nephrotoxic compounds and succinylacetone (which probably plays an important role in neurotoxicity). NTBC treatment leads to rapid improvement in hepatic and renal problems and it prevents neurological dysfunction in most patients. Also, in those who have started on NTBC treatment at a young age the risk of early development of HCC is reduced [82]. NTBC is established as an alternative to transplantation.

Plasma tyrosine concentrations increase with NTBC treatment. In tyrosinaemia type II high plasma tyrosine concentrations are the probable cause of the oculocutaneous manifestations and may also be

associated with the mental retardation reported in some patients [77]. To reduce the risks linked with high plasma tyrosine concentrations, patients on NTBC are treated with a low tyrosine/low phenylalanine diet (in practice a low protein diet).

Dietary management for NTBC treated patients

The aim of dietary treatment is to maintain plasma tyrosine concentrations below 600 μmol/l and above 200 μmol/l (normal reference range 30–120 μmol/l).

Natural protein intake is reduced, thereby limiting tyrosine and phenylalanine intakes. Intake is altered according to plasma tyrosine concentrations. The amount of natural protein tolerated varies between patients. It has been reported to decrease from a peak of 1.8–2.4 g protein/kg/day at four to five months to around 1 g protein/kg/day in late infancy [83]. Thereafter, once the patient has stabilised, the total protein intake usually varies little irrespective of age, except during growth spurts. The natural protein intake is measured as 1 g protein exchanges, i.e. the weight of food which provides 1 g of protein (Table 15.20).

A supplement of tyrosine/phenylalanine-free amino acids is usually given, even if the allowance of natural protein provides the safe level of intake for growth. There are no set recommendations in the UK for amounts of amino acid supplement to give so these are either extrapolated from the PKU guidelines (Table 15.5) or together with natural protein intake calculated to provide 10–12% of energy intake. Table 15.5 gives guidelines for total protein intake as protein equivalent from amino acid supplement plus phenylalanine exchanges (natural protein). Generous intakes of the amino acid supplement should help minimise disturbance of flux of amino acids across the blood–brain barrier [70, 84]. Several amino acid supplement (protein substitute) products of varying composition, appropriate for different age groups, are available for children with tyrosinaemia (Table 15.21). The supplement is given as a divided dose, preferably three times per day with natural protein at main meals.

Low plasma phenylalanine concentrations have been observed in patients with tyrosinaemia type I on restricted tyrosine/phenylalanine intakes [85]. If plasma phenylalanine concentrations remain low they may become rate-limiting for protein synthesis and plasma tyrosine levels will remain high. It is therefore

Table 15.20 Basic list of 1 g protein exchange foods for low protein diets

	Food	Weight (g) = 1 exchange		Food	Weight (g) = 1 exchange
Infant formula	SMA Gold	65		Lentils	
	Premium	70		boiled	12
	Farley's First	65		raw	5
	Aptamil First	65		Peas	15
				Mange tout	30
Milk and dairy	Cow's milk	30 ml		Sweetcorn	35
	Single cream	40 ml			
	Double cream	60 ml	**Vegetables**†	Asparagus	30
	Yoghurt*	20		Brussels sprouts	35
	Ice-cream*	30		Broccoli tops	30
	Milk chocolate*	12		Cauliflower	30
	Plain chocolate*	20		Okra	40
				Spinach	45
Potatoes and	Potato (boiled)	55			
starchy	Jacket potato (flesh only)	45	**Cereals**	Cornflakes*	10
vegetables†	Jacket potato (flesh and skin)	25		Rice Krispies*	15
				Sugar Puffs*	20
	Chips (fresh, frozen)	25		Weetabix*	10
	Roast potato	35		Oatmeal	10
	Crisps	15		Rice	
	Sweet potato	90		raw	15
	Plantain	125		boiled	45
	Yam	125		Macaroni (white) (boiled)	35
				Spaghetti (white) (boiled)	30
Pulse	Baked beans*	20		Semolina (raw)	10
vegetables	Beans			Flour (white)	10
	aduki, broad, butter, haricot, black-eye, mung, red and white kidney			Flour (wholemeal)	8
			Breads	White, wholemeal, brown*	12
	boiled	12		Rolls – soft, crusty*	10
	raw	5		Nan*	12
	Chick peas			Pitta*	10
	boiled	12			
	raw	5			

* For manufacutered foods the weight for one exchange will be more accurate if calculated from the nutritional label on the food. The figures given can be used as a guide.
† The weight of one exchange is for cooked weight unless stated otherwise.

Source of data: Royal Society of Chemistry, Ministry of Agriculture, Fisheries and Food. *McCance and Widdowson's 'The Composition of Foods'*, 5th edn. London: The Stationery Office, 1991.

important to monitor phenylalanine levels and give supplements as necessary. Ideally the phenylalanine supplement should be given as a divided dose along with the amino acid supplement.

An adequate energy intake must be supplied for normal growth and to prevent endogenous protein catabolism causing increased tyrosine concentrations. Energy comes from protein exchanges and the amino

acid supplement; additional energy is provided by the following groups of foods which are allowed freely in the diet:

- Foods naturally low in or free of protein – fruits and some vegetables (Table 15.22); sugar and fats (Table 15.17)
- Manufactured low protein foods (Table 15.7)

Table 15.21 Manufactured products used in treatment of tyrosinaemia

Product	Amino acids g/100 g	Protein equiv. g/100 g	Energy kcal/100 g	kJ/100 g	Carbohydrate g/100 g	Fat g/100 g	Vitamins and minerals	Dilution	Osmolality mOsm/kg	Comment
XPhen, Tyr Analog[a]	15.5	13	475	1990	54	23	Full range	15%	353	Infant formula. Reconstituted 1 scoop to 30 ml
XPhen, Tyr, Met Analog[b]	15.5	13	475	1990	54	23	Full range	15%	353	Infant formula. Reconstituted 1 scoop to 30 ml
XPhen, Tyr Maxamaid[a]	30	25	309	1311	51	<0.5	Full range	1 to 5	782	Suitable from 1 year of age. Can be given as a drink or paste
XPhen, Tyr, Met Maxamaid[b]	30	25	309	1311	51	<0.5	Full range	1 to 5	782	Suitable from 1 year of age. Can be given as a drink or paste
XPhen, Tyr Maxamum[a]	47	39	297	1260	34	<0.5	Full range	1 to 5	1181	Suitable from 8 years of age. Can be given as a drink or paste
XPT, Tyrosidon	93	77	326	1386	4.5	0	Calcium and phosphorus only		363	Usually given as a paste
XPTM, Tyrosidon	93	77	326	1386	4.5	0	Calcium and phosphorus only		365	Usually given as a paste

[a] Contains a full range of essential and non-essential amino acids except phenylalanine and tyrosine
[b] Contains a full range of essential and non-essential amino acids except phenylalanine, tyrosine and methionine
[c] Requires complete vitamin and mineral supplementation
XPhen, Tyr Maxamum and XTyr Maxamum are other formulations which can be produced if required.
All products are manufactured by Scientific Hospital Supplies and approved by the Advisory Committee Borderline Substances for prescription on FP10.
Other products for tyrosinaemia are manufactured by Milupa and Ross Laboratories but are not currently available in the United Kingdom.

- Energy supplements such as glucose polymer and fat emulsions.

Vitamin and mineral supplements are essential because of the limited intake of foods which would normally provide these. Additional vitamins and minerals can be supplied from either the amino acid product (XPhen, Tyr Analog, Maxamaid or Maxamum) or, if using the pure amino acid mix, from a separate vitamin and mineral supplement as described for PKU and MSUD (p. 246). The diet and supplements should together provide the RNI [71] for all vitamins and minerals.

Dietary management of the newly diagnosed infant

The newly diagnosed infant may be acutely unwell with liver failure. It may be necessary to decrease tyrosine and phenylalanine to a very low intake and give a generous amount of the amino acid supplement

Table 15.22 Fruits and vegetables with a low protein content

Fruit

(protein content less than 1.0 g protein/100 g)

Apples	Grapes	Paw paw
Apricots (not dried)	Grapefruits	Passion fruit
Bananas (1 small daily)	Guavas	Peaches
Bilberries	Kiwi fruits	Pears
Blackberries	Lemons	Pineapple
Blackcurrants	Limes	Plums
Cherries	Lychees	Pomegranate
Clementines	Mandarins	Raisins
Cranberries	Mangoes	Raspberries
Currants	Melons (all types)	Rhubarb
Damsons	Mulberries	Satsumas
Figs (not dried)	Nectarines	Strawberries
Gooseberries	Olives	Sultanas
	Oranges	Tangerines

Commercial baby fruit jars/tins which contain ≤0.5 g protein/100 g – allow freely

Fruit juices usually contain around 0.5 g protein/100 ml

Vegetables

(protein content of less than 1.0 g protein/100 g)

Artichokes	Cress	Parsley
Aubergines	Cucumber	Parsnip
Beans – French/green/runner	Fennel	Peppers
Beansprout	Gherkins	Pumpkins
Beetroot	Gourd	Radishes
Cabbage	Leeks	Spring greens
Carrots	Lettuces	Swedes
Celeriac	Marrows	Tomatoes
Celery	Mushrooms	Turnips
Chicory	Onions	Watercress
Courgettes		

Sources: Royal Society of Chemistry, Ministry of Agriculture, Fisheries and Food. *McCance and Widdowson's 'The Composition of Foods'*, 5th edn. London: The Stationery Office, 1991.

XPhen, Tyr Analog for the first few days, to help reduce production of toxic metabolites. Natural protein can then be introduced as either breast milk or infant formula. The intake is determined by plasma tyrosine levels, aiming to maintain these between 200 and 600 µmol/l. If breast feeding, a measured volume of XPhen, Tyr Analog will be given before most breast feeds to suppress intake of breast milk and thus tyrosine/phenylalanine intake. If infant formula is providing natural protein (tyrosine and phenylalanine), this is given as an evenly divided dose (usually six feeds), throughout the 24 hour period and followed by XPhen, Tyr Analog on demand.

NTBC will be commenced at a dose of 1 mg/kg/day. Some patients may have a significant degree of cholestasis so an additional fat soluble vitamin supplement such as Ketovite tablets and liquid may be required initially. Renal tubular dysfunction leads to increased losses of phosphate, and prevention of rickets usually requires the administration of both a phosphate supplement and 1-alpha-hydroxycholecalciferol (or 1,25-dihydroxycholecalciferol). There may also be increased losses of both bicarbonate and potassium in the urine, which necessitates supplements of these electrolytes. The renal problems will improve with NTBC so these supplements may only be needed in the early stages of treatment, and care should be taken to avoid vitamin D toxicity (e.g. hypercalcaemia).

Feeding the infant and child with tyrosinaemia type I

The diet for infants and children is provided by a measured intake of natural protein, the amino acid supplement (free from phenylalanine and tyrosine) and very low protein foods to appetite.

The guidelines given for the progression of the diet from infancy to and during childhood in MSUD (p. 259) can be applied to tyrosinaemia but using 1 g protein exchanges and the XPhen, Tyr range of products. The section on practical aspects of low protein diets later in this chapter will also provide useful information (p. 276).

Monitoring the diet

The diet is monitored by clinical examination, biochemical assessment, anthropometric measurement and dietary assessment. The diet is reviewed regularly to ensure adequate intakes of all nutrients: total protein intake (amino acid supplement/protein substitute and natural protein (Table 15.5)), vitamins, minerals and trace elements. Periodic biochemical assessment is important. Plasma amino acids are measured; the plasma tyrosine concentration is used to determine natural protein intake. If plasma tyrosine is around 600–700 µmol/l protein, intake is decreased by 1–2 g protein; if less than 200 µmol/l, the diet is increased by 1 g of protein. The plasma amino acid profile is also used to check that all other essential amino acids do not fall below the normal reference range, in particular phenylalanine.

Dietary management during illness

A formal emergency regimen is not normally used in these patients when unwell. However, it would seem prudent to encourage the child to continue to take the amino acid supplement and/or a high energy intake from CHO drinks, to reduce catabolism and thus prevent plasma tyrosine concentrations from increasing to high levels. High tyrosine levels have been reported to cause eye lesions in tyrosinaemia type II during illness [86].

TYROSINAEMIA TYPE II: RICHNER-HANHART SYNDROME

In tyrosinaemia type II there is accumulation of tyrosine due to deficiency of hepatic tyrosine aminotransferase (Fig. 15.3). Crystals of tyrosine are found intracellulary and these cause inflammation. The main clinical features are corneal erosions and plaques, palm and sole erosions and hyperkeratosis. Mental retardation has been reported in some patients [77]. At presentation plasma tyrosine concentrations are usually greater than $1000 \mu mol/l$ (normal reference range $30–120 \mu mol/l$).

Dietary management

Tyrosinaemia type II is treated with a low phenylalanine, low tyrosine diet to reduce high plasma tyrosine concentrations. The principles of dietary management for type I tyrosinaemia can be applied to type II. Methionine restriction is not necessary. On institution of diet, the skin and eye problems usually improve rapidly. The optimum level for maintenance of plasma tyrosine remains unknown. Reported cases have maintained plasma levels between 500 and $1000 \mu mol/l$ [86, 87]. The degree of dietary restriction is usually determined by the clinical response. Usually the oculocutaneous abnormalities resolve and do not recur provided the plasma tyrosine level is kept below $800 \mu mol/l$. It is not certain whether this degree of restriction will completely prevent neurological complications. It is our practice to aim to keep plasma tyrosine below $600 \mu mol/l$.

During intercurrent illness, although severe metabolic decompensation does not occur, it may be beneficial to give high CHO drinks similar to the standard emergency regimen drinks (p. 287), to prevent large increases in plasma tyrosine concentrations which have been reported to cause eye lesions during illness [86].

HOMOCYSTINURIA

Classical homocystinuria (HCU) is due to deficiency of the enzyme cystathionine β synthase (CBS). This results in increased plasma concentrations of methionine, homocysteine and other sulphur-containing metabolites (mixed disulphides) and low levels of plasma cysteine, cystathionine and serine. There are several other inherited metabolic disorders which lead to homocystinuria with a raised plasma homocysteine, but with normal to low methionine levels. These are caused by defects in the remethylation pathway by which homocysteine is normally converted to methionine (methionine synthase deficiency) or are due to inherited disorders of the vitamins (B_{12}, folic acid) involved in the metabolic pathways of homocysteine metabolism (Fig. 15.4).

The commonest cause of HCU is due to CBS deficiency and treatment involves dietary therapy. HCU was first described in 1962 [88]. It is inherited as an autosomal recessive trait. The defect is in the CBS gene protein and at least 64 mutations have been identified [89]. The worldwide incidence of HCU is approximately 1 in 344 000 [90], but there are large population differences with the incidence at least 1 in 65 000 in Ireland [91].

HCU may be diagnosed from screening in the neonatal period. However, few centres specifically screen for the disorder and because plasma methionine levels may not be significantly increased in newborns with HCU, a significant proportion will only be diagnosed following the onset of clinical symptoms. Individuals who have HCU are clinically normal at birth. Without early diagnosis and treatment there will be a gradual onset of the clinical features of HCU which are multisystemic [92], including:

- Ocular system – causing lens dislocation, myopia, glaucoma
- Skeletal system – causing osteoporosis, scoliosis, elongation and thinning of the long bones, marfanoid appearance
- Vascular system – causing thromboembolisms
- Central nervous system – causing developmental delay, learning difficulties, electroencephalogram changes, epilepsy, psychiatric disturbance.

The complications of HCU are due to the significantly raised plasma homocysteine levels. Homocysteine is present in the plasma in several forms [93]:

- Homocysteine (reduced form)⎫ free homocysteine
- Homocystine (disulphide of ⎬ (20–30%)
  homocysteine) ⎭

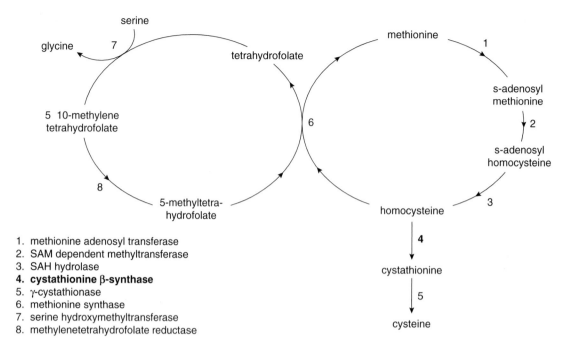

Fig. 15.4 Metabolic pathways of homocysteine metabolism.

1. methionine adenosyl transferase
2. SAM dependent methyltransferase
3. SAH hydrolase
4. **cystathionine β-synthase**
5. γ-cystathionase
6. methionine synthase
7. serine hydroxymethyltransferase
8. methylenetetrahydrofolate reductase

- Mixed disulphide homocysteine–cysteine
- Protein-bound homocysteine (70–80%).

The plasma total homocysteine (tHcy) concentration is the sum of all the different forms. Normally in plasma, free homocysteine (fHcy) is undetectable and tHcy <15 μmol/l.

Classical HCU can be classified into two forms, as follows.

Pyridoxine responsive HCU

The enzyme CBS requires pyridoxal-5-phosphate, formed from pyridoxine (vitamin B_6), as its co-factor. A significant number of CBS deficient individuals show clinical and biochemical response to pharmacological doses of pyridoxine, up to 500 mg/day [94]. The defect in these cases is still within the CBS protein and not a disorder of pyridoxine metabolism.

All individuals diagnosed as having classical HCU should be given a trial with pharmacological doses of pyridoxine. Worldwide up to 50% of cases of CBS deficiency HCU are pyridoxine responsive showing a decrease in plasma methionine and almost complete elimination of homocysteine from plasma and urine [95]. There are population differences with a much smaller percentage showing pyridoxine responsiveness in certain populations, e.g. Britain and Ireland. In CBS deficiency, folic acid requirements are probably increased due to an increased use of the remethylation pathway. It is therefore essential to also give additional folic acid, 5 mg daily, and to ensure that plasma vitamin B_{12} levels (required for folate metabolism) are adequate. In those individuals with pyridoxine responsive HCU, treatment with pyridoxine and folic acid can prevent further deterioration in symptoms except for advanced eye disease [94].

Pyridoxine non-responsive HCU

In this group plasma homocysteine levels do not fall following pharmacological doses of pyridoxine. Treatment strategies aim at reducing homocysteine levels by:

- Decreasing the intake of the substrate methionine by use of a methionine restricted diet to reduce plasma methionine and homocysteine levels

- Utilising alternative pathways to remove homocysteine by giving betaine (a methyl donor) which remethylates homocysteine back to methionine and so reduces plasma homocysteine levels.

Treatment aims and biochemical monitoring

Good long term biochemical control in HCU can prevent the onset of complications in early diagnosed individuals and can curtail further progression of the disorder in late diagnosed cases [94]. Formerly methods of biochemical monitoring available have only been for the measurement of free homocysteine (fHcy). Only more recently has measurement of total homocysteine (tHcy) become more routine. From follow-up of patients treated over many years a life-long median fHcy <11 µmol/l significantly reduces the probability of developing complications [91]. Data on acceptable tHcy is not yet available. In the normal population tHcy levels are 5–15 µmol/l [96]. Free homocysteine is only detectable when tHcy >60 µmol/l. Until there is more data available on tHcy levels and clinical outcome both plasma fHcy and tHcy need to be monitored.

Treatment aims will be dependent on the form of classical HCU and the treatment regimen in use (Table 15.23). In addition to the monitoring of plasma homocysteine, methionine and cysteine levels, vitamin B_{12} and folate status should be assessed as low levels of these could cause inadequate response to treatment due to their intimate roles in homocysteine metabolism.

Dietary management of classical HCU

The aim of dietary treatment is to reduce plasma methionine levels to within or slightly above the normal age related reference range, decrease plasma homocysteine levels and increase plasma cysteine levels to within the normal range (Table 15.23).

The principles of dietary management are as follows.

Reduce methionine intake by using a protein restricted diet

As methionine is an essential amino acid an allowance must be included in the diet. A methionine exchange system is used, predominantly consisting of foods of low biological protein value. One exchange contains 20 mg methionine, or approximately 1 g natural protein (Table 15.24). Where information on methionine content is not available, e.g. manufactured foods, the protein content is used.

Methionine intake varies between individuals. Among our group methionine intake naturally falls within a range of 160–900 mg per day with a median value of 230 mg/day. The methionine allowance should be spread throughout the day.

Supplement intake of amino acids with a methionine-free protein substitute

A protein substitute which is free from methionine is essential in ensuring an adequate total protein intake as the dietary allowance of natural protein will not provide sufficient total protein for normal growth. The protein substitute used should contain cystine as this amino acid is normally formed from methionine but becomes deficient in HCU due to the metabolic block. A number of methionine-free, cystine enriched protein substitutes are available (Table 15.25). Currently the amino acid requirements recommended for PKU

Table 15.23 Biochemical monitoring in classical HCU

	Plasma methionine	Plasma cysteine	Plasma homocysteine Free	Total
B_6 responsive	Normal range	Normal range	0–10 µmol/l	? <50 µmol/l
B_6 non-responsive – diet alone	Normal range	Normal range*	<10 µmol/l	? <80 µmol/l
B_6 non-responsive + betaine	High (up to 1000 µmol/l)	Normal range*	<10 µmol/l	? <80 µmol/l

* Individuals treated with low methionine diet and methionine-free protein substitute can at times have low cysteine levels even though the protein substitutes are supplemented with cystine. This may be due to poor solubility of cystine which may remain behind in the drinking vessel.

Table 15.24 20 mg methionine exchanges (1 g protein) for use in HCU

Food	Weight (g)*	Food	Weight (g)*
Dairy products		Chips	35
Cow's milk	20 ml	Canned new	100
Aptamil First	50 ml**	Instant mash (powder)	15
Cow & Gate Premium	55 ml**	Crisps	20
SMA Gold	***		
Farley's First	55 ml**	*Vegetables*	
Single cream	30 ml	Baked beans (canned)	35
Whipping cream	35 ml	Broad beans (boiled)	75
Double cream	30 ml	Broccoli tops (boiled)	45
Custard	20 ml	Brussels sprouts (boiled)	75
Yoghurt (natural/fruit/flavoured)	20	Cauliflower (boiled)	65
		Mushrooms (raw)	35
Cereals		Mushrooms (fried)	25
All Bran	10	Peas (canned garden)	45
Cornflakes	10	Peas (canned processed)	35
Muesli	10	Spinach (boiled)	20
Oatmeal (raw)	10	Sweetcorn (canned)	35
Puffed Wheat	10	Yam (raw)	70
Ready Brek	10	Yam (boiled)	85
Rice Krispies	15		
Shredded Wheat	10	*Fruit*	
Sugar Puffs	20	Apricots (dried)	85
Weetabix	10	Avocado	30
		Banana	100
Rice (raw)	15	Currants	35
Rice (boiled)	40	Dates (dried)	75
		Figs (dried)	70
Potatoes		Nectarine	55
Boiled, mashed (no milk)	85	Peach	85
Baked (flesh only)	50	Raisins	55
Baked (flesh + skin)	60	Sultanas	35
Roast	45		

*   weight to nearest 5 g
**   manufacturer's data, March 2000
***   data available from manufacturer
Source: Paul AA, Southgate DAT, Russell J First supplement to McCance and Widdowson's *The Composition of Foods*. London: The Stationery Office, 1979

[11] are also used in HCU (Table 15.5). These recommended protein intakes are high compared with normal recommended intakes for protein [71] to take into account the synthetic nature of the protein (as amino acids), the effect of this on their bioavailability and the aim of preventing protein catabolism and promoting protein synthesis. The protein substitute should be given in divided doses through the day, usually together with the methionine exchanges at main meals.

Achieve adequate energy intake to prevent protein catabolism and achieve normal growth

Dietary energy is provided by:

- Foods naturally low or free from protein (methionine) – fruits and vegetables (Table 15.26), sugars and fats (Table 15.17)
- Specially manufactured low protein (low methionine) foods, e.g. flour, bread, breakfast cereals, pasta, biscuits (Table 15.7)
- Energy supplements – glucose polymers, fat emulsions.

Provide adequate vitamins, minerals and trace elements

Because of the limited range of foods allowed in the diet it is essential to supplement the diet with the full

Table 15.25 Methionine-free protein substitutes used in HCU

Product	Amino acids (g per 100 g)	Protein equiv. (g/100 g)	Energy (kcal/kJ)	Carbohydrate (g per 100 g)	Fat (g per 100 g)	Vitamins and minerals
XMet Analog	15.5	13	475 (1986)	54	23	full range
XMet Maxamaid	30	25	309 (1292)	51	<0.5	full range
XMet Maxamum	47	39	297 (1241)	34	<0.5	full range
XMet Amino Acid Mix	93	77	326 (1363)	4.5	Nil	calcium and phosphorus*

* requires complete vitamin and mineral supplementation
All products manufactured by Scientific Hospital Supplies International. All are ACBS approved and available on FP10 prescription in the UK.

range of vitamins, minerals and trace elements to achieve the reference nutrient intakes for age [71]. Many of the methionine-free protein substitutes will provide these (Table 15.25). If the methionine-free protein substitute does not contain vitamins, minerals or trace elements a separate supplement is necessary, e.g. Paediatric Seravit, or Forceval Junior capsules together with a separate calcium supplement.

Again due to increased use of the remethylation pathway, an additional pharmacological dose of folic acid, 5 mg daily, is also prescribed to ensure adequate supply of folate.

Management of the early diagnosed infant and child with HCU

Infants with HCU who fail to respond to a pharmacological dose of pyridoxine are commenced on dietary therapy. Initially all natural protein (methionine) intake is stopped and the infant is fed entirely on a methionine-free infant formula, XMet Analog, aiming to give approximately 2.5 g methionine-free protein (3 g amino acids)/kg body weight/day and normal energy requirements for age. After 48 hours a measured amount of natural protein as normal infant formula is reintroduced, usually initially to provide 120 mg methionine per day (personal practice). The normal infant formula is divided equally between several feeds (four to five times daily) with XMet Analog offered to appetite after each feed. The quantity of normal infant formula is adjusted according to subsequent plasma methionine and homocysteine levels, aiming to keep within the desirable limits (Table 15.23).

As yet there has been no published practical ex-

Table 15.26 Fruits and vegetables with low methionine content

Fruit
Fresh, frozen, or tinned in syrup (less than 15 mg methionine and/or less than 1 g protein per 100 g)

Apple	Grapes	Pawpaw
Apricot	Guava	Pear
Blackberries	Kiwi fruit	Pineapple
Clementine	Lemon	Plum
Cherries	Lychees	Pomegranate
Cranberries	Mandarin	Raspberries
Damson	Mango	Rhubarb
Fruit salad	Melon	Satsuma
Figs – green, raw	Olives	Strawberries
Gooseberries	Orange	Tangerine
Grapefruit	Passion fruit	Water melon

Vegetables
Fresh, frozen or tinned (less than 20 mg methionine and/or less than 1 g protein per 100 g)

Artichoke*	Endive*	Peppers
Asparagus	Garlic	Plantain
Aubergine	Gherkin	Pumpkin
Beans – French, green	Gourd*	Radish
Beansprouts*	Fennel	Spring greens
Beetroot*	Leek*	Swede
Cabbage	Lettuce	Sweet potato
Carrot	Marrow	Tomato
Celery	Mustard and cress	Turnip
Chicory	Onion	Watercress*
Courgette*	Spring onion	
Cucumber	Parsley	

* Contain more than 20 mg methionine and/or 1 g protein per 100 g but are generally eaten in small quantities

Source: Paul AA, Southgate DAT, Russell J First supplement to McCance and Widdowson's *The Composition of Foods*. London: The Stationery Office, 1979; Royal Society of Chemistry, Ministry of Agriculture, Fisheries and Food. McCance and Widdowson's *The Composition of Foods*, 5th edn. London: The Stationery Office, 1991.

perience of breast feeding an early diagnosed infant with classical HCU. In theory it should be possible for such an infant to be breast fed using the principles employed in PKU. The infant would be given a measured amount of methionine-free infant formula at the start of a feed and then breast fed on demand. The prescribed quantity of methionine-free infant formula would be increased or decreased according to blood methionine/homocysteine levels in order to manipulate the amount of breast milk the infant takes.

Weaning

- Solids are usually introduced at the normal age for weaning of between 4 and 6 months. Initially solids of a low protein content (free foods), e.g. fruits, vegetables and low protein rusk, are used (Table 15.26).
- Once the infant is accepting low protein solids regularly then methionine (protein) containing solids are gradually introduced with a corresponding reduction in the normal infant formula allowance until protein-containing solids make up all the methionine allowance. The protein-containing methionine exchanges are given before the XMet Analog feeds. Once all the methionine allowance is provided from solids the exchanges are divided between the main meals.
- Use of the manufactured low protein foods is encouraged as part of the weaning process to accustom the child to them as they will become important in providing variety and a source of energy in the diet.
- From around 1 year of age a more concentrated methionine-free protein substitute, XMet Maxamaid, is introduced. This can be given as a drink or more concentrated as a paste. If there are concerns about achieving an adequate total protein intake before 1 year of age then XMet Maxamaid may be introduced earlier, or additional methionine-free amino acids (XMet Amino Acid Mix) added into the XMet Analog.

During childhood the methionine allowance remains fairly constant. Periods of rapid growth may temporarily increase methionine tolerance. The intake of low protein foods gradually increases according to appetite to ensure an adequate energy intake. The quantity of the methionine-free protein substitute prescribed should be reviewed regularly and increased to meet the protein requirements for age (Table 15.5). From around 8 years of age XMet

Maxamum, which is more concentrated in protein, can be introduced.

Dietary treatment must continue for life in order to prevent the development of late complications of HCU.

Management of illness

During intercurrent infections general advice is given to minimise protein catabolism and therefore prevention of an excessive rise in plasma homocysteine levels:

- Encouragement of the usual intake of methionine-free protein substitute – without force feeding as this can lead to refusal once well
- Reduction of methionine exchanges – in practice a reduced appetite leads to reduced methionine intake
- Generous use of non-protein energy, e.g. high carbohydrate drinks.

A strict emergency regimen is not essential as acute metabolic decompensation does not occur.

Dietary management in later diagnosed cases

Individuals diagnosed late after the onset of clinical symptoms, or as a result of investigation following a sibling being diagnosed with classical HCU, are started on a methionine restricted diet. Initially a diet restricting methionine intake to 200 mg/day is started, together with an age appropriate methionine-free protein substitute (Table 15.25) to make up the total protein requirement for age (Table 15.5). If, from diet history, the normal dietary protein intake prior to diagnosis has been exceptionally high, a larger methionine allowance may be given. Subsequent methionine allowance is adjusted in the light of plasma methionine and homocysteine levels so as to achieve acceptable levels (Table 15.23).

Dietary compliance in this group can in some cases be difficult to achieve because they are used to a normal unrestricted diet. Most will have learning difficulties and so understanding the need for such a radical change in diet can be difficult to achieve. Individuals may cheat with high protein foods and take extra methionine exchanges, or refuse the methionine-free protein substitute. These problems need to be addressed. A positive family attitude and support from the multidisciplinary team, including clinical psychologist, are important if dietary treatment is to succeed. In some late diagnosed individuals in whom all attempts to give the methionine-free protein substitutes have failed, a modified low protein diet using the minimum safe level of protein intake [97] (so protein catabolism and poor growth may be minimised) is used in conjunction with oral betaine therapy (see below).

Betaine therapy

Betaine is a methyl donor and promotes the remethylation reaction of homocysteine to methionine (Fig. 15.5). Thus plasma methionine levels are significantly increased although this is not universal and plasma homocysteine levels fall [98, 99]. The use of oral betaine can be useful in improving biochemical control in circumstances where dietary compliance is poor, e.g. adolescents, adults and those late diagnosed. Compliance with betaine is not always good and it is unlikely to be able to replace dietary therapy [94].

Maternal HCU

CBS deficiency HCU in women appears to be associated with a higher incidence of spontaneous abortion, but there is little evidence of other adverse effects on the fetus [95]. As there is no data on the effect of betaine in pregnancy our current practice is to discontinue betaine and 'tighten up' on diet to control plasma homocysteine levels. Uncontrolled homocysteine levels are probably a greater risk to the mother than the fetus. In one woman betaine was discontinued and dietary methionine intake reduced by 40% of normal to achieve satisfactory biochemical control; there was a slight increase in methionine tolerance towards the end of the pregnancy (pers. exper.).

ORGANIC ACIDAEMIAS AND UREA CYCLE DISORDERS

LOW PROTEIN DIET FOR THE MANAGEMENT OF UREA CYCLE DISORDERS AND ORGANIC ACIDAEMIAS – PRACTICAL ASPECTS

Protein requirements

Low protein diets must provide at least the minimum amount of protein, nitrogen and essential amino acids to meet requirements for normal growth. Safe levels of protein intakes (Table 15.27) and requirements

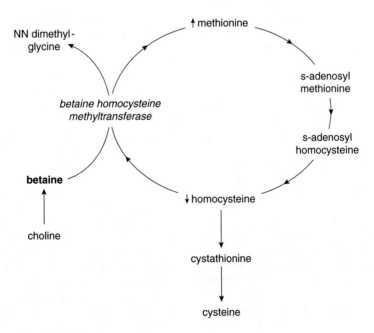

Fig. 15.5 Methyl group donation by betaine

Table 15.27 Safe level of protein intake for infants, children and adolescents

Age	Safe level (g protein/kg/day)	
	*	**
0–1 months	—	2.69
1–2	—	2.04
2–3	—	1.53
3–4	1.86	1.37
4–5	1.86	1.25
5–6	1.86	1.19
6–9	1.65	1.09
9–12	1.48	1.02
1–1.5 years	1.26	1.0
1.5–2	1.17	0.94
2–3	1.13	0.92
3–4	1.09	0.9
4–5	1.06	0.88
5–6	1.02	0.86
6–9	1.01	0.86
9–10	0.99	0.86
Girls		
10–11	1.0	0.87
11–12	0.98	0.86
12–13	0.96	0.85
13–14	0.9	0.84
14–15	0.9	0.81
15–16	0.87	0.81
16–17	0.83	0.78
17–18	0.8	0.7
Boys		
10–11	0.99	0.86
11–12	0.98	0.86
12–13	1.0	0.88
13–14	0.97	0.86
14–15	0.96	0.86
15–16	0.92	0.84
16–17	0.9	0.83
17–18	0.86	0.81

* Energy and protein requirements. Report of a joint FAO/WHO/UNU Expert Consultation. WHO Technical Report no. 724, Geneva, 1985.

** Dewey KG *et al.* Protein requirements of infants and children. *Eur J Clin Nutr*, 1996, **50** (Suppl 1) 119–50.

for essential amino acid intake were set by FAO/WHO/UNU in 1985 [97]. These safe levels are based on an intake of high biological value (HBV) protein foods, milk and hen's egg, with 100% digestibility, thus ensuring an adequate intake of all essential amino acids. It is important to be aware that the safe levels of protein intakes have been calculated as the mean requirement +2 SD of the requirement, so as to meet or exceed the requirements of most individuals. Therefore for some individuals, a protein intake which is below the safe intake may be adequate for growth. These recommendations have recently been reviewed and it is suggested the safe levels of protein intakes have been set too high [100]. Revised estimates are given (Table 15.27). These figures can certainly be used as a guide for very low protein diets.

Ideally the protein source in low protein diets should be mainly from HBV protein, but this is not common practice because a greater variety of foods and a higher energy intake per gram of protein can be provided from low biological value (LBV) protein foods. Children on low protein diets who frequently consume a limited range of LBV protein foods may be at risk of one or more essential amino acids becoming rate-limiting for protein synthesis. It is therefore important that a variety of LBV protein foods (e.g. potato, cereals, rice, pasta, pulses) are taken to ensure an adequate intake of all essential amino acids. If the protein prescription is generous enough, more HBV proteins should be included to improve the protein quality of the diet.

Protein tolerance will vary depending on residual enzyme activity of the specific disorder, growth rate, age and sex. During early infancy growth is at a maximum so protein requirements per kg body weight are greatest at this time. If the child has had a period of slow growth, protein intake may need to be temporarily increased during the following period of catch-up growth. Protein requirements may also be temporarily increased if a child has had repeated intercurrent infections with inadequate protein intakes.

Protein exchanges and free foods

Protein intake from LBV protein foods is measured by an exchange system, i.e. one exchange equals the amount of food which provides 1 g of protein (Table 15.20). This allows greater variety in the diet as foods can be substituted for each other and still provide a similar protein content. Nowadays most manufactured foods have nutritional labelling with the protein content expressed as grams of protein/100 g and sometimes also grams of protein per portion. Parents are taught how to interpret the food label and calculate exchanges.

For manufactured foods one exchange (1 g protein) is calculated as:

- $100 \div$ (g protein per 100 g of food)
- If more than 1 g protein is desired this is multiplied by that number of exchanges.

Ideally the protein intake should be evenly distributed between main meals and some for snacks. Protein food exchanges should be weighed, at least initially. Digital scales which weigh in 2 g increments are recommended. If parents are unable to cope with the concept of protein exchanges or weighing, then a set menu with handy measures for foods is used.

The energy provided by exchange foods can range greatly, e.g. an exchange of baked beans provides 20 kcal (84 kJ) and crisps 110 kcal (462 kJ). It may be helpful, particularly if the child has a poor appetite, to give parents advice on choosing protein exchanges which are more energy dense and provide more than 60 kcal (252 kJ) per exchange.

Energy

Low protein diets may not provide sufficient energy because the intake of many foods is restricted. This must be avoided as an inadequate energy intake causes poor growth and poor metabolic control with endogenous protein catabolism resulting in increased production of toxic metabolites, e.g. ammonia in urea cycle disorders.

Concerns have been expressed about possible inadequate intakes of essential fatty acids (EFAs) in patients on low protein diets [101]. It is therefore important that energy from fat also provides the requirements for EFAs; at least 1% of energy intake should come from linoleic acid and 0.2% from α-linolenic acid [71]. Low protein diets and modular feeds should be assessed for EFA content.

Dietary energy can be provided by both the protein exchanges and the following groups of foods which are allowed without restriction in the diet:

- Foods naturally low in or free of protein – sugar and fats (Table 15.17), fruits and some vegetables (Table 15.22)
- Specially manufactured low protein foods, e.g. bread, pasta, biscuits (Table 15.7)
- Energy supplements such as glucose polymer, fat emulsions.

Manufactured low protein foods are not always popular with this group of patients. Children with urea cycle disorders usually obtain sufficient energy from normal foods and obviously prefer to eat these. Children with disorders of propionate metabolism often have poor appetite and are tube fed, hence they usually depend on energy supplements as their main energy source.

Vitamins, minerals and trace elements

Vitamin and mineral supplements are almost always essential as intake will be severely limited due to the protein restriction. An adequate intake of vitamins A and C and folic acid could be provided from fruit and vegetables but iron, zinc, copper, calcium and B vitamins are most likely to be deficient. Together the diet and supplement should provide at least the reference nutrient intakes (RNI) for vitamins and minerals [71]. The amount required will vary and needs to be assessed for the individual. The supplement is best given as a divided dose to enhance absorption.

Paediatric Seravit provides a comprehensive vitamin and mineral supplement (except for sodium, potassium and chloride). It can be added to the infant formula in the required dose. For older children it can be given as a drink or paste combined with a drink (because it is hyperosmolar). To mask the unpleasant flavour of Paediatric Seravit it can be added to fruit juice, squash, low protein milk with milk shake flavouring or mixed with honey, jam or fruit purée. It can be mixed with food such as breakfast cereal but it then becomes important that all the food is eaten. For older children Forceval Junior Capsules or Forceval Capsules with additional calcium often replace Paediatric Seravit as the vitamin and mineral supplement. It is important to be aware that Forceval does not contain calcium, sodium, potassium, chloride, inositol and choline and contains only small quantities of magnesium. These and alternative vitamin and mineral supplements have also been reviewed in the PKU and MSUD sections (pp. 245, 246, 257).

Monitoring low protein diets

Protein and mineral deficiencies have been reported in patients with inborn errors of metabolism on restricted protein intakes. This type of diet, comprising mainly LBV proteins, is often used in children with organic acidaemias and urea cycle disorders,

Table 15.28 Protein-free modular feed

	Energy (kcal)	(kJ)	CHO (g)	Protein (g)	Fat (g)	Sodium (mmol)	Potassium (mmol)
55 g Maxijul	209	888	52	—	—	0.5	0.1
40 ml Calogen	180	756	—	—	20	0.2	—
12 g Paediatric Seravit	36	151	9	—	—	—	—
25 ml Normasol						3.9	
5.0 ml KCl solution							10.0
Plus water to 600 ml							
Totals	425	1785	61	—	20	4.6	10.1
Per 100 ml	71	298	10.2	—	3.3	0.8	1.7

therefore protein and amino acid intakes need to be carefully monitored. This should be done by clinical examination (skin and hair, looking specifically for signs of protein deficiency such as skin rashes), anthropometric measurements, biochemical assessment (quantitative amino acids, albumin and electrolytes) and regular dietary assessment. Periodic assessment of plasma status of vitamins, minerals and trace elements is important (Table 1.6).

Infants and children – low protein diets

Breast milk or a whey-based infant formula should provide the main protein source for infants. If demand breast feeding provides too much protein, intakes can be reduced by giving a supplementary bottle feed before some or all breast feeds of either:

- A modular protein-free feed for urea cycle disorders and organic acidaemias (Table 15.28)
- A specialised infant formula free from precursor amino acids (i.e. does not contain the amino acids which cannot be metabolised, e.g. XMTVI Analog for propionic or methylmalonic acidaemia.

Scientific Hospital Supplies have recently produced Energivit, a protein-free feed which could also be used, but this is not available on prescription. A protein-free diet powder 80056 is produced by Mead Johnson Nutritionals; this can be made available on request, but it is not prescribable on FP10.

If a whey-based infant formula is used, the amount is adjusted to provide at least the safe level of protein intake for age (Table 15.27) or more if clinically indi-

cated. Additional fluid, energy, vitamins and minerals are added to make it a nutritionally adequate feed. The aim is to produce a feed which gives the RNI for all vitamins and minerals [71] and is comparable to a normal infant formula. An example of a low protein infant feed is shown in Table 15.29. The protein-free modular feed described above can also be fed to appetite if the infant has had the prescribed protein intake from infant formula and is still hungry.

Weaning is commenced at the usual time between 4 and 6 months of age. The first solids given are 'protein-free' such as fruit or low protein vegetable purée, low protein rusk, e.g. Aminex, or commercial baby foods containing <0.5 g protein/100 g, so that if they are refused the total protein intake is not affected. Once these are accepted protein-containing solids are introduced from either commercial baby foods or home cooked foods such as potato, vegetables or cereals. The energy content of protein exchanges can be increased by adding butter/margarine to savoury foods and sugar to desserts. It is best to have a flexible approach as to when the protein food should be given; some infants may take this best before (if not too hungry) or between feeds.

One gram of protein from infant formula is replaced by 1 g of protein from solids. This is less easy to regulate in the breast fed infant as the protein intake is not known. Therefore an aim for total protein intake (usually the safe level of intake) is set and as protein exchanges are introduced the number of breast feeds is reduced to compensate. It is important to ensure that an adequate energy intake is provided by exchanges and free foods, otherwise breast feeds will not be reduced sufficiently. In both the bottle and breast fed infant this process is continued

Table 15.29 Low protein feed for 3 month old male infant, weight 5 kg

	Energy		CHO	Protein	Fat	Sodium	Potassium
	(kcal)	(kJ)	(g)	(g)	(g)	(mmol)	(mmol)
80 g SMA Gold	419	1760	45	9.6	23	4.4	11.3
40 g Glucose Polymer e.g. Maxijul	152	638	38	—	—	0.4	<0.2
2 g Paediatric Seravit	6	25	1.5	—	—	—	—
Plus water to 750 ml							
Totals	577	2423	85	9.6	23	4.8[c]	11.3[c]
per 100 ml	77	323	11.3	1.3	3.1	0.6	1.5
per kg	115	485	—	1.9	—	1.0	2.3
DRV per kg 0–3 months[a]	115–100	480–420		2.1		2.0	3.4
Minimum protein requirement[b]				1.86			

[a] Dietary reference values [71]

[b] FAO/WHO/UNU safe level of protein intake (Table 15.27)

[c] Additional sodium and potassium may be necessary (some medicines provide electrolytes)

throughout the first year of life or so and is dictated by what the infant can manage, until all the protein is provided by solid food. Ideally the protein exchanges should be evenly distributed between main meals. During this changeover period it is important to ensure that vitamin and mineral intakes are adequate. The vitamin and mineral supplement is increased and may even have to be introduced to the breast fed infant with the progressive change to solids, as these foods are a poorer source of nutrients than infant formula and breast milk.

Throughout childhood the protein intake is increased to provide at least the safe level of protein intake (Table 15.27) for age or more if clinically indicated. This is given in conjunction with an adequate energy, vitamin and mineral intake for age. It is important to ensure the child consumes a variety of LBV protein foods. HBV foods can also provide some of the protein in the diet. Useful foods include: thin sliced meats (ham, chicken or turkey), cheeses (Dairylea cheese triangles, Philadelphia cream cheese, Boursin), hot dog sausages, fish fingers, eggs, fromage frais and yoghurt (choosing the highest energy varieties). The energy content of the diet can be increased by frying foods, adding butter oil, or double cream (1 g protein and 270 kcal (1080 kJ) per 60 ml) to savoury foods such as pasta, rice or potato. Sugar, glucose polymer or double cream can be added to desserts. High CHO drinks are encouraged, such as Lucozade or Ribena, and often glucose polymer is added to drinks to a final concentration of 15–25% CHO,

depending on age. Low protein milks (Tables 15.7, 15.30) can be used to make milkshakes and desserts and can be poured on cereals. If the child does not consume all the daily protein allowance as food, it should be replaced with fluids; cow's milk with added glucose polymer to 15–20% CHO is often the simplest way to do this. Another useful alternative is to give a juice supplement such as Fortijuce which provides 1 g protein and 30 kcal (125 kJ) per 25 ml. Table 15.30 provides an example of a low protein diet.

Some patients, particularly those with disorders of propionate metabolism, refuse to eat or have a very limited intake of solid food. They will depend on feeds given by mouth or tube feeds to provide most of their low protein diet. A modular feed would be designed to meet the nutritional needs of the child and the specific disorder. An example of a low protein feed is shown in Table 15.31.

DISORDERS OF PROPIONATE METABOLISM

The disorders of propionate metabolism, methylmalonic acidaemia (MMA) and propionic acidaemia (PA) share common biochemical and clinical features due to accumulation of propionyl-CoA (Fig. 15.2) which is formed from catabolism of the four essential amino acids, isoleucine, valine, threonine and methionine, but about half is derived from other sources.

PA is due to a defect of propionyl-CoA carboxylase

Table 15.30 Low protein diet (20 g), for 6 year old girl, weight 18 kg

	Protein (g) (using 1 g protein exchanges)
Breakfast	
20 g Cornflakes and sugar	2
Protein-free milk*	
36 g (1 slice) bread	3
Butter, jam, honey, marmalade	
100 ml pure fruit juice + 10 g glucose polymer	
Mid AM	
15 g (1) chocolate digestive biscuit	1
1 can Lucozade	
Packed lunch	
36 g (1 slice) bread	3
Butter, tomato and mayonnaise	
30 g (1 packet) crisps	2
Portion fresh fruit	
200 ml carton Ribena	
Mid afternoon	
25 g milk chocolate	2
Squash + 150 ml water + 20 g glucose polymer	
Evening meal	
25 g (1) fried fish finger	3
50 g chips	2
15 g peas	1
Carrots and butter	
30 g ice cream	1
Tinned fruit	
Bed time	
Protein-free milkshake	
or Squash + 150 ml water + 20 g glucose polymer	
Daily	
8 g Paediatric Seravit	
Fluoride drops	

* Protein-free milk alternatives:
  15 g Duocal and water to 100 ml
  10 g glucose polymer or sugar, 10 ml Calogen + water to 100 ml
  low protein milk (Table 15.7)

which causes high plasma and urinary propionate levels and excretion of multiple organic compounds, including methylcitrate and 3-hydroxypropionate. MMA is caused by a defect of either methylmalonyl-CoA mutase-apoenzyme causing reduced (mut⁻) or absent (mut°) activity or alternatively a defect in the synthesis of its co-factor 5′-deoxyadenosylcobalamin. Impairment results in accumulation of methyl-malonic acid and the compounds found in propionic acidaemia. These disorders vary widely in severity depending on the degree of enzyme deficiency. Some MMA patients are completely responsive to co-factor vitamin B_{12}, and require no dietary treatment except for an emergency regimen during intercurrent illness.

Both disorders can present in the neonatal period or early infancy with a severe metabolic acidosis (although not always) [102], poor feeding, vomiting, lethargy, hypotonia and dehydration; or in early childhood with less severe symptoms including failure to thrive and developmental delay [103].

The prognosis of MMA and PA is generally not good [104, 105, 106, 107]. The mechanisms of toxicity are complex and not well understood, but propionate and its metabolites appear to be implicated. Early onset of PA is associated with poor intellectual outcome and early death, while late onset may be complicated by a severe disabling movement disorder [108]. Others report a similar high mortality but in both early and late onset patients, with better neurological outcome for late onset patients [107]. Severe MMA (mut°) is associated with developmental retardation and early death [104]. Cobalamin responsive patients have a much better long term outcome. In both early and late onset MMA patients, there is increased risk of developing new neurological symptoms with age; these normally develop following episodes of acute metabolic decompensation [109]. Other more recently recognised complications in both disorders include cardiomyopathy [110] and pancreatitis [111], and in MMA also chronic renal failure [105, 112].

As outcome on conventional therapy is poor, alternative forms of therapy are now being used, including liver and combined liver and kidney transplant although these are associated with significant risk.

Sources of propionate

It is important to appreciate that propionate is formed from three main sources, not just from amino acid catabolism. Estimates of the contributions of these sources are:

(1) Around 50% is derived from the catabolism of the precursor amino acids, isoleucine, valine, threonine and methionine [113].
(2) Around 25% is produced from anaerobic bacterial fermentation in the gut [113]. Oral adminis-

Table 15.31 Low protein tube feed for a 4 year old girl, weight 15 kg

	Energy		CHO	Protein	Fat	Sodium	Potassium
	(kcal)	(kJ)	(g)	(g)	(g)	(mmol)	(mmol)
550 ml Paediasure	556	2335	60.5	15.4	27.5	14.3	15.4
170 g Maxijul	646	2713	161.5	—	—	1.5	0.2
60 ml Calogen	270	1134	—	—	30.0	0.2	—
8.0 g Paediatric Seravit	24	102	6.0	—	—	—	—
100 ml Normasol						15.4	
8.0 ml KCl solution							16.0
Plus water to 1200 ml							
Totals	1496	6283	228	15.4	57.5	31.4	31.6
Per 100 ml	125	524	19	1.3	4.8	2.6	2.6
Per kg	100	420		1.0		2.1	2.1
DRV 4–6 years*	1460	6120		1.1			
Safe level of protein intake**				1.0			

* Dietary reference values [71]
** FAO/WHO/UNU safe level of protein intake (Table 15.27)

tration of the antibiotic Metronidazole will reduce gut bacteria propionate production, but the long term efficacy of this therapy is still being studied [114].

(3) Probably around 25% is derived from the oxidation of odd-numbered long chain fatty acids (C15 and C17) [115] and other metabolites. These odd chain fatty acids are synthesised by the normal pathway of fatty acid synthesis but propionyl CoA acts as the primer instead of acetyl CoA, hence the additional odd number of carbons in the chain [116].

Dietary management

The aims of dietary treatment are to reduce production of propionate by both the restriction of precursor amino acids using a low protein diet and avoidance of fasting to limit oxidation of odd-chain fatty acids. The precursor amino acids (isoleucine, valine, threonine and methionine) do not accumulate in plasma in these disorders. It is therefore not possible to use the measurement of plasma levels of these amino acids to determine the intake of natural protein. Dietary protein intake can therefore only be restricted to the safe level of intake for growth (Table 15.27). Too low a protein intake can have serious effects, such

as poor growth, skin rashes, hair loss, vomiting and metabolic decompensation. Dietary protein is increased according to age, weight, clinical condition and quantitative plasma amino acid concentrations, ensuring that diet always provides at least the safe level of protein intake.

Practical aspects of low protein diets and feeds have been discussed earlier in this chapter. There are no published reports of babies with these disorders being breast fed. However, the author does have recent experience of one patient with early-onset MMA who was exclusively breast fed (once stabilised) for the first 4 months and maintained good metabolic control.

To improve the quality of low protein diets, some centres supplement the diet with synthetic amino acids which are free from the precursor amino acids. These can take the form of infant formula, drink mixes or pure amino acids, e.g. XMTVI Analog, Maxamaid, Maxamum or Amino Acid Mix. However, the long term value of these supplements remains uncertain. Metabolic balance can be achieved without them, and they are unpalatable and difficult to administer to children who have poor appetite unless they are tube fed. One study of two patients with MMA showed that although there was increased nitrogen retention when the low protein diet was supplemented with precursor-free amino acids, there was no improvement in growth or decrease in methyl-malonate excretion [117].

It is recommended that long fasts are avoided to limit the production of propionate from the oxidation of odd-numbered long chain fats [118]. Mobilisation of fatty acids can be suppressed by the use of regular three to four hourly daytime feeding and overnight tube feeding. Currently, overnight tube feeding is used universally although many receive this because of feeding problems. In one patient with MMA, uncooked cornstarch was used to minimise lipolysis at night [119].

Impaired renal function is a common complication in non-B_{12} responsive MMA, manifesting initially with a urinary concentrating and acidification defect due to renal tubular dysfunction [120]. Glomerular failure develops later [121] with progression to chronic then end-stage renal failure (ESRF). Supplements of sodium bicarbonate are often needed both to replace sodium losses and reduce acidosis. Increased urinary methylmalonate excretion also increases electrolyte losses.

The low protein diet used for MMA is also appropriate dietary treatment for those who develop chronic renal failure. It is also important to ensure a good energy intake and maintenance of adequate fluids. Further dietary manipulations may also be necessary with the progression towards ESRF, such as limiting the intake of phosphate and potassium and reducing protein intake further. Haemodialysis can cause symptomatic and biochemical improvement in ESRF [122]. Protein restriction remains necessary on dialysis, but the intake may be slightly increased compared with intake pre-dialysis (personal experience of two patients).

Anorexia and feeding problems with degrees of severity are almost invariably present and irreversible in the children with more severe variants. The causative factors are unclear, but increased plasma propionate is a possibility [114]. Enteral feeding via nasogastric tube or, more recently, button gastrostomy is often essential to provide an adequate dietary intake, to prevent metabolic decompensation, and to help the parents cope with a child who is difficult to feed.

A variety of feeding problems have been observed. In general those with more severe disease have worse problems. Food and fluid refusal is often acquired during the course of the disease and is frequently associated with repeated intercurrent infections. Many children have a poor appetite for solid food and often the diet is provided solely from oral fluids. Some will only eat a few selected foods, occasionally changing the type of foods that they will eat. Some are difficult feeders; parents complain of children being slow, fussy, retching or self-inducing vomiting with foods.

Dietary management of illness

During intercurrent infections patients are at risk of developing metabolic acidosis and encephalopathy. Development of new neurological signs has been reported in MMA following episodes of acute metabolic decompensation [109].

To help prevent this the standard emergency regimen (ER) (p. 287) is given: a high CHO intake from glucose polymer is given orally and/or via a tube at frequent two hourly intervals both day and night or as a continuous tube feed. This will reduce protein catabolism and lipolysis and hence propionate production. The usual protein intake is stopped for the minimum time possible to prevent protein deficiency which could greatly exacerbate the effects of illness. It is normally reintroduced early (within 2–3 days) and over a period of 1–4 days depending on the clinical condition of the child. Obviously, a more rapid reintroduction of protein is beneficial. Practical advice on protein reintroduction is given in the section on ERs. Continuation of an adequate energy intake is important throughout this period.

Inadequate nutrition in these disorders leads to catabolism, making the metabolic disturbance worse. If a child is unable to be re-established on their normal diet and protein intake within a few days, or is experiencing repeated intercurrent infections with inadequate protein intake, then an early resort to parenteral nutrition becomes essential. Parenteral nutrition can reverse the catabolic spiral and improve the metabolic state. If parenteral nutrition is indicated a normal amino acid solution can be used, but the amount is limited to provide only the child's usual protein intake [123]. This may need to be increased further in a malnourished patient.

In addition to the standard ER, metronidazole is given to reduce gut propionate production, and carnitine (100 mg/kg/day) to increase the removal of propionyl groups as propionyl carnitine in the urine. In MMA a generous fluid intake and sodium bicarbonate are needed to prevent dehydration and reduce acidosis. Additional potassium may also be necessary.

Treatment of the newly diagnosed patient

The newly diagnosed patient may be very sick in intensive care with severe acidosis and/or hyperammonaemia requiring ventilation and dialysis (to remove ammonia and toxic compounds). The aim of dietary treatment is to provide a high energy feed to reverse catabolism. Initially a glucose polymer solution (10–15% CHO) is given and a fat emulsion is added in 1–2% increments as tolerated. Provision of an adequate energy intake may initially be difficult because of imposed fluid restrictions in the ventilated child. Intravenous fluids of 10% dextrose will contribute to the total energy intake. Electrolytes (sodium and potassium) are added to the feed to provide normal requirements for age, taking into account any contribution of these from intravenous fluids and medicines such as sodium bicarbonate and sodium benzoate (which is used by some centres for the treatment of hyperammonaemia in these disorders). However, in MMA electrolyte requirements may be increased because of increased urinary losses. The feed is usually administered as frequent 2 hourly bolus feeds or continuous nasogastric feeds.

Protein is reintroduced with the minimum of delay once the acute metabolic derangement, including the acidosis, has been corrected and the plasma ammonia is less than or around 100 μmol/l (normal <40 μmol/l). Protein is usually commenced with 0.5 g protein/kg body weight/day from infant formula and increased to the final safe level of protein intake (Table 15.27) within a few days. Vitamins and minerals should be added to the feed if there is a delay in introducing or increasing protein intake. Paediatric Seravit can be used for this purpose. Table 15.29 provides an example of a nutritionally complete low protein infant feed.

If the baby is being breast fed the mother should be encouraged to express until the baby becomes more metabolically stable, then breast feeding can be reintroduced. Protein-free feeds may need to be given in combination with breast feeds while metabolic control is being established.

ISOVALERIC ACIDAEMIA

Isovaleric acidaemia (IVA) is caused by a deficiency of isovaleryl-CoA dehydrogenase which blocks the catabolism of leucine at the level of isovaleryl-CoA and causes it to accumulate (Fig. 15.2). IVA can

present in neonates (acute form) or in older children (chronic intermittent form). The neonate subsequently follows the chronic intermittent course.

During remission the majority of isovaleryl-CoA is conjugated to isovalerylglycine which is non-toxic and is excreted in large amounts in urine. Isovaleryl-CoA is also conjugated to carnitine to form isovaleryl carnitine which is also excreted in the urine. However, during acute episodes the natural capacity of this detoxification pathway is exceeded and isovaleryl-CoA is deacylated to produce large amounts of toxic isovaleric acid which may cause an overwhelming illness [124]. The outcome of IVA is variable, ranging from normal psychomotor development to severe mental retardation [125].

Dietary management

The aim of dietary treatment is to limit dietary leucine intake and minimise formation of isovaleric acid. Sufficient leucine must be given for normal growth requirements. Leucine does not accumulate in plasma so it is not possible to use measurement of this to determine protein intake.

Usually a modest protein restriction (2 g/kg in infants and young children decreasing to between 1.5 and 1 g/kg in older patients) combined with an adequate energy intake, is sufficient to limit the production of isovaleric acid in the well child. Higher protein intakes than this may be tolerated by some patients (personal experience). Although patients are not on very low protein diets it is still important to ensure that an adequate intake of all vitamins and minerals is provided. Practical management of low protein diet and feeds has been given earlier in this chapter. Most children with isovaleric acidaemia have a reasonable appetite but major feeding problems do occur in some. In addition to diet, patients are treated with glycine (250 mg/kg/day) and carnitine (100 mg/kg/day) to increase conjugation and hence reduce isovaleric acid levels, particularly during periods of metabolic decompensation [124, 126, 127].

Dietary management during illness

During intercurrent infections protein catabolism will greatly increase production of isovaleric acid and patients are at risk of developing acidosis. To help prevent this, the standard emergency regimen (p. 287) of frequent high CHO drinks day and night is given.

Protein intake is stopped temporarily and reintroduced early within 1–3 days maximum and over a period of 1–4 days depending on the clinical condition of the child. Practical advice on protein reintroduction is provided in the ER section. Oral or intravenous glycine and carnitine should continue to be given as part of the emergency regimen and the doses may need to be increased temporarily.

GLUTARIC ACIDURIA TYPE I

Glutaric aciduria type I (GA I) is caused by a deficiency of the enzyme glutaryl-CoA dehydrogenase in the catabolic pathway of the amino acids lysine, hydroxylysine and tryptophan. This results in the accumulation of glutaric, 3-hydroxyglutaric and glutaconic acids in body fluids and tissues [128]. Typically babies with GA I usually appear normal in the first months of life, although many will have macrocephaly. The majority of patients present between 6 and 18 months following an intercurrent illness such as a respiratory or gastrointestinal illness which precipitates to an acute encephalopathic crisis. Patients are consequently left with a severe dystonic-dyskinetic disorder that is similar to cerebral palsy and ranges from extreme hypotonia to choreathetosis to rigidity and spasticity [129]. Intellectual function is generally preserved initially. A minority of patients have a more insidious onset with no obvious encephalopathic episode preceeding the development of the movement disorder. Some patients with genetically proven GA I do not develop neurological disease at all [131].

Dietary management

The dietary manangement of GA I is controversial as the clinical value of this has not been proven. Dietary practice varies between centres; low protein and low lysine and tryptophan diets [130] are used in the treatment of both symptomatic and presymptomatic patients with GA I and some (including this centre) use either a modest or no protein restriction and just recommend avoiding a high intake. It is known that protein restriction cannot reverse neurological damage which has already occurred and dietary protein restriction alone is not sufficient to prevent brain injury [131, 132]. Much more important is the need to prevent catabolic states such as intercurrent infections by use of an emergency regimen (see below) to minimise brain damage.

Feeding problems are common in this group of patients and include chewing and swallowing difficulties due to dyskinesia and reflux and vomiting due to truncal hypotonia. The extent of these feeding problems are related to the severity of the neurological disease, with acute onset being much worse than insidious onset. Tube feeding is often essential to maintain an adequate energy intake and to achieve satisfactory growth. Fundoplication (and insertion of gastrostomy) may be necessary in some patients for treatment of gastro-oesophageal reflux and vomiting.

Assessing energy requirements in this group of patients can be difficult; the worst patients cannot walk so should need less energy, but energy expenditure is reported to often be increased due to high muscle tone and dystonic movements and to disturbances in temperature control [129]. In our patient group provision of a near normal energy intake for age has resulted in satisfactory weight gain provided there were no problems with vomiting and gastro-oesophageal reflux. In one patient with spasticity and rigidity, the energy requirement for normal growth was very low: around 50% of normal for age.

Dietary management of illness

Prompt management of intercurrent illness is critical in GA I to prevent neurological damage in presymptomatic patients and further injury in symptomatic patients. At the first sign of illness or loss of appetite (or usual feeds not being tolerated) the standard emergency regimen (p. 287) of frequent high CHO drinks or tube feeds is given to minimise catabolism. If the child does not tolerate the ER it is crucial they are admitted to hospital without delay for intavenous therapy of 10% dextrose. Carnitine should also be given orally or if not tolerated, intravenously. Once the child begins to improve, their usual diet is reintroduced and additional glucose polymer drinks/feeds are given particularly at night until the child has fully recovered and returned to their normal regimen. Parents will need guidance on how to do this.

UREA CYCLE DISORDERS

The urea cycle has two main functions – it converts waste nitrogen compounds into urea (excreted by the kidney) and it is the biosynthetic pathway of arginine. Inborn errors at each step of the pathway have been identified (Fig. 15.6). The urea cycle disorders are

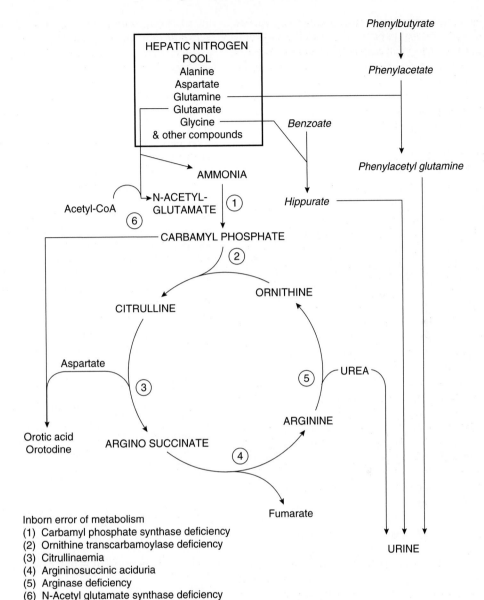

Fig. 15.6 Hepatic nitrogen metabolism

inherited as autosomal traits apart from ornithine transcarbamoylase deficiency (OTC), which is an X-linked trait, and the most common of these disorders. Arginase deficiency is distinct from the other disorders and will be discussed separately.

Deficiencies of these enzymes result in waste nitrogen accumulating as ammonia and glutamine, which are neurotoxic and may cause a severe encephalopathy. These disorders can present at any age from the neonatal period throughout childhood. The onset of symptoms often coincides with an intercurrent infection or an increase in dietary protein intake although many of these patients self-select a low protein diet. A diet history can be very revealing.

The clinical presentation varies depending on the age of onset. Loss of appetite, poor feeding and vomiting are common in all ages. In the newborn there is often respiratory distress with signs of hyperpnoea, seizures and collapse. In the later onset patients confusion, headache, disorientation, abnormal behaviour, ataxia, focal neurologial signs or coma can occur and in some there is also delayed physical growth and developmental delay [133].

The outlook for patients who present in the newborn period is very poor [134]. In late-presenting patients almost all have some degree of learning and neurological disability [135]. Those who are treated prospectively have a much better outcome. The urea cycle disorders are treated by:

- Restriction of dietary protein intake to decrease the need to excrete waste nitrogen
- Medicines which utilise alternative pathways for the excretion of waste nitrogen
- Arginine supplements.

Medicines

Sodium benzoate and phenylbutyrate increase waste nitrogen excretion by using alternative pathways to the urea cycle (Fig. 15.6) [136]. Phenylbutyrate is more effective than sodium benzoate as a vehicle for nitrogen excretion. Phenylbutyrate is metabolised *in vivo* to form phenylacetate which is conjugated with glutamine to form phenylacetylglutamine. This is then excreted so that 2 moles of nitrogen are excreted for each mole of phenylbutyrate given. Sodium benzoate is conjugated with glycine to form hippurate so that 1 mole of nitrogen is excreted for each mole of sodium benzoate given. Although phenylbutryate is twice as effective it is less palatable and more expensive than sodium benzoate. Both can be administered orally or intravenously (IV) and are usually prescribed in doses of up to 250 mg/kg body weight/day, divided between three or four doses. Parents are innovative in finding methods of masking the unpleasant flavour of these medicines. Some ideas are milk shake flavourings, jam, honey, yoghurt, peppermint essence and fruit purées. Sodium benzoate is available in powder, syrup or tablet form and phenylbutyrate as coated granules or tablets which are more readily taken.

In N-acetylglutamate synthase (NAGS) deficiency, N-acetylglutamate, the activator of carbamyl-phosphate synthase (CPS) is not formed. Patients are treated with carbamylglutamate which is an orally active form of N-acetylglutamate.

Arginine

Arginine becomes an essential or semi-essential amino acid in urea cycle disorders because its synthesis is greatly reduced [137]. In ornithine carbamyl transferase (OCT) and CPS deficiency arginine supplements of 100–170 mg/kg body weight/day are given to replace that which would normally be formed. Alternatively in OCT, in order to meet the arginine requirements, supplements of citrulline can be given as it is rapidly converted to arginine via the intact part of the urea cycle. Also, citrulline contains one less nitrogen atom than arginine, thereby reducing waste nitrogen production, but it is much more expensive than arginine.

In citrullinaemia and arginosuccinic aciduria (ASA), large doses of arginine up to 700 mg/kg/day are given to replenish ornithine supply. The carbon skeleton of ornithine is needed for the formation of citrulline and arginosuccinic acid which accumulate and are excreted in citrullinaemia and ASA respectively. Arginosuccinic acid is more effective than citrulline as it carries two waste nitrogen atoms and has a higher renal clearance. Arginine increases the concentrations of both citrulline and arginosuccinic acid, the full consequence of which is unknown. However, this appears to be less toxic than the accumulation of ammonia and glutamine.

Arginine can be administered orally or intravenously. It is available in powder or tablet form for oral use. It is given as a divided dose and usually in conjunction with the other medicines.

Dietary management – low protein diet

Urea cycle disorders are treated with a low protein diet to reduce the accumulation of waste nitrogen. A normal energy intake for age is provided to ensure normal growth and to prevent endogenous protein catabolism with consequent metabolic decompensation.

For those with severe defects the dietary protein intake is usually reduced to the safe level (Table 15.27), but patients with milder defects will tolerate a higher protein intake. Practical management of the low protein diet is given earlier in this chapter. If the child is unable to take a sufficient intake orally, nasogastric or gastrostomy feeding must be used to prevent metabolic decompensation (most children will feed orally if metabolic control is good). Regular feeding and avoidance of prolonged fasts is recommended to help maintain good biochemical control as plasma glutamine and ammonia concentrations will increase with fasting and endogenous protein catabolism.

Essential amino acid supplements

For some children an essential amino acid (EAA) supplement is incorporated as part of the total protein intake. This is beneficial because, by limiting the intake of non-essential amino acids, waste nitrogen is utilised to synthesise these and hence nitrogen destined for excretion as urea will be reduced.

EAA supplements are often given first when the blood biochemistry cannot be corrected by altering the medicines because the child is either on maximum doses of medicines or refusing to take more. There is no set dose of EAA supplement. The amount prescribed usually varies between 0.2 and 0.5 g/kg/day, given as a divided dose between two or three meals. EAA supplements can also be used to improve the biological value of a low protein diet which may be lacking in one or more essential amino acids. This may occur if the protein is provided from a limited range of low biological value (LBV) protein foods.

EAA supplements are often used during the stabilisation period in newly diagnosed patients (see below). Details of EAA supplements are provided in Table 15.32.

Low protein diet – monitoring

Regular measurements of plasma ammonia and quantitative amino acids including glutamine are essential for the management of urea cycle disorders. Monitoring 3–4 monthly is recommended for most patients who are stable but it may need to be done more frequently if the child is not well. A 24 hour profile of plasma ammonia and glutamine is helpful in patients who are difficult to manage. Alterations to dietary protein, essential amino acid intakes and medicines are based on the results of these investigations 15.33). High concentrations of glutamine and ammonia in plasma may not only mean that protein intake is too high; similar results will be obtained during periods of chronic catabolism so growth and clinical status must also be considered when interpreting these results.

Good biochemical control may be difficult to achieve during periods of slow growth before and particularly after puberty [138]. When the adolescent stops growing there may be a period of instability because protein is no longer needed for growth; protein intake and medicines may require adjustment to restore stability.

Glutamine Poor appetite is observed in some children [139] with high glutamine levels implicated as a cause. It is thought that glutamine causes an increased influx of tryptophan (the precursor of serotonin) into the brain and promotes serotonin synthesis. Serotonin increases a feeling of satiety [138]. If plasma

Table 15.32 Essential amino acid products used in urea cycle disorders

Product	Amino acids (g/100 g)	Protein equivalent (g/100 g)	Energy (kcal (MJ) 100 g)	CHO (g/100 g)	Fat (g/100 g)	Vitamins and minerals	Comments
Dialamine[a]	30	25	360 (1.5)	65[b]	nil	[c]	Orange flavoured. Suitable from 6 months. Can be added to a feed, drink or given as a paste
Essential Amino Acid Mix[a]	94.5	79	316 (1.3)	nil	nil	nil	Suitable for infants under 6 months

[a] A powdered mixture of essential amino acids (including cystine and histidine)
[b] Contains a mixture of glucose polymer and sugar
[c] Contains vitamin C and trace amounts of sodium, potassium, chloride, calcium, phosphorus and magnesium

Both products are manufactured by Scientific Hospital Supplies. Other products are manufactured by Milupa and Ross Laboratories but are not available in the United Kingdom.

Table 15.33 Outline of management decisions for urea cycle disorders (excluding arginase deficiency)

Ammonia μmol/l normal reference range <40	Glutamine μmol/l normal reference range 400–800	Quantitative plasma amino acids	Action
>80–100	>800	low	Increase medicines* Increase natural protein or essential amino acids Increase arginine in ASA and citrullinaemia**
>80–100	>800	normal	Increase medicines* Increase arginine in ASA and citrullinaemia** No change to diet
<80	400–800	low	No change to medicines* Increase natural protein
<80	400–800	normal	No change to medicines or diet

* Medicines – sodium benzoate and/or phenylbutyrate
** If plasma arginine is high, arginine dose is not increased. If plasma citrulline or arginosuccinic acid is too high, arginine is not increased

glutamine is maintained within the normal range then, in some children, appetite may improve.

Management of the newly diagnosed patient

Neonates with hyperammonaemia will be very sick, requiring ventilation and often haemofiltration or haemodialysis (to remove ammonia). The aim of dietary treatment is to provide a high energy feed to prevent catabolism. Initially a glucose polymer solution (10–15% CHO) is given; a fat emulsion may be added to this feed in 1–2% increments as tolerated. It is often difficult to provide sufficient energy because of restricted fluid intake in the ventilated child. Fluids are usually initially provided by intravenous 10% dextrose and medicines to control hyperammonaemia (sodium benzoate, phenylbutyrate and arginine). Enteral fluids will be gradually increased as 10% dextrose is decreased. Electrolytes, sodium and potassium are added to the feed to provide normal requirements for age, taking into account any contribution of these from intravenous fluids and medicines, e.g. sodium benzoate and phenylbutyrate.

Protein needs to be reintroduced promptly to prevent protein catabolism with further metabolic decompensation. Once the plasma ammonia falls to around 100 μmol/l or less, some natural protein is introduced from infant formula, usually 0.25–0.5 g/kg body weight/day and increased daily to the full allow-ance (around 2 g/kg/day) over a period of 3–4 days. Protein requirement is likely to be higher than this if the neonate has had no protein for several days and has been on haemodialysis. Plasma ammonia is monitored at least once per day during protein reintroduction. Guidelines for low protein feeds are given on p. 276. Occasionally it can be difficult to reintroduce protein without inducing hyperammon-aemia; in these instances an essential amino acid sup-plement, e.g. Essential Amino Acid Mix (Table 15.32) is used and will be replaced with natural protein once the patient is more stable. It is also important to ensure sufficient energy is being provided to prevent hyperammonaemia and promote anabolism. Energy requirements will often be greater than normal because of low intakes both pre-diagnosis (poor feeding and vomiting) and during the initial days of stabilisation. If the baby is being breast fed the mother should be encouraged to express until the baby is more stable, then breast feeding can be rein-troduced. Protein-free feeds may be required in addi-tion to breast feeds to achieve good metabolic control.

For patients who present later in infancy or during childhood with hyperammonaemia the principles of initial dietary treatment are the same; a protein-free, high energy diet and medicines are given initally and protein is reintroduced to the safe level of intake (Table 15.27) over 3–4 days once the plasma ammonia concentration has decreased and the patient is more stable.

Management of illness

During intercurrent illness, protein catabolism may cause rapid accumulation of ammonia and glutamine. The standard emergency regimen (p. 287) is used to prevent these effects of illness. Protein intake is stopped temporarily and regular two hourly drinks of glucose polymer are given. The usual doses of sodium benzoate, phenylbutyrate and arginine are administered. If necessary during acute illness the benzoate and phenylbutyrate dose can be temporarily increased to 500 mg/kg/day. Protein is usually reintroduced within 2–3 days and over a period of 1–4 days depending on the child's clinical condition. Practical advice on protein reintroduction is given in the emergency regimen section later in this chapter.

If the child does not tolerate oral fluids and medicines, 10% dextrose and medicines are given intravenously. Oral fluids can usually be recommenced within 24–48 hours, with a gradual changeover from intravenous to oral, thus ensuring an adequate energy intake. Plasma ammonia and quantitative amino acids should be measured regularly. Once the plasma ammonia is less than 80–100 µmol/l, protein is gradually reintroduced over a period of 2–4 days. If hyperammonaemia is induced during protein reintroduction an essential amino acid supplement is used and energy intake is increased.

ARGINASE DEFICIENCY

Arginase deficiency (Fig. 15.6) is a rare disorder whose presentation is distinct from the other urea cycle defects. It is characterised by a progressive spastic tetraplegia, seizures and developmental regression [133]. Hyperargininaemia and a mild hyperammonaemia occur due to defective hydrolysis of arginine. The mechanisms responsible for the neurological damage are not yet completely understood, but arginine and its guanidino metabolites are possible neurotoxins [140, 141]

Dietary management

Arginase deficiency is treated with a low protein diet, sodium benzoate and phenylbutyrate. The aim is to maintain plasma arginine levels at less than 200 µmol/l (normal reference range 40–120 µmol/l) and a near normal plasma ammonia (normal range <40 µmol/l).

All dietary nitrogen has the potential to be converted to arginine, this source being considerably greater than the small amount of arginine which is naturally present in protein. In the past, in order to restrict the nitrogen intake, diets comprised an EAA supplement with a very limited intake of natural protein. Nowadays, by giving sodium benzoate and phenylbutyrate a more generous intake of natural protein is possible while still maintaining acceptable plasma arginine and ammonia levels. These medicines reduce available nitrogen destined for arginine synthesis by increasing its excretion via alternative pathways to the urea cycle (Fig. 15.6). Protein intake is restricted to the safe level (Table 15.27), and is provided by a combination of natural protein and an EAA supplement. The precise composition of protein intake must be determined by the balance of requirements for growth and the medicines necessary for good biochemical control. The practical management of the low protein diet and EAA supplementation are provided on pages 274 and 285 respectively.

The diet is monitored by regular measurements of plasma ammonia, plasma arginine and the other amino acids quantitatively.

During intercurrent illness the standard emergency regimen of a protein-free high energy intake from frequent carbohydrate drinks is used to prevent hyperargininaemia and hyperammonaemia. This should be implemented promptly to prevent irreversible deterioration [141]. Sodium benzoate and phenylbutyrate should be given orally or intravenously.

EMERGENCY REGIMENS

For some inborn errors of intermediary metabolism, intercurrent infections combined with a poor oral intake and fasting, will precipitate severe metabolic decompensation. To help prevent this, the child's usual diet is stopped (although this often occurs naturally because of reduced appetite) and an emergency regimen (ER) is given. In some disorders the ER is combined with additional specific therapy (refer to respective disorders).

The aim of the ER is to provide an exogenous energy source to:

- Reduce production of potentially toxic metabolites from either protein catabolism and/or lipolysis in disorders such as organic acidaemias (e.g. glutaric

Table 15.34 Emergency regimens

Age (yrs)	Glucose polymer concentration %CHO	Energy/100 ml		Osmolality (mOsm/kg H$_2$O*)	Daily volume	Feeding frequency
		(kcal)	(kJ)			
0–0.5	10	40	167	103	150–200 ml/kg	Initially two to three
0.5–1	12	48	202		120–150 ml/kg**	hourly, night and
1–2	15	60	250	174	1200 ml	day
2–6	20	80	334	245	1200–1600 ml	
6–10	20	80	334	245	1600–2000 ml	
>10	25	100	418	342	2000 ml	

*   Data provided by Scientific Hospital Supplies International Limited
** Maximum fluid intake of 1200 ml daily.

aciduria type I), fatty acid oxidation defects (e.g. medium chain acyl-CoA dehydrogenase deficinency)

- Prevent hypoglycaemia in disorders such as ketotic hypoglycaemia or glycogen storage disease type I.

The standard ER is essentially the same for all disorders. A solution of glucose polymer is given as the main energy source because it is simple to administer and is usually well tolerated. These solutions alone will not provide the estimated average requirement for energy [71]. Fat emulsions can be added as an additional energy source, but these may be less well tolerated, particularly in the child who is vomiting. Fat is contraindicated in disorders of fatty acid oxidation.

The carbohydrate (CHO) concentration of the ER and fluid volumes given depend on the age of the child (Table 15.34). Too concentrated a solution of glucose polymer will be hyperosmolar, cause diarrhoea and exacerbate the effects of illness. To improve palatability the glucose polymer solution can be flavoured with squash, taking care not to exceed the recommended CHO concentration per 100 ml. Alternatively glucose polymer powder can be added to fruit juice or carbonated drinks to the required concentration of CHO. Parents are taught to make these drinks using handy scoop measurements. For children who are unfamiliar with the taste of glucose polymer drinks it is worthwhile having a trial of different drinks when they are well to ascertain what they will take and to familiarise the parents with reconstitution of these in a non-emergency situation. Lucozade contains 17–18% CHO and Ribena in a carton 15% CHO; these drinks are convenient because they are ready to use, portable and can be

stored for use in an emergency situation at nursery or school.

During gastrointestinal illness an oral rehydration solution (ORS) supplemented with glucose polymer to provide extra energy, usually to a concentration of 10 g CHO per 100 ml, is used. The osmolality of such feeds needs to be considered [142]; ORS with glucose polymer added to a final concentration of 10 g CHO per 100 ml has an osmolality around 320 mOsmol/kg H$_2$O.

To reduce the period of fasting and optimise energy intake the ER is initially fed at frequent two hourly intervals night and day. In some circumstances it may be better to give small very frequent sips of the ER. Such frequent overnight feeding (two hourly) can be difficult to achieve, particularly for patients without nasogastric tubes and more realistic targets should be considered.

The ER is normally commenced at home at the first signs of illness and is given orally or enterally. It is useful to teach the parents of patients who refuse to drink when they are unwell how to feed their child nasogastrically at home. If the child persistently vomits the ER or is obviously not recovering, then a hospital admission for stabilisation with intravenous (IV) therapy is usually necessary. Dextrose 10% is given by peripheral drip or more concentrated dextrose can be administered through a central line. When oral fluids are reintroduced there is a gradual changeover from IV to oral feeding, thus ensuring an overall adequate energy intake. If oral or enteral feeds are unable to be re-established then an early resort to parenteral nutrition is indicated for some disorders [143]; refer to specific disorders.

The basic ER of glucose polymer must not be continued for long periods of time because it does not provide adequate nutrition. Poor growth and nutritional deficiencies will occur in patients on low protein diets, who have repeated infections and are frequently on the ER. If so, it may be necessary to increase protein intake temporarily when the child is well to compensate for inadequate intakes of protein while on the ER.

As the child improves normal diet is reintroduced. With the exception of low protein diets the ER is often just replaced with the child's usual diet within 1–2 days. During the recovery phase if the child's appetite is reduced it is important to give additional ER drinks or feeds to maximise energy intake and prevent further metabolic decompensation.

For patients on low protein diets, the protein intake is stopped for the shortest time possible (1–3 days maximum). Protein, whether from feed or diet, is reintroduced by increasing the daily amount, providing one quarter, one half and three quarters of the usual intake, resuming the normal allowance by the fourth day. If on diet, additional ER drinks are given throughout the reintroduction period (usually less frequently) to maximise energy intake. If on feeds, additional glucose polymer is added to the infant formula or low protein tube feed to the same concentration as the ER. If the child's usual feed contains more CHO than the ER it will be increased up to this concentration (over the 4 days). If the feed normally contains fat and vitamins and minerals these too will be increased over the same 4 days. This reintroduction period will be done more rapidly over fewer days if clinically indicated. In milder illnesses protein intake is generally not regraded. The child's usual feeding frequency is also gradually resumed as tolerated.

Instructions for parents

Treatment of intercurrent infections can be an anxious and difficult time for parents. To make this easier, parents are taught a three staged plan telling them what to do and when [144]. This type of approach can also help reduce episodes of metabolic decompensation and hospital admissions.

(1) If the parents are unsure whether their child is showing the first signs of illness (pallor, lethargy, irritability) then an ER drink is given as a precaution. Clinical observations are reported to be generally better than biochemical measurements for detecting decompensation; subtle changes in behaviour are usually the earliest signs of this and are most easily detected by parents [145]. The child's clinical state is then reviewed regularly within 1–2 hours.

(2) If on reassessment the child has improved, the normal diet is resumed; if however the child has deteriorated or shown no signs of improvement the full ER is commenced for a period of 24–48 hours. The parents are instructed how to reintroduce the usual diet.

(3) If the child is not tolerating the ER (i.e. refusing ER drinks, vomiting or becoming encephalopathic) then the child is admitted to hospital.

The parents are taught to recognise signs of encephalopathy such as disorientation and poor responsiveness, accompanied by a glazed look.

REFERENCES

1 Costello PM, Beasley MG, Tillotson SL, Smith I Intelligence in mild atypical phenylketonuria. *Eur J Pediat*, 1994, **153** 260–63.

2 Woo SLC, diLella AG, Marvit J, Ledley FD Molecular basis of phenylketonuria and somatic potential gene therapy. *Cold Spring Symposia on Quantitative Biology*, 1986, **LI**, 395–401.

3 Smith I The hyperphenylalaninaemias. In: Lloyd JK, Scriver CR (eds) *Genetic and Metabolic Disease in Paediatrics.* London: Butterworths, 1985, pp. 166–210.

4 Aoki K, Wada Y Outcome of the patients detected by newborn screening in Japan. *Acta Paediatr Jpn*, 1988, **30** 429–34.

5 Jervis GA Studies on phenylpyruvic oligophrenia. The position of the metabolic error. *J Biol Chem*, 1947, **169** 651–6.

6 Udenfriend S, Cooper JR The enzymatic conversion of phenylalanine to tyrosine. *J Biol Chem*, 1952, **194** 503–11.

7 Woolf LI, Vulliamy DG Phenylketonuria with a study of the effect upon it of glutamic acid. *Arch Dis Childh*, 1951, **26** 487–94.

8 Bickel H, Gerrard J, Hickmans E Influence of phenylalanine intake on phenylketonuria. *Lancet*, 1953, **2** 812.

9 Scriver CR, Kaufman S, Eisensmith RC, Woo SLC The hyperphenylalaninemias. In: Scriver CR, Beaudet AL, Sly WS, Valle D (eds) *The Metabolic and Molecular Bases of Inherited Disease*, vol 1. New York: McGraw-Hill, 1995, pp. 1015–75.

10 Ledley FD, Levy HL, Woo SLC Molecular analysis of the inheritance of phenylketonuria and mild hyperphenylalaninemia in families with both disorders. *New Eng J Med*, 1986, **314** 1276–9.

11 Hilton MA, Sharpe JN, Hicks LG, Andrews BF A simple method for detection of heterozygous carriers of the gene for classical phenylketonuria. *J Pediatr*, 1986, **109** 601–4.

12 Medical Research Council Working Party on Phenylketonuria. Recommendations on the dietary management of phenylketonuria. *Arch Dis Childh*, 1993, **68** 426–7.

13 Kaufman S, Holtzman NA, Milstein S, Butler IJ, Krumholtz A Phenylketonuria due to a deficiency of dihydropteridine reductase. *New Eng J Med*, 1975, **293** 785–90.

14 Kaufman S, Berlow S, Summer GK, Milstein S, Schulman J, Orloff S, Spielberg S, Pueschel S Hyperphenylalaninemia due to a deficiency of biopterin. A variant form of phenylketonuria. *New Eng J Med*, 1978, **299** 673–9.

15 Leeming RJ, Blair JA, Rey F Biopterin derivatives in atypical phenylketonuria. *Lancet*, 1976, **1** 99–100.

16 Pollitt RJ Amino acid disorders. In: Holton J (ed) *The Inherited Metabolic Diseases*. Edinburgh: Churchill Livingstone, 1994, pp. 67–113.

17 Smith I, Cook B, Beasley M Review of neonatal screening programme for phenylketonuria. *Brit Med J*, 1991, **303** 333–5.

18 Waisbren SE, Zaff J Personality disorder in young women with treated phenylketonuria. *J Inher Metab Dis*, 1994, **17** 584–92.

19 Tyfield LA, Meredith AL, Osborn MJ, Primavesi R, Chambers TL, Holton JB, Harper PS Genetic analysis of treated and untreated phenylketonuria in one family. *J Med Genet*, 1990, **27** 564–8.

20 Medical Research Council Working Party on Phenylketonuria. Phenylketonuria due to phenylalanine hydroxylase deficiency: an unfolding story. *Brit Med J*, 1993, **306** 115–19.

21 Weglage J, Fünders B, Wilken B, Schubert D, Ullrich K School performance and intellectual outcome in adolescents with phenylketonuria. *Acta Paediatr*, 1993, **81** 582–6.

22 Smith I, Beasley MG, Ades AE Intelligence and quality of dietary treatment in phenylketonuria. *Arch Dis Childh*, 1990, **65** 472–8.

23 Smith I, Beasley MG, Ades AE Effect on intelligence of relaxing the low phenylalanine diet in phenylketonuria. *Arch Dis Childh*, 1991, **66** 311–16.

24 Holtzman NA, Kronmal RA, van Doorninck W, Azen C, Koch R Effect of age at loss of dietary control on intellectual performance and behaviour of children with phenylketonuria. *New Eng J Med*, 1986, **314** 593–8.

25 Thompson AJ, Smith I, Brenton D, Youl BD, Rylance G, Davidson DC, Kendall B, Lees AJ Neurological deterioration in young adults with phenylketonuria. *Lancet*, 1990, **336** 602–5.

26 Smith I, Lobascher ME, Stevenson JE, Wolff OH, Schmidt H, Grubel-Kaiser S, Bickel H Effect of stopping low-phenylalanine diet on intellectual progress of children with phenylketonuria. *Brit Med J*, 1978, **2** 723–6.

27 Hudson FP, Mordaunt VL, Leahy I Evaluation of treatment begun in first 3 months of life in 184 cases of phenylketonuria. *Arch Dis Childh*, 1970, **45** 5–12.

28 Güttler F, Guldberg P The influence of mutations on enzyme activity and phenylalanine tolerance in phenylalanine hydroxylase deficiency. *Eur J Pediatr*, 1996, **155** S6–10.

29 Acosta PB, Wenz E, Williamson M Nutrient intake of treated infants with phenylketonuria. *Amer J Clin Nutr*, 1977, **30** 198–208.

30 Wendel U, Ullrich K, Schmidt H, Batzler U Six year follow up of phenylalanine intakes and plasma phenylalanine concentrations. *Eur J Pediatr*, 1990, **149** S13–16.

31 Lyman FL, Lyman JK Dietary management of phenylketonuria with Lofenalac. *Arch Pediatr*, 1960, **77** 212.

32 Thompson S *Protocol for the use of XP Maxamaid in the Dietary Management of Phenylketonuria*. Liverpool: SHS, 1997.

33 NSPKU (1999) Dietary information for the treatment of phenylketonuria. 1999/2000 revision. Gateshead: National Society for Phenylketonuria.

34 MacDonald A *Diet and phenylketonuria*. PhD thesis, Birmingham University, 1999.

35 van Spronsen FJ, van Dijk T, Smit GPA, Van Rijn M, Reijngoud D-J, Berger R, Heymans HSA Phenylketonuria: plasma responses to different distributions of the daily phenylalanine allowance over the day. *Pediatrics*, 1996, **97** 839–44.

36 van Spronsen FJ, van Rijn M, Van Dijk T, Smit GPA, Reijngoud D-J, Berger R, Heymans HSA Plasma phenylalanine and tyrosine responses to different nutritional conditions (fasting/post-prandial) in patients with phenylketonuria: effect of sample timing. *Pediatrics*, 1993, **92** 570–73.

37 Motil KJ, Matthews DE, Bier DM, Burke JF, Munro HN, Young VR Whole body leucine and lysine metabolism: response to dietary protein intake in young men. *Amer J Physiol*, 1981, **240** E712–21.

38 Schoeffer A, Herrmann M-E, Brösicke HG, Mönch E Influence of single dose amino acid mixtures on the nitrogen retention in patients with phenylketonuria. *J Nutr Med*, 1994, **4** 415–18.

39 MacDonald A, Rylance G, Hall SK, Asplin D, Booth IW Does a single blood specimen predict quality of control in PKU? *Arch Dis Childh*, 1997, **78** 122–6.

40 Prince AP, McMurry MP, Buist NRM Treatment

products and approaches for phenylketonuria: improved palatability and flexibility demonstrate safety, efficacy and acceptance in US clinical trials. *J Inher Metab Dis*, 1997, **20** 486–98.

41 Allen JR, McCauley JC, Waters DL, O'Connor J, Roberts DC, Gaskin KJ Resting energy expenditure in children with phenylketonuria. *Am J Clin Nutr*, 1995, **62** 797–801.

42 Galli C, Agostoni C, Mosconi C, Riva E, Salari C, Giovannini M Reduced plasma C-20 and C-22 polyunsaturated fatty acids in children during dietary intervention. *J Pediatr*, 1991, **119** 562–7.

43 Giovanni M, Biasucci G, Agostoni C, Luotti D, Riva E Lipid status and fatty acid metabolism in phenylketonuria. *J Inher Met Dis*, 1995, **18** 265–72.

44 Lipson A, Masters H, O'Halloran, Thompson S, Coveney J, Yu J The selenium status of children with phenylketonuria: results of selenium supplementation. *Aust Paediatr J*, 1988, **24** 128–31.

45 Wilke BC, Vidailhet M, Favier A, Guillemin C, Ducros V, Arnaud J, Richard MJ Selenium, glutathione peroxidase (GSH-Px) and lipid peroxidation products before and after selenium supplementation. *Clinica Chimica Acta*, 1992, **207** 137–42.

46 Greeves LG, Carson DJ, Craig BG, McMaster D Potentially life-threatening cardiac dysrhythmia in a child with selenium deficiency and phenylketonuria. *Acta Paediatr Scand*, 1990, **79** 1259–62.

47 Bodley JL, Austin VJ, Hanley WB, Clarke JTR, Zlotkin S Low iron stores in infants and children with treated phenylketonuria: a population at risk for iron-deficiency anaemia and associated cognitive deficits. *Eur J Pediatr*, 1993, **152** 142–3.

48 Bohles H, Ullrich K, Endres W, Behbehani AW, Wendel U Inadequate iron availability as a possible cause of low serum carnitine concentrations in patients with phenylketonuria. *Eur J Pediatr*, 1991, **150** 425–8.

49 Hanley WB, Feigenbaum ASJ, Clarke JTR, Schoonheyt WE, Austin VJ Vitamin B_{12} deficiency in adolescents and young adults with phenylketonuria. *Eur J Pediatr*, 1996, **155** S145–7.

50 National Society for Phenylketonuria Medical Advisory Panel. Management of PKU. Gateshead: NSPKU, 1999.

51 Green A, Isherwood D Reference data excluding neonates. In: Clayton BE, Round JM (eds) *Clinical Biochemistry and the Sick Child*. Oxford: Blackwell Science, 1994, pp. 523–39.

52 Gregory DM, Sovetts D, Clow CL, Scriver CR Plasma free amino acid values in normal children and adolescents. *Metabolism*, 1986, **35** 967–9.

53 Scriver CR, Gregory DM, Sovetts D, Tissenbaum G Normal plasma-free amino acid values in adults: the influence of some common physiological variables. *Metabolism*, 1985, **34** 868–73.

54 Hanley WB, Linsao L, Davidson W, Moes CAF Malnutrition with early treatment of phenylketonuria. *Paediatr Res*, 1970, **4** 318–27.

55 Biasucci G Randomised controlled trial of a long chain polyunsaturated fatty acid (LC-PUFA) supplemented phenylalanine free infant formula. International Metabolic Dietitians' Group, York: Study for the Society of Inborn Errors of Metabolism, 1999.

56 MacDonald A, Rylance G, Asplin D, Harris G, Booth IW Abnormal feeding behaviours in phenylketonuria. *J Hum Nut Diets*, 1997, **10** 163–70.

57 Schultz B, Bremer HJ Nutrient intake and food consumption of adolescents and young adults with phenylketonuria. *Acta Paediatr*, 1995, **84** 743–8.

58 Francis D Diets for Sick Children. Oxford: Blackwell Science, 1987.

59 Weetch EI, MacDonald A, Wadsworth J, Laing S, White F Fruit and vegetables in PKU: phenylalanine analysis re-visited. International Metabolic Dietitians' Group. *A compilation of papers presented at the first dietitians' meeting at the Society for the Study of Inborn Errors of Metabolism*, Cardiff 1996, 10–14, 1997.

60 Holland B, Welch AA, Unwin ID, Buss DH, Paul AA Southgate DAT *McCance and Widdowson's The Composition of Foods*, 5th edn. Royal Society of Chemistry and Ministry of Agriculture, Fisheries and Food. London: The Stationery Office, 1991.

61 Clark B, MacDonald A, Lilburn M, Watling R A novel approach for the prescription of protein substitutes for phenylketonuria. *Proceedings of the VI International Congress: Inborn Errors of Metabolism*, Milano, Italy. Poster No 15, 1994.

62 Wardley BL, Taitz LS Clinical trial of a concentrated amino acid formula for older patients with phenylketonuria (Maxamum XP). *Eur J Clin Nut*, 1988, **42** 81–6.

63 Kecskemethy HH, Lobbregt D, Levy HL The use of gelatin capsules for ingestion of formula in dietary treatment of maternal phenylketonuria. *J Inher Metab Dis*, 1993, **16** 111–18.

64 Daner D, Elsas L Disorders of branched chain amino acid and keto acid metabolism. In: Scriver CR *et al.* (eds) *The Inherited Metabolic Basis of Inherited Disease*, 6th edn. New York: McGraw-Hill, 1989.

65 Hilliges C, Awiszus D, Wendel U Intellectual performance of children with maple syrup urine disease. *Eur J Paed*, 1993, **152** 144–7.

66 Nord A, Doornick W, Greene C Developmental profile of patients with maple syrup urine disease. *J Inher Metab Dis*, 1991, **14** 881–9.

67 Treacy E *et al.* Maple syrup urine disease: interrelations between branched-chain amino, oxo and hydroxy acids; implications for treatment; associations with CNS dysmyelination. *J Inher Metab Dis*, 1992, **15** 121–35.

68 Kaplan P *et al*. Intellectual outcome in children with maple syrup urine disease. *J Pediatr*, 1991, **119** 46–50.

69 Wendel U Disorders of branched-chain amino acid metabolism. In: Fernandes J, Saudubray J, Tarda K (eds) *Inborn Metabolic Diseases, Diagnosis and Treatment*. Berlin: Springer-Verlag, 1990.

70 Pratt OE The needs of the brain for amino acids and how they are transported across the blood-brain barrier. In: Belton NR, Toothill C (eds) *Transport and Inherited Disease*. Boston: MTP Press, 1981, pp. 87–122.

71 Department of Health Report on Social Subjects No 41. *Dietary Reference Values for Food, Energy and Nutrients for the United Kingdom*. London: The Stationery Office, 1991.

72 Jouvet P *et al*. Continuous venovenous haemodiafiltration in the acute phase of neonatal maple syrup urine disease. *J Inher Metab Dis*, 1997, **20** 463–72.

73 Thompson G *et al*. Protein and leucine metabolism in maple syrup urine disease. *Am J Physiol*, 1990, **258** 654–60.

74 Giarcoia GP, Berry GT Acrodermatitis enteropathica-like syndrome secondary to isoleucine deficiency during treatment of maple syrup urine disease. *AM J Dis Child*, 1993, **147** 954–6.

75 Schwahn B *et al*. Diurnal changes in plasma amino acids in maple syrup urine disease. *Acta Paediatr*, 1998, **87** 1245–6.

76 Thompson G, Francis D, Halliday D Acute illness in maple syrup urine disease: dynamics of protein metabolism and implications for management. *J Paediatr*, 1991, **119** 35–41.

77 Mitchell GA, Lambert M, Tanguay RM Hypertyrosinaemia. In: Scriver *et al*. (eds) *The Metabolic and Molecular Basis of Inherited Disease*, 7e. New York: McGraw-Hill, 1995, pp. 1077–106.

78 Mitchell G *et al*. Neurologic crisis in hereditary tyrosinaemia. *N Engl J Med*, 1990, **322** 432–7.

79 van Spronsen FJ *et al*. Hereditary tyrosinaemia type I: a new clinical classification with difference in prognosis on dietary treatment. *Hepatology*, 1994, **20** 1187–91.

80 Michaels K, Matalon R, Wong K Dietary treatment of tyrosinaemia type I. *J Am Diet Assoc*, 1978, **73** 507–14.

81 Lindstedt S *et al*. Treatment of hereditary tyrosinaemia type I by inhibition of 4-hydroxyphenylpyruvate dioxygenase. *Lancet*, 1992, **340** 813–17.

82 Lindstedt S, Holme E Tyrosinaemia type I and NTBC (2-(2-nitro-4-trifluoromethylbenzoyl)-1,3-cyclohexanedione). *J Inher Metab Dis*, 1998, **21** 507–17.

83 van Wyk KG, Clayton PT Dietary management of tyrosinaemia type I. In: *International Metabolic Dietitians Group, 2nd dietitians meeting SSIEM*, Gothenberg, Sweden, 1997.

84 Fernstrom JD, Fernstrom MH Dietary effects on tyrosine availability and catecholamine synthesis in the central nervous system: possible relevance to the control of protein intake. *Proc Nut Soc*, 1994, **53** 419–29.

85 Wilson CJ *et al*. Phenylalanine supplementation improves the phenylalanine profile in tyrosinaemia. *J Inher Metab Dis*, in press.

86 Barr D, Kirk J, Laing S Outcome in tyrosinaemia type II. *Arch Dis Childh*, 1991, **66** 1249–50.

87 Halvorsen S Tyrosinemia. In: Fernandes J, Saudubray J, Tada K (eds) *Inborn Metabolic Disease: Diagnosis and Treatment*. Berlin: Springer-Verlag, 1990.

88 Carson NAJ, Neill DW Metabolic abnormalities detected in a survey of mentally backward individuals in Northern Ireland. *Arch Dis Childh*, 1962, **37** 505.

89 Kraus JP Biochemistry and molecular genetics of cystathionine β synthase deficiency. *Eur J Paediatr*, 1998, **157** (suppl 2) S50–53.

90 Mudd SH, Levy HL, Skovby F Disorders of transsulfuration. In: Scriver CR, Beaudet AL, Sly WS, Valle D (eds) *The Metabolic and Molecular Basis of Inherited Disease*, 7th edn. McGraw-Hill: New York, 1995, pp. 1279–368.

91 Yap S, Naughten E Homocystinuria due to cystathionine β synthase deficiency in Ireland: 25 years experience of a newborn screened and treated population with reference to clinical outcome and biochemical control. *J Inher Metab Dis*, 1998, **21** 738–47.

92 Andria G, Sebastio G Homocystinuria due to cystathionine β synthase deficiency and related disorders. In: Fernandes J, Saudubray, van den Berghe G (eds) *Inborn Metabolic Disorders – Diagnosis and Treatment*, 2nd edn. Berlin: Springer-Verlag, 1996, pp. 177–82.

93 Moat SJ, Bonham JR, Tanner MS *et al*. Recommended approaches for the laboratory measurement of homocysteine in the diagnosis and monitoring of patients with hyperhomocysteinaemia. *Ann Clin Biochem*, 1999, **36** 372–9.

94 Walter JH, Wraith JE, White FJ *et al*. Strategies for the treatment of cystathionine β synthase deficiency: the experience of the Willink Biochemical Genetics Unit over the past 30 years. *Eur J Paediatr*, 1998, **157** (suppl 2) S71–6.

95 Mudd SH, Skovby F, Levy HL *et al*. The natural history of homocystinuria due to cystathionine β synthase deficiency. *Am J Hum Genet*, 1985, **37** 1–31.

96 Ueland PM, Refsum H *et al*. Total homocysteine in plasma or serum, methods and clinical application. *Clin Chem*, 1993, **39** 1764–9.

97 *Energy and protein requirements*. Report of a joint FAO/WHO/UNU Expert Consultation. WHO Geneva: WHO, 1985.

98 Smolin LA, Benevenga NJ, Berlow S The use of betaine for the treatment of homocystinuria. *J Pediatr*, 1981, **99** 467–72.

99 Wilcken DEL, Wilcken B, Dudman NPB, Tyrrell PA Homocystinuria – the effects of betaine in the treatment of patients not responsive to pyridoxine. *N Engl J Med*, 1983, **309** 448–53.

100 Dewey KG *et al.* Protein requirements of infants and children. *Eur J Clin Nut*, 1996, **50** (suppl 1) 119–50.

101 Sanjurjo P, Ruiz JI, Montejo M Inborn errors of metabolism with a protein-restricted diet: effect on polyunsaturated fatty acids. *J Inher Metab Dis*, 1997, **20** 783–9.

102 Walter JH, Wraith JE, Cleary MA Abscence of acidosis in the initial presentation of propionic acidaemia. *Arch Dis Childh*, 1995, **72** 197–9.

103 Rosenberg L, Fenton W Disorders of propionate and methylmalonate metabolism. In: Scriver CR *et al.* (eds) *Inherited Metabolic Basis of Disease*, 6e. New York: McGraw-Hill, 1989.

104 Matsui S, Mahoney M, Rosenberg L The natural history of the inherited methylmalonic acidaemias. *N Engl J Med*, 1987, **38** (15) 857–61.

105 Baumgarter ER, Viardot C Long-term follow-up of 77 patients with isolated methylmalonic acidaemia. *J Inher Metab Dis*, 1995, **18** 138–42.

106 van der Meer SB *et al.* Clinical outcome of long-term management of patients with vitamin B_{12}-unresponsive methylmalonic acidaemia. *J Paediatr*, 1994, **125** 903–8.

107 van der Meer SB *et al.* Clinical outcome and long-term management of 17 patients with propionic acidaemia. *Eur J Pediatr*, 1996, **155** 205–10.

108 Surtees R, Matthews E, Leonard J Neurologic outcome of propionic acidaemia. *Pediatr Neurol*, 1992, **8** 333–7.

109 Nicolaides P, Leonard JV, Surtees R Neurological outcome of methylmalonic acidaemia. *Arch Dis Childh*, 1998, **78** 508–12.

110 Massoud A, Leonard J Cardiomyopathy in propionic acidaemia. *Eur J Pediatr*, 1993, **152** 441–5.

111 Kahler SG *et al.* Pancreatitis in patients with organic acidaemias. *J Pediatr*, 1994, **124** 239–43.

112 Molteni KH *et al.* Progressive renal insufficiency in methylmalonic acidaemia. *Pediatr Nephrol*, 1991, **5** 323–6.

113 Thompson G *et al.* Sources of propionate in inborn errors of propionate. *Metabolism*, 1990, **39** 1133–7.

114 Thompson G *et al.* The use of metronidazole in management of methylmalonic and propionic acidaemias. *Eur J Pediatr*, 1990, **149** 792–6.

115 Sbai D *et al.* Possible contributions of odd-chain fatty acid oxidation to propionate production in methylmalonic and propionic acidaemia. *Paedatr Res*, 1992, **31** 188A.

116 Wendel U Abnormality of odd-numbered, long-chain fatty acids in erythrocyte membrane lipids from patients with disorders of propionate metabolism. *Pediatr Res*, 1989, **25** 147–50.

117 Ney D *et al.* An evaluation of protein requirements in methylmalonic acidaemia. *J Inher Metab Dis*, 1985, **8** 132–42.

118 Sbai D *et al.* Contribution of odd-chain fatty acid oxidation to propionate production in disorders of propionate metabolism. *Am J Clin Nutr*, 1994, **59** 1332–7.

119 Wasserstein MP *et al.* Successful pregnancy in severe methylmalonic acidaemia. *J Inher Metab Dis*, 1999, **22** 788–94.

120 D'Angio C, Dillon M, Leonard J Renal tubular dysfunction in methylmalonic acidaemia. *Eur J Pediatr*, 1991, **150** 259–63.

121 Walter JH, Dillon MJ, Leonard JV *et al.* Chronic renal failure in methylmalonic acidaemia. *Eur J Pediatr*, 1989, **148** 344–8.

122 van't Hoff WG, Dixon M, Taylor J *et al.* Combined liver-kidney transplant in methylmalonic acidaemia. *J Pediatr*, 1998, **132** 1043–4.

123 Sperl W *et al.* Parenteral administration of amino acids in disorders of branched chain amino acid metabolism. *J Inher Metab Dis*, 1994, **17** 753–4.

124 Sweetman L Branched chain organic acidurias. In: Scriver CR *et al.* (eds) *The Metabolic Basis of Inherited Disease*, 6e. New York: McGraw-Hill, 1989.

125 Berry G, Yudkoff M, Segal S Isovaleric acidaemia: medical and neurodevelopmental effects of long-term therapy. *J Paediatr*, 1988, **113** 58–63.

126 Naglak M *et al.* The treatment of isovaleric acidaemia with glycine supplement. *Pediatr Res*, 1988, **24** 9–13.

127 Fries MH *et al.* Isovaleric acidaemia: response to a leucine load after 3 weeks of supplementation with glycine, l-carnitine, and combined glycine-carnitine therapy. *J Pediat*, 1996, **129** 449–52.

128 Goodman SI, Frerman FE Organic acidaemias due to defects in lysine oxidation: 2-ketoadipic acidaemia and glutaric acidaemia. In: Scriver CR *et al.* (eds) *The Metabolic and Molecular Basis of Inherited Disease*, 7e. New York: McGraw-Hill, 1995, pp. 1451–60.

129 Baric I *et al.* Diagnosis and management of glutaric aciduria type I. *J Inher Metab Dis*, 1998, **21** 326–40.

130 Monavari AA, Naughten ER Prevention of cerebral palsy in glutaric aciduria type I by dietary management. *Arch Dis Childh*, 2000, **82** 67–70.

131 Superti-Furga A, Hoffman GF Glutaric aciduria type I (glutaryl-CoA-dehydrogenase deficiency): advances and unanswered questions. *Eur J Paediatr*, 1997, **156** 821–8.

132 Hoffman GF, Zschocke J Glutaric aciduria type I: from clinical diversity to successful therapy. *J Inher Metab Dis*, 1999, **22** 381–91.

133 Brusilow S, Harwich A Urea cycle enzymes. In: Scriver CR *et al.* (eds) *The Metabolic Basis of Inherited Disease*, 6e. New York: McGraw-Hill, 1989.

134 Leonard JV Urea cycle disorders In: Fernandes J, Saudubray JM, van den Berghe G (eds) *Inborn*

Metabolic Diseases, Diagnosis and Treatment, 2e. Berlin: Springer-Verlag, 1995, pp. 167–76.

135 Feillet F, Leonard JV Alternative pathways for urea cycle disorders. *J Inher Metab Dis*, 1998, **21** (suppl 1) 101–111.

136 Brusilow S, Tinker J, Batshaw ML Amino acid acylation: a mechanism of nitrogen excretion in inborn errors of urea synthesis. *Science*, 1980, **207** 659–61.

137 Brusilow S Arginine, an indispensable amino acid for patients with inborn errors of urea synthesis. *J Clin Invest*, 1984, **74** 2144–8.

138 Bachman C Ornithine carbamyl transferase deficiency: findings, models and problems. *J Inher Metab Dis*, 1992, **15** 578–91.

139 Hyman S *et al.* Behaviour management of feeding disturbances in urea cycle and organic acid disorders. *J Paediatr*, 1987, **111** 558–62.

140 Lambert M *et al.* Hyperargininaemia; intellectual and motor improvement related to changes in biochemical data. *J Pediatr*, 1991, **118** 420–24.

141 Prasad AN *et al.* Argininemia: a treatable genetic cause of progressive spastic diplegia simulating cerebral palsy: case reports and literature review. *J Child Neurol*, 1997, **12**, 301–9.

142 Verber I, Bain M Glucose polymer regimens and hypernatraemia. *Arch Dis Childh*, 1990, **65** 627–8.

143 Morris AAM, Leonard JV Early recognition of metabolic decompensation. *Arch Dis Childh*, 1997, **76** 555–6.

144 Dixon M, Leonard J Intercurrent illness in inborn errors of intermediary metabolism. *Arch Dis Childh*, 1992, **67** 1387–91.

145 Morris AAM, Dixon MA Parenteral nutrition for patients with inherited metabolic diseases. In: *British Inherited Metabolic Disease Group Newsletter*, 1997 Issue 13.

FURTHER READING

Brusilow S Inborn errors of urea synthesis. In: *Genetic and Metabolic Disease in Paediatrics*. London: Butterworths, 1985.

Maestri N, McGowan K, Brusilow S Plasma glutamine concentration; a guide in the management of urea cycle disorders. *J Paediatr*, 1992, **121** (2) 259–61.

USEFUL ADDRESSES

National Society for Phenylketonuria (NSPKU)
7 Lingey Lane, Wardley, Gateshead, Tyne & Wear NE10 8BR.
Climb (Children living with inherited metabolic diseases)
The Quadrangle, Crewe Hall, Weston Road, Crewe, Cheshire CW1 6UR.

CHAPTER 16

Disorders of Carbohydrate Metabolism

GLYCOGEN STORAGE DISEASE TYPE I

Glucose-6-phosphatase has a central role in glucose production, catalysing the final common pathway for endogenous glucose synthesis from glycogenolysis and gluconeogenesis (Fig. 16.1). The enzyme glucose-6-phosphatase is normally expressed in liver, kidney and intestine. Glycogen storage disease type I (GSD I) is caused by either deficiency of glucose-6-phosphatase itself (type Ia) or of the glucose-6-phosphate transport system (type Ib) [1]. The clinical manifestations include growth retardation and hepatomegaly (due mainly to fatty infiltration of the liver). Increased glycolytic flux leads to lactic acidosis and hyperlipidaemia, with triglycerides being more markedly elevated than cholesterol [2]. Additionally in type Ib, there is neutropenia and impaired neutrophil function which increases susceptibility to bacterial infections, particularly of the skin and respiratory tract [2]. A chronic inflammatory bowel disease similar histopathologically to Crohn's disease is also seen [3].

Complications have been reported: renal dysfunction, hepatic tumours (mostly benign adenoma, but with the potential for malignant transformation), osteoporosis and polycystic ovaries in females [4].

Dietary management

The aim of dietary treatment is to promote normal growth by maintaining a normal blood glucose level. This will also improve the secondary metabolic abnormalities, but it is recognised that these cannot be completely normalised [5]. Infants and children are administered a frequent supply of exogenous glucose both day and night at least until they have stopped growing. Glucose requirements are calculated from basal glucose production rates in normal children [6]. It is important to be aware that these requirements for glucose decrease with age (Table 16.1). Dietary energy is provided as follows: 60–70% from carbohydrate (CHO), 20–25% from fat and 10–15% from protein. Fat intake is decreased to compensate for increased carbohydrate intake.

Provision of carbohydrate to GSD I patients has altered over the years. Traditionally frequent CHO feeding was given day and night. In 1976, Greene *et al.* reported the intensive regimen of regular drinks of glucose polymer by day and continuous nasogastric feeding at night [7]. In 1984 Chen *et al.* introduced uncooked cornstarch to the diet to provide a source of slow-release glucose [8]. Most centres now use a combination of continuous overnight feeding and two hourly feeding using glucose polymers, or uncooked cornstarch during the daytime, or uncooked cornstarch throughout the 24 hour period (p. 299).

Some centres restrict fructose and galactose in the diet because these sugars are not converted to glucose via the gluconeogenic pathway but, instead, increase lactate production [9]. However, a mildly elevated blood lactate level of up to 4.0 mmol/l is considered acceptable because lactate provides an alternative source of energy to the brain and therefore has a protective effect against fuel depletion [10]. Consequently many feel that the restriction of these sugars is not essential and that regular provision of glucose is the more important dietary manoeuvre.

Replacement of saturated fat with polyunsaturated fat is recommended by some in an attempt to improve the hyperlipidaemia [11], but this is less important than supplying a frequent CHO intake. Despite persistent hyperlipidaemia, no evidence of premature arteriosclerosis has yet been observed [12, 13, 14].

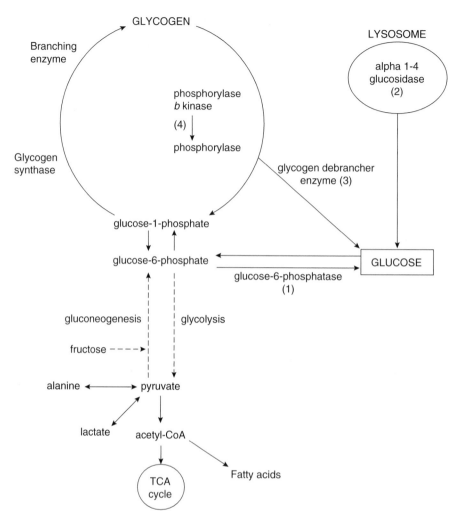

(1) Glycogen storage disease type I
(2) Glycogen storage disease type II
(3) Glycogen storage disease type III
(4) Phosphorylase system deficiencies

Fig. 16.1 Pathway of liver glycogen metabolism

Glucose requirements

Glucose intakes for children with GSD I are calculated to be similar to normal hepatic glucose production [6, 15]. Glucose requirements (g/kg/hour) decrease with age (Table 16.1). Although we use these figures as a guide when planning the diet it is our practice to use total CHO intake (g CHO/kg/hour), i.e. all sugars, not just glucose and starch, as the fuel source rather than just grams of glucose/kg/hour. It is important to ensure that only the required amount of glucose is administered at night and as 2 hourly daytime CHO drinks because large quantities of exogenous glucose will exacerbate swings in blood

Table 16.1 Glucose requirements based on glucose production rates [6]

Age	Glucose: mg per kg per minute	Glucose: grams per kg per hour	
		Day	Night
Infants	8–9	0.5	0.5
Toddlers and children	5–7	0.3–0.4	0.3–0.4
Adolescents and adults	2–4 at night		0.2–0.25

Table 16.2 Infant feeding regimen GSD type I. 5 kg infant: aim 0.5 g carbohydrate per kg per hour

	Fluid (ml)	Energy (kcal)	(kJ)	CHO (g)	Protein (g)	Fat (g)
SMA Gold	840	546	2282	60	12.6	30
Amount/kg	170	110	456	12.0	2.5	
Amount/kg/hr				0.5		
Amount/hr				2.5		

Daily feed distribution:
Day: Oral feeds 70 ml
   8.30 AM, 10 AM, 12 noon, 2 PM, 4 PM, 6 PM = 420 ml
Night: Continuous nasogastric feeds 35 ml
   every hour from 8 PM finishing at 8 AM = 420 ml
   Bolus nasogastric feeds – 20 ml at 8 PM and 8 AM
   (extra to calculated fluid requirement)

glucose levels and make patients more prone to hypoglycaemia [16]. Obesity is a problem for some GSD patients and hence another reason for avoiding excessive glucose intakes. Equally important is the need to provide adequate glucose as insufficient amounts will lead to high plasma lactate levels and growth retardation. Achieving optimum biochemical control is difficult. For some patients it may be beneficial to measure blood glucose at home; however, this is not perceived to be essential for daily management.

Nasogastric feeding

Continuous nasogastric feeding is used to provide glucose overnight. Careful management of this is necessary because it can render the patient more sensitive to hypoglycaemia [5]. Indeed, fatalities have been reported because of unplanned cessation in delivery of the glucose feed, and the pump feed not being switched on [17, 18]. It is therefore essential that the paediatric feed pump accurately controls flow rate and alarms if there is electrical or mechanical pump failure. The tubing used for the delivery system and nasogastric tube needs to be secure [18]. Parents need thorough teaching and must be adept and confident with the enteral feeding system prior to home use. Gastrostomy feeding is a suitable alternative to nasogastric feeding.

When commencing the continuous overnight tube feed an oral or bolus feed is given if the child has not been fed for 2 hours. On discontinuation of the night feed it is extremely important that the child is fed within 15 minutes to avoid hypoglycaemia [5]. In practice, usually a small bolus feed is given immediately on cessation of the night feed and then the child is fed again after 30 minutes.

Diet for infants

Infants often present between 4 and 8 months of age. Initially CHO requirements (0.5 g CHO/kg/ hour) can be provided by infant formula fed at normal fluid volumes of 150–200 ml/kg. Additional glucose polymer is not always necessary. Regular two hourly feeding during the day and continuous nasogastric feeds by night are needed to maintain normoglycaemia. During the daytime infants may demand feed and take more than 0.5 g CHO/kg/hour; however, the night feed should be maintained at the CHO requirement of 0.5 g CHO/kg/hour.

At the beginning and end of the night feed, an oral or bolus feed providing sufficient glucose to last for 30 minutes is given. An example of an infant's feed regimen is shown in Table 16.2.

Weaning is commenced at the normal time between 4 and 6 months of age, and a regular intake of starchy foods is recommended, e.g. baby rice, rusk, potato. As the intake of starchy food increases it can replace the infant feed at main meals as the source of glucose for the following two hours. As relatively small quantities of food provide the glucose requirements a complicated CHO food exchange system is not necessary. It is usually sufficient just to teach parents which foods provide CHO and to include these at main meals. However, for those infants and children who have poor appetites or are fussy eaters a list of foods which

Table 16.3 Example of a diet for a 10 month old infant with GSD type I
Weight 8 kg, providing 0.5 g carbohydrate per kg per hour (4 g CHO per hour)

Time	Food or drink	Total CHO (g)	Grams CHO per kg per hr*	Protein (g)	Energy (kcal)	(kJ)
8.15 AM	1 Weetabix	10.0	0.9	1.7	50	209
	100 ml SMA Gold	7.2		1.5	65	272
10.00 AM	15 ml concentrated baby juice diluted to 100 ml	9.0	0.5	—	36	150
12.00 midday	Minced beef, vegetable	—		6.0	60	250
	Small potato	10.0	1.6	1.0	40	167
	100 g yoghurt	15.0		5.0	80	334
2.00 PM	90 ml SMA Gold + glucose polymer to 10% CHO	9.0	0.5	1.3	68	284
4.00 PM	1 slice bread + butter	12.0		2.2	70	292
	Ham filling	—	1.3	4.0	30	125
	Small banana	10.0		0.5	40	167
6.00 PM	90 ml SMA Gold + glucose polymer to 10% CHO	9.0	0.5	1.3	68	284
8.00 PM to 8.00 AM finish	30 ml hourly for 12 hours SMA Gold + glucose polymer to 13% CHO	47.0	0.5	5.4	317	1325
8.00 PM and 8.00 AM	15 ml bolus SMA Gold + glucose polymer to 13% CHO	3.9		1.0	26	109
Totals		142		30.0	950	3968
% Energy intake		60%		13%		

* The portion size of carbohydrate foods (appropriate for age) will make the carbohydrate content of main meals in excess of the specified requirement of 0.5 g per kg per hour

provide appropriate amounts of CHO can prove extremely useful. Certainly the practice of feeding every 2 hours can cause feeding problems in some children. This often begins to improve when uncooked cornstarch is introduced as the interval between feeding times can be increased.

As more energy is derived from solids, the infant should take smaller volumes of feeds. To ensure adequate intake of CHO, glucose polymer is added to the infant feed to give a final concentration of 10–15% CHO. From 9 months onwards, some of the infant feeds can be replaced by CHO drinks such as baby juices with added glucose polymer or glucose polymer solution. However, it is important that the daily intake of infant formula should not fall to less than 500–600 ml because it continues to provide a major source of nutrients in the older baby's diet. Care must be taken to avoid giving drinks which are too concentrated in CHO content because of high osmolality precipating diarrhoea. Intermittent diarrhoea or loose stools does occur in some patients, but the cause is not completely understood [19, 20]. A maximum concentration of 12–15% CHO is recommended in older infants. An example of a weaning diet is shown in Table 16.3.

Diet for children

During the daytime a source of CHO continues to be given at 2 hourly intervals either from a meal or snack containing CHO or a CHO drink. The portion size of CHO foods (appropriate for age) will make the CHO content of main meals in excess of the specified requirement (0.3 to 0.5 g CHO/kg/hour). In between meal snacks or drinks should aim to provide only the specified requirement of CHO as excessive amounts may reduce appetite for main meals and cause excess weight gain. Parents are given information on different drinks and snacks that supply only the required amount of glucose. Starchy foods such as potato, rice, pasta, bread and cereals are encouraged in preference to sugary foods because these are more slowly digested to produce glucose.

From one year of age the night feed is often changed to a solution of glucose polymer provided that the requirement for other nutrients is supplied by the daytime diet. As the child gets older more concentrated glucose polymer solutions are used: 15% CHO in 1–2 year olds, 20% CHO in 2–6 year olds, 25% up to a maximum of 30% CHO for older children. Occasionally a paediatric enteral feed is administered at night in preference to glucose polymer alone, particularly when growth and nutrient intakes are inadequate. If the child has not eaten for 2 hours a bolus or oral feed will be given at the start of the night feed, providing sufficient glucose for 30 minutes. On cessation of the night feed a bolus feed (same as the pre-night feed) is given. As many children with GSD I find it difficult to eat breakfast due to being fed overnight, a CHO drink (plus cornflour for some patients) is usually given 30 minutes after stopping the feed.

Children with GSD I can be at risk of vitamin and mineral deficiencies, particularly if a high percentage of the CHO intake is provided as glucose polymer and cornstarch. Inadequate calcium intakes have been reported in GSD I patients who were demonstrated to have reduced bone mineral density [21]. Vitamin and mineral intakes should be regularly assessed.

Additional CHO may be required by some children when doing strenuous or prolonged exercise. Ideally this should be given as starchy food in advance of the exercise.

Cornstarch therapy

Uncooked cornstarch (UCCS) as cornflour is slowly digested, primarily by pancreatic amylase to release glucose. When compared with glucose polymer feeding, a smoother blood glucose profile is produced and less glucose is required [22]. Satisfactory glycaemia has been reported to last from 4 to 9 hours after ingestion [8, 22]. However, a more recent study reported only achieving satisfactory glycaemia for a median of 4.25 hours (range 2.5–6) [23].

UCCS can obviate the need for 2 hourly feeding. It is administered at regular intervals throughout the day (and night for some patients) in doses which approximate the basal glucose production rate. In practice the amount of UCCS given per dose is: 2 g/kg body weight in young children, decreasing to around 1.5 g/kg in older children; 1 g/kg in adolescents who have stopped growing. In obese children lower doses are given. Usually a dose of UCCS is required every 4–6 hours but this is based on the results of the UCCS load test (see below).

UCCS can be introduced around 2 years of age. In younger children it may not be adequately digested to maintain a normal blood glucose because pancreatic amylase activity only reaches adult levels between 2 and 4 years of age, although its activity is reported to be induced by oral starch [11]. Success has been reported with UCCS in children under 2 years of age using smaller more frequent doses [24, 25, 26].

Cornflour is given raw; cooking or heating disrupts the starch granules by hydrolysis and thus makes it much less effective. To increase palatability of UCCS it can be mixed with different drinks such as milk, squash, carbonated drinks or with cold food such as ice cream, yoghurt, fruit purée, thin cold custard, or mixed with milk then poured on cereal. If mixed with food it gives more bulk for the child to eat. Some studies have reported that mixing UCCS with sugary drinks makes it less effective [8, 22, 27].

When initiating UCCS treatment, a fasting 'cornflour load test' is done in hospital to assess the child's metabolic response by serial measurement of blood glucose and lactate. These biochemical results are used to determine the frequency and quantity of UCCS given. Prior to this, UCCS will have been introduced at home to test its palatability and acceptance. The dose of UCCS is gradually increased to 2 g/kg at one meal, beginning with 5 g and increasing by 5 g every week to the required dose. Some patients may experience side effects such as diarrhoea, abdominal distention and flatulence but these are usually transient. Two hourly feeding will continue during this intoductory period of UCCS.

The dose and frequency of UCCS needs to be

Table 16.4 Example of a diet for a 7 year old child with GSD type I. Weight 25 kg; aim 0.3 g carbohydrate per kg per hour overnight

Time	Food or drink	
7.30 AM	**Breakfast** including: CHO foods, e.g. breakfast cereal, bread, chapatti, pitta bread 50 g cornflour mixed with 100 ml water + squash	2 g per kg
12.30 PM	**School dinner** including: CHO foods, e.g. potato, rice, pulses, biscuits (crackers or semi-sweet), fruit 50 g cornflour mixed with milk	2 g per kg
5.30 PM	**Evening meal** including: CHO foods, e.g. potato, pasta, bread, fruit, yoghurt 25 g cornflour mixed with 50 ml milk	1 g per kg
8.00 PM to 7.00 AM	20% glucose polymer 40 ml hourly	Provides 0.3 g CHO per kg per hour overnight
8.00 PM and 7.00 AM	20 ml bolus of 20% glucose polymer	

reviewed regularly taking into consideration growth velocity, frequency of hypoglycaemia and biochemical results. Ideally patients should have a 24 hour glucose and lactate profile, and UCCS load test every 1–2 years. An example of a diet incorporating UCCS is given in Table 16.4. When planning the regimen it is important to be aware that cornflour takes around 30 minutes to start releasing glucose. The diet usually comprises 2–3 doses of UCCS during the daytime. A lower dose may be given in the evening if there is a relatively short time interval between this time, the evening meal and the night feed.

In children, continuous overnight nasogastric feeding is usually continued until they have stopped growing. However some families prefer to use UCCS at night as it is less complicated and more socially acceptable than tube feeding, but the main disadvantage of this for young children is the need to wake at around 4–6 hourly intervals, thereby interrupting sleep. Parents will also need to wake up to give the UCCS and rely on an alarm clock to do so.

After puberty some form of nocturnal glucose therapy needs to continue to prevent fasting hypoglycaemia and biochemical abnormalities [28]. The adolescent should be reassessed at this time to determine their fasting tolerance. It is our recent experience that discontinuing the overnight tube feed is difficult even when growth ceases, as UCCS does not maintain normoglycaemia for sufficiently long periods. Further work on optimising starches for GSD treatment is still needed.

A comparative study of long term management of both forms of treatment, UCCS versus continuous nocturnal nasogastric glucose feeds, reported no significant differences in physical growth and biochemical parameters, but growth in height was still not optimal [29]. Inadeqate growth in height has also been reported in a study of long term continuous glucose therapy with cornstarch begun in infancy [26].

Cornflour and glucose polymer are approved by the Advisory Committee Borderline Substances for prescription on FP10.

Hypoglycaemia

It is inevitable that hypoglycaemia will occasionally occur. Parents need to recognise early warning signs such as sweating, irritability or drowsiness. They should respond to these by immediately giving a CHO drink and, on recovery, some starchy foods. Hypostop (p. 132) is another extremely useful alternative for treatment of hypoglycaemia.

Cornflour is not a suitable treatment for hypoglycaemia because it releases glucose slowly.

Illness

During intercurrent infections, the frequent supply of glucose must be maintained to prevent hypoglycaemia and lactic acidosis. At least the basal glucose requirement must be given and an adequate intake of fluids. Often a change in dietary regimen is needed because of loss of appetite. During the daytime, two hourly glucose polymer drinks or continuous tube feeds of glucose polymer will often replace either the usual two hourly dietary regimen, or UCCS. If the child has diarrhoea and is vomiting, an oral rehydration solution supplemented with glucose polymer to a maximum of 10% CHO is given. If the child does not tolerate the intensive glucose polymer regimen then a hospital admission for intravenous therapy becomes essential. Severe, symptomatic hypoglycaemia can develop rapidly in this situation and intravenous treatment needs to start with minimal delay. The child's usual dietary regimen can be re-introduced during the recovery period.

GSD type Ib

The dietary treatment of patients with type Ib is the same as for GSD I. However, the additional problems seen in type Ib may necessitate further dietary manipulation. Mouth ulcers are a feature of type Ib and can make oral feeding difficult and painful. Meals and snacks may need to be temporarily replaced with nutritionally complete fluid supplements and if necessary these can be given via the enteral route. An elemental feed is sometimes used if the bowel is inflamed and bleeding.

GLYCOGEN STORAGE DISEASE TYPE III

Glycogen storage disease type III (GSD III) is characterised by abnormal activity of the glycogen debranching enzyme in various tissues including liver and muscle (Fig. 16.1). This enzyme has two activities: it transfers three glucose residues to a neighbouring glycogen chain and hydrolyses the branch-point directly to glucose. The debranching enzyme can be absent in liver and muscle (GSD type IIIa) or just in liver (GSD type IIIb) or have defects in its transferase activity in liver and muscle (GSD IIId) [2]. The production of glucose from glycogenolysis is greatly limited due to debrancher deficiency. However, the gluconeogenic pathway is functional for endogenous glucose production and this prevents the developement of profound hypoglycaemia during fasting, although it can still occur.

Patients can present either in infancy with symptoms similar to GSD I (hepatomegaly and hypoglycaemia), or later in childhood with poor growth and hepatomegaly due to both glycogen and fat accumulation. Spontaneous catch-up growth does however occur during puberty [30]. Type IIIa and IIId patients can also suffer from myopathy and develop cardiomyopathy but these are mainly problems found in adults, although some children do tire easily with exercise. The outlook for those with GSD IIIb appears to be good.

Dietary management

The main aims of dietary treatment in GSD III are to promote normal growth and prevent hypoglycaemia. Controversy surrounds which dietary therapy

is best for patients. Either CHO intake can be increased to provide a continuous supply of glucose (similar to GSD I) or protein intake can be increased to rely on gluconeogenesis as the main source of glucose. A high protein diet has been recommended because patients with GSD III may have increased gluconeogenic activity associated with decreased circulating levels of the gluconeogenic substrates alanine and lactate [31, 32, 33]. This increased demand for gluconeogenesis and loss of muscle amino acids may be a contributory factor to the myopathy seen in some patients with type IIIa. Use of a high protein diet and night feed has been reported to be beneficial in improving muscle strength in patients with a myopathy [31]. However, whole-body protein turnover has been shown not to be altered in a GSD IIIa patient and consequently questions the role of a high-protein diet [34]. Alternatively, provision of a regular, high CHO intake can be used to maintain normoglycaemia and reduce the need for production of glucose via gluconeogenic substrates [35]. Hence this treatment may be as effective as the high protein diet. One study has compared uncooked cornflour (UCCS) diet to a high protein diet and shown unchanged glycaemic control, liver function tests and lipid profiles in both regimens, but better growth and reduced liver spans when using UCCS. However, two patients with muscle involvement showed increased creatine phosphate kinase levels on UCCS diet [36].

The choice of dietary management for children with GSD III will also vary depending on the severity of the disorder. The diet needs to be individually tailored to the child's specific requirement.

High CHO diet

Infants who present early with hypoglycaemia and poor fasting tolerance require a more intensive dietary regimen with increased CHO, the same as for GSD I (p. 297). At night, continuous nasogastric feeding is used and regular two hourly feeding or uncooked cornstarch during the daytime. There is greater emphasis on increased protein intake compared with GSD I. Children with GSD III may be able to replace nocturnal feeds with uncooked cornstarch before they have stopped growing if their fasting tolerance is greater then 6 hours. This can happen between 4 and 9 years. It is important to monitor carefully the energy distribution of the diet because overtreatment with too high an energy intake from CHO can cause rebound hypoglycaemia [37].

High protein diet

If a high protein diet is used, it is recommended that this provides 20–25% energy intake from protein, 50–55% from CHO and 20–25% from fat [31, 33]. No studies of high protein diets have been reported in infants or young children. Such a high protein intake may not be tolerated or warranted in this age group. A gradual increase in protein intake with age or if there is evidence of myopathy may be more appropriate.

For infants, protein powders such as Maxipro can be added to infant or follow-on formula milks to provide around 3 g protein/100 ml, but additional glucose polymer will also be needed. These milks can be used for both the day and night feeds. From 1 year of age, cow's milk with added protein powder and/or glucose polymer can replace the infant formula feeds. A paediatric enteral feed could be used but this may provide too much energy and not the optimal energy ratio of protein and CHO.

Children who have a good appetite and enjoy milk may possibly achieve sufficient protein intake from high protein foods but protein supplements are invariably necessary. Practical guidelines for a high protein, high starch, low fat diet are given in Table 16.5. A variety of high protein supplements are available. Often the choice of supplement is determined by what the child will happily take. Pure protein powders, such as Maxipro or Vitapro, are versatile and can be fairly easily incorporated into drinks or food. They are often preferable to some of the high protein drink or dessert supplements because these are too high in energy content. Table 16.6 provides a list of high protein, lower energy supplements suitable for children. If it is not possible to achieve such a high protein intake, a lower protein with a higher CHO intake is certainly an acceptable alternative.

For children with milder disorders a high starch or high protein diet with regular daytime meals and a late-night snack or dose of cornflour may be sufficient dietary treatment.

Alcohol

Adolescents and adults must be made aware that alcohol is a potent inhibitor of gluconeogenesis and even quite moderate amounts may reduce glucose production. Alcohol intake should be limited and must always be taken in combination with food [38].

Table 16.5 High protein, high starch, low fat diet for glycogen storage disease type III

High protein, low fat foods
One serving of high protein food at three main meals and bedtime snack. Generous intakes of milk or high protein drinks (Table 16.6) should be given

Milk	Semi-skimmed or skimmed milk, milk puddings, e.g. rice, custard, semolina, fromage frais + yoghurt (low fat)
Meat	Lean red meat (<10% fat content), trim off all visible fat
Poultry	White meat in preference to dark meat
Fish	White fish instead of oily
Cheese	Low fat cheese, e.g. cottage, Edam type, half fat Cheddar, quark
Pulses	Beans, lentils, peas, sweetcorn
Eggs	Egg white in preference to yolk
Meat alternatives	Tofu, Quorn

Carbohydrate foods (starch and sugar)
Starch foods At least one serving at three main meals and include at bedtime snack, e.g. bread, chapatti, pitta, cereal, potato, rice, pasta, fruit, plain biscuits or crackers, tea cake, muffins, scones

Sugar These foods are allowed but should be kept to a minimum, e.g. table sugar, sweets, cakes, ice cream, preserves

Fats
High fat foods should be used sparingly, e.g. butter, margarine, vegetable oil, animal fats, cream (double, whipping, single), imitation cream, mayonnaise, salad dressings
Avoid fried or roasted foods. Spread butter or margarine thinly on bread

Snack foods
Most children choose high fat or sugary snack foods, e.g. crisps, nuts, sweets, chocolate
Low fat, high protein, high carbohydrate snack foods should be used instead, e.g. yoghurt, fromage frais, sandwich with protein filling, crackers and cheese, glass of milk

Illness

Children with GSD III are at risk of hypoglycaemia and therefore during illness a frequent supply of glucose must be maintained. The guidelines given for management of intercurrent illness in GSD I can also be used for patients with GSD type III (p. 300).

GLYCOGEN STORAGE DISEASE TYPE II

GSD type II is caused by deficiency of acid maltase (alpha 1–4 glucosidase) (Fig. 16.1). It is a generalised

Table 16.6 High protein drinks

	Protein	Energy/100 ml		
	(g/100 ml)	(kcal)	(kJ)	Comments
Build-up + skimmed milk (i)	6.0	79	330	Milk based Various flavours
Fortimel	10	100	420	Milk based Various flavours
Protein Forte	10	100	420	Milk based Various flavours
Skimmed Milk + Vitapro (ii)	6.3	45	272	Milk based

(i) 13 g Build-up plus 100 ml skimmed milk
(ii) 4 g Vitapro plus 100 ml skimmed milk

lysosomal storage disorder in which deficiency of lysosomal acid maltase leads to accumulation of glycogen. The infantile form (Pompe's disease) is associated with poor prognosis and early death. The childhood form is less severe and progresses more slowly. There is generalised muscle weakness, which can eventually lead to cardiorespiratory insufficiency and cause death between the second and fourth decade [2]. At present there is no effective treatment for any form of GSD II.

A high protein diet providing 25% dietary energy from protein is reported to improve muscle strength, by reducing protein catabolism, and to delay the downward course of the childhood form [39, 40]. The long term value of this diet is not proven. Fat and carbohydrate intakes are decreased so that each provides 35–40% of energy intake to compensate for increased protein intake.

Dietary protein intake is increased in a similar manner to GSD III (p. 302). High protein, low fat foods are encouraged and high protein supplements, such as drinks or pure protein powders, are invaluable in increasing protein intake.

Trials of enzyme replacement therapy are currently taking place [41].

THE PHOSPHORYLASE SYSTEM

Deficiencies of the phosphorylase system (Fig. 16.1), of which phosphorylase *b* kinase is most prevalent,

have similar symptomatology to but are much milder than GSD III [2]. In these disorders glycogen degradation is reduced but gluconeogenesis is functional for endogenous glucose production. Children present with hepatomegaly and growth retardation but catch-up growth usually occurs before puberty [42]. Hypoglycaemia is generally mild and usually only occurs after prolonged fasting or infection [11]. Most adults will be entirely asymptomatic with a normal life expectancy.

Many patients do not require specific dietary treatment. Nevertheless, general dietary advice on provision of increased intakes of protein and starch and avoidance of prolonged fasts particularly during illness would be appropriate. To reduce the period of overnight fasting a late night bedtime snack rich in protein and starch should be given. However, for some patients more aggressive treatment with uncooked cornstarch (p. 299) may be necessary both to prevent low blood glucose levels and improve growth. Since alcohol is a potent inhibitor of gluconeogenesis, it is recommended that these patients only drink in moderation and preferably in combination with food [38].

INBORN ERRORS OF GALACTOSE METABOLISM

There are three inborn errors of galactose metabolism: deficiencies of the enzymes galactokinase, uridine diphosphate galactose-4-epimerase and galactose-1-phosphate uridyl transferase which result in the inability to metabolise the monosaccharide galactose (Fig. 16.2).

Galactosaemia

Of the defects in this pathway, classical galactosaemia is by far the most common disorder with an incidence of 1 in 45 000 in the UK [43]. It is caused by a deficiency of the enzyme galactose-1-phosphate uridyl transferase which catalyses the reaction that converts galactose-1-phosphate (gal-1-p) to glucose-1-phosphate and uridine diphosphate galactose (UDP-galactose) (Fig. 16.2). The latter is the substrate for the incorporation of galactose into complex glycoproteins and glycolipids. Absence of transferase causes the accumulation of gal-1-p, galactitol and galactonic acid.

As galactose is a constituent of breast milk and

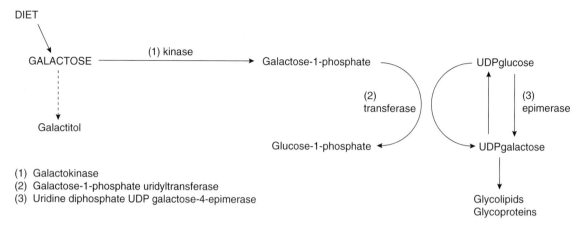

Fig. 16.2 Pathways of galactose metabolism

most infant formulas, the majority of infants present in the first week of life. The most common features are jaundice, failure to thrive, hepatomegaly, diarrhoea, vomiting and cataracts, with improvement on IV fluids. It is thought that the accumulation of gal-1-p is responsible for the acute symptoms and galactitol for the formation of cataracts.

Dietary management

The main treatment of this disorder is exclusion of dietary galactose (Table 16.7). The diet needs to be continued for life and without any relaxation. However, complete elimination of galactose is virtually impossible because of traces of galactose and galactolipids, particularly in plant foods. Despite the early introduction of diet and continuation of good dietary control, long term complications of galactosaemia are increasingly recognised. These include learning difficulties, speech abnormalities, growth retardation and ovarian dysfunction in females [44, 45]. Recent evidence suggests there is endogenous production of galactose and this may be responsible for these long term problems [46].

On minimal galactose diet the symptoms rapidly regress. The red cell gal-1-p level initially falls rapidly and then more slowly to an 'acceptable' low, but it is not possible to reduce this to zero which would be the value for a normal individual. Treated patients usually have a gal-1-p level below the 'acceptable' figure of 0.57 μmol per gram haemoglobin, but levels often fluctuate. It is not completely clear what is

responsible for this variation. Gal-1-p is often used as a marker for dietary compliance, but its limitations should be recognised. Caution should be applied when interpreting red blood cell gal-1-p levels; a given value reflects only galactose intake in the previous 24 hours, and no correlation with long term clinical outcome has been shown [47].

Sources of galactose

The main source of galactose in the diet is the disaccharide lactose (milk sugar). Lactose is hydrolysed in the gut to form galactose and glucose. Galactose is then transported across the epithelial cells and enters the portal vein to undergo further metabolism in the liver (Fig. 16.2).

The source of lactose in the diet is milk. Therefore to exclude galactose all milk, milk products and manufactured foods containing milk need to be avoided. Another potential source of galactose is from the oligosaccharides, raffinose, stachyose and verbacose which are found predominantly in pulses and legumes. However it is thought unlikely that galactose is absorbed from these sources as the small intestine does not contain the alpha-galactosidase enzyme that is required to split galactose from the oligosaccharide [48]. Instead they are fermented to produce volatile fatty acids in the large intestine. It has been suggested that in the presence of diarrhoea the small intestine can be colonised with bacteria capable of releasing α-linked galactosides [49]. Nowadays most UK centres do not exclude galactosides. Foods containing galac-

Table 16.7 Minimal galactose and lactose diet. Lactose-free foods are listed. Manufactured foods which contain or could contain milk or milk derivatives are shown in italics. For suitable lactose-free manufactured foods refer to the Galactosaemia Support Group 'Lactose free booklets' (GSG list)

Milk, milk products and milk derivatives
These should all be avoided – refer to Table 16.10

Soya milk and soya products
Infant soya formula
Liquid soya milk – calcium enriched (not before 1 year of age)
Soya cheese, soya yoghurt, soya ice-cream, soya desserts

Fats and oils
Milk-free margarine
Many margarines and low fat spreads contain milk – refer to GSG list
Vegetable oils
Lard, dripping, suet

Meat and fish
Meat, poultry, fish, shellfish (fresh or frozen)
Ham and bacon (lactose may occasionally be used as a flavour enhancer – see ingredient label)
Fish fingers
Quorn
Tofu
Many meat or fish products such as sausages, burgers, pies, breaded or battered foods or in sauce will not be suitable – refer to GSG list

Eggs

Cereal, flour, pasta
All grains: wheat, oats, corn, rice, barley, maize, sago, rye, tapioca
Pasta, spaghetti, macaroni, dried noodles, cous cous
Tinned pasta such as spaghetti hoops may contain cheese – refer to GSG list
Flour: plain, self-raising, cornflour, rice flour, soya flour
Custard powder, semolina
Carob

Breakfast cereals
Most are suitable, e.g. Weetabix, Cornflakes, Rice Krispies
A few cereals may contain chocolate or milk derivatives – refer to GSG list

Bread and yeast products
Most bread is suitable
Milk bread and nan bread contain milk – avoid
Pitta, chapatti
Muffins, crumpets, teacakes some may not be suitable – refer to GSG list

Cakes, biscuits, crackers
Many cakes, biscuits and crackers contain milk in some form – refer to GSG list

Desserts
Sorbet, jelly, soya desserts, soya ice-cream, soya yoghurt
Home-made soya milk custard or rice pudding
Most desserts contain milk in some form – refer to GSG list

Fruit
All fresh, frozen, tinned or dried fruit

Vegetables
All fresh, frozen, tinned or dried vegetables
Most dried and tinned pulses, e.g. red kidney beans, chick peas, lentils
Baked beans and ready made vegetable dishes such as coleslaw, potato salad – refer to GSG list

Savoury snacks
Plain crisps, popadom
Nuts, peanut butter
Flavoured crisps may not be suitable because they contain cheese or lactose as a filler in the flavouring – refer to GSG list for suitable flavoured crisps
Dry roasted nuts and popcorn – refer to GSG list

Seasonings, gravies
Pepper, salt, pure spices and herbs, mustard
Marmite, Bovril, Bisto
Gravy granules and stock cubes – refer to GSG list

Sauces, spreads, pickles, dips
Pickles in vinegar, most chutney, tomato ketchup
White and cheese sauce made with milk – avoid
Chocolate spread – avoid
Many sauces, spreads and dips will be suitable – refer to GSG list

Soups
Tinned, packet, carton soups – refer to GSG list

Sugar, sweet spreads
Sugar, glucose, fructose
Pure artificial sweeteners
Powdered and tablet artificial sweeteners may contain lactose – refer to GSG list
Jam, syrup, honey, marmalade, lemon curd

Confectionery
Boiled sweets, most mints, marshmallow, plain fruit lollies, chewing gum
Milk chocolate, most plain chocolate, butterscotch and fudge – avoid
All other sweets, plain or carob chocolate, toffee – refer to GSG list

Drinks
Soya milk
Milk shake syrup or powders
Fizzy drinks, squash, fruit juice
Cocoa, tea, coffee
Drinking chocolate – refer to GSG list
Instant milk drinks and malted milk drinks – avoid

Miscellaneous – used in baking
Baking powder, yeast, gelatine, marzipan

Flavourings
Lactose may be used as a 'carrier' for flavourings particularly in crisps and similar snack foods. In sweets lactose is rarely used for this purpose except in some dairy flavours. All flavourings in the GSG list have been checked to ensure they are lactose-free

Eating out
The GSG list provides information on lactose-free foods for some popular restaurants

Table 16.8 Dietary sources of galactosides and nucleoproteins

Galactosides	Peas, beans, lentils, legumes, chick peas, dahls, grams, spinach
	Texturised vegetable protein
	Soya (other than soya protein isolates), soya beans, soya flour
	Cocoa, chocolate
	Nuts
Nucleoproteins	Offal – liver, kidney, brain, sweetbreads, heart
	Eggs

Table 16.9 Milk substitutes for use in galactosaemia

Infant formula	Protein source	Calcium (mmol per 100 ml)
InfaSoy	soya-protein isolate	1.3
Wysoy	soya-protein isolate	1.7
Prosobee	soya-protein isolate	1.6
Farley's Soya formula	soya-protein isolate	1.4
Isomil Powder	soya-protein isolate	1.7
Galactomin 17*	sodium and calcium caseinate	2.1
Pregestimil*†	casein hydrolysate	1.6
Enfamil Lactofree*	milk protein	1.4
AL110	caseinates	1.5

All infant formulas are approved by the Advisory Committee Borderline Substances for prescription on FP10. Enfamil Lactofree and Pregestimil are not specifically listed for disorders of galactose metabolism
* Galactomin 17 contains up to 6.5 mg galactose per 100 ml
  Pregestimil contains 8.7 mg galactose per 100 ml
  Enfamil Lactofree contains 1.3–2 mg galactose per 100 ml
  AL110 contains <3 mg galactose per 100 ml
† Contains medium chain triglyceride

tosides that were previously restricted were drawn mainly from a list compiled by a group of paediatric dietitians in 1978, reported at a Galactosaemic Workshop in 1982 [50] (Table 16.8). However, even this list was compiled from tenuous sources. An extensive search of the literature can substantiate only some of these reported foods as containing galactosides [51]. This list could still be used if restriction of galactosides was perceived to be necessary.

More recent work by Gross and Acosta [52] indicates that plants, including fruit and vegetables, may contain significant sources of galactose in the form of free galactose, plant cell wall galactans and beta-1,4–linked galactosyl residues in chloroplast membranes of green plant tissue (galactolipids). These galactans and galactolipids might be hydrolysed by beta-galactosidase, present in the small intestine, to liberate galactose. More investigation has been recommended by the authors before the diets of galactosaemic children are restricted further.

Traditionally, foods which are rich in nucleoproteins were also excluded from the diet because of them being a possible source of galactose; again this is far from proven. These foods were also listed at the 1982 Galactosaemic Workshop [50] (Table 16.8). Once again most UK centres do not, nowadays, avoid nucleoproteins.

Milk substitutes

Breast feeding and cow's milk-based infant formulas are contraindicated for the galactosaemic infant because they contain lactose. Infant soya formulas (Table 16.9) are the feeds of choice; they are lactose-free and oligosaccharides are removed during manufacture. Only in those with severe liver disease would a protein hydrolysate formula containing MCT, such

as Pregestimil, be used. It should be noted that some of the accepted milk substitutes used in galactosaemia do contain small amounts of lactose, and therefore galactose, as it is virtually impossible to completely remove this during manufacture.

Milk and milk products normally provide the main source of calcium in children's diets. For the galactosaemic child an infant soya milk can continue to be used to provide calcium, but as the content is relatively low an additional medicinal supplement may still be needed. From 1 year a commercial liquid soya milk can be used but these soya milks are not a good source of vitamins and minerals, so continuation of an infant soya formula may be more appropriate if appetite is poor. Those which contain calcium provide on average 3.5 mmol/100 ml, for example Sainsbury's UHT soya milk (calcium enriched), Tesco's calcium enriched soya milk, Vandemoortele's Provamel calcium enriched soya milk. Some manufacturers also produce soya yoghurts and desserts which contain calcium; these can be a useful additional or alternative source of calcium to soya milk. As children often develop a dislike for the taste of soya milks, medicinal calcium supplements are required. Care must be taken to ensure that these are galactose-free. It is important to check the diet regularly to ensure that the reference nutrient intake [53]

Table 16.10 Milk, milk products and milk derivatives

Milk and milk products

Cow's milk, goat milk, sheep milk
Cheese, cream, butter
Ice-cream, yoghurt, fromage frais, creme fraiche
Chocolate

Milk derivatives

Skimmed milk powder, milk solids, milk protein, non-fat milk solids,
    separate milk solids
Whey, hydrolysed whey protein, margarine or shortening containing whey,
    whey syrup sweetener, hydrolysed whey sugar, vegetarian whey
Casein, caseinates, hydrolysed casein, sodium caseinate, calcium
    caseinate
Buttermilk, butterfat, butter oil, milk fat, animal fat (may be butter), ghee,
    artificial cream
Cheese powder

Lactose as a filler may be used in:
Flavourings
Table-top or tablet artificial sweeteners

Table 16.11 Non-milk derivatives

Lactic acid E270, sodium lactate E325, potassium lactate E325, calcium
    lactate E327
Lactitol, lactalbumin, lactoglobulin, lycasin, stearoyl lactylates, glucona-
    delta-lactose, monosodium glutamate, cocoa butter, non-dairy cream

for calcium is always being achieved, particularly during adolescence, when requirements are high. There is evidence of inadequate bone mineralisation in patients with galactosaemia and inadequate calcium intake may be a causative factor [54, 55].

Milk products and milk derivatives

Milk is processed to make several different foods: cheese, yoghurt, butter, cream (Table 16.10). These products need to be avoided in a minimal galactose diet. Often, they are added to manufactured foods such as biscuits, desserts and pasta, which therefore need to be excluded. Even when milk is processed and separated into component parts both the protein fractions, casein, and in particular whey, still contain lactose. Therefore these milk derivatives (protein or fat-based) must be excluded from the diet to ensure it is lactose-free.

Difficulties frequently arise with manufactured foods because milk derivatives often occur in a form which is not instantly recognisable as milk, e.g. casein, hydrolysed whey protein. It is imperative that parents are taught to interpret food labels for the presence of these products. Unfortunately reading the label will not always provide a conclusive answer as UK labelling does not require the listing of all compound

ingredients (if the compound ingredient forms less than 25% of the final product its individual constituents need not be declared [56]). This makes it very difficult to guarantee from the ingredient label that the food is milk-free. Also, it is not a legal requirement for all foods to have ingredient labels, e.g. those found in a baker's or butcher's shop. These may need to be avoided because of limited information concerning their composition. Conversely confusion may also occur with words which might alert parents to thinking milk is an ingredient when this is not the case (Table 16.11).

Lactose is sometimes used as a filler or carrier and is found in medicines especially tablets, some artificial table-top or tablet sweeteners and flavourings. Historically lactose has been regarded as a carrier for monosodium glutamate (MSG). However, after extensive investigation this has been proven unlikely and foods containing MSG can be included in the diet.

Many of these difficulties of interpreting food labels have been overcome since 1995 when the Galactosaemia Support Group (GSG) employed a dietitian to produce lactose-free manufactured food lists. Lactose-free food lists are produced for general use and for feeding babies and are updated biannually. Members of GSG automatically receive copies of these lists and food information updates. GSG produce another useful booklet, *A Glossary of Terms for use with a Milk-Free Diet in Galactosaemia*, which gives definitions of ingredients found in manufactured foods, some of which are sources of lactose.

Alcohol

In adolescents with galactosaemia, avoidance of alcohol is often recommended because alcohol inhibits galactose metabolism [57]. However, if the pathway is blocked the restriction of alcohol has little logic. UK practice varies and most centres do allow alcohol in moderation.

Heterozygote mothers – dietary treatment

There is no clear evidence that the outcome of pregnancy in heterozygote mothers is better for those infants whose mothers have been on a strict low galactose diet and those who have not [58, 59]. Despite this a restricted milk intake may still be recommended by some.

Galactokinase deficiency (Fig. 16.2)

The clinical manifestations of galactokinase deficiency are much less severe than in classical galactosaemia. Cataracts are the main feature and there is no liver disease or developmental delay. The dietary treatment is the same as for galactosaemia, i.e. galactose avoidance. Gitzelmann [48] has suggested that the degree of galactose avoidance can be less strict but recognises that no systematic study has been done.

UDPgalactose 4-epimerase deficiency (Fig. 16.2)

Two forms of epimerase deficiency exist; only the severe form which is extremely rare requires dietary treatment. Epimerase forms UDPgalactose from UDPglucose. Theoretically a complete absence of galactose from the diet and lack of UDPgalactose formation would result in an inability to form complex glycoproteins and glycolipids. It has, however, been suggested that glycoprotein and glycolipid production is sufficient, presumably as a result of some residual epimerase activity in the liver [60]. It may therefore be unnecessary to provide galactose. Of the five cases reported in the literature, a galactose supplement was given initially then stopped in two patients without obvious detrimental effect [61, 62, 63].

The optimal dietary therapy of patients with epimerase deficiency is not known. A galactose restricted diet is essential, but whether or not a small supplement of galactose is needed is not clear.

HEREDITARY FRUCTOSE INTOLERANCE

Hereditary fructose intolerance (HFI) is caused by a deficiency of the enzyme fructose-1,6 bisphosphate aldolase (aldolase B) in the liver, kidney and small intestine. This enzyme is an essential step in the metabolism of fructose (Fig. 16.3).

Symptoms will only develop when the child is given fructose. In the UK exposure to fructose is uncommon prior to weaning as breast milk and infant formula are fructose-free. During the introduction of solid food sources of fructose become abundant from fruits, vegetables and commercial baby foods. While the clinical picture and dietary history should enable a diagnosis of HFI to be made in older patients, the diagnosis can be more difficult in young patients. However, even in older patients symptoms may be minimal because they develop an aversion to sweet tasting foods and self-select a low fructose diet. Nevertheless, these children may still be given fructose from unexpected sources such as medicines.

In the infant and young child the main clinical symptoms include poor feeding, vomiting, abdominal distention and failure to thrive. Hypoglycaemia may develop after exposure to fructose. Continued exposure to fructose causes severe liver failure, proximal renal tubular dysfunction and specific metabolic disturbances [64]. None of these problems are specific and the key to diagnosis is a very accurate clinical and dietary history.

The main treatment of HFI is strict exclusion of fructose, sucrose and sorbitol from the diet. This results in a rapid improvement of symptoms. The long term prognosis is good although hepatomegaly and fatty changes in the liver may persist [65]. The diet needs to be continued for life without relaxation as even small amounts of fructose have been shown to be harmful [66]. Abdominal pain and vomiting can occur if a child on the diet is accidentally exposed to fructose.

Sources of fructose

Fructose in the diet comes from fructose, sucrose and sorbitol. Fructose is absorbed by a carrier mediated process across the small intestine and then enters the liver to undergo further metabolism (Fig. 16.3). The disaccharide sucrose is cleaved in the small intestine by sucrase-isomaltase to form a molecule of both glucose and fructose. Sorbitol, a sugar alcohol, diffuses slowly across the intestinal absorptive surface with only 10–30% being absorbed. In the liver it is rapidly converted via sorbitol dehydrogenase to fructose. Another potential source of fructose is from the trisaccharide raffinose and the tetrasaccharide

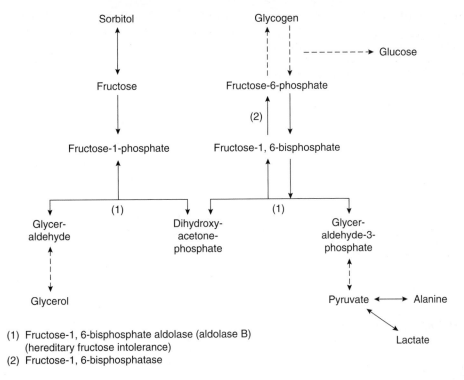

(1) Fructose-1, 6-bisphosphate aldolase (aldolase B)
     (hereditary fructose intolerance)
(2) Fructose-1, 6-bisphosphatase

Fig. 16.3 Fructose metabolism

stachyose; however it is thought unlikely that these are hydrolysed to any significant extent in the small intestine and therefore little of the fructose is absorbed. Fructans such as inulin are widespread in various plants, e.g. artichokes [67]. Again these are not absorbed; instead they undergo bacterial fermentation in the colon.

There has been an increase in the use of commercially prepared sugar alcohols as artificial sweeteners which are potential sources of fructose. Isomalt is a mixture of two disaccharide alcohols, glucose–sorbitol and glucose–mannitol. During digestion in the small intestine it is hydrolysed to 50% glucose, 25% sorbitol and 25% mannitol. Lycasin is a glucose syrup in which all glucose units with free aldehyde groups have been reduced by hydrogenation to sorbitol. The product consists of sorbitol, hydrogenated oligo- and higher polysaccharides. Oligofructose is obtained from inulin through enzymatic hydrolysis, producing a mixture of chains of fructose molecules of varying chain length (2 to 20 molecules). Commercial syrups of oligofructose contain small amounts of fructose and sucrose.

Minimal fructose, sucrose, sorbitol diet

The aim of dietary treatment of HFI is complete elimination of fructose, sucrose and sorbitol, but it is not possible to exclude these sugars completely (Table 16.12). In practice it is not possible to get the intake of fructose from all sources to be less than 1 to 2 g per day. The normal average daily intake of fructose (including contribution from sucrose) in unaffected infants has been reported as 20 g per day [68]. Obviously intakes in older children on normal diets would be much greater and could easily be of the order of 100 g per day.

Fructose is the natural sugar present in fruit, vegetables and honey. Sucrose is also found in fruit and vegetables but a much greater source is from sugar cane or beet. These are refined to produce table sugar which is used extensively in food manufacture as a sweetener and bulking agent. Sugar is a major ingredient in cakes, biscuits, desserts and soft drinks. Many other commercial foods (e.g. stock cubes, tinned meats, bottled sauces and savoury snack biscuits) contain sugar but are much less obvious sources.

Table 16.12 Minimal fructose, sucrose and sorbitol diet (<2 g/day)

Foods allowed	Foods to avoid
Sugars, sweeteners and preserves	
Glucose, glucose polymers, glucose syrup, dextrose, lactose, starch, maltose, maltodextrin, malt extract	Sugar or sucrose (cane or beet) – white, brown, caster, icing
Saccharin, aspartame	Fruit sugar, fructose, laevulose
	Honey, treacle, molasses
	Sorbitol, Lycasin, Isomalt
	Golden syrup, corn syrup, invert syrup, high-fructose or isoglucose syrups, hydrogenated glucose syrup
	Jam, marmalade, lemon curd
Fruit	
Avocado, rhubarb (occasionally)	All other fruit and fruit products
Vegetables	
(cooked, boil and discard water)	Beetroot, Brussels sprouts, carrots, gherkins, green beans, kohl rabi, okra, onion, parsnip, peas, pepper, plantain, shallots, spring onion, squash, sweetcorn, sweet potato, tomato, tomato purée
*Group 1 (< 0.5 g fructose/100 g)**	
Celery, globe artichokes, mange-tout, mushrooms, spinach, watercress	
Beans: haricot, mung, red kidney	Beans – green, French, runner,
Dried split peas, lentils	Baked beans, tinned vegetables with added sugar, mayonnaise or salad cream, coleslaw
Potato: old potato, plain potato crisps, (potato waffle, potato croquette – check food label)	Flavoured crisps
*Group 2 (0.5–1.0 g fructose/100 g)**	Pickles, chutney
Aubergine, asparagus, beansprouts, broccoli, cabbage, cauliflower, courgette, cucumber, fennel, artichoke, leeks, lettuce, marrow, new potato, pumpkin, radish, spring greens, swede, turnip	
Beans: black-eye, broad, butter, soya	
Marrowfat peas, processed peas canned in water, chick peas	
Milk	
Infant formula milk, cow's milk, unsweetened evaporated milk, Coffeemate, dried milk powder	Flavoured milk, condensed milk, milk shake powders and syrups
Cream	Liquid soya milk
Cheese, plain cottage cheese	Aerosol cream
Natural yoghurt	Cheese with added ingredients, e.g. nuts, fruit
	Fruit and flavoured yoghurt, fromage frais
	Ice-cream
Eggs	
Allowed	
Meat and poultry	
All fresh meat and poultry	Processed meats which have added sucrose, e.g. meat pastes, frankfurters, salami, paté, sausages, tinned meat
If processed read label to check for added sucrose, fructose or honey	Tendersweet meats, e.g. ham,
	Honey cured meats
	Ready-made meat meals – possible sources are the gravy, sauces, vegetables, breadcrumbs, batter, pastry
Meat substitutes	
Soya meat, Tofu, Quorn	
Fish	
Fresh and frozen fish, shell fish, fish tinned in brine, oil or water	Fish tinned in tomato sauce, fish paste, fish cakes, fish fingers
	Ready-made fish meals – possible sources are the sauce, vegetables, breadcrumb, batter, pastry
Flour and cereals	
Flour (white in preference to wholemeal), buckwheat, cornflour, custard powder, sago, semolina, tapioca, oatmeal, barley	Bran, wheatgerm
Flaky pastry, shortcrust pastry (not sweetened)	

Table 16.12 *Continued*

Foods allowed	Foods to avoid

Pasta and rice

Spaghetti, macaroni, other pasta (white in preference to wholemeal) | Pasta tinned in tomato sauce
Noodles, egg noodles | Pot Noodle
Rice (white in preference to brown)

Breakfast cereals

Porridge, Puffed Wheat, Ready Brek, Shredded Wheat | Most manufactured breakfast cereals

Bread and crackers

White bread (pre-packed) | Wholemeal bread, sweetened breads, e.g. malt bread, soda bread, currant
Bakers' bread – check if sugar is added to dough mixture | bread
Cream crackers, Matzo crackers, water biscuits, Ryvita (not sesame), | Savoury snack biscuits
plain rice cakes
Crumpets

Cakes, biscuits and pastries

Home-made using permitted ingredients and sweeteners | All cakes, biscuits and pastries

Desserts

Home-made using permitted ingredients, e.g. custard sweetened with | Most desserts, e.g. jelly, meringue, mousse, gateaux, fruit pie or crumble,
glucose, choux pastry | ice-cream, yoghurts

Fats and oils

Butter, margarine, vegetable oils, lard, suet

Drinks

Lucozade (not fruit flavour), soda water, mineral water (without fruit | Fruit juices, vegetable juices, fruit squash, fizzy drinks, diabetic squash
flavour) | containing sorbitol or fructose, tonic water
Squashes and fizzy drinks flavoured with only saccharin or aspartame (free | Drinking chocolate, malted milk drinks
from sugar, sorbitol, fruit flavourings or comminuted fruits) | Instant tea mixes, coffee essence
Tea, coffee, cocoa

Confectionery

Lucozade Sport Glucose Energy tablets – original only | Sweets, chocolate, toffee, jelly, ice lollies, chewing gum, diabetic sweets
Dextrosol – glucose tablets | (sweetened with fructose or sorbitol)
  | Some glucose tablets, e.g. orange flavour Lucozade tablets

Gravies, sauces and soups

Marmite, Bovril | Gravy granules, stock cubes
White or cheese sauce made with milk, flour, fat and cheese only | Bottled sauces and dressings, e.g. tomato ketchup, horseradish sauce,
  | mint sauce, soy sauce
  | Sauce mixes, e.g. sweet and sour, curry
  | Mayonnaise, salad cream
  | All soups (packet, tinned or fresh)

Herbs, spices, nuts and seeds

Pure herbs, mustard and spices, salt, pepper | Nuts, peanut butter, marzipan
Sesame seeds
Pumpkin and sunflower seeds maximum of 10 g per day total

Baking products

Baking powder, bicarbonate of soda, yeast, arrowroot, food colourings, food
essences, gelatine

---

* Total fructose content of vegetables is calculated as fructose plus $\frac{1}{2}$ sucrose.

NB
- Always read the label of manufactured food to check for sucrose, fructose, sorbitol or the artificial sweeteners lycasin or isomalt
- Check toothpaste for sorbitol

Analysis of fructose and sucrose content of foods

1 *Cereals and Cereal Products – The Third Supplement to McCance and Widdowson's 'The Composition of Foods'* 4e, 1988.
2 *Milk and Milk Products and Eggs – The Fourth Supplement to McCance and Widdowson's 'The Composition of Foods'* 4e, 1989.
3 *Vegetables, Herbs and Spices – The Fifth Supplement to McCance and Widdowson's 'The Composition of Foods'* 4e, 1991.
4 *Fruit and Nuts – The First Supplement to McCance and Widdowson's 'The Composition of Foods'* 5e, 1992.
Publishers of above: Holland B, Unwin ID, Buss DH, The Royal Society of Chemistry and Ministry of Agriculture, Fisheries and Food, The Stationery Office.

Indeed, very few manufactured foods are suitable for inclusion in the diet. Flavourings can be another potential trace source of sucrose and fructose as these sugars are sometimes used as carriers for flavouring compounds.

Only vegetables which have a very low fructose content and contain predominantly starch can be included in the diet, but in restricted amounts (Table 16.12). Fructose from vegetables should not exceed 1.0–1.5 g per day as small amounts of fructose from cereals will increase the total intake to the 2 g maximum. Permitted vegetables have been divided into two groups (with a fructose content of 0.5 g per 100 g and 0.5–1.0 g per 100 g) to give a wider choice. It is important to note the difference in fructose content between raw and cooked vegetables. Cooking causes a loss of free sugars, consequently cooked vegetables have a lower fructose content and are recommended in preference to raw. New potatoes have a higher fructose content than old (0.65 g/100 g versus 0.25 g/100 g). Sucrose content of stored potatoes has previously been reported to both decrease and increase on storage [69, 70]; however, no further analysis is available to resolve this issue. Wholemeal flour contains more fructose than white because the germ and bran contain sucrose. Similarly other wholegrain foods (e.g. brown rice, wholemeal pasta) contain more sucrose than the refined varieties. No accurate analysis for the fructose content of bread is available; however it would appear prudent to choose white in preference to wholemeal. Bread has previously been restricted in the diets of children with HFI. Nowadays this restriction is probably unnecessary because most flour improvers for bread making do not contain sugar. If the bread does contain sugar it has to be declared on the ingredient label. Caution should be applied where richer doughs are used (e.g. in soft rolls) because often the flour improver does contain sugar in these instances. Bread bought from craft bakers may also contain sugar, and bakers are under no legal obligation to declare this information to the consumer.

Sorbitol is used as an artificial sweetener and bulk sweetener, particularly in diabetic foods and drinks; these foods must be avoided. Isomalt and lycasin are used as alternative sweeteners, predominantly being used in confectionery. Isomalt may also be found in baked goods, breakfast cereals, desserts, snack foods and jam. These need to be avoided because of their sorbitol content. Sucrose, sorbitol and artificial sweeteners are often used as excipients or as flavour improvers in medicines, tablets and syrups. Parents need to be made aware of this and know to check with a pharmacist about the suitability of medicines.

Intravenous fructose and sorbitol are potential lethal sources of fructose; these are rarely used in the UK, but are more commonly used in Europe [71].

Starch, glucose and lactose can be included in the diet. Glucose can be used as an alternative sweetener to sucrose and can also provide a useful source of energy. The relative sweetness of glucose is only half that of sucrose, so additional sweetening may be needed in baked goods. Some intense sweeteners, e.g. Sweetex, can be successfully added to cooked food; others, e.g. aspartame, decompose on heating and are therefore not suitable for baking. However, extra sweetening may not be necessary or desirable as children with HFI dislike and avoid sweet tasting foods. Glucose is not prescribable on FP10 for treatment of HFI.

Nutritional problems

Children with HFI are at risk of vitamin C and possible folic acid deficiency due to the exclusion of the major dietary sources of these vitamins, i.e. fruits and vegetables. A suitable medicinal supplement (e.g. Vitamin C Powder from Boots the Chemist) should be prescribed to meet the RNI [53]. Lack of dietary fibre may also be a problem. This could be overcome by including pulses and oats, which contain only very small amounts of fructose, in the diet.

FRUCTOSE-1,6-BISPHOSPHATASE DEFICIENCY

In the fasting state, glycogen initially provides the major fuel source for glucose production. As the duration of fast extends and glycogen stores are depleted, glucose is synthesised via gluconeogenesis from lactate, glycerol and the gluconeogenic amino acids such as alanine. A deficiency of fructose-1,6-bisphosphatase (Fig. 16.3) blocks the gluconeogenic pathway and, as a result, during fasting patients develop hypoglycaemia and a marked lactic acidosis with ketosis.

Fructose-1,6-bisphosphatase deficiency may present in the newborn period or, in older children, during intercurrent infections associated with prolonged fasting [64]. Once diagnosed, these life threatening acute episodes can be prevented with careful treatment. The prognosis is good, with normal growth and development.

Dietary treatment

The aims of the dietary management of fructose-1,6-bisphosphatase deficiency are to:

- provide good glycogen reserves
- prevent hypoglycaemia
- reduce the need for gluconeogenesis.

This can be achieved by avoidance of prolonged fasts and provision of regular meals, with a high intake of carbohydrate from starch. Patients should be carefully assessed for fasting tolerance, which should improve with age. The majority of children will be well controlled without the need for fructose restriction when they are well. Nevertheless, it is inadvisable for them to have a very high intake of fructose as this may cause hypoglycaemia and lactic acidosis. During illness fructose must be completely avoided.

Diet when well

The young infant is fed at four hourly intervals during the day and night. Even when weaning is well established, a late night and early morning feed is still given to reduce the duration of overnight fasting.

The older child is given regular meals containing a high carbohydrate intake from starch to provide a constant supply of 'slow-release' glucose. Fasting overnight is not normally a problem provided a starchy bedtime snack and early breakfast is given. A high intake of fructose as sucrose in cakes, biscuits, confectionery and sugary drinks is discouraged.

Alcohol inhibits gluconeogenesis and if taken in excess in healthy adolescents can precipitate hypoglycaemia. Alcohol should therefore be taken in moderation and only with food.

Diet during illness

Poor appetite and fasting are common in the sick child. In the child with fructose-1,6-bisphosphatase deficiency it is critical to prevent such prolonged fasts because the gluconeogenic pathway for production of glucose is blocked. During intercurrent illnesses an exogenous source of glucose must be supplied. The standard emergency regimen (p. 287) must be given during times of illness to reduce the risk of hypoglycaemia and lactic acidosis. Fructose, sucrose and sorbitol must be excluded because these will exacerbate the metabolic derangement. Fat should be avoided during decompensation as glycerol may exacerbate the illness. Emergency regimen drinks are restricted to those which are glucose-based: glucose polymer and low calorie squash (sorbitol-free) or Lucozade (original variety). Medications must be free of fructose, sucrose and sorbitol. Some patients may decompensate rapidly, becoming very ill with marked acidosis. The impact can be reduced by giving sodium bicarbonate up to 4 mmol/kg body weight/day. If there are signs of metabolic acidosis the patient's condition must be assessed in hospital. Once the child improves, normal diet can be resumed, with a gradual reintroduction of fructose and sucrose-containing foods. During the recovery period extra glucose polymer drinks should continue to be given, particularly at night.

REFERENCES

1 Burchell A, Waddell I Identification, purification and genetic deficiencies of the glucose-6-phosphatase system transport proteins. *Eur J Pediatr*, 1993, **152** (Suppl 1) 14–17.

2 Hers H, Van Hoof F, de Barsy T Glycogen storage diseases. In: Scriver CR *et al.* (eds.) *The Metabolic Basis of Inherited Disease*, 6e. New York: McGraw-Hill, 1989.

3 Roe T *et al.* Inflammatory bowel disease in glycogen storage disease type IB. *J Paediatr*, 1986, **109** 55–9.

4 Lee PJ, Leonard JV The hepatic glycogen storage diseases – problems beyond childhood. *J Inher Metab Dis*, 1995, **18** 462–72.

5 Stanley CA, Mills J, Baker L Intragastric feeding in type I glycogen storage disease: factors affecting the control of lacticacidaemia. *Pediatr Res*, 1981, **15** 1504–8.

6 Bier D *et al.* Measurement of true glucose production rates in infancy and childhood with 6,6-diodeuteroglucose. *Diabetes*, 1977, **26** 1016–23.

7 Green H *et al.* Continuous nocturnal nasogastric feeding for management of type I GSD. *New Eng J Med*, 1976, **294** 423–5.

8 Chen Y, Cornblath M, Sidbury J Cornstarch therapy in type I glycogen storage disease. *New Eng J Med*, 1984, **310** 171–5.

9 Fernandes J The effect of disaccharides on the hyperlacticacidaemia of glucose-6-phosphatase-deficient children. *Acta Paediatr Scand*, 1974, **63** 695–8.

10 Fernandes J, Berger R, Smit P Lactate as a cerebral metabolic fuel for glucose-6-phosphatase deficient children. *Pediatr Res*, 1984, **18** 335–9.

11 Fernandes J The glycogen storage disease. In: Fernandes J, Saudubray JM, Tada K (eds.) *Inborn Metabolic Diseases, Diagnosis and Treatment.* Berlin: Springer-Verlag, 1990.

12 Fernandes, J, Alaapovic P, Wit J Gastric drip feeding in patients with glycogen storage disease type I: its effects on growth and plasma lipids and apolipoproteins. *Pediatr Res*, 1989, **25** 327–31.

13 Schmitz G, Hohage H, Ullrich K Glucose-6-phosphate; a key compound in glycogenosis I and favism leading to hyper- or hypolipidaemia. *Eur J Pediatr*, 1993, **152** (Suppl 1) 77–84.

14 Lee PJ *et al.* Hyperlipidaemia does not impair vascular endothelial function in glycogen storage disease Ia. *Atherosclerosis*, 1994, **110** 95–100.

15 Schwenk WF, Haymond WM Optimal rate of enteral glucose administration in children with glycogen storage disease type I. *New Eng J Med*, 1986, **314** 1257–8.

16 Collins J *et al.* Glucose production rates in type I glycogen storage disease. *J Inher Metab Dis*, 1990, **13** 195–206.

17 Leonard J, Dunger D Hypoglycaemia complicating feeding regimens for glycogen storage disease. *Lancet*, 1978, **11** 1203–4.

18 Dunger DB, Sutton P, Leonard JV Hypoglycaemia complicating treatment regimens for glycogen storage disease (letter). *Arch Dis Childh*, 1995, **72** 274–5.

19 Fine R, Kogut M, Donnell G Intestinal absorption in type I glycogen storage disease. *J Pediatr*, 1969, **75** 632–5.

20 Milla P *et al.* Disordered intestinal function in glycogen storage disease. *J Inher Metab Dis*, 1978, **1** 155–7.

21 Lee PJ *et al.* Bone mineralisation in type I glycogen storage disease. *Eur J Pediatr*, 1995, **154** 483–7.

22 Smit G *et al.* The dietary treatment of children with type I glycogen storage disease with slow release carbohydrate. *Pediatr Res*, 1984, **18** 879–81.

23 Lee PJ, Dixon MA, Leonard JV Uncooked cornstarch – efficacy in type I glycogenosis. *Arch Dis Childh*, 1996, **74** 546–7.

24 Hayde M, Widhalm K Effects of cornstarch treatment in very young children with type I glycogen storage disease. *Eur J Pediatr*, 1990, **149** 630–33.

25 Ogata T *et al.* Effect of cornstarch formula in an infant with type I glycogen storage disease. *Acta Paediatr Jpn*, 1988, **30** 547–52.

26 Wolfsdorf JI, Crigler JF Effect of continuous glucose therapy begun in infancy on the long-term clinical course of patients with type I glycogen storage disease. *J Pediatr Gastroenteral Nutr*, 1999, **29** 136–43.

27 Sidbury J, Chen Y, Roe L The role of raw starches in the treatment of type I glycogenosis. *Arch Intern Med*, 1986, **146** 370–73.

28 Wolfsdorf JI, Crigler JF Biochemical evidence for the requirement of continuous glucose therapy in young adults with type I glycogen storage disease. *J Inher Metab Dis*, 1994, **17** 234–41.

29 Chen YT *et al.* Type I glycogen storage disease: nine years of management with cornstarch. *Eur J Pediatr*, 1993, **152** (Suppl 1) 56–9.

30 Dunger DB, Leonard JV, Preece MA Patterns of growth in the hepatic glycogenoses. *Arch Dis Childh*, 1984, **59** 657–60.

31 Slonim A, Coleman R, Moses W Myopathy and growth failure in debrancher enzyme deficiency: improvement with high protein nocturnal enteral therapy. *J Paediatr*, 1984, **105** (6) 906–11.

32 Slonim AE *et al.* Reversal of debrancher deficiency myopathy by use of high-protein nutrition. *Ann Neur*, 1982, **11** 420–22.

33 Slonim AE *et al.* Amino acid disturbances in type III glycogenosis: differences from type I glycogenosis. *Metabolism*, 1983, **32** 70–74.

34 Bodamer OAF, Mayatepek E, Leonard JV Leucine and glucose kinetics in glycogen storage disease type IIIa. *J Inher Metab Dis*, 1997, **20** 847.

35 Gremse D, Bucuvalas J, Balisteri W Efficacy of cornstarch therapy in type III glycogen storage disease. *Am J Clin Nutr*, 1990, **52** 671–4.

36 McCallion N *et al.* Uncooked cornflour (UCF) compared to high protein diet in the treatment of glycogen storage disease type III. *J Inher Metab Dis*, 1998, **21** (Suppl 2) 93.

37 Lee PJ, Ferguson C, Alexander FW Symptomatic hyperinsulinism reversed by dietary manipulation in glycogenosis type III. *J Inher Metab Dis*, 1997, **20** 612–13.

38 Collins JE *et al.* The effect of ethanol on glucose production in phosphorylase *b* kinase deficiency. *J Inher Metab Dis*, 1989, **12** 312–22.

39 Slonim E *et al.* Improvement of muscle function in acid maltase deficiency by high protein therapy. *Neurology*, 1983, **33** 34–8.

40 Umpleby M *et al.* Protein turnover in acid maltase deficiency before and after treatment with a high protein diet. *J Neurosurgery Psychiatry*, 1987, **50** 587–92.

41 DiMauro S, Bruno C Glycogen storage diseases of muscle. *Curr Opin Neurol*, 1998, **11** 477–84.

42 Smit GPA *et al.* The long term outcome of patients with glycogen storage diseases. *J Inher Metab Dis*, 1990, **13** 411–18.

43 Honeyman M *et al.* Galactosaemia: results of the British Paediatric Surveillance Unit Study 1988–90. *Arch Dis Childh*, 1993, **69** 339–41.

44 Waggoner DD, Buist NR, Donnell GN Long-term prognosis in galactosaemia: results of a survey of 350 cases. *J Inher Metab Dis*, 1990, **13** 802–18.

45 Schweitzer S *et al.* Long-term outcome in 134 patients with galactosaemia. *Eur J Pediatr*, 1993, **152** 36–43.

46 Berry GT *et al.* Endogenous synthesis of galactose in

normal men and patients with hereditary galactosaemia. *Lancet*, 1995, **346** 1073–4.

47 Walter JH *et al.* Recommendations for the management of galactosaemia. *Arch Dis Childh*, 1999, **80** 93–6.

48 Gitzelmann R, Auricchio S The handling of soya alpha-galactosides by a normal and a galactosaemic child. *Paediatr* 1965, **36** 231.

49 Gitzelmann R Disorders of galactose metabolism. In: Fernandes J, Saudubray JM, Tada K (eds.) *Inborn Metabolic Diseases*. Berlin: Springer-Verlag, 1990.

50 Clothier CM, Davidson DC Galactosaemia workshop. *Hum Nutr: Appl Nutr*, 1983, **37a** 483–90.

51 Southgate DAT *et al.* Free sugars in foods. *J Hum Nutr*, 1978, **32** 335–47.

52 Gross KC, Acosta PB Fruits and vegetables are a source of galactose. *J Inher Metab Dis*, 1991, **14** 253–8.

53 Department of Health Report on Health and Social Subjects No 41. *Dietary Reference Values for Food Energy and Nutrients for the United Kingdom*. London: The Stationery Office, 1991.

54 Matthai S *et al.* Bone mineral density in galactosaemia. Inborn error review series, Scientific Hospital Supplies, 1997, No 7.

55 Kaufman FR *et al.* Effect of hypogonadism and deficient calcium intake on bone density in patients with galactosaemia. *J Pediatr*, 1993, **123** 365–70.

56 *The Food Labelling Regulations*, No 1305. London: The Stationery Office, 1984.

57 Brandt NJ How long should galactosaemia be treated? In: *Inherited Disorders of Carbohydrate Metabolism*. Lancaster: MTP Press, 1980.

58 Irons M *et al.* Accumulation of galactose-1-phosphate in the galactosaemic fetus despite maternal milk avoidance. *J Paediatr*, 1985, **107** 261–3.

59 Jacobs C *et al.* Dietary restriction of maternal lactose intake does not prevent accumulation of galactitol in the amniotic fluid of fetuses affected with galactosaemia. *Prenantal Diagnosis*, 1998, **8** 641–5.

60 Kingsley DM *et al.* Structure and function of low density lipoprotein receptors in epimerase deficient galactosaemia. *New Eng J Med*, 1986, **314** 1257–8.

61 Holton JB *et al.* Galactosaemia: a new severe variant due to uridine diphosphate galactose-4-epimerase deficiency. *Arch Dis Childh*, 1981, **56** 885–7.

62 Sardharwalla IB *et al.* A patient with a severe type of epimerase deficiency galactosaemia. *Abstracts of the 25th SSIEM Annual Symposium*, 1987, 91.

63 Walter JH *et al.* Generalised uridine diphosphate galac-tose-4-epimerase deficiency. *Arch Dis Childh*, 1999, **80** 374–6.

64 Gitzelmann R, Steinmann B, Van den Berghe G Disorders of fructose metabolism. In: Scriver CR *et al.* (eds.) *The Metabolic Basis of Inherited Disease*, 6e. New York: McGraw-Hill, 1989.

65 Odièvre M *et al.* Hereditary fructose intolerance in childhood: diagnosis, management and course in 55 patients. *Am J Dis Childh*, 1978, **132** 605–8.

66 Oberhaensli R *et al.* Study of hereditary fructose intolerance by the use of magnetic resonance spectroscopy. *Lancet*, 1987, (24 Oct) 931–4.

67 Rumessen J *et al.* Fructans of Jerusalem artichokes: intestinal transport, absorption, fermentation and influence on blood glucose, insulin and C-peptide responses in healthy subjects. *Am J Clin Nutr*, 1990, **52** 675–81.

68 Mills A, Tyler H *Food and Nutrient Intakes of British Infants aged 6 to 12 Months*. London: Ministry of Agriculture, Fisheries and Foods, The Stationery Office, 1992.

69 Francis D Galactosaemia, fructosaemia and favism – dietary management. In: *Diets for Sick Children*, 4e. Oxford: Blackwell Science, 1987.

70 Bell L, Sherwood W Current practices and improved recommendations for treating hereditary fructose intolerance. *J Am Diet Assoc*, 1987, **87** (6) 721–31.

71 Collins J Metabolic disease, time for fructose solutions to go. *Lancet*, 1993, **341** 600.

FURTHER READING

Coleman R *et al.* Glycogen debranching enzyme deficiency: long term study of serum enzyme activities and clinical features. *J Inher Metab Dis*, 1992, **15** 869–81.

Moses S Pathophysiology and dietary treatment of the glycogen storage diseases. *J Paediatr Gastroenterol Nutr*, 1990, **11** 155–74.

Manir A, Rellos P, Cox TM Hereditary fructose intolerance. *J Med Genet*, 1998, **35** 353–65.

USEFUL ADDRESSES

Association for Glycogen Storage Disease (UK)
9 Lindop Road, Hale, Altrincham, Cheshire WA15 9DZ.

Galactosaemia Support Group
31 Cotysmore Road, Sutton Coldfield, West Midlands B75 6BJ.

CHAPTER 17

Disorders of Fatty Acid Oxidation

Long chain fatty acids form a major fuel source in most tissues of the body, particularly during fasting. They are also the principal energy source of cardiac and skeletal muscle in the resting state and during prolonged exercise.

Fat metabolism begins in adipose tissue with the release of free fatty acids from triglycerides into the blood stream. These are then transported to the tissues bound to albumin. Long chain fatty acids enter the mitochondria via a carnitine dependent pathway and are broken down by the spiral of beta-oxidation (Fig. 17.1). Every turn of the spiral involves four steps, catalysed by several enzymes of different chain-length specificities. In addition to producing energy, each turn of the spiral shortens the fatty acid by two carbon atoms and produces a molecule of acetyl-CoA. The latter is either metabolised in the tricarboxylic acid cycle, or converted in the liver to ketone bodies for use as a fuel by other tissues such as cardiac and skeletal muscle and brain (after prolonged fasting). Medium chain fatty acids are absorbed from the intestine into the hepatic portal vein and enter mitochondria in hepatocytes by carnitine independent as well as carnitine dependent pathways [1].

A number of disorders of the mitochondrial fatty acid oxidation pathway have now been described. These vary in severity and may present at any time from the neonatal period to adulthood [2]. In infancy the clinical picture is one of acute encephalopathy often accompanied by a 'hypoketotic hypoglycaemia'. Additionally in long chain fatty acid oxidation defects, neonates and infants often have a cardiomyopathy and adults have muscle problems. Patients with long chain 3-hydroxy acyl-CoA dehydrogenase deficiency may develop additional complications of a pigmentary retinopathy and peripheral neuropathy. The clinical features of these disorders are thought to be the result of both the reduction of oxidation of fatty acids and the accumulation of toxic intermediates.

Treatment of fatty acid oxidation disorders is primarily by diet, which varies with the disorders. The main aim is to minimise the oxidation of fatty acids by use of an emergency regimen when ill, avoidance of fasting and in more severe defects by also limiting the intake of dietary fat. With the exception of medium chain acyl-CoA dehydrogenase deficiency most disorders of fatty acid oxidation are rare and experience of dietary treatment is therefore limited.

Acyl-CoA dehydrogenases

The first step of beta-oxidation is catalysed by an acyl-CoA dehydrogenase. There are four separate enzymes which metabolise fatty acids of different chain length, with some overlapping substrate specificity [2], as follows.

Fatty acid chain length specificity

Very long chain acyl-CoA dehydrogenase	C22 down to C14
Medium chain acyl-CoA dehydrogenase	C12 down to C4
Short chain acyl-CoA dehydrogenase	C6 and C4

The long chain acyl-CoA dehydrogenase enzyme is primarily involved with oxidation of branched-chain fatty acids.

Medium chain acyl-CoA dehydrogenase deficiency

Medium chain acyl-CoA dehydrogenase (MCAD) deficiency is the most common of the fatty acid

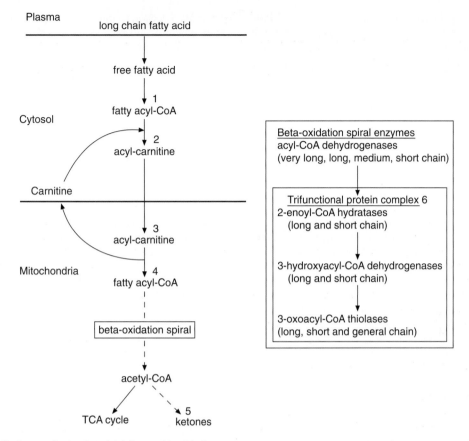

Fig. 17.1 Pathway of mitochondrial fatty acid oxidation
Enzymes involved
1 – Acyl-CoA synthase
2 – Carnitine palmitoyl transferase I (CPT I)
3 – Carnitine acylcarnitine translocase (CAT)
4 – Carnitine palmitoyl transferase II (CPT II)
5 – 3-Hydroxy-3-methylglutaryl-CoA lyase deficiency (or 3-hydroxy-3-methylglutaric aciduria)
6 – Trifunctional protein complex is composed of long-chain-enoyl-CoA hydratase, long chain 3-hydroxyacyl-CoA dehydrogenase (LCHAD) and long-chain 3-oxothiolase
TCA – tricarboxylic acid cycle

oxidation defects with an estimated incidence of up to 1 in 10 000 in some regions of the UK [3]. It is also relatively common in some European populations. MCAD deficiency usually presents between 6 months and 4 years but neonatal onset can also occur [4, 5, 6]. The typical picture is of encephalopathy with hypoketotic hypoglycaemia, precipitated by metabolic stress such as fasting, gastrointestinal illness or respiratory infections. Without treatment patients will progress ultimately to coma with high mortality.

Between episodes the patients are usually completely well.

Dietary management

Children with MCAD deficiency have impaired oxidation of medium chain fatty acids (MCFA) which are predominantly derived from long chain fatty acids. However, under basal conditions the oxidation of MCFA has been reported to be near normal due to overlapping enzyme substrate specificity [7]. The well child can therefore be on a normal diet without restriction of long chain fat. It is nevertheless important to avoid prolonged fasts as fatty acid oxidation rates increase as the period of fasting is extended. In infants fatty acid oxidation rates are higher after a shorter duration of fast, therefore frequent feeding is recommended. Current practice is for young infants to be fed 3–4 hourly around the clock, with a maximum fast of 6–8 hours for 6 to 9 month old infants and 8–10 hours for 10 to 12 month old infants. Children should have regular meals containing starch, such as bread, potato, pasta, rice or cereals. Missed meals should be replaced by a sugary or glucose polymer-based drink. A bedtime snack and breakfast are essential meals to minimise the duration of the overnight fast (a maximum of 12 hours is suggested).

Medium chain triglycerides (MCT) occur in only a few foods and are not present in sufficient quantities to cause a problem. Coconut is the only exception (9 g MCT/100 g), but small amounts in the well child are acceptable. Some specialised dietetic products such as Pregestimil, Pepti-Junior, Monogen, Frebini and Paediasure and some low birthweight infant formulas contain a high percentage of MCT and must not be given.

The following guidelines should be followed when treating a child with MCAD deficiency:

- Prolonged fasts should be avoided
- A late night snack should be given
- Breakfast must not be missed
- Missed meals should be replaced
- Meals containing starch should be given regularly
- Dietetic products containing MCT must be avoided.

Neonatal deaths have been reported in MCAD deficiency [8]. If an infant is at risk of MCAD deficiency it is essential that they receive adequate feeds and are not starved during the first few days of life. This is particularly important for the breast fed infant who may take longer to establish feeding than the formula fed infant. Supplementary feeds may be required until breast feeding is established or MCAD deficiency excluded.

Diet during illness

In contrast to the diet advised for the well child, a much stricter dietary regimen is needed during illness. It is critical to inhibit the mobilisation of fatty acids which would result in the production of toxic fatty acid metabolites and precipitate overwhelming illness. If the child is unwell and has a reduced appetite, the standard emergency regimen (ER) of very frequent feeds, day and night, of glucose polymer should be given without delay (p. 287). Long chain fat intake should be excluded from the diet during the acute period and MCT is strictly contraindicated. As the child improves, the normal diet can be resumed but extra ER drinks should be given, particularly during the night, until the child is fully recovered and eating well. If the ER is not tolerated then the child should have rapid access to their local paediatric services, avoiding casualty, so there is no delay in starting an intravenous infusion of 10% dextrose. Management decisions should be based on the child's clinical state. Monitoring of blood glucose at home is not recommended because hypoglycaemia is a relatively late finding during illness in MCAD deficiency [9].

Long chain fatty acid oxidation disorders

The long chain fatty acid oxidation disorders include:

- *Defects in the carnitine dependent pathway* Carnitine palmitoyl transferases I and II (CPT I and CPT II), carnitine acylcarnitine translocase (CAT) and the transporter for uptake of carnitine across the cell membrane (OCTN2)
- *Defects of beta-oxidation* Very long chain acyl-CoA dehydrogenase deficiency (VLCAD) and trifunctional protein (TFP) complex in which the long chain 3-hydroxy acyl-CoA dehydrogenase enzyme resides (LCHAD deficiency) (Fig. 17.1).

The clinical features of CPT I deficiency resemble those of MCAD deficiency (except that some patients have a renal tubular acidosis during infancy). The other disorders of long chain fatty acid oxidation are substantially more severe. The presenting clinical picture is usually one of collapse, coma and fasting hypoglycaemia in the neonatal period. There is also a risk of cardiomyopathy and episodes of rhabdomyolysis; indeed, in cases of partial CPT II deficiency, exercise-induced rhabdomyolysis is usually the only clinical problem. These features are probably attributable to impaired energy production and a toxic effect of accumulated fatty acids and long chain acyl-CoA intermediates in the mitochondria.

Dietary management

Patients with defects of the transporter for cellular carnitine uptake (OCTN2) usually show an excellent response to carnitine (50 mg/kg twice daily) and require little dietary modification.

Dietary management is similar for all the other long chain disorders, except that the use of MCT may need to be limited in the defects of the carnitine dependent pathway [1, 10]. The main aim of dietary treatment is to minimise fatty acid oxidation. Since fatty acids for oxidation are derived from both dietary fat and adipose tissue, it is necessary to restrict the intake of dietary fat (minimal long chain fat) and to institute frequent feeding with a high carbohydrate intake to reduce production of fatty acids from adipose tissue.

The safe upper limit for long chain fat intake is not known and this will obviously vary with the severity of the disorder. In patients with VLCAD and TFP defects (including LCHAD), medium chain fats provide a useful energy source and may have other beneficial effects [11]. Dietary MCT is rapidly converted to ketone bodies, which are thought to inhibit the mobilisation of fatty acids from adipose tissue and the oxidation of fatty acids by cardiac muscle. For disorders of the carnitine dependent pathway, MCT intake may need to be limited (or even, perhaps, avoided in severe defects) since entry of medium chain triglycerides into mitochondria is partly carnitine dependent [1, 10, 12].

Since long chain fat intake is minimal, essential fatty acid (EFA) supplements are required. At least 1% of total energy intake should come from linoleic acid and 0.2% from alpha-linolenic acid [13]. Deficiency in plasma of the long chain polyunsaturated fatty acid, docosahexaenoic acid (DHA) has been reported and it has been suggested that this might be responsible for the pigmentary retinopathy seen in LCHAD deficient patients [14]. Other patients with retinopathy have, however, had normal plasma and red cell DHA levels (pers. comm. Leonard & Morris).

Frequent feeding is recommended to reduce lipolysis, with three hourly feeding during the day and continuous nasogastric or gastrostomy feeding overnight. If this is not possible, the child should be woken for feeds during the night. In children over the age of 2 years uncooked cornstarch can provide 'slow-release glucose' and may allow the interval between feeds to be extended. Before use the metabolic response to cornstarch should be assessed since this varies between patients.

The following provides a guide to the typical energy distribution and long chain fat intake of the diet for long chain disorders:

- 70–75% energy from carbohydrate
- 10–15% energy from protein
- up to 20% energy from medium chain fat (depending on the disorder)
- 1.2–2% energy from EFAs.

Long chain fat intake (including EFAs):

- Infants   <3 g/day
- 1–3 years   up to 6 g/day
- 4–8 years   up to 8 g/day
- 8–12 years   up to 12 g/day

Dietary management of long chain beta-oxidation disorders

Infants

Infants need a minimal long chain fat (LCT), high carbohydrate feed with frequent feeding. This can be provided by Monogen, a nutritionally complete infant formula with minimal LCT (Table 17.1). Monogen contains MCT, so it is important to establish if MCT can be oxidised before using this feed. A modular feed without fat (long or medium chain) may need to be used initially until the diagnosis is confirmed. Skimmed milk powder or a whey protein powder, e.g. Maxipro, can be used as the protein base with glucose polymer and additional minerals and vitamins to provide recommended intakes. EFAs should also be

Table 17.1 Nutritional content per 100 ml standard dilution (17.5%) of Monogen

Energy	74 kcal (310 kJ)
Protein	2 g
Carbohydrate	12 g
Fat – MCT (93%)	1.86 g
– LCT (7%)	0.14 g
Linoleic acid	0.09 g
Alpha-linolenic acid	0.02 g

Reconstitution: 1 scoop (4.5 g) added to 25 ml or 1 oz of water provided if the infant remains on a modular feed for several days.

The newly diagnosed infant is likely to be on intravenous (IV) 10% dextrose. While oral or nasogastric feeds are being introduced, IV fluids should be gradually reduced so that an adequate energy intake is maintained and further metabolic decompensation is prevented. The initial feeds given may vary depending on the clinical situation but should, if possible, provide 10 g carbohydrate/100 ml (10% CHO). Once the infant is well and established on full feeds of Monogen these should be given three hourly during the daytime and as a continuous feed overnight. The night feed can be commenced 2 hours after the last three hourly day feed was given and probably be stopped 2 hours before the first oral feed in the morning. The actual amount of glucose required overnight to minimise lipolysis is not known. For older infants current practice is to provide 0.5 gCHO/kg/hour which will equal basal glucose production rates (p. 297) and should therefore minimise lipolysis. This amount will easily be exceeded in the young infant who is being fed Monogen throughout the day and night at normal fluid requirements.

Weaning is commenced at the normal age of 4–6 months. Solids should have a minimal fat content (around 2 g/day) and be high in CHO. Rice cereal, potato and fruit are suitable as first weaning foods. Once these have been introduced low fat, high protein foods can also be given, e.g. turkey, white fish, lentils and low fat yoghurt. Commercial baby foods can be included in the diet but need to be limited to those which have a low fat content (Table 17.2).

As the amount of solid food increases this can replace some of the three hourly Monogen day feeds. If the child has a poor appetite parents will need guidance on the amount of food needed at a meal to replace the feed, at least 0.5 g CHO/kg/hour × three hourly to give sufficient CHO until the next feeding time is suggested. Infants who eat well will easily exceed this amount of CHO at a meal.

Monogen can continue to be given overnight, but nearer 1 year of age the feed volume can be decreased and glucose polymer added to provide the required amount of CHO (0.5 g CHO/kg/hour). A daily intake of 600 ml of Monogen will be needed to provide an adequate intake of fat soluble vitamins. Table 17.2 provides a suggested menu plan for infants.

Monogen will provide an adequate intake of EFAs when it is fed at 150 ml/kg, and provides the sole source of nutrition, but once solids are being taken

Table 17.2 Minimal long chain fat (<3 g) weaning diet: sample menu

8AM **Breakfast**	*Commercial baby cereal mix with Monogen
11AM	Monogen feed
1.00PM **Lunch**	Purée turkey, chicken (white only), white fish or lentils Purée potato Purée vegetables *Commercial baby savoury foods
4.00PM **Tea**	Purée fruit and sugar or *commercial baby fruit dessert Very low fat yoghurt or fromage frais Milk pudding (custard, cornflour, ground rice) made with Monogen
7.00PM	Monogen
9.00PM to 6.00AM	Continuous overnight feed of Monogen 30 ml per hour provides 0.5 g CHO/kg/hour for a 7 kg infant

Extra feeds of Monogen or baby juice can be given with meals

* Commercial baby foods
  Allow freely: wet baby foods ≤0.5 g fat/100 g and dried baby foods ≤2 g/100 g.
  Allow one serve per day: wet baby foods 0.5–1.0 g/100 g or dried baby foods 2–5 g/100 g.
  Walnut oil – refer to text for dose (p. 320).

Table 17.3 Walnut oil – essential fatty acid composition

1 ml walnut oil provides:	
Energy	8.4 kcal 35 kJ
Fat	0.93 g
Linoleic acid	0.55 g
Alpha-linolenic acid	0.12 g
Ratio n6 : n3 fatty acids	4.5

Analysis provided by Scientific Hospital Supplies International Limited.

and the volume decreases an additional source is needed. Walnut oil provides a good source of EFAs at an acceptable ratio and allows a minimum amount of long chain fat to be given (Table 17.3). To provide the suggested requirement of EFAs the dose of walnut oil needed is 0.1 ml per 56 kcal (234 kJ) of the estimated average requirement of energy for age [13], subtracting the energy provided by Monogen feeds. It is adminstered as a single dose and given as a medicine from a spoon or via the feeding tube. In the UK walnut oil can be purchased from most large chain supermarkets. It should be stored as recommended to avoid peroxidation.

Children

Children need to continue on a minimal fat, high CHO diet, with an energy distribution as previously outlined, with frequent feeding. During the daytime 3–4 hourly feeding and at night continuous overnight tube feeds are necessary to minimise lipolysis. The amount of glucose given overnight should at least equal basal glucose production rates for age (around 0.3 to 0.5 g CHO/kg/hour). The night feed can be changed to a glucose polymer solution. Monogen and glucose polymer could also be continued but the volume of Monogen should be limited so it does not provide too high an energy intake and interfere with daytime appetite. Alternatively, uncooked cornstarch (cornflour) could be given during the night. A hospital admission is recommended if initiating this treatment so that fasting tolerance can be assessed. The results of these studies are used to plan how frequently a dose of cornflour needs to be given (our experience with a few patients has shown this to be around six hourly). Doses of cornflour used are 2 g/kg in young children and 1 g/kg in older children and this is usually mixed with Monogen or skimmed milk.

The minimal fat diet is provided mainly by starchy foods and very low fat sources of protein such as white fish, white chicken or turkey meat, or pulses (Table 17.4). It is best to give the necessary high CHO intake from starchy foods (e.g. rice, pasta, potato, bread, cereals) as these will be more slowly digested than sugary foods. However, it is recognised that not all children can manage such a bulky diet and sugar containing foods such as jelly, low fat ice-cream, cake or biscuits, should form part of their diet. Nowadays there are many very low fat alternatives to regular high fat foods such as crisps, sauces, desserts, ice-cream and cheeses which can also be incorporated into the diet. To allow a greater variety of foods parents need to be given guidance on interpreting food labels for fat content and on understanding the many and potentially misleading descriptions used about the fat content of food, e.g. reduced fat, low fat, virtually fat free, 90% fat free.

MCT oil can be incorporated into the diet to increase palatability and provide an alternative source of energy. Also, some MCT is stored in adipose tissue

and can be used as an energy source [15]. MCT oils available in the UK contain predominantly C8 and C10 fatty acids and are suitable for children with long chain beta-oxidation defects. MCT oil has a low smoke point compared with other cooking oils. Care must therefore be taken to ensure it does not burn or become overheated as it develops a bitter taste and unpleasant odour. The optimium cooking temperature for MCT is 160°C. MCT oil can be used for cooking and baking, e.g. cakes, biscuits and pastry.

Supplements of fat soluble vitamins (A, D and E) will be needed unless the child remains on 600 ml of Monogen. Intakes of iron, zinc and B_{12} should be regularly calculated as these can be low on minimal fat diets. Forceval Junior Capsules can provide an adequate intake of fat soluble vitamins and minerals. EFAs can be provided from Monogen and walnut oil, as described above for infants.

Disorders of the carnitine dependent pathway

The dietary management of these disorders is the same as for long chain beta-oxidation defects (see above) with the exception of MCT. Since patients with disorders of the carnitine pathway may have impaired uptake of medium chain fatty acids, it has been recommended that their MCT intake should be limited and carefully monitored [1, 10, 12]. If MCT is restricted, more energy will need to be given from CHO. Monogen may not be a suitable feed and a minimal fat modular feed with less MCT may be indicated. Skimmed milk powder or a whey protein powder can be used as the protein base with glucose polymer to the required amount of CHO (e.g. 12–15%) and vitamins, minerals and EFAs to provide the suggested intakes [13]. MCT emulsion such as Liquigen could be added to the individual patient's tolerance. Scientific Hospital Supplies have recently produced a Fat Free Module Feed which could also be used, but this is not available on prescription. For older children use of MCT oil in cooking may need to be restricted.

Diet during illness for long chain fatty acid oxidation disorders

If the child becomes unwell and has a reduced appetite the standard emergency regimen (ER) of very frequent feeds, day and night, of glucose polymer should be given (p. 287). These can be given

Table 17.4 Minimal long chain fat diet

	Foods allowed	Foods to avoid
Milk	Skimmed milk, condensed skimmed milk Natural yoghurt, very low fat yoghurt and fromage frais Low fat cottage cheese *95% fat free cheeses Quark (skimmed milk soft cheese) Low fat ice-cream	Full fat and semi-skimmed milk. Cream Full fat yoghurt and fromage frais Full and half fat cheeses †Ice-cream
Egg	Egg whites	Egg yolks
Fish	White fish (no skin), e.g. haddock, cod, sole, plaice Crab, crabsticks, tuna, prawns, shrimps, lobster	Oily fish, e.g. sardines, kippers, salmon, mackerel Fish in breadcrumbs, batter, sauces, pastry
Poultry	*Chicken,*turkey (white breast meat, no skin)	Chicken, turkey (dark meat and skin), basted poultry, duck Chicken in breadcrumbs, batter, sauces, pastry
Meat	*Lean red meat (<5% fat content)	Fatty meat, sausages (normal and low fat), burgers, meat paste, paté, salami, pies
Meat substitutes	Soya mince, *Quorn, *tofu	
Pulses	Peas, e.g. chick peas, split peas, lentils Beans, e.g. red, white, borlotti, black-eyed	
Fats/oils	Medium chain triglyceride oil as permitted	Butter, margarine, low fat spread, vegetable oils, lard, dripping, suet, shortening
Pasta and rice	Spaghetti, macaroni, other pasta, noodles, cous cous, rice (white)	Wholemeal pasta, pasta in dishes, e.g. macaroni cheese, carbonara, Brown rice, egg noodles
Flours and cereals	Flour (white), cornflour, custard powder, semolina, sago, tapioca	Flour (wholemeal), soya flour, oats, bran Foods made with flour which contain fat, e.g. pastry, sauces, cake, biscuits, batter, breadcrumb coatings
Breakfast cereals	Most are suitable Wholewheat cereals, e.g. Weetabix, bran flakes are higher in fat content than non-wholewheat cereals, e.g. Rice Krispies, cornflakes	Cereals with nuts, e.g. muesli All-bran, Ready Brek
Bread and crackers	*White bread, white pitta, crumpets, muffins Some crackers have a low fat content, e.g. rice cakes, Matzos, Ryvita (not sesame)	Wholemeal, wholegrain breads, naan bread, chapatti made with fat, croissant, oatcakes, cheese crackers, †crackers
Cakes and biscuits and pastry	Only those made from low fat ingredients 95% fat free cakes and biscuits	†Cakes, †biscuits, buns, pastry for sweet and savoury foods, e.g. apple pie, quiche
Desserts	Jelly, meringue, sorbet, very low fat ice-cream, skimmed milk puddings, e.g. rice, custard	Most desserts, e.g. whole milk puddings, trifle, cheesecakes, gateaux, †mousse, fruit pie or crumble
Fruit	Most varities – fresh, frozen, tinned, dried	Avocado pears, olives
Vegetables	All vegetables and salad Very low fat crisps	Chips, †crisps, †low fat crisps, roast potato, potato or vegetable salad in mayonnaise or salad dressing, †coleslaw
Herbs and spices	Pickles, chutney Herbs, spices, salt, pepper	
Nuts Seeds		Nuts, peanut butter, seeds, e.g. sesame, sunflower
Sauces and gravies	Tomato ketchup, brown sauce, soy sauce, Marmite, Oxo, Bovril, very low fat gravy mixes Fat-free dressings and mayonnaise Minimal fat sauces (jars, tins, packets)	†Gravy granules, †stock cubes Salad cream, mayonnaise, oil and vinegar dressings †Sauce mixes (jars, tins, packets)

Table 17.4 *Continued*

	Foods allowed	Foods to avoid
Soups	Some low calorie and 'healthy eating type' soups are very low fat	Most soups, cream soups
Confectionery	Boiled sweets, jelly sweets, fruit gums, pastilles, marshmallow, mints, ice-lollies	Chocolate, chocolate covered sweets, toffee, fudge, butter mints
Sugars and preserves	Sugar, golden syrup, jam, marmalade, honey, treacle	Lemon curd, chocolate spread
Baking products	Baking powder, bicarbonate of soda, yeast, arrowroot, essences, food colouring	
Drinks	Fruit juice, squash, fizzy drinks, milkshake flavourings, tea, coffee	†Instant chocolate drinks, cocoa, malted milk type drinks, e.g. Horlicks

* Intake of these foods may need to be restricted because of their fat content.
† These foods in the 'avoid list' often have very low fat equivalents which can be included in the diet.

via the tube if refused orally. It is important to stress the early use of the ER to inhibit the mobilisation of fatty acids as decompensation may be rapid. Long chain fat is strongly contraindicated and if the diet contains MCT it is best avoided initially. As the child improves, the normal diet can be resumed. While the normal diet is being reintroduced it is essential to maximise energy intake and continue with frequent feeding, usually two to three hourly by day and continuous tube feeds overnight.

Patients with cardiomyopathy should probably be admitted during any intercurrent illness since there is a risk of deteriorating cardiac function. Families should also be warned to look for dark urine, since illness can precipitate rhabdomyolysis with myoglobinuria and, occasionally, acute renal failure. As in MCAD, blood glucose monitoring by parents is not recommended since hypoglycaemia is a relatively late finding and treatment should be initiated long before this develops [9].

Multiple acyl-CoA dehydrogenase deficiency

Multiple acyl-CoA dehydrogenase deficiency (MADD) or glutaric aciduria type II is caused by defects in the electron transfer flavoprotein pathway which carries electrons to the respiratory chain from the six flavin-dependent acyl-CoA dehydrogenases. Defects in this pathway will therefore affect the oxidation of fatty acids (long, medium and short) as well as the oxidation of branch chain organic acids and lysine and tryptophan. MADD can present either as

a severe neonatal form or a milder later onset form. Neonatal onset cases are associated with cardiomyopathy and often with congenital malformations, such as renal cysts. All forms of the disorder can cause muscle weakness and episodes of hypoglycaemic encephalopathy. Some mild cases show a clinical and biochemical response to riboflavin (100–200 mg/day). These patients usually present with progressive weakness as young adults, though there may be a long history of vague symptoms such as abdominal migraine [16].

Dietary management

In severe neonatal cases with congenital malformations, no treatment is effective or appropriate. At the other end of the spectrum, some patients respond completely to riboflavin and no dietary modification is necessary. The mild variants are treated with a modest restriction of protein and fat, since MADD affects the oxidation of some amino acids in addition to fatty acids. Designing an appropriate diet can be difficult and the degree of restriction needs to be individually tailored to the patient. Regular feeding with a high CHO intake is recommended to reduce lipolysis. Overnight fasting might be a problem. It may be sufficient to give a late-night bedtime snack; however, some might require a more frequent feeding regimen. Uncooked cornflour could be used in older children to provide a source of 'slow-release glucose' and reduce the need for frequent feeding. It is essential to assess tolerance individually (p. 299). Medium chain fatty acids are best avoided in MADD deficiency.

Dietary guidelines are to provide:

- 65–70% energy from carbohydrate
- 8–10% energy from protein
- 20–25% energy from fat
- frequent feeding to tolerance.

During illness the standard emergency regimen of very frequent feeds, day and night, of glucose polymer should be given to minimise endogenous protein catabolism and lipolysis (p. 287). These should be given via a tube if not managed orally. Long chain fats should be avoided during the acute period. The usual diet can be introduced during the recovery period, but it is important to continue with frequent feeding and additional glucose polymer feeds until the normal diet is resumed.

3-Hydroxy-3-methylglutaryl-CoA lyase deficiency

Children with 3-hydroxy-3-methylglutaryl-CoA lyase deficiency (HMGCoA lyase deficiency or 3-hydroxy-3-methylglutaric aciduria) effectively have defects in two metabolic pathways. The final step of the catabolic pathway of leucine is deficient and the last step of ketone synthesis. The latter means acetyl-CoA from fatty acid oxidation is not converted to ketone bodies. Patients normally present either in the early neonatal period or later between 3 and 11 months of age with episodes of illness characterised by vomiting, lethargy, hypotonia, hypoglycaemia and a metabolic acidosis (with a notable absence of ketones) which may progress to coma [17].

Dietary management

Dietary treatment probably necessitates a restriction of both dietary protein and fat, as the accumulated toxic metabolites are derived from leucine catabolism and the ketone body synthesis pathway. However, fat restriction has been shown to be more effective in reducing the abnormal metabolite production [18] and only a modest protein restriction is necessary. Medium chain triglycerides are contraindicated. It is also important to avoid prolonged fasts to reduce fatty acid oxidation. Infants need to be fed at regular intervals. Tolerance to fasting may need to be individually assessed when considering how long the infant/toddler can safely fast for overnight. Older children

can be on a more relaxed diet but it is important to give regular meals (including a bedtime snack) and a high CHO intake from starch. Missed meals should be replaced with a high CHO drink.

Dietary guidelines are to provide:

- 8–10% energy from protein
- 25% energy from fat
- 65% energy from carbohydrate.

During intercurrent infections the standard emergency regimen (p. 287) is used to reduce protein catabolism and lipolysis, hence limiting the production of toxic metabolites from both defective pathways. During the recovery phase the usual protein and fat intake can be reintroduced over a period of a few days.

REFERENCES

1 Schaefer J *et al.* Characterisation of carnitine palmitoyltransferases in patients with a carnitine palmitoyl transferase deficiency: implications for diagnosis and therapy. *J Neurol Neurosurg Psychiatry*, 1997, **62** 169–76.

2 Roe C, Coates P Mitochondrial fatty acid oxidation disorders. In: Scriver C *et al.* (eds) *The Metabolic and Molecular Basis of Inherited Disease*, 7e. New York: McGraw Hill, 1995, pp. 1501–34.

3 Seddon HR *et al.* Regional variations in medium-chain acyl-CoA dehydrogenase deficiency (letter). *Lancet*, 1995, **345** 135–6.

4 Iafolla AK, Thompson RJ, Roe CR Medium-chain acyl-CoA dehydrogenase deficiency: clinical course in 120 affected children. *J Paediatr*, 1994, **124** 409–15.

5 Touma EH, Charpentier C Medium-chain acyl-CoA dehydrogenase deficiency. *Arch Dis Childh*, 1992, **67** 142–5.

6 Wilcken B, Hammond J, Silink M Mortality and morbidity in medium chain acyl-coenzyme A dehydrogenase deficiency. *Arch Dis Childh*, 1994, **70** 410–12.

7 Heales SJR *et al.* Production and disposal of medium-chain fatty acids in children with medium-chain acyl-CoA dehydrogenase deficiency. *J Inher Metab Dis*, 1994, **17** 74–80.

8 Wilcken B, Carpenter KH, Hammond J Neonatal symptoms in medium chain acyl-coenzyme A dehydrogenase deficiency. *Arch Dis Childh*, 1993, **69** 292–4.

9 Morris AAM, Leonard JV Early recognition of metabolic decompensation. *Arch Dis Childh*, 1997, **76** 555–6.

10 Parini R *et al.* Medium chain triglyceride loading test in

carnitine-acylcarnitine translocase deficiency: insights on treatment. *J Inher Metab Dis*, 1999, **22** 733–9.

11 Morris AAM, Turnball DM Fatty acid oxidation defect in muscle. *Curr Opin Neurol*, 1998, **11** 485–90.

12 Chalmers RA *et al*. Mitochondrial carnitine-acyl carnitine translocase deficiency presenting as sudden neonatal death. *J Pediatr*, 1997, **131** 220–25.

13 Department of Health Report on Health and Social Subjects No 41. *Dietary Reference Values for Food Energy and Nutrients for the United Kingdom*. London: The Stationery Office, 1991.

14 Harding CO *et al*. Docosahexaenoic acid and retinal function in children with long-chain 3-hydroxyacyl-CoA dehydrogenase deficiency. *J Inher Metab Dis*, 1999, **22** 276–80.

15 Sarda P *et al*. Storage of medium chain triglycerides in adipose tissue of orally fed infants. *Am J Clin Nutr*, 1987, **45** 399–405.

16 Frerman FE, Goodman SI Nuclear-encoded defects of the mitochondrial respiratory chain including glutaric acidaemia type II. In: Scriver C *et al*. (eds) *The Metabolic and Molecular Basis of Inherited Disease*, 7e. New York: McGraw Hill, 1995, pp. 1611–29.

17 Sweetman L, Williams JC Branched chain organic acidurias. In: Scriver C *et al*. (eds) *The Metabolic and Molecular Basis of Inherited Disease*, 7e. New York: McGraw Hill, 1995, pp. 1387–422.

18 Walter J, Clayton P, Leonard J Case report, 3-hydroxy-3-methylglutaryl-CoA lyase deficiency. *J Inher Metab Dis*, 1986, **9** 286–8.

USEFUL ADDRESS

LCHAD & VLCAD Parent Support Group
118 Hull Road, Anlaby, East Yorkshire HU10 6UB.

SECTION 6

Lipids

CHAPTER 18

Lipid Disorders

There are three main types of lipid in the body: triglycerides, cholesterol and phospholipids. They are transported in the serum bound to specific proteins called apolipoproteins to form the four major lipoprotein families (Table 18.1). Each of these lipoproteins contain a different amount of cholesterol and triglyceride and have different functions:

- *Chylomicrons* carry dietary triglycerides from the intestine to peripheral tissues
- *Very low density lipoproteins (VLDL)* are synthesised by the liver and carry excess triglycerides produced by the liver to other tissues
- *Low density lipoproteins (LDL)* are formed from VLDL and transport cholesterol from the liver to the peripheral tissues
- *High density lipoproteins (HDL)* transport excess cholesterol from the cells to the liver for excretion in the bile.

Disorders of lipid metabolism which are managed by dietary intervention can be classified into those in which serum lipoproteins are deficient or absent (hypolipoproteinaemia) or those in which they are increased (hyperlipoproteinaemia) (Tables 18.2 and 18.3). The nature of the lipid disorder should be determined by measurement of serum lipoprotein fractions as well as total serum cholesterol and triglycerides.

Hyperlipoproteinaemia, secondary to diabetes, nephrotic syndrome or glygogen storage disease, is treated by management of the underlying disease and specific dietary measures are not usually necessary. The dietary management of the primary disorders which are genetically inherited are reviewed. A brief description of the biochemical defect of each disorder is given; more detailed information on the biochemistry can be found in the references at the end of the chapter.

THE HYPOLIPOPROTEINAEMIAS

All the primary hypolipoproteinaemias (Table 18.2) are rare and only abetalipoproteinaemia and occasionally hypobetalipoproteinaemia require dietary management.

ABETALIPOPROTEINAEMIA

This is an autosomal recessive disorder characterised by the virtual absence of VLDL, LDL and chylomicrons from plasma. It is thought that abetalipoproteinaemia is due to defects in the processing of β apoproteins or impairment of the assembly or secretion of triglyceride rich proteins [1]. The clinical features of abetalipoproteinaemia are diverse. The presenting clinical feature is usually severe fat malabsorption seen in the neonatal period as steatorrhoea and failure to gain weight. This is accompanied by low plasma levels of vitamins E, A and K. Other features are acanthocytosis of red blood cells, neurological lesions and ocular manifestations, predominantly retinitis pigmentosa.

The onset of neurological symptoms may be during the first year of life; ophthalmic symptom onset is variable but may begin during the first decade. The neurological and ophthalmic manifestations appear to be secondary to defects of transport of vitamin E; vitamin A deficiency may also contribute to retinopathy [1, 2]. Despite the inability to secrete chylomicrons there does appear to be some

Table 18.1 Composition of lipoproteins

Lipoprotein class	Principal lipids	Major apolipoproteins
Chylomicrons	Dietary triglycerides	A,B,C
VLDL	Endogenous triglycerides	B,C,E
LDL	Cholesterol ester and cholesterol	B
HDL	Cholesterol ester and phospholipid	A

Table 18.2 Classification and treatment of hypolipoproteinaemias

Primary disorder	Lipoprotein class	Treatment
Abetalipoproteinaemia	Chylomicrons LDL	Very low fat diet Vitamin A, E, K supplements MCT not recommended
Hypobetalipoproteinaemia	LDL	None usually indicated Low fat diet if steatorrhoea is a problem

MCT-Medium chain triglycerides

Table 18.3 Classification of hyperlipoproteinaemias

Primary disorder	Lipoprotein class
Familial hyperchylomicronaemia (type I)	Chylomicrons
Familial hypercholesterolaemia (type IIa)	LDL
Familial combined hyperlipidaemia (type IIb)	LDL VLDL
Familial type III hyperlipidaemia (broad beta disease)	IDL
Familial hypertriglyceridaemia (type IV)	VLDL
Familial hyperlipoproteinaemia (type V)	Chylomicrons

IDL-Intermediate density lipoprotein

absorption of long chain fatty acids [3]. These are probably transferred to the liver as free fatty acids. Levels of essential fatty acids are low in plasma and tissue although clinical deficiency is not reported.

Treatment results in catch-up growth and further growth and development are normal.

Dietary management

The gastrointestinal symptoms respond to a low fat diet. The degree of fat restriction is determined by individual tolerance which increases with age and intake and can vary from 5 g/day in infants to 20 g/day in an older child. Although clinical deficiency of essential fatty acids has not been reported, a proportion of dietary fat should be provided as essential fatty acids (EFAs). Recommendations are that for infants, children and adults linoleic acid should provide at least 1% of the total energy, and alpha linolenic acid at least 0.2% of the total energy [4]. It should be borne in mind that these are minimum requirements for EFAs and their absorption will be impaired. At present there is no specific guidance for EFA supplementation in abetalipoproteinaemia and individual tolerance of total fat limits the amount of supplement which can be given. Individual monitoring of essential fatty acid status is recommended in order to optimise EFA supplementation.

Medium chain triglyceride (MCT)

Fatty acids derived from MCT do not require chylomicrons for absorption as they are transported via the hepatic portal system. Reports of hepatic fibrosis have, however, been associated with the use of MCT in abetalipoproteinaemia and its use is not recommended [5].

Infancy

In infancy a low fat modular feed can be formulated (Table 18.4) using a protein source, e.g. Maxipro, Vitapro or skimmed milk powder, glucose polymer and an essential fatty acid source, e.g. walnut oil or soya oil. A long chain fat (LCT) emulsion (Calogen) can then be added to tolerance. This feed will require vitamin, mineral and trace element supplementation, which should be tailored to meet individual requirements.

Weaning

Weaning foods should be introduced at the usual age of 4–6 months. Very low fat foods are suitable,

Table 18.4 Minimal fat feed for infants for use in abetalipoproteinaemia

Per 100 ml	Energy		Protein (g)	CHO (g)	Fat (g)	Sodium (mmol)	Potassium (mmol)
	(kJ)	(kcal)					
2 g Maxipro	33	8	1.6	Trace	Trace	0.1	0.2
15 g Glucose polymer	225	60	0	14	0	Trace	Trace
Water to 100 ml							
Total	258	68	1.6	14	Trace	0.1	0.2

1 Fat can be added to tolerance using an LCT emulsion (e.g. Calogen), and the glucose polymer can be decreased accordingly.

2 Vitamins, minerals, trace elements and electrolytes must be supplemented to ensure individual requirements are met.

3 A source of essential fatty acids is required to be added to the feed

e.g. baby rice, fruit, vegetables and pulses (p. 320). The infant should continue to take a reasonable volume of feed to ensure nutritional requirements are met.

Childhood and adolescence

It is necessary to continue with the use of glucose polymers to ensure sufficient energy is taken and normal growth and development are achieved. With increasing age children may maintain energy intakes by regular consumption of carbohydrate foods, e.g. sugar, sweets, jam, fizzy drinks, bread, pasta, potatoes and rice.

Many low fat products, e.g. biscuits, cakes and savoury foods, can be made by adapting standard recipes. Regular dietary assessment should be undertaken throughout life to ensure the diet remains nutritionally adequate.

Vitamins A, E and K

The following therapeutic doses are recommended [6]:

- Vitamin A   7000 µg/day to maintain normal plasma concentrations
- Vitamin E   100 mg/kg/day. Concentrated preparations now permit the convenient administration of these doses
- Vitamin K   5–10 mg/day.

These supplements should be in a water miscible form. It is not necessary to supplement vitamin D in this way.

THE HYPERLIPOPROTEINAEMIAS

The main types of primary hyperlipoproteinaemia are summarised in Table 18.3 and the typing system advocated by the World Health Organisation is used. The two most commonly encountered in childhood are familial hyperchylomicronaemia (type I) and familial hypercholesterolaemia (type IIa). These two are discussed in detail. The other disorders, familial combined hyperlipidaemia (type IIb), familial type III hyperlipidaemia, familial hypertriglyceridaemia (type IV) and familial hyperlipoproteinaemia (type V) are rarely expressed in childhood and treatment is therefore not described.

FAMILIAL HYPERCHYLOMICRONAEMIA (TYPE I)

The manifestation of the clinical features of this rare disorder varies greatly and often the child is asymptomatic. The asymptomatic child may be diagnosed by a chance finding of turbid plasma when a blood sample is taken for some other reason, or the finding of hepatomegaly or lipaemia retinalis in an older child. Alternatively, the child may present with attacks of acute abdominal pain due to pancreatitis and/or eruptive xanthomata and hepatosplenomegaly. The classical disorder is due to a molecular defect in the activity of the enzyme lipoprotein lipase. There is a group of patients who have a distinct molecular abnormality in the apolipoprotein CII activator of the lipoprotein lipase enzyme complex. These patients tend to present later than those with classical lipoprotein lipase deficiency [7]. It is inherited as an autosomal recessive trait. There is a failure to clear chylomicrons at the normal rate which leads to an accumulation in the serum and there is a gross elevation of triglycerides (35–115 mmol/l, normal fasting level 0.5–2.2 mmol/l), and moderate elevation of cholesterol. There is no current evidence that the high triglyceride levels are associated with an increased risk of atherosclerosis in later life. Growth and development are normal and clinical deficiency of linoleic acid has not been reported.

Dietary management

The aim of the dietary treatment is to relieve the symptoms. Restriction of fat to 5 g/day will result in optically clear fasting serum and lowering of serum triglycerides. However, it is difficult to maintain this restriction long term, and fat intake is determined by tolerance. Triglycerides will remain high but as the condition is not associated with premature atherosclerosis there is no need for severe dietary restriction.

Acute episodes

During attacks of acute abdominal pain, a fat-free diet should be given (<5 g LCT a day) (Table 12.9). This will produce a rapid decrease in serum triglyceride levels within 5–7 days. A suitable feed for an infant is shown in Table 18.4. Older children should have frequent high carbohydrate drinks and very low fat foods as tolerated.

Long term management

Fat   Fat intake can be gradually increased to tolerance, which is usually around 20–30 g a day, although there is individual variation. Tolerance does not seem to increase with age. The fat should be equally distributed between meals. The serum triglyceride level will increase, but the restriction should be sufficient to avoid attacks of acute pancreatitis or the development of xanthomata. In infants a LCT emulsion

(Calogen) can then be added to the low fat feed (Table 18.4) to tolerance.

Medium chain triglycerides   MCT emulsion (Liquigen) can also be used to provide additional energy. Several MCT based formulas are available (Table 6.19).

The amount of LCT in some of these feeds may be too high for the acute phase. Feeds containing MCT should always be introduced slowly and care should be taken to ensure that the feed provides sufficient essential fatty acids [8].

In older children MCT oils and emulsions can also be used to provide extra energy and to improve the palatability of the diet. They should always be introduced slowly. MCT oils and emulsions can be used in cooking and baking.

Energy   Energy requirements can be met by the use of MCT, refined carbohydrates, and glucose polymers if necessary.

Vitamins and minerals   In infants on modular feeds, supplementation of the feeds is essential. MCT-based complete infant formula feeds should provide adequate intakes provided sufficient volume is taken. Older children should have a supplement of fat-soluble vitamins.

FAMILIAL HYPERCHOLESTEROLAEMIA (TYPE IIA)

Familial hypercholesterolaemia (FH) is the most common primary lipoprotein disorder of childhood and is inherited as an autosomal dominant trait. It is characterised by an elevated plasma LDL concentration and deposition of LDL cholesterol in tendons, skin (xanthomas) and arteries (atheromas). The primary defect is a mutation in the gene for the LDL receptor in the hepatic and extra-hepatic cells. This results in a reduction in the rate of removal of plasma LDL which is then deposited in the cells producing xanthomas and atheromas. The incidence of homozygous FH is 1 in 1 000 000. It is characterised by severe hypercholesterolaemia (plasma cholesterol levels approximately 16–26 mmol/l) and coronary heart disease which begins in childhood; death from myocardial infarction frequently occurs before the age of 20 years. Cholesterol levels in children are generally considered to be normal up to a level of

5 mmol/l. Reference ranges will differ, however, between laboratories, and plasma cholesterol levels will change throughout childhood due to the influences of growth and puberty. Homozygotes for FH are generally resistant to dietary treatment, and radical therapy such as plasma LDL apheresis or liver transplantation may be considered. The incidence of heterozygous FH is approximately 1 in 500 and is one of the most common inborn errors of metabolism. Plasma cholesterol levels are typically 9–14 mmol/l from birth. Tendon xanthomas and coronary atherosclerosis usually develop after 20–30 years [9]. For the purpose of this chapter diet therapy will refer to the treatment of heterozygous FH.

Screening

Routine screening for FH is not currently undertaken. The recommendations of the British Hyperlipidaemia Association are as follows [10]:

- The use of selective screening based on a family history of FH or of premature coronary artery disease (premature defined as <50 years for men and <55 years for women)
- Measurement of non-fasting total cholesterol as a suitable screening test. If >5.5 mmol/l, then measure fasting total cholesterol, HDL cholesterol and triglyceride
- In a child under 16, total cholesterol >6.7 mmol/l and LDL cholesterol >4.0 mmol/l on two occasions more than one month apart should be considered abnormal
- Screening should not be carried out before 2 years of age but hypercholesterolaemia should be diagnosed before 10 years of age
- Affected children should be referred for specialist care.

Dietary management

The aim of dietary management is to lower total serum and LDL cholesterol in an attempt to decrease the risk of cardiovascular disease in later life.

Energy intake

This should be based on age, weight and activity levels [4]. Obesity itself is a risk factor for coronary heart disease and if present then weight reduction must be the primary goal of diet therapy.

Total fat intake

The principal aim of the diet traditionally used in the treatment of FH has been to reduce the total dietary fat to 30–35% of total energy intake. This is achieved by avoidance of fried foods and those known to be high in fat. In addition, low fat dairy products, i.e. skimmed or semi-skimmed milk, low fat cheese and yoghurt are advocated. Lean meat is usually advised to be taken only once per day, using beans, pulses, poultry and fish as protein sources in preference. Eggs may be included as part of the total fat allowance.

Compliance with this dietary treatment is often poor due to its potentially bulky nature and low satiety value. In addition, energy from carbohydrate is substituted for fat resulting in a reduction in both HDL and LDL cholesterol [11]. This reduces total plasma cholesterol levels but leaves the LDL:HDL ratio unaffected and may not reduce the risk of coronary heart disease [12].

Saturated fatty acids (SFAs)

SFAs are limited to provide less than 10% of the total energy intake. There is much clinical and experimental evidence which shows that a diet high in SFAs is associated with increased plasma cholesterol concentrations.

Dietary cholesterol

Uncertainty remains as to whether dietary cholesterol requires restriction. In support of a restriction it is suggested that saturated fat downregulates the LDL receptor especially when cholesterol is concurrently present. Conversely there is the view that there is a negative feedback mechanism on the synthesis of cholesterol by the intake of dietary cholesterol. Where dietary cholesterol restriction is practised, foods low in saturated fat but high in dietary cholesterol, e.g. prawns and liver, are also excluded from the diet.

Polyunsaturated fatty acids (PUFAs)

PUFAs lower LDL cholesterol but there are concerns regarding their safety if used excessively. It is generally recommended that their intake should not exceed 10% of the total energy intake [4].

Monounsaturated fatty acids (MUFAs)

MUFAs have been shown to have a hypocholesterolaemic effect when substituted for SFAs in the diet. Replacing energy with MUFAs rather than carbohydrate does not result in a reduction in plasma HDL [13]. Significant reductions in coronary heart disease have also been shown using increased consumption of MUFAs from rapeseed margarine in a group of people after myocardial infarction [14]. There are many other reports of the beneficial effects of the Mediterranean diet which is high in MUFAs. Replacing energy lost from SFAs by MUFAs is currently used in some treatment centres. Anecdotally compliance with diet is reported to be better than that of a low total fat diet. The long term consequences of this type of diet therapy for children with FH are unknown and practice should perhaps be treated with caution until more information regarding its use has been gathered.

Garlic, oats and soy protein

A systematic review of trials in the general population suggested that garlic may exert a cholesterol lowering effect; however, the evidence is not reliable due to flaws in these trials. Systematic reviews of studies in the general population evaluating oat and soy protein consumption showed a cholesterol lowering effect [15].

Fat soluble vitamins

If a low fat diet is to be used then fat soluble vitamin supplementation may be required.

In order to examine the evidence for diet therapy in children with FH a systematic review is planned to be carried out and published on the Cochrane Library in 2000/2001. Readers are advised to access this once published [16].

Effectiveness and compliance

Dietary treatment can be expected to lower plasma cholesterol levels by 10–20%. Compliance with diet is often poor as the children feel well and cannot moti-

vate themselves to keep to a diet to avert symptoms which may not present clinically for 20 years or more. Inevitably compliance is always greater in families where there has been a parental death from coronary heart disease.

Drug therapy

Dietary intervention should always be the first line of treatment. The introduction of drugs will be influenced by plasma cholesterol concentration and family history. In the majority of cases long term management will be by a combination of drugs and diet. The only drugs currently licensed for children are Fenofibrate and Ion exchange resins (Cholestyramine and Colestipol). Resins are available as powders and can be mixed as a drink or with food. They are poorly tolerated by patients, but if used require the prescription of fat soluble vitamins and folate [17].

Since the late 1980s a new class of cholesterol lowering drugs – the statins (HMG CoA reductase Inhibitors) – have become available which can dramatically reduce plasma LDL cholesterol concentrations. They are not licensed for use in children.

Follow-up

Children with FH should ideally be seen in a combined adult/paediatric clinic to ensure dietary advice is uniform and to encourage the incorporation of advice into the family meal plan.

Emphasis should also be placed on the reduction of other risks for coronary heart disease, i.e. avoidance of smoking, increasing exercise, watching weight and managing stress.

REFERENCES

1 Kane JP, Havel RJ Disorders of the biogenesis and secretion of lipoproteins. In: Scriver CR *et al*. (eds) *The Metabolic and Molecular Basis of Inherited Disease*, 7e. New York: McGraw-Hill, 1995.
2 Desjeux JF Congenital transport defects. In: Walker *et al*. (eds) *Paediatric Gastrointestinal Disease*, 2e. St Louis: Mosby, 1996.
3 Hoghwinkel GJM, Brwyn GW Congenital lack of betalipoproteins. A study of blood phospholipids in a patient and his family. *J Neurol Sci*, 1996, 3 374.
4 Department of Health Report on Health and Social Subjects No. 41. *Dietary Reference Values for Food*,

Energy and Nutrients for the United Kingdom. London: The Stationery Office, 1991.

5 Illingworth DR, Connor WE, Miller RG Abetalipoproteinaemia: report of two cases and review of therapy. *Arch Neurol*, 1980, **37** 659.

6 Muller DPR, Lloyd JK, Wolf OH Vitamin E and neurological function. *Lancet*, 1983, **1** 225–8.

7 Nyham WL, Ozand PT *Atlas of Metabolic Diseases*. London: Chapman and Hall, 1998.

8 FAO/WHO *Dietary Fats and Oils in Human Nutrition*. Rome: FAO of the United Nations, 1980, pp. 21–37.

9 Goldstein JL, Hobbs H, Brown M Familial hypercholesterolaemia. In: Scriver CR *et al.* (eds) *The Metabolic and Molecular Basis of Inherited Disease*, 7e. New York: McGraw-Hill, 1995.

10 Wray R, Neil H, Rees J Screening for hyperlipidaemia in childhood. Recommendations of the British Hyperlipidaemia Association. *J R Coll Physicians*, London, 1996, Mar–Apr **30** 115–18.

11 Durrington PN Dietary fat and coronary heart disease. In: Poulter N, Sever P, Thom S (eds) *Cardiovascular Disease. Risk factors and intervention*. Oxford: Radcliffe Medical Press, 1993.

12 Clarke R, Frost C, Collins R *et al.* Dietary lipids and blood cholesterol: quantitative meta-analysis of metabolic ward studies. *Brit Med J*, 1997, **314** 112–17.

13 Colquhoun DM, Moores D, Somerset SS *et al.* Comparison of the effects on lipoproteins of a diet high in monounsaturated fatty acids enriched with avocado and a high carbohydrate diet. *Am J Clin Nutr*, 1992, **56** 671–7.

14 De Longeril M, Renaud S, Mamelle N *et al.* Mediterranean alpha linolenic acid rich diet in secondary prevention of coronary heart disease. *Lancet*, 1993, **343** 1454–9.

15 NHS Centre for Reviews and Dissemination. University of York. *Effective Health Care, Cholesterol and Coronary Heart Disease: Screening and Treatment*. Latimer Trend & Co. Ltd., 1998, **4** 1.

16 *The Cochrane Database of Systematic Reviews* (database on disk and CD Rom). The Cochrane Collaboration: Oxford: Update Software, Summertown Pavillion, Summertown, Oxford, England.

17 Tonstad S, Kudtzan J, Sivertsom M *et al.* Efficacy and safety of cholestyramine treatment in peripubertal and prepubertal children with familial hypercholesterolaemia. *J Paediatr*, 1996, **129** 4–7.

USEFUL ADDRESS

The Family Heart Association
7 North Road, Maidenhead, Berks SL6 1PE.

Peroxisomal Disorders

CHAPTER 19

Refsum's Disease

Heredopathia atactica polyneuritiformis (Refsum's disease) is a rare inborn error of lipid metabolism inherited as an autosomal recessive trait. The chief characteristics are retinitis pigmentosa, peripheral neuropathy, and cerebellar ataxia. Other manifestations can include nerve deafness, anosmia, ichthyosis, cardiac abnormalities and skeletal abnormalities.

Patients accumulate phytanic acid (3,7,11,15-tetramethyl hexadecanoic acid) in plasma and body tissues, and it is this which distinguishes Refsum's disease from many other neurological disorders. This unusual 20-carbon branched chain fatty acid is normally rapidly degraded in the human body. The major mechanism involves an initial alpha-hydroxylation step followed by decarboxylation before the beta-oxidation analogous to that found in the oxidation of straight chain fatty acids. Patients with Refsum's disease have an enzyme deficiency which prevents the initial alpha-oxidation, probably in the alpha-hydroxylation step itself [1]. The onset of symptoms is usually slow and diagnosis is often not made until the second to fifth decade of life, although some patients have been diagnosed in early childhood [2, 3, 4]. There is usually no developmental or mental retardation, but this has been reported in a child where symptoms presented at 7 months. It is possible this child was exposed to phytanate *in utero* [4].

Phytanic acid is exogenous in origin, and treatment is aimed at reducing plasma and tissue levels by means of a diet low in phytanic acid and free phytol, which must be followed for life. Reduction of plasma phytanic acid levels significantly improves peripheral nerve function, ichthyosis and cardiac arrhythmias; it cannot, however, reverse the damage done to the sensory nerves although further deterioration can be arrested. It is thought that in the case of young children early diagnosis and treatment could delay or prevent the development of these irreversible lesions.

Steinberg and Gibberd *et al.* provide an overall review of Refsum's disease [3, 5].

PEROXISOMAL DISORDERS

Patients with global peroxisomal defects can also show raised plasma levels of phytanic acid. These conditions, e.g. infantile Refsum's, Zelwegger syndrome and neonatal adrenoleukodystrophy, must be distinguished from 'true' Refsum's disease (HAP). While patients with HAP appear to have an isolated phytanic acid alpha-hydroxylase deficiency, infantile Refsum's disease is associated with many more defective metabolic functions including that of very long chain fatty acids, especially C:26. These metabolic defects result in severe clinical symptoms, including mental and physical retardation, which present in infancy [4, 6–9].

A low phytanic acid diet may be requested for children with infantile Refsum's disease and some improvement in behaviour has been claimed [10].

Reference values for plasma phytanic acid

Normal	0–33 µmol/l
	(usually <10)
Heterozygote for HAP	0–130 µmol/l
Peroxisomal disease	0–320 µmol/l
HAP after 1 year treatment	16–1000 µmol/l
HAP untreated	990–6400 µmol/l

DIET FOR TREATMENT OF REFSUM'S DISEASE (HAP)

The aims of dietary treatment are:

- To avoid dietary sources of phytanic acid and free phytol

- To encourage suitable weight gain and guard against weight loss (phytanic acid moves between body fat stores and plasma; when weight loss occurs plasma levels will rise causing exacerbation of symptoms)
- To ensure an adequate intake of all nutrients.

Dietary sources of phytanic acid

Phytanic acid derives from phytol, which is a part of the chlorophyll molecule. It is found in the fats of ruminant animals (cows, sheep and goats) and also of fish. The average western diet will provide between 50 mg and 100 mg per day [11].

Free phytol in food is absorbed and metabolised to phytanic acid by humans and, therefore, would present an additional source in the diet. Most phytol in food, however, is bound to chlorophyll which is poorly absorbed by humans [12]. The free phytol content of a typical western diet has been found to be less than 10% of the preformed phytanic acid [11]. The phytanic acid and free phytol content of some foods have been reported from various sources [11, 13–19]. Varying values have been obtained for similar foods. This reflects the difficulty of the estimation and the variation to be expected when allowing for changes in the diet of the animals, food processing

methods (especially oils) and the composition of commercial food ingredients.

Little information is available on the phytol content of individual foods [3, 11, 20]. Again, published values show variation, reflecting perhaps the changes in food processing or the presence of other branched chain substances. Initially, many fruits and vegetables were excluded from the diet as a potential source of phytol: this meant that vitamin supplements were necessary and the diet was extremely restricted and unpalatable. In 1998 it was shown that fruit and vegetables could be introduced into the diet without any deterioration in clinical condition [20] and these are now permitted.

Patients with Refsum's disease have a residual capacity to metabolise phytanic acid by an alternative pathway, possibly involving ω-oxidation. Opinions as to the efficacy of this vary between 10 and 30 mg per day for adults [3]. Accordingly, diets were devised to provide less than 10 mg phytanic acid per day based on published food analyses. Recent analysis of foods has demonstrated the variability of these values and foods are now simply placed in one of three groups. Actual values will be found in the literature [11, 13–19].

Table 19.1 lists foods as presenting low risk, moderate risk and high risk for phytanic acid content based on recent analysis. Patients are advised to:

Table 19.1 Sources of phytanic acid in food

Low risk (no phytanic acid, allowed freely)	Moderate risk (up to 10 mg per serving)	High risk (more than 10 mg per serving)
Cereals and cereal products Wheat, rice, maize, oats, sago, tapioca Crispbreads, bran cereals Biscuits containing only vegetable and hydrogenated vegetable oils, e.g. Sainsbury Rich Tea		Biscuits with animal fat, e.g. shortbread
Dairy products Very low fat cottage cheese <1% fat	Half fat cottage cheese	Butter Margarines containing butter or animal fats
Fat-free fromage frais Skimmed milk and powder Very low fat yoghurt <1% fat Soya milks Soya based yoghurts, e.g. Berrydales Non-dairy ice cream, e.g. Walls' Vanilla Blue Ribbon, containing only vegetable fats Eggs	Semi-skimmed milk Low fat yoghurt	All cheeses including goat, sheep, cheese spreads, processed cheese Full fat milk. Sheep, goat milks, evaporated milk Sheep and goat milk yoghurts, cream, Elmlea Infant formulas containing animal fats and fish oils Dairy ice cream

Table 19.1 *Continued*

Low risk (no phytanic acid, allowed freely)	Moderate risk (up to 10 mg per serving)	High risk (more than 10 mg per serving)
Fats and oils		
Margarines and spreads containing only vegetable oils and hydrogenated vegetable oils, e.g. Flora, Tomor, Tesco soya		Margarines and spreads containing animal fats, e.g. Clover, Vitalite
Oils: corn, sunflower, safflower, soya, olive, rapeseed, arachis		Butter
Lard		Beef suet
Fish		
	Coley, cod (no skin), smoked haddock, tuna, crab, prawns	Plaice. All fatty fish, e.g. herring, mackerel, sardines, salmon fresh and canned
		Fish oils, e.g. Maxepa, cod-liver oil
		Fish in sauces (boil in bag)
Meat	Rabbit	Beef and offal
Pork, pig liver, pig kidney		Lamb and offal
Ham, bacon		Goat (not analysed)
Chicken, chicken liver, turkey, duck		Beefburgers, sausages (not analysed)
		All meat products (not analysed)
Vegetarian meat substitutes		
Soya based TVP products, e.g. Protoveg soya chunks, Sosmix		
Tofu		
Plain Quorn mycoprotein		
Vegetables		
Root vegetables, potatoes, crisps cooked in all vegetable oil, e.g. Golden Wonder, Sainsbury lower fat		Beef, cheese, prawn flavour crisps (not analysed)
Dried beans and pulses		
Green vegetables		
Fruit	Dried fruit (possible phytol content)	
All fresh and canned fruit		
Nuts	Walnuts	
Almonds, peanuts, coconut, Brazil, peanut butter	Skins of nuts (possible phytol)	
Tahini (sesame)		
Miscellaneous	Tea in large amounts (phytol content)	
Beverages – coffee, cocoa, drinking chocolate		
Supplements – See Table 19.2		
Chicken Oxo, Bisto, Marmite		Beef Oxo
Clear vegetable soups		Cream soups
Confectionery		
Sugar based sweets containing no fat, e.g. boiled sweets, fruit gums, jellies, Turkish delight, marshmallows		Milk chocolate, e.g. Mars Bars, Dairymilk
Plain chocolate with no butter fat, e.g. Waitrose continental plain chocolate		Plain chocolate with butter, e.g. Terry's, Sainsbury plain
Carob, e.g. Plamil raw sugar confection		

- Habitually choose low risk foods
- Avoid high risk foods altogether
- Limit their intake of moderate risk foods to one single choice per day, and perferably not every day.

Treatment on diagnosis

A child presenting with classical Refsum's disease may be anorexic and vomiting, making it very difficult to establish feeding. If plasma phytanic acid levels are very high, plasma exchange may be performed. It is still of vital importance, however, to feed the child since any weight loss mobilises body fat stores, releasing further phytanic acid into the blood and exacerbating symptoms. If the child is not able to take adequate nutrition orally, then total or supplementary nasogastric feeding should be instituted as a matter of urgency.

Most commercial enteral feeding products are free from animal fats (and hence phytanic acid) and are, therefore, suitable for use. Products available are listed in Table 19.2 together with the origin of the vegetable oils used. The choice of feed should be made commensurate with the age and requirements of the child.

If the child is able to eat, the diet should be devised to provide enough energy for growth appropriate for age and chosen from low risk foods (Table 19.1).

Suitable nutritional supplements will almost certainly need to be prescribed to promote weight gain at the beginning of treatment. Their use can be discontinued at the discretion of the dietitian when the child is eating suitable foods in adequate amounts and is clinically stable.

Supplements

Those whose lipid source is solely vegetable oils are suitable for a low phytanic acid diet; those containing fats from animal sources are not suitable since these are likely to be from cow's milk or hydrogenated fish oils, both of which contain phytanic acid.

It has been suggested that oils which are high in linoleic acid are preferable since this has a faster metabolic turnover and would prevent further release of body stores of phytanic acid [13, 14]. Sunflower and safflower oils have therefore been favoured. The recent concern with $\omega6:\omega3$ ratio of essential fatty acids (EFAs) perhaps points to the use of rapeseed and soya oils. Table 19.2 lists suitable supplements and the vegetable oil used where this is known.

Fresubin (Fresenius) has been used successfully for adults and is suitable for children above 6 years of age, although it may be used with care in younger children. It is prescribable for patients with Refsum's disease.

Table 19.3 Infant formulas free from animal fats

Manufacturer	Product
Cow & Gate	Premium
	Plus
	Step-up
	InfaSoy
	Pepti-Junior
Farley	Farley's Follow-on Milk
Mead Johnson	Pregestimil
	Prosobee
Milupa	Forward
	Prejomin
Scientific Hospital Supplies	Caprilon
	Galactomin 17, 19
	Monogen
	Neocate
	Pepdite[+], MCT Pepdite 2+
SMA Nutrition	SMA Gold
	SMA White
	SMA Low Birthweight
	SMA High Energy
	SMA Lactofree
	Progress
	Wysoy

Table 19.2 Tube and sip feed products free from animal fats

Product	Fat source
Fresubin	Soya
Fresubin Isofibre	Soya, MCT
Ensure Plus	Canola, sunflower high oleic
Osmolite	Canola, sunflower, MCT
Paediasure	Soya, MCT, sunflower
Fortisip Nutrison Nutrini	Vegetable oil

Maintenance diet and long term management

Dietary treatment (sometimes together with plasma exchange) will usually lower plasma phytanic acid within a matter of weeks. The child will then be put on a diet low in phytanic acid and phytol which must be followed for life. Initially, the child is restricted to low risk foods only (Table 19.1). As the condition improves, one food from the moderate risk group may be allowed occasionally at the discretion of the physician. High risk foods must be avoided altogether. Attention to satisfactory growth (or weight maintenance in older children) is essential, since any weight loss mobilises stored phytanic acid. With rigorous adherence to diet these stores can be gradually eliminated.

Special care is needed during infection or other intercurrent illness to maintain nutritional status and liquid supplements may need to be used at these times.

In general the diet, if chosen from a variety of permitted foods, should be adequate in all nutrients. The exclusion of many saturated fats from animal sources shifts the diet of these patients towards a much higher polyunsaturated to saturated fat ratio than that of the general population. This means that the dietitian should check that there is an adequate intake of antioxidant nutrients, especially vitamin E. Although most oils do contain vitamin E, it is prudent to recommend the use of fat spreads which have extra vitamin E added, e.g. Flora (Van den Berg Ltd).

The inclusion of convenience and manufactured foods in the diet of patients with Refsum's disease requires extreme vigilance in reading the ingredients list on food labels. The guidance of the dietitian can be very helpful here. Many commercial fats used in desserts and baked goods contain fish oils which are a rich source of phytanic acid.

Patients are advised to look for and *avoid* the following: butter, cream, animal fats, full cream milk, cheese, butter oil, ghee, beef, lamb, suet, milk fat, fish, fish products, fish oils.

Foods labelled as suitable for vegans are quickly and easily identified as safe. Most large retail food shops now issue lists of vegan foods on request. These are updated at regular intervals.

DIETARY TREATMENT OF INFANTILE REFSUM'S DISEASE

Infantile Refsum's disease is a global peroxisomal disease which, unlike classic Refsum's, presents in infancy with more widespread biochemical deficiencies including raised plasma phytanic acid and abnormal levels of very long chain fatty acids. There are also physical and mental abnormalities [3, 7, 8, 9, 21, 22]. Despite the more complex nature of this condition some paediatricians will prescribe a low phytanic acid diet. Some improvement has been claimed in lowering plasma phytanate but not for other parameters [8].

Infant feeding

If the mother is breast feeding this should be encouraged since human breast milk does not contain phytanic acid unless the mother is affected. Infant formulas should contain no animal fats (milk, beef etc.) since the amount of phytanic acid in these is variable and could be significant. Soya based milks are acceptable.

Suitable infant feeds free from animal fats are given in Table 19.3. The formulation of infant feeds is constantly being changed in line with new research. Concern about essential fatty acids has led to the introduction of milk fats and fish oils into some formulas. The ingredients should always be checked before use.

Nuts and seed oils (especially peanuts/arachis oil) have been shown to contain hexacosanoic acid (C26 : 0). The use of feeds containing medium chain triglyceride (MCT) oils, and which are also free of phytanic acid, might be of some benefit to infantile Refsum's patients although this is, at present, untested in practice.

Solid food

The choice of weaning foods should be based on those shown in Table 19.1. Only low risk foods should be used. Proprietary baby foods should be checked for the presence of 'milk solids', milk fat, butter, cream, cheese, beef and beef fat, lamb and fish. These ingredients should be avoided.

Products labelled as suitable for vegans will again be suitable.

Since children with infantile Refsum's syndrome also have abnormal metabolism of very long chain fatty acids (VLCFA) especially C26, as in adrenoleukodystrophy (ALD), they might benefit from the dietary treatment applied in ALD.

REFERENCES

1 Verhoeven N *et al*. Phytanic acid alpha oxidation in man. Resolution of the complete pathway. Society for the Study of Inborn Errors conference, York 1998. *J Inher Met Dis*, 1998, **21** (Suppl 2) 212.

2 Dickson N *et al*. A child with Refsum's disease, successful treatment with diet and plasma exchange. *Develop Med Child Neurol*, 1989, **31** 92–7.

3 Steinberg D Refsum disease. In: Scriver CR *et al*. (eds) *Metabolic Basis of Inherited Disease*, 7e. New York: McGraw-Hill, 1995.

4 Herbert MA, Clayton PT Phytanic acid alpha-oxidase deficiency (Refsum disease) presenting in infancy. *J Inher Met Disease*, 1994, **17** 211–14.

5 Gibberd FB *et al*. Heredopathia atactica polyneuritiformis: Refsum's disease. *Acta Neurol Scand*, 1985, **72** 1–17.

6 Stokke O, Skjeldal O, Hoie K Disorders related to the metabolism of phytanic acid. *Scand J Clin Lab Invest*, 1986, **46** (Suppl 184) 3–10.

7 Poulos A, Sharp P, Whiting G Infantile Refsum's disease (phytanic acid storage disease): a variant of Zellwegger's syndrome? *Clinical Genetics*, 1984, **26** 579–86.

8 Poulos A *et al*. Accumulation and defective β-oxidation of very long chain fatty acids in Zellwegger's syndrome, adrenoleukodystrophy, and Refsum's disease variants. *Clin Gen*, 1986, **29** 397–408.

9 Poll-The BT, Saudebray JM *et al*. Infantile Refsum's disease: an inherited peroxisomal disorder. Comparison with Zellwegger's syndrome and neonatal adrenoleukodystrophy. *Europ J Pediatr*, 1987, **146** 477–83.

10 Robertson EF *et al*. Treatment of infantile phytanic acid storage disease: clinical, biochemical and ultrastructural findings in two children treated for two years. *Europ J Pediatr*, 1988, **147** 133–42.

11 Steinberg D *et al*. Refsum's disease, a recently characterised lipidosis involving the nervous system. *Ann Intern Med*, 1967, **66** 365–95.

12 Baxter J Absorption of chlorophyll phytol in normal man and in patients with Refsum's diseases. *J Lipid Res*, 1968, **9** 636–41.

13 Masters-Thomas A *et al*. Heredopathia atactica polyneuritiformis (Refsum's disease). 1 Clinical features and dietary management. *J Hum Nutr*, 1980, **34** 245–50.

14 Masters-Thomas A *et al*. Heredopathia atactica polyneuritiformis (Refsum's disease). 2 Estimation of phytanic acid in foods. *J Hum Nutr*, 1980, **34** 251–4.

15 Steinberg D Phytanic acid storage disease (Refsum's disease). In: Stanbury JB (ed.) *Metabolic Basis of Inherited Disease*, 5e. New York: McGraw-Hill, 1983.

16 Ackman RG, Harrington M Fishery products as components of diets restricted in phytanic acid for patients with Refsum's syndrome. *J Canad Diet Assoc*, 1975, **36** 50–53.

17 Ackman RG, Hooper SN Isoprenoid fatty acids in the human diet: distinct geographical features in butterfat and importance in margarines based on marine oils. *Can Inst Food Tec J*, 1973, **6** 159–65.

18 Lough AK The phytanic acid content of the lipids of bovine tissues and milk. *Lipids*, 1977, **12** 115–19.

19 Brown PJ *et al*. Diet and Refsum's disease. The determination of phytanic acid and phytol in certain foods and the application of this knowledge to the choice of suitable convenience foods in Refsum's disease. *J Hum Nutr Diet*, 1993, **4** 295–305.

20 Coppack SW *et al*. Can patients with Refsum's disease safely eat green vegetables? *Brit Med J*, 1988, **296** 828.

21 Poulos A, Sharp P Plasma and skin fibroblast C26 fatty acids in infantile Refsum's disease. *Neurology*, 1984, **34** 1606–9.

22 Wanders RJ, Heyman HS, Schutgens RB, Poll-The BT, Saudebray JM, Tager JM *et al*. Peroxisomal functions in classical Refsum's disease: comparison with the infantile form of Refsum's disease. *J Neurological Sciences*, 1988, **84** 147–55.

CHAPTER 20

X-linked Adrenoleukodystrophy

X-linked adrenoleukodystrophy (X-ALD) is a serious, progressive, peroxisomal inherited disorder. It is associated with central nervous system demyelination, peripheral nerve abnormalities, primary adrenal cortical insufficiency (Addison's disease) and frequently primary hypogonadism. There is an accumulation of very long chain saturated fatty acids (VLCFA), especially the 26-carbon acid hexacosanoic acid, in membrane and tissues [1]. This is due to an impaired capacity to β-oxidise these fatty acids [2] due to a deficiency of the peroxisomal enzyme lignoceroyl-CoA ligase [3]. The X-ALD gene, identified in 1993, encodes a peroxisomal membrane protein (adrenoleukodystrophy protein: ALDP) that belongs to the ATP binding cassette transporter super-family [4].

X-ALD affects only males, although a small number of female carriers may develop a milder form of the disease. The disorder has been reported in all races. The incidence is unknown but the lowest estimated birth incidence is 1 per 100 000 [5, 6, 7]. There are at least six known clinical phenotypes or subtypes of X-ALD of which the most frequently reported are childhood cerebral X-ALD and adrenomyeloneuropathy (AMN). At present, there is no evident correlation between mutations of the ALD gene and the different neurological phenotypes [2, 8]. Relative frequencies, age of onset and features of the different phenotypes are given in Table 20.1.

DIETARY TREATMENT

A detailed account of diet therapy and its evolution is given in the first edition of this book. The current diet is summarised in Table 20.2 and consists of:

- Lorenzo's oil
- Glycerol trioleate oil for cooking
- Low fat diet
- Vitamin and mineral supplementation
- Essential fatty acids
- Energy supplementation.

Success of Lorenzo's oil and diet therapy

The clinical benefit of Lorenzo's oil as a treatment in X-ALD is still unknown, but results of trials reported so far are disappointing. Lorenzo's oil is capable of reducing plasma C26:0 to normal in up to 86% of patients [9] within one month of diet therapy. It reduces C26:0 concentrations in the plasma, adipose tissue and liver, but not in the brain [10, 11], indicating that little erucic acid crosses the blood–brain barrier. It has not been shown to halt the neurological progression in the cerebral forms of childhood X-ALD [12, 13, 14]. However a retrospective analysis of the efficacy of Lorenzo's oil in boys with the childhood cerebral X-ALD indicated that there was slight but significant slowing of progression of symptoms and delay of death [15]. There is also evidence that Lorenzo's oil has no effect in adult patients with AMN [6, 12, 16]. Aubourg demonstrated in an open trial with 14 men with AMN that there was no clinically relevant benefit from dietary treatment with Lorenzo's oil [16].

Even with asymptomatic boys and patients with milder phenotypes, the initial results are not promising. In a trial at Birmingham Children's Hospital, the therapy failed to prevent the onset of cerebral childhood X-ALD in four out of eight boys who were all asymptomatic and under the age of ten years at the start of therapy [17]. In a further study of 22 patients with milder phenotypes of X-ALD, Lorenzo's oil

Table 20.1 Clinical phenotypes of X-ALD (adapted from van Geel *et al.* 1997 [8])

Clinical phenotype	Age of presentation (years)	Relative frequency (%)	Features	Progression
Childhood cerebral ALD	3–10	31–57	Behavioural disturbances, poor school performance, visual loss, deafness, melanoderma, dysarthria, seizures, spastic tetraplegia, progressive dementia, Addison's disease	Rapid, rarely slowly
Adolescent ALD	10–21		Similar to childhood cerebral ALD	Rapid, rarely slowly
Adult cerebral ALD	>21	1–3	Similar to childhood cerebral ALD	Rapid, sometimes slowly
AMN	>18	25–40	Leg stiffness, progressive spastic paraparesis of the lower extremities, ataxia, testicular insufficiency, scanty scalp hair	Slowly, sometimes rapidly
Addison's only	>2	8–14	Fatigue, hypotension, diffuse or focal bronzing of skin	—
Pre- or asymptomatic ALD	—	4–10	Risk of developing neurological symptoms high, but some patients remain asymptomatic in their 60s	—

neither improved neurological function nor arrested progression of the disease [9]. Follow-up for at least 12 months indicated that disability status score increased mildly in 16 patients with neurological symptoms. Furthermore, one patient with Addison's only and one patient with AMN developed cerebral demyelination and another patient with Addison's only developed AMN [9].

Lack of concurrent control groups, variable natural history of X-ALD, short length of follow-up and small study groups have hampered studies evaluating Lorenzo's oil in asymptomatic X-ALD. As a result, data on 100 boys with biochemically proven, asymptomatic X-ALD from eight centres was shared at a Society for the Study of Inborn Errors of Me-tabolism meeting in 1994. Although a number of boys deteriorated during therapy, there was insufficient data for statistically significant conclusions to be drawn [17]. This led to the formation of the ALD-International Research Group, which has established an international register, including 201 boys with asymptomatic X-ALD who have been treated with Lorenzo's oil. It was estimated that by December 2000 there would be sufficient data on the 'study group' to statistically evaluate the outcome on Lorenzo's oil compared with untreated individuals [17].

Complications with Lorenzo's oil

A number of side effects have been noted with Lorenzo's oil including mild increases in liver enzymes [9, 17], thrombocytopenia [17, 18, 19, 20], gastrointestinal complaints [9], gingivitis [9] and a reduction of plasma essential fatty acids [17]. Generally, the platelet reduction does not appear severe enough to warrant discontinuation of diet therapy in the majority of the patients, but careful monitoring is recommended.

OTHER TREATMENTS

In addition to Lorenzo's oil, a number of other treatments are being evaluated in X-ALD. These include:

- *Lovastatin*: A lipid lowering drug that inhibits 3-hydroxy-3-methyl glutaryl-coenzyme. It normalises the levels and metabolism of VLCFAs in the plasma of X-ALD patients [21].
- *Phenylbutyrate*: This reduces the levels of VLCFAs in the brain and adrenal gland in the X-ALD mouse model [22].
- *Bone marrow transplant*: Haematopoietic stem cell transplantation is the treatment of choice in boys

Table 20.2 Summary of diet therapy used in ALD

Lorenzo's oil	Glycerol trioleate oil (GTO)	Low fat diet	Vitamin and mineral supplementation	Essential fatty acids	Energy supplements
Description 4 parts GTO: 1 part glycerol trierucate (GTE)	*Description* Rich in oleic acid; free of C26:0	*Description* Give 20–25% of dietary energy as fat (try not to exceed total intake of 40% energy from fat)	*Description* Diet low in fat-soluble vitamins and commonly trace elements	*Description* Diet is low in essential fatty acids Lorenzo's oil leads to reduced levels of omega 6 and omega 3 fatty acids	*Description* Energy intake may be low
Dose 20% of energy intake: some boys need less than this to normalise C26:0 levels	*Dose* No set dose	NB. No other dietary restrictions are necessary	*Type of supplements* Give comprehensive vitamin and mineral supplement, e.g. Forceval Junior vitamin and mineral supplement or Paediatric Seravit	*Type of supplements* Give 1–2% of total energy from essential fatty acid supplement. It should provide a source of linoleic acid and alpha-linolenic acid in the ratio 4:1 to 10:1, e.g. walnut oil	*Type of supplements* Useful ACBS energy supplements include glucose polymers, glucose drinks (liquid Polycal, liquid Maxijul, Calsip) and fortified fat-free fruit juice drinks (Fortijuce, Provide Xtra, and Enlive)
Administration Give 2–3 times daily. Give neat as a medicine, or mixed with skimmed milk and flavouring or fruit juice. Can also be mixed with very low fat yoghurt Not ACBS prescribable	*Administration* Use for frying potatoes, fish, and meats, preparation of GTO margarine, salad dressings Not ACBS prescribable		*Monitoring* Vitamin and mineral status must be monitored annually		

ACBS = Advisory Committee on Borderline Substances

with early symptoms and/or deteriorating magnetic resonance imaging (MRI) [17]. It is not recommended for patients with advanced disease. In patients with early neuropsychological deterioration, it has been shown to reverse or stabilise abnormalities on cerebral MRI [23, 24] and may result in stability of mental ability.

REFERENCES

1 Ho JK, Moser H, Kishimota Y, Hamilton JA Interactions of a very long chain fatty acid with model membranes and serum albumin. Implications for the pathogenesis of adrenoleukodystrophy. *J Clin Invest*, 1995, **96** 1455–66.

2 Korenke GC, Roth C, Krasemann E, Hufner M, Hunneman DH, Hanefield Variability of endocrinological dysfunction in 55 patients with X-linked adrenoleucodystrophy: clinical, laboratory and genetic findings. *Eur J Endocrinol*, 1997, **137** 40–47.

3 Moser HW Clinical and therapeutic aspects of adrenoleukodystrophy and adrenomyeloneuropathy. *J Neuropathol Exp Neuro*, 1995, **54** 740–45.

4 Mosser J, Douar AM, Sarde CO, Kioschis P, Feil R, Moser H, Poustka AM, Mandel JL, Aubourg P Putative X-linked adrenoleukodystrophy gene shares unexpected homology with ABC transporters. *Nature*, 1993, **361** 726–30.

5 Moser HW, Smith KD, Moser AB X-linked adrenoleukodystrophy. In: Scriver CR *et al.* (eds) *The Metabolic and Molecular Bases of Inherited Disease*. New York: McGraw-Hill, 1995, pp. 2325–49.

6 van Geel BM, Assies J, Weverling GJ, Barth PG Predominance of the adrenomyeloneuropathy phenotype of X-linked adrenoleukodystrophy in the Netherlands: a survey of 30 kindreds. *Neurology*, 1994, **44** 2343–6.

7 Sereni C, Paturneau-Jouas M, Aubourg P, Baumann N, Feingold J Adrenoleukodystrophy in France: an epidemiological study. *Neuroepidemiology*, 1993, **12** 229–33.

8 van Geel BM, Assies J, Wanders RJ, Barth PG X-linked adrenoleukodystrophy: clinical presentation, diagnosis,

and therapy. *J Neurol Neurosurg Psychiatry*, 1997, **63** 4–14.

9 van Geel BM, Assies J, Haverkort EB, Koelman JH, Varbeetan B, Wanders RJ, Barth PG Progression of abnormalities in adrenomyeloneuropathy and neurologically asymptomatic X-linked adrenoleukodystrophy despite treatment with Lorenzo's oil. *J Neuro Neurosurg Pscyhiatry*, 1999, **67** 290–99.

10 Rasemussen M, Moser AB, Borel J, Moser HW Brain, liver, and adipose tissue erucic and very long chain fatty acid levels in adrenoleukodystrophy patients treated with glyceryl trierucate and trioleate oils (Lorenzo's oil). *Neurochem Res*, 1994, **19** 1073–82.

11 Poulos A, Gibson R, Sharp P, Beckman K, Grattan-Smith P Very long chain fatty acids in X-linked adrenoleukodystrophy brain after treatment with Lorenzo's oil. *Ann Neurol*, 1994, **36** 741–6.

12 Moser HW, Moser AB, Smith KD, Bergin A, Borel J, Shankroff J, Stine OC, Merette C, Ott J, Krivit W *et al.* Adrenoleukodystrophy: phenotypic variability and implications for therapy. *J Inherit Metab Dis*, 1992, **15** 645–54.

13 Uziel G, Bertini E, Bardelli P, Rimoldi M, Gambetti M Experience on therapy of adrenoleukodystrophy and adrenomyeloneuropathy. *Dev Neurosci*, 1991, **13** 274–9.

14 Asano J, Suzuki Y, Yajima S, Inoue K, Shimozawa N, Kondo N, Murase M, Orii T Effects of erucic acid therapy on Japanese patients with X-linked adrenoleukodystrophy. *Brain Dev*, 1994, **16** 454–8.

15 Moser HW Adrenoleukodystrophy: natural history, treatment and outcome. *J Inherit Metab Dis*, 1995, **18** 435–47.

16 Aubourg P, Adamsbaum C, Lavallard-Rousseau MC, Rocchiccioli F, Cartier N, Jambaque I, Jakobezak C, Lemaitre A, Boureau F, Wolf C *et al.* A two-year trial of oleic and erucic acids (Lorenzo's oil) as treatment for adrenomyeloneuropathy. *N Engl J Med*, 1993, **329** 745–52.

17 Alger S, Green A, Kohler W, Sokolowski P, Moser H Proceedings of the 4th International Workshop of the Adrenoleukodystrophy International Research Group (ALD-IRG), University of York, 3 September 1998. *J Inher Metab Dis*, 2000, **23**.

18 Zierz S, Schroder R, Unkrig CJ Thrombocytopenia induced by erucic acid therapy in patients with X-linked adrenoleukodystrophy. *Clin Investig*, 1993, **71** 802–5.

19 Crowther MA, Barr RD, Kelton J, Whelan D, Greenwald M Profound thrombocytopenia complicating dietary erucic acid therapy for adrenoleukodystrophy. *Am J Hematol*, 1995, **48** 132–3.

20 Kickler TS, Zinkham WH, Moser A, Shankroff J, Borel J, Moser H Effect of erucic acid on platelets in patients with adrenoleukodystrophy. *Biochem Mol Med*, 1996, **57** 125–33.

21 Singh I, Pahan K, Khan M Lovastatin and sodium phenylacetate normalize the levels of very long chain fatty acids in skin fibroblasts of X-adrenoleukodystrophy. *FEBS Lett*, 1998, **426** 342–6.

22 Kemp S, Wei HM, Lu JF, Braiterman LT, McGuinness MC, Moser AB, Watkins PA, Smith KD Gene redundancy and pharmacological gene therapy: implications for X-linked adrenoleukodystrophy. *Nat Med*, 1998, **4** 1261–8.

23 Loes DJ, Stillman AE, Hite S, Shapiro E, Lockman L, Latchaw RE, Moser H, Krivit W Childhood cerebral form of adrenoleukodystrophy: short-term effect of bone marrow transplantation on brain MR observations. *Am J Neuroradiol*, 1994, **15** 1767–71.

24 Shapiro EG, Lockman LA, Balthazor M, Krivit W Neuropsychological outcomes of several storage diseases with and without bone marrow transplantation. *J Inherit Metab Dis*, 1995, **18** 413–29.

SECTION 8

Childhood Cancers

CHAPTER 21

Nutritional Support: Leukaemias, Lymphomas and Solid Tumours

Childhood cancers differ from those seen in adults in both type and outcome [1]. In comparison with therapies used to treat adults, multimodal therapy and combination chemotherapy have been effective in vastly improving the outlook for children with cancer. Children have tumours that are chemotherapy responsive and they tolerate chemotherapy better than adults do [2]. Children differ metabolically as well and continued growth and development is desired throughout therapy that often spans several years. Therefore, with more curable children being treated for what is much of the time a chronic disease, the more children there are who are subject to the nutritional problems caused by their disease and treatment.

Malnutrition and cancer cachexia are a frequent consequence of paediatric cancer and therapy. A clear understanding of the metabolic alterations in the presence of malignancy which leads to cachexia and the value of maintaining nutritional equilibrium are a valuable part of managing these children. Nutritional support may enhance therapy, decrease complications, improve immunologic status and hopefully improve survival [3].

TYPES OF CANCERS SEEN IN CHILDHOOD

The types of cancers seen in children can be divided into three main groups:

- Leukaemias
- Lymphomas
- Solid tumours

Leukaemias

Leukaemia is the commonest neoplastic disease of infancy and childhood, accounting for 30–45% of all childhood cancers [4, 5]. Acute lymphoblastic leukaemia (ALL) is the commonest form of the disease in childhood, followed by acute myeloid leukaemia (AML) and then chronic myeloid leukaemia (CML). The cure rate (i.e. five year survival without relapse) is 65–70% with ALL and 50% with AML [5].

The leukaemias are fatal unless treated. At presentation pallor, fever, fatigue and aches and pains are the commonest features. Haemorrhage, apart from easy bruising, is not common unless infection is present. Enlargement of the spleen and lymph nodes may be present [4].

Lymphomas

Lymphomas account for 9–15% of all childhood cancers [4, 5]. In children the types of lymphomas seen are virtually limited to three types [6]:

- Hodgkin's disease which affects the lymph glands causing them to enlarge
- Non-Hodgkin's lymphoma (NHL) which is a monoclonal neoplastic proliferation of lymphoid cells, usually B or T cells. It is more malignant than Hodgkin's
- Burkitt's lymphoma which is a malignant lymphoma of poorly differentiated lymphoblastic type masses of immature lymphoid cells.

Solid tumours

Solid tumours account for 40% of childhood cancers [4, 7]. The most common solid tumours seen in children are [4, 7]:

- Brain tumours, of which medulloblastoma is the most common. It is a tumour arising in the posterior fossa.

- Wilm's tumour, also known as nephroblastoma, which is a congenital highly malignant kidney tumour and can be bilateral.
- Neuroblastoma, which is another highly malignant tumour arising from the adrenal medulla from tissue of sympathetic origin. It can also arise from some parts of the abdominal, thoracic, pelvic or cervical chains of sympathetic ganglia.
- Rhabdomyosarcoma, which is a malignant tumour of striated muscle most commonly found in the orbital region, nose, mouth or pharynx.
- Osteosarcoma, which is a malignant tumour arising from bone. Any bone can be affected, but it usually occurs in the legs.
- Ewing's sarcoma, which is a very malignant tumour that can develop anywhere in the body, but usually starts in the bones, most commonly the pelvis, upper arm or thigh. It can develop in the soft tissue near bones.
- Primitive neuroectodermal tumour (PNET), which is a highly malignant tumour of neuro-epithial origin and can be thought of as being similar to a Ewing's sarcoma.

Incidence rates and survival rates for these tumours are given in Table 21.1 and Fig. 21.1.

THE AETIOLOGY OF MALNUTRITION IN CHILDREN WITH CANCER

To a certain extent the problems of malnutrition seen in children with cancer are no different from the problems of any child who has an inadequate intake for demand. The incidence of malnutrition in paediatric oncology patients ranges from 6 to 50% depending on the type, stage and location of the tumour [8, 9]. Malnutrition is more severe with aggressive tumours in the later stages of malignancy, occuring in up to 37.5% of newly diagnosed patients with metastatic disease [10]. The initial nutritional problems resulting from the tumour may soon be compounded by iatrogenic nutritional abnormalities, the consequence of the treatment and its complications; metabolic and psychological factors also play a role [11].

Malnutrition at diagnosis may be more common than previously thought due to nutritional assessment being based on measurement of height and weight, which may not be appropriate for assessing children with cancer. Many children with cancer have large

tumour masses which inevitably add to their body weight, therefore weight to height ratios are distorted and, consequently, are unlikely to be a sensitive indicator of malnutrition. Height is also a poor indicator, as the history of ill health in children with cancer is usually brief, therefore height for age, an index of chronic malnutrition, is unlikely to be depressed. The use of arm anthropometry gives a more reliable indication of the presence of malnutrition at diagnosis and indicates that malnutrition is more common at diagnosis than previously realised [12].

Metabolic factors

Cancer cachexia is complex and multifactorial. It includes weight loss, anorexia, organ dysfunction and tissue wasting associated with significant alterations in protein, carbohydrate and lipid metabolism. Recently there has been more attention to the role of the cytokines, tumour necrosis factor (TNF), interleukin-1 [IL-1], interleukin-6 [IL-6], and interferon-γ [IFN-γ], in cancer cachexia [13]. These cytokines are secreted by macrophages and lymphocytes and are thought to represent a host defence reaction to tumour cell invasion. In healthy adult human volunteers, the administation of TNF induced changes characteristic of cancer cachexia, including increased energy expenditure, increased acute phase protein synthesis, lipolysis, muscle proteolysis and anorexia [13, 14]. The effects of IL-1 are similar to those of TNF and in animals result in a hypermetabolic response and anorexia [13]. IL-6 has been found to be elevated in some cancer patients, causing an ongoing acute phase protein response [13, 15]. However, there is little evidence that individually these cytokines actually play a major role in cancer patients but the possibility of an indirect or synergistic involvement cannot be ruled out [13].

The normal response to starvation is to conserve energy (decreased energy expenditure) and protein reserves (decreased proteolysis and gluconeogenesis) at the expense of endogenous carbohydrate and fat stores (increased glycogenolysis and lipolysis). However, in the tumour-induced host the result is a cascade of metabolic events that are typically characteristic of the acute metabolic stress response. In addition to glycogenolysis and lipolysis, this response includes a marked increase in energy expenditure (hypermetabolism), proteolysis and gluconeogenesis

Table 21.1 UKCCSG registrations for children aged under 15, by diagnostic group, 1977–98

Diagnosis	Diag year																						Total
	77	78	79	80	81	82	83	84	85	86	87	88	89	90	91	92	93	94	95	96	97	98	
ALL	95	230	233	255	250	287	287	292	299	290	311	327	328	368	359	369	392	376	379	380	356	113	6576
ANLL	20	55	56	30	53	55	43	60	62	65	61	63	73	64	65	54	75	80	68	82	74	18	1276
Hodgkin's disease	19	39	31	47	40	50	42	42	50	60	31	40	33	42	43	59	46	49	65	57	60	13	958
NHL	27	58	54	62	55	56	50	68	66	68	70	84	74	81	76	88	79	73	95	72	87	17	1460
PNET	8	32	27	32	40	29	50	28	39	33	48	43	48	56	58	72	57	72	67	65	63	17	984
Neuroblastoma	27	44	45	60	85	77	72	79	72	77	99	111	96	116	102	93	89	86	92	100	94	25	1741
Retinoblastoma	2	3	8	5	6	8	21	21	30	35	45	29	42	33	43	49	62	45	40	35	42	5	609
Wilm's tumour	19	55	42	55	48	63	69	64	63	69	84	76	69	94	72	76	81	91	68	85	86	23	1452
Osteosarcoma	1	10	23	13	22	20	20	13	16	22	19	23	14	23	20	20	36	30	45	37	28	6	461
Ewing's sarcoma	7	10	25	23	24	19	25	24	22	21	22	21	26	22	25	20	21	20	28	23	19	6	453
Rhabdomyosarcoma	17	28	36	48	49	51	59	59	67	50	69	56	53	67	69	61	78	55	64	65	52	15	1160

ANLL – acute non-lymphoblastic anaemia
United Kingdom Children's Cancer Study Group Scientific Report, 1998

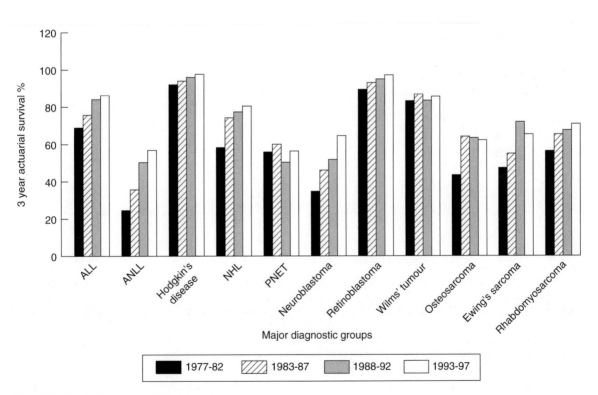

Fig. 21.1 Survival rates in childhood cancers

(protein catabolism). This response results in an accelerated depletion of endogenous energy and substrate stores in the face of decreased exogenous fuel substrate provision [3].

Alterations in carbohydrate metabolism associated with malignancy are characterised by decreased glucose tolerance, increased glucose uptake and increased lactate production [13, 16]. Lactate is metabolised through the Cori cycle to regenerate glucose, and this process has been associated with a 10% increase in energy expenditure in cancer patients [13, 16].

Abnormalities in protein metabolism are also present with total protein turnover being accelerated due to an increase in both protein synthesis and degradation. This results in a reduction in skeletal muscle mass and hypoalbuminaemia, both of which are common in cancer patients [13].

Alterations in lipid metabolism include increased lipolysis and fatty acid oxidation. Increased rates of glycerol and fatty acid turnover have been shown in weight losing versus weight stable cancer patients [17].

Malignant cachexia appears to result mainly from the increased metabolic demands imposed by the tumour burden itself, coupled with the acute stress response that malignancy evokes in the host. Generally, as the tumour burden increases, especially with metastases, the catabolism of endogenous substrate reserves increases, resulting in increased weight loss and compromise of organ function. Malnutrition results in further reduction of endogenous reserves, therefore reducing the host's ability to compensate for increased metabolic demands and placing the patient at higher risk of cachexia.

Complications of disease and treatment

Most of the malnutrition seen is a direct consequence of the disease progression and treatment. Table 21.2

Table 21.2 Side effects relating to treatment seen in paediatric oncology patients

Side effect		Causative chemotherapeutic agent
Infection	Both chemotherapy and radiotherapy are known immune depressants; malnutrition also has an effect on immunity. The malnourished child with cancer and an uncontrolled infection can further deteriorate nutritionally from the side effects of cancer and infection leading to a vicious cycle	
Diarrhoea	This is the commonest side effect and can be due to mucositis and consequent malabsorption; tumour infiltration of the bowel; infection and prolonged use of antibiotics. Children are especially sensitive to the effects of drugs and radiotherapy to the intestinal tract	Actinomycin, Adriamycin, Methotrexate (high dose) Cytosine
Nausea and vomiting	This is another common side effect and some of the chemotherapy drugs are powerful inducers of vomiting	Actinomycin, Adriamycin, Carboplatin, Cisplatinum, Cyclophosphamide, Ifosfamide, Cytosine, Etoposide, Procarbazine
Stomatitis mucositis	Stomatitis or mucosal damage is a common side effect of chemotherapy and can be severe enough to prevent an adequate oral intake	Actinomycin, Adriamycin, Daunorubicin, Epirubicin, Bleomycin, Melphalan, Methotrexate
Renal damage and nutrient loss	A large number of chemotherapy drugs cause renal damage and hence significant protein and mineral losses	Cisplatin, Cyclophosphamide, Ifosfamide
Dysgeusia	This is often seen in advanced cancers, but is more often seen in adults	
Xerostomia	Xerostomia and poor oral hygiene can both be serious deterrents to an adequate oral intake	
Constipation	Occasionally this can be a problem in children with cancer	Vincristine

shows the side effects which result in an increased risk of malnutrition.

Psychological factors

Learned food aversion associated with treatment has been demonstrated in children with cancer and part of this behaviour is the phenomenon of anticipatory vomiting [18, 19]. Parents can often become preoccupied with getting their children to eat. However, this preoccupation may reduce the child's appetite further, causing them to rebel against the parent and purposely not eat.

IDENTIFICATION OF NUTRITIONAL RISK

Criteria for identifying children with cancer who are malnourished differ; however determination of the nutritional risk of the child with cancer can be associated with the diagnosis of certain tumours and stages of the disease [20] (Table 21.3) [21]. The following criteria can be used to identify children with cancer who are likely to require supplementary nutritional support [3]:

Table 21.3 Types of childhood cancers associated with high or low nutritional risk

High nutritional risk	Low nutritional risk
Advanced diseases during initial intense treatment	Good prognosis acute lymphoblastic leukaemia
Stages III and IV Wilm's tumour and unfavourable histology Wilm's tumour	Non-metastatic solid tumours
Stages III and IV neuroblastoma	Advanced diseases in remission during maintenance treatment
Ewing's sarcoma	
Pelvic rhabdomyosarcoma	
Some non-Hodgkin's lymphoma	
Multiple relapse leukaemia	
Acute non-lymphoblastic leukaemia	
Some poor prognosis acute lymphoblastic leukaemia	
Medulloblastoma	

- Total weight loss of >5% relative to pre-illness body weight
- Weight for height <90%
- Serum albumin <32 mmol/l (in absence of recent acute metabolic stress within the last 14 days)
- A decrease in current percentile for weight (or height) of two percentiles
- Adipose energy reserves as determined by triceps skinfold thickness <5th percentile for age and gender
- Voluntary food intake <70% of estimated requirements for 5 days for well-nourished patients
- Anticipated gut dysfunction due to treatment for >5 days for well-nourished patients
- High nutritional risk patients based on tumour type and oncology treatment regimens
- Bone marrow transplant as a treatment for any tumour.

The consequences of malnutrition are multiple and include a poorer outcome compared with children who are well nourished at diagnosis [8]. Malnutrition contributes to a reduced tolerance to therapy. Dose adjustments in chemotherapy have been seen most frequently in patients during a time of malnutrition [9]. Compromised nutritional status before initiation of therapy is associated significantly with relapse in solid tumour patients [22]. There also appear to be differences in the metabolism of chemotherapy agents between adequately nourished and inadequately nourished patients [23]. Malnutrition is associated with a higher risk of infectious complications and higher infection rates have been documented in malnourished children [10]. The risk of opportunistic infection also appears to be increased in malnourished children with cancer.

NUTRITIONAL SUPPORT

The main aims of nutritional support are to reverse the malnutrition seen at diagnosis, to prevent the malnutrition associated with treatment and to promote weight gain and growth rather than weight maintenance [24].

One of the questions that is often addressed in feeding cancer patients is the possibility that the nutrients given to replete the host may stimulate further growth of tumour mass [16]. Clinical studies of children with malignancy receiving nutritional support have failed to demonstrate increase in tumour growth or decreased survival despite improved host nutritional status [8]. Children have increased requirements for growth and development which must be met despite extended periods of cancer treatment. Therefore nutritional support should be considered a major part of therapy in order to prevent or reverse the effects of protein energy malnutrition and to increase the wellbeing of the child. If this is achieved then the aim of nutritional support has been reached even if the overall prognosis remains the same.

Oral feeding

In patients with a low nutritional risk, unless complicated by factors such as relapse, sepsis or major abdominal procedures, oral feeding is the best method if they are able to consume sufficient nutrients. However, the majority will need high energy supplements and specific advice on eating problems related to the side effects of their treatment (Table 21.4). Ideally there should be flexibility with regard to menu choice, meal times and parental involvement. Unfor-

Table 21.4 Advice on nutritional problems associated with cancer and its treatment [25]

Problem	Suggested dietary advice	Problem	Suggested dietary advice
Loss of appetite	Offer small frequent meals/snacks 5–6 per day Avoid rich fatty foods A soft diet may be better tolerated Avoid drinking just before and during mealtimes		Sucking fruit drops or boiled mints may stimulate saliva production Keep foods moist by using butter, sauces, cream, yoghurt, gravy
Nausea	Offer small amounts of food at a time Cold food may be better tolerated Avoid fatty or greasy foods Offer dry foods, e.g. crackers, plain biscuits or toast Avoid very sweet foods Avoid hot and spicy foods Serve meals attractively Avoid favourite foods as the child may then develop a permanent dislike for them Sips of a cool, fizzy drink may help, e.g. soda water or ginger ale	Taste changes and loss of taste	If the child complains of a 'metallic' taste when eating meat, then try poultry, fish, eggs or cheese instead Experiment using herbs and spices to flavour food Try cold sharp foods Offer foods familiar to and liked by the child Flavour gravy with Bovril, Marmite, soy and sweet and sour sauces Vary the colour and texture of the foods Emphasise the aroma of food
Vomiting	Give mouth washes to help to remove the taste Avoid fluids or food until vomiting is controlled and then introduce clear fluids Avoid favourite foods Dry foods may be better tolerated	Diarrhoea	Avoid foods high in fibre Ensure the child continues to drink plenty, but avoid chilled drinks straight from the fridge Avoid any specific foods known to aggravate the diarrhoea
Sore mouth/throat	Offer soft, moist foods, e.g. mashed potato, scrambled egg, custard, yoghurt, ice cream If severe blended/puréed foods may be more appropriate Use straws for drinking Keep foods moist by using butter, sauces, cream or yoghurt Avoid citrus fruits and fruit juices, spicy or salty foods Avoid rough or very dry foods	Intermittent constipation	Encourage foods high in fibre and plenty of fluids
		Malabsorption	A low fat, low residue or lactose-free diet as appropriate for the type of malabsorptive problem In some cases the enteral route will need to be avoided and the child will require total parenteral nutrition
Dry mouth	Offer frequent drinks Crushed ice or cubes to suck may be useful	Food aversion	Avoid favourite foods prior to chemotherapy Give carbohydrate based meals prior to chemotherapy rather then protein based meals Avoid making a big issue of the child's nutritional intake

tunately in the hospital environment this is not always possible. Fluids and foods consumed should be recorded accurately in order to assess nutrient intake.

Advice with regard to the use of high energy foods and small frequent meals should be given routinely to parents for when the child is at home. Advice on the use of supplements should be given and how to modify them in order to improve their palatability is useful as it is often found in this group of patients that their appetites for certain tastes change very frequently.

Enteral nutrition

Whenever nutritional intervention is indicated it is highly preferable to use the enteral route. Enteral nutrition has numerous practical and psychological advantages over parenteral nutrition, including a low risk of infection and other catheter related complications, more normal play activities, and a lifestyle that provides a positive way for both parent and child to be involved in the child's care. In addition enteral feeding is more economical [8].

Studies report that nasogastric supplementary feeding benefits children with cancer and that it is practical, acceptable and tolerated in children with newly diagnosed advanced malignancy who are commencing intensive treatment protocols. It has been shown to improve their energy intake and wellbeing and to result in a significant improvement in nutritional status as measured by mid upper arm circumference [26]. Even in children undergoing bone marrow transplant where the nutritional insult is complex, as is its management, enteral nutrition when tolerated is effective in limiting the nutritional insult, leading to a better response and fewer complications [27, 28].

Generally a whole protein feed will be tolerated. However, following chemotherapy a hydrolysate or elemental feed may be more appropriate if malabsorption occurs. If the child has had total parenteral nutrition he may not tolerate a whole protein feed initially when transferring to enteral feeding, so again a hydrolysate feed may be useful (Table 6.6).

The majority of children receiving enteral feeding will require it throughout their intense treatment, but once they go onto maintenance treatment their appetites generally improve and a conscious effort should be made to try and wean them off their feeds. When deciding to feed the child with cancer by the enteral route, it is also important to establish whether

he has minimal gastrointestinal complaints and that the passing of the tube will not cause bleeding due to a low platelet count. Continuing support is essential.

Parenteral nutrition

Parenteral nutrition should be reserved for those whose enteral feeding regimens cannot provide adequate nutrients, or for those patients with abnormal gastrointestinal function related either to their tumour or following chemotherapy or radiotherapy treatments.

Parenteral nutrition is both safe and effective in children with advanced cancer; in those who are already malnourished or likely to become so, it may be the most effective feeding method [29]. Parenteral nutrition alone or in combination with enteral nutrition continues to be used frequently in paediatric cancer patients. It has been shown to reverse malnutrition, improve immunologic status, improve muscle function, decrease cancer therapy related complications and improve survival. Parenteral nutrition that delivers 90% of the recommended daily amount for energy and protein has been shown to reverse preexisting malnutrition in children with late stage malignancies and recurrent leukaemia or lymphoma who require aggressive toxic anti-cancer therapy [30]. Several studies have documented fewer drug treatment delays caused by marrow suppression and fewer drug dose reductions in patients who maintain good nutritional status while receiving parenteral nutrition [24, 31].

In children undergoing bone marrow transplant where the gastrointestinal damage is complex and can have profound nutritional consequences, parenteral nutrition should be used in children with severe oral mucositis, in patients unable to tolerate enteral nutrition due to diarrhoea and/or vomiting and in those with graft verus host disease involving the gut [32, 33].

Although parenteral nutrition is an appropriate method of renourishing children with cancer, some patients may not benefit from parenteral nutritional support because of overwhelming medical problems which may limit fluid and nutrient intake, or because of interruptions of nutrient delivery or because of rapidly progressive disease. During the peroid of toxicity associated with intense oncologic treatment, when the child is generally dependent on parenteral nutritional support for an adequate nutrient intake, a

Table 21.5 Effect of chemotherapy drugs on electrolytes

Electrolyte affected	Side effect	Chemotherapy drug
Potassium	Muscular weakness Confusion Cardiac arrhythmias	Ifosfamide Cyclophosphamide Cisplatin Carboplatin
Phosphate	Anorexia, weakness, bone pain, joint stiffness Further symptoms include muscle weakness, tremor, paraesthesia, confusion and coma	Ifosfamide Cyclophosphamide Cisplatinum Carboplatin
Calcium	Tetany Fitting Lethargy Osteomalacia	Ifosfamide
Magnesium	Muscle weakness Fasciculation Tetany Vertigo Depression	Cisplatin

small frequent amount may be given enterally [34]. This may be as little as 5 ml per hour of a hydrolysate or elemental feed. This may help to protect the mucosal barrier and possibly decrease bacterial translocation.

Metabolic complications of parenteral nutrition are well documented and are not significantly different between children with malignancies and other children requiring nutritional support. Monitoring of the patient's weight, fluid balance and biochemical parameters is essential. It is extremely important to check electrolyte levels daily, especially if the child is receiving a course of chemotherapy containing drugs which impair renal function, e.g. Ifosfamide and Cyclophosphamide. In this case, certain electrolytes will be required above normal maintenance level (Table 21.5).

BENEFITS OF NUTRITIONALLY SUPPORTING THE CHILD WITH CANCER

Nutritional support to prevent loss of lean body mass is an integral part of treatment of paediatric oncology patients. A multidisciplinary team approach, of which the dietitian is a key member, is the best way of providing safe, appropriate and effective nutritional support for this group of patients.

The benefits from nutritional support are inherently important, independent of potential benefit related to survival. Proper nutritional support in children with cancer has value in improving growth and wellbeing. Current data suggests that chemotherapy-induced bone marrow suppression may be attenuated and chemotherapy tolerance improved with the use of adequate nutritional support in children with advanced cancers [11].

NUTRITION AND THE CHILD WITH CANCER UNDERGOING BONE MARROW TRANSPLANT

Bone marrow transplant (BMT) is now widely used in children with malignancies and non-malignancies. Bone marrow transplant is indicated for patients with high risk leukaemia or for patients with leukaemia who have disease recurrence. These patients undergo an allogenic transplant using donor (related or unrelated) marrow. Some children with solid tumours, e.g. stage IV neuroblastoma and stage IV rhabdomyosarcoma, may undergo high dose therapy, usually Melphalan, supported with a peripheral blood stem-cell transplant. This is the latest development in BMT and involves the return of the patient's own stem cells.

The priming chemotherapy used causes severe nausea, vomiting and oral ulceration and BMT in children is associated with diarrhoea, protein-losing enteropathy, hypoalbuminaemia and trace element deficiencies [27]. Transient intestinal failure following BMT is a common clinical problem as unlike other organ/tissue transplantation, BMT often requires the use of total body irradiation in addition to immunosuppression. Cells with a rapid turnover, such as haemopoietic cells and immature enterocytes, are well recognised as highly susceptible to the effects of radiation and chemotherapy [32].

The aetiology of nutritional compromise caused by chemotherapy and total body irradiation is complex and nutritional support in this group of patients is challenging. In addition to this the patient is severely neutropenic and needs to keep to a clean diet in order to prevent gastrointestinal infection from foodborne pathogens [35]. The provision of a clean diet is described elsewhere (Chapter 2).

ALTERNATIVE DIETS

There are various alternative or 'fad' diets advised by religious or philosophical groups which claim to treat or cure cancer and are used either in conjunction with or instead of conventional cancer treatments. Examples include the Bristol diet, the Kelly anticancer diet and the Macrobiotic diet.

Most of these diets claim to rid the body of unnatural chemicals and to restore the efficiency of and strengthen the body's immune system by maximising the mineral, vitamin and enzyme systems. They are usually strictly vegetarian or vegan and, ideally, organic. The diets exclude all animal products, salt and refined carbohydrate and allow only small quantities of fat. They often involve taking large amounts of vitamin and mineral supplements. They are therefore very bulky, low in energy, low in protein and totally inappropriate for most children, let alone the child with cancer. Children with a loss of appetite, nausea and vomiting will find it extremely difficult to eat a high fibre, raw food diet.

These diets are also very time consuming and costly to prepare and the high doses of vitamins and minerals may be harmful. Any parent contemplating putting a child on such a diet should be advised strongly against it.

The benefits of nutritional support for the child with cancer are extremely important. Proper nutritional support can improve growth and organ function and appears to improve treatment tolerance and quality of life.

REFERENCES

1 Van Eys J Nutritional therapy in children with cancer. *Cancer Res*, 1977, **87** 2457–61.
2 Van Eys J Malnutrition in pediatric oncology. In: Newell GR (ed.) *Nutrition and Cancer: Etiology and Treatment*. New York: Raven Press, 1981.
3 Andrassy RJ Nutritional support of the pediatric oncology patient. *Nutrition*, 1998, **14** 124–9.
4 Eden OB Paediatric oncology. *Hospital Update*, 1983, March, 779–88.
5 United Kingdom Children's Cancer Study Group *Scientific Report*. London: UKCCSG, 1998.
6 Bury CL *Paediatric Pathology*, 2e. Berlin: Springer-Verlag, 1989.
7 Mott MG Paediatric malignancy: tumour types. *Medicine*, 1995, 460–63.
8 Donaldson SS A study of nutritional status in paediatric cancer patients. *Am J Dis Childh*, 1981, **135** 1107–12.
9 Van Eys J Malnutrition in children with cancer: incidence and consequences. *Cancer*, 1979, **43** 2030–35.
10 Smith DE Malnutrition at diagnosis of malignancy in childhood; common but mostly missed. *Eur J Pediatr*, 1991, **150** 318–22.
11 Mauer AM *et al.* Special nutritional needs of children with malignancies – a review. *J Parent Ent Nutr*, 1990, **14** 315–23.
12 Smith DE *et al.* Malnutrition in children with malignant solid tumours. *J Hum Nutr Diet*, 1990, **3** 303–309.
13 Tidsdale MJ Cancer cachexia; metabolic alterations and clinical manifestations. *Nutrition*, 1997, **13** 1–7.
14 Starnes HF *et al.* Tumour necrosis factor and the acute metabolic response to tissue injury in man. *J Clin Invest*, 1988, **82** 1321–4.
15 Falconer JS *et al.* Cytokines, the acute phase response, and resting energy expenditure in cachetic patients with pancreatic cancer. *Ann Surg*, 1994, **219** 325.
16 Rossi-Fanelli F *et al.* Abnormal substrate metabolism and nutritional strategies in cancer management. *J Parent Ent Nutr*, 1991, **15** 680–83.
17 Shaw JHF *et al.* Fatty acid and glycerol kinetics in septic patients and patients with gastrointestinal cancer: the response to glucose infusion and parenteral feeding. *Ann Surg*, 1987, **205** 368–71.
18 Bernstein IL Learned taste aversions in children receiving chemotherapy. *Science*, 1978, **200** 1302–3.
19 Bernstein IL Physiological and psychological mechanisms of cancer anorexia. *Cancer Res*, 1982, **42** 715s–720s.
20 Rickard KA The value of nutritional support in children with cancer. *Cancer*, 1986, **52** 587–90.
21 Rickard KA Advances in nutrition care of children with neoplastic disease – a review of treatment, research and application. *J Am Diet Assoc*, 1986, **86** 1666–75.
22 Rickard KA Effect of nutritional staging on treatment delays and outcome in stage IV neuroblastoma. *Cancer*, 1983, **52** 587–92.
23 Van Eys J Nutrition in the treatment of cancer in children. *J Am Coll Nutr*, 1984, **3** 159–68.
24 Rickard KA Effectiveness of enteral and parenteral nutrition in the management of children with Wilm's tumours. *Am J Clin Nutr*, 1980, **56** 2881–7.
25 *EAT* Paediatric Dietetic Department, St James's University Hospital, Leeds, 1999.
26 Smith DE An investigation of supplementary nasogastric feeding in malnourished children undergoing treatment for malignancy: results of a pilot study. *J Hum Nutr Diet*, 1992, **5** 85–91.
27 Papadopoulou A Enteral nutrition after bone marrow transplant. *Arch Dis Childh*, 1997, **77** 131–6.
28 Papadopoulou A Nutritional support in children undergoing bone marrow transplant. *Clin Nutr*, 1998, **17** 57–63.
29 Rickard KA Short and long term effectiveness of enteral and parenteral nutrition in reversing or pre-

venting protein–energy malnutrition in advanced neuroblastoma. *Cancer*, 1985, **56** 2881–7.

30 Rickard KA Reversal of protein energy malnutrition in children during treatment of advanced neoplastic disease. *Ann Surg*, 1979, **190** 777–81.

31 Yokoyama S Use of parenteral nutrition in pediatric bone marrow transplantation. *Nutr*, 1989 **5** 27–30.

32 Papadopoulou A *et al.* Gastrointestinal and nutritional sequelae of bone marrow transplant. *Arch Dis Childh*, 1996, **75** 208–13.

33 Papadopoulou A Nutritional considerations in children undergoing bone marrow transplant. *J Clin Nutr*, 1998, **52** 863–71.

34 Chellis MJ *et al.* Cost effectiveness of early enteral feeding in the critically ill child. *Crit Care Med*, 1994, **2** 147.

35 Henry L. Immunocompromised patients and nutrition. *Prof Nurse*, 1997, **12** 655–9.

USEFUL ADDRESS

Cancer Link Directory of Cancer Self Help Support 1999
Available from Cancer Link, 11–21 Northdown Street, London N1 9BW.

SECTION 9

Eating Disorders and Obesity

CHAPTER 22

Eating Disorders

INTRODUCTION

Eating disorders are psychiatric disorders (generally considered to be emotional disorders) in which abnormalities of eating are the main behavioural symptoms. Hand-in-hand with abnormal eating behaviours go characteristic fears or beliefs, the so-called 'core psychopathology' of eating disorders. As with other psychiatric disorders, the diagnosis of an eating disorder depends on the presence of specific thoughts or ideas, *and* associated behavioural disturbance outside the range of what might be considered normal behaviour. These criteria distinguish the eating disorders from other abnormal eating behaviours, in which psychological disturbance may be present but is usually secondary, not primary. For example, low self-esteem and depression may be associated with obesity, but obesity is not a psychiatric disorder.

The most widely recognised and well-described eating disorders are anorexia nervosa and bulimia nervosa. In both the sufferer has an extreme preoccupation with her (usually) weight and/or shape and a specific 'morbid' fear of weight gain. In anorexia nervosa the associated behavioural disturbances are methods for achieving weight loss. Most commonly this is through dietary restriction, often coupled with excessive exercise – the so-called 'restrictive subtype' of anorexia nervosa [1]. Alternatively weight loss can be achieved by means of purging behaviours, such as self-induced vomiting, or laxative or diuretic abuse – the so-called 'binge-purge subtype'.

In bulimia nervosa the same fears and beliefs about weight and shape exist, but the behavioural characteristics differ. The sufferer submits to intense cravings for large quantities of food – a binge – eaten over a short period of time. 'Bulimia' means 'the hunger of an ox'. The binge is then followed by extreme guilt about eating (because of fear of weight gain). The sufferer will attempt to compensate for the additional calorie load through one or more 'compensatory behaviours', either self-induced vomiting and purgative abuse (binge-purge subtype) or periods of fasting and exercising (restrictive subtype). An additional psychological feature of bulimia nervosa is the sufferer's sense of being unable to control her eating behaviour. There is clearly a lot of overlap between anorexia nervosa and bulimia nervosa, and indeed up to a third of bulimia nervosa sufferers have had a previous episode of anorexia nervosa. Sufferers of bulimia nervosa are usually in the normal or slightly overweight range; if they were severely underweight they would be diagnosed as suffering from anorexia nervosa – binge-purge subtype.

More recently a third disorder has been described, 'binge-eating disorder' (BED). In BED the sufferer has binge episodes, a sense of lack of control over food intake and a preoccupation with weight and shape, but does not utilise compensatory behaviours following a binge episode. Thus overall dietary intake is in excess of normal, and sufferers are usually overweight. BED is in the process of validation as a separate diagnostic entity, but this type of behaviour is well described as one form of psychological disturbance associated with obesity.

There are a number of other disturbances of eating recognised as being severe enough to constitute disorder. These 'syndromes' are of uncertain status, in terms of whether they are disorders in their own right or merely associated features of other disorders. Nonetheless the International Classification of Diseases [2] includes in its eating disorders section, in addition to anorexia nervosa and bulimia nervosa, overeating leading to obesity as a reaction to distressing events (*not* psychological disturbance as a consequence of obesity); vomiting associated with other psychological disturbances (e.g. dissociative disorders, hypochondriacal disorders or when emotional factors in pregnancy contribute); and other eating disorders such as pica and psychogenic loss of appetite.

In children there are a number of eating behaviours which are not currently classified at all, but which are nonetheless manifestations of, or cause, extreme psychological distress. There is no international consensus on how to name these behaviours or how they should be classified. The terms used in this chapter are therefore descriptive, but we have found them to be useful and meaningful in a clinical context working with children in the middle childhood and early adolescent age range. Work is underway to validate the categories described [3].

EATING DISORDERS IN A DEVELOPMENTAL CONTEXT

Eating is a key behaviour in developmental terms. Failure to make the transitions from milk through liquids to solids would raise suspicion of an organic or developmental disorder, or the possibility of severe abuse and neglect. Once established on solids, the developmental tasks are centred on increasing self-regulation on behalf of the child, with the gradual transition of control and responsibility for food intake from the parent to the child. Thus by the age of eight or so, although a parent is the food provider, a children will usually feed themselves, choose which of the provided food they will eat (by and large), and ask for more or stop eating when full (self-regulate quantity).

This process of transfer of responsibility is a careful balance of timing and encouragement – too much parental regulation and the child may rebel; too much autonomy for the child and he or she may not be able to cope. As such the transition from feeding to eating is highly susceptible to tension and conflict, particularly over issues of autonomy and control. It is also a point of communication between a child and his or her parent, and as such can be a method for communicating distress or anxiety. In younger children we tend to call disorders where eating behaviour reflects disturbed communication or emotional distress of this kind, feeding disorders (conventionally requiring onset before the age of 6 years). In adolescents and adults we call them eating disorders. The eating disturbances of middle childhood lie somewhere between the eating disorders and the feeding

disorders of early childhood, and share some features of each.

When eating behaviour becomes the focus for distress or of significant harm (such as failure to thrive), help may be sought through a variety of means. Often a dietitian will be the first port of call, and it is important to be able to recognise the ways in which psychological distress can manifest through eating, and consider how to address these difficulties when encountered in clinical practice.

ANOREXIA NERVOSA

Both anorexia nervosa and bulimia nervosa are predominantly disorders of teenage girls and young women. However, anorexia nervosa can occur in boys and in children as young as 7 years. Both disorders are relatively common, with anorexia nervosa occurring in almost 1% of teenage girls. In the USA anorexia nervosa is now the third commonest chronic illness of adolescence [4]. While the figures in the UK are not quite so high, certain populations are more at risk – for example girls in high achieving academic environments, and in high risk professions such as modelling and dancing. The prevalence of anorexia nervosa is probably not increasing [5], although the severity of the disorder may be [6]. Many of the complications of anorexia nervosa are related to the duration of illness and age of onset [7], and thus early diagnosis is important, particularly in growing children. The peak age of onset is around the time of completion of puberty (13–15), although pre-pubertal onset anorexia nervosa is by no means uncommon.

The essential features of anorexia nervosa are:

- Weight loss (or failure of weight gain in growing children) sufficient for there to be physiological signs of underweight

In post-menarchal girls, this means enough for periods to have stopped for more than three menstrual cycles. In younger girls and in boys, signs of endocrine dysfunction would be failure to progress in puberty and slowing of linear growth. Both these signs can take months to become manifest. In practice a child whose weight is not rising or is falling over a period of months can be assumed to be losing significant weight. The diagnostic criteria have a cut-off for weight of a body mass index (BMI) of

17.5, or of 85% ideal body weight (see 'Nutritional Assessment' section in Chapter 1). Rapid weight loss is a poor prognostic sign and should be treated urgently.

- Avoidance of food

This may be evident simply as not eating (restraint) or by more surreptitious means such as hiding food, exercising to 'burn off' food, or purging (vomiting or laxative use). Sufferers may also indulge in rituals and compulsions to control their eating.

- Morbid preoccupation with weight and/or shape

The reason for avoiding food is a fear of weight gain and the changes in body shape that may accompany it. The individual may acknowledge this fear directly. Sometimes it may be inferred only by the specific avoidance of fattening foods. Thus the anorectic will often know more than their parents and even professionals about the calorific content of foods. In boys and young men the form of the preoccupation may differ slightly. For example, females with anorexia nervosa see their stomach and thighs as particularly fat, whereas boys may be more concerned about their chest size and musculature.

Recognising anorexia nervosa

Eating disorders rarely present directly to specialists. In one series of 48 children presenting with determined food avoidance, 52% spent some time on a general paediatric ward [8] before referral to a child psychiatry team. Atypical presentations and a particular lack of awareness that these conditions can arise in young children and boys may lead to delay in referral, diagnosis and treatment [9, 10].

The patient with anorexia nervosa is not usually hard to recognise. The contrast between the sufferer's emaciated state and her irritable reluctance to acknowledge any difficulties or concern is a good indicator. The protest that she is 'naturally thin' is not borne out by her low pulse rate, low blood pressure and cold, often blue, hands and feet. She may not present herself, but will be there at the behest of a family member, a friend, or because concerns have been expressed at school. While the sufferer may not want to be ill, she has an even greater desire not to be made to eat. She will therefore tend to avoid situations where her eating difficulties are most manifest, for example, eating in public or social groups, and will avoid situations where she may be confronted about her weight. Adolescent patients typically present wearing many layers of clothes in all seasons, partly from a wish to hide their body and partly from feeling cold. Younger children, however, may not be self-conscious about their low weight, and even seem to wish to display it at times.

If there is some doubt, the simplest discriminator is food. When food intake is increased to counteract the effects of starvation, the anorexia nervosa sufferer will need to increase food avoiding behaviours, and/or will demonstrate greater distress/protest about eating. On a hospital ward this behaviour becomes evident very quickly. Or it may become clear that there is a big discrepancy between what the sufferer is thought to be eating and what the weight tells you they must really be eating.

Having recognised the patient with anorexia nervosa, direct challenge or confrontation is unlikely to be helpful. Reasonable aims for a first meeting would be as follows.

- Give provisional information, based on observations

For example, calculate BMI or % BMI. Body mass index (BMI) is not a linear constant in childhood and adolescence [11], and calculation of the % weight for height or % BMI is better [12]. Alternatively BMI can be plotted on centile charts, as for weight and height. A Cole's slide rule for calculating % BMI or a BMI chart can be obtained from the Child Growth Foundation. Clinically, however, rate of weight loss may be more important than a single % BMI measurement.

- Agree a system of weight monitoring, and a plan of action for if the weight falls

The weight may be monitored (usually weekly) by a parent, school nurse, GP or any other responsible adult. It should not be known only to the sufferer. Admission to hospital should be requested for patients with a BMI of 13, or a % BMI of 70% or below.

- Give information about literature or other sources of help for both sufferers and families

The following are useful texts, although their use has not been evaluated as an adjunct to treatment: *Anorexia nervosa: a survival guide for friends, families and sufferers* [13], and *A Parents' Guide to Eating Disorders* [14]. In the UK, the Eating Disorders Association provides information, has a helpline, and publishes a newsletter.

• Decide who needs to know

For children under 16 parents need to be informed. It is usual for medical responsibility to lie with the sufferer's GP, even if ongoing monitoring or outpatient treatment is being offered elsewhere.

Overview of treatment issues

Whatever the eating disorder, the child's needs are essentially the same – to be able to eat enough to grow and develop normally, and to find a way of addressing her/his emotional needs through a medium other than food. Debate continues over which to tackle first: the eating behaviour or the emotional symptoms. A similar debate exists for the sufferer – 'the problem isn't really about eating' versus 'I can't bear to eat'. In young patients, parents may focus on eating behaviour while the child/adolescent has another agenda. The main concern is that both are addressed.

In childhood food related issues are usually addressed first for a number of reasons. Firstly, children can dehydrate and physically decompensate very quickly. Secondly, responsibility for food intake will often lie with the parents and can therefore be established more quickly than when the patient needs to become self-motivated. Thirdly, as mentioned, the risk of complications such as growth failure, pubertal arrest and failure of bone accretion are related to age of onset and duration of illness. In a growing child anorexia nervosa can have significant impact in as little as 6 months.

A multidisciplinary approach is essential because of the need to address the medical, nutritional and therapeutic needs of the young person and her family. Such an approach also minimises the risk of isolating the professional or their being drawn into colluding with the sufferer. Collusion is not uncommon, as the most difficult part of managing anorexia nervosa is agreeing mutually acceptable goals for treatment. Failure to agree goals, or failure to reach treatment goals (e.g. BMI remains below 17.5 for 3 months or more) are good indications for referral to a specialist eating disorders team. A number of specialist services exist nationwide, although availability of services for children and young adolescents is more patchy. Anorexia nervosa is a disorder that can be treated under the Mental Health Act 1983 or under the Children Act 1989, if necessary. Specialist teams rarely, if ever, need to force-feed patients.

The mainstay of treatment for anorexia nervosa is various forms of psychotherapy, the type and intensity varying with the age of the sufferer and the chronicity of the problem. For patients under the age of 18 with an illness of less than 3 years duration, family therapy is the treatment of choice [15, 16]. There is no empirical evidence to suggest that families cause eating disorders, although there is no doubt that family functioning can become severely distorted as a result of the illness. Behavioural techniques are not much use in isolation, and at worst can be punitive. Despite this, they continue to form the basis of treatment on some inpatient wards.

Vitamin supplements are not generally advised, and energy is best directed at encouraging a 'normal diet eaten normally', with weight gain at a rate of $\frac{1}{2}$ to 1 kg per week.

Osteoporosis is a recognised complication of prolonged anorexia nervosa. Traditional methods of oestrogen supplementation are not helpful, although they may be useful for damage limitation in persistent anorexia nervosa by preventing further bone loss [17]. Calcium supplements may help where intake is low, although evaluation suggests the impact is minimal. Vitamin D is usually unnecessary as patients are not usually deficient. See Weaver *et al.* [18] for a review of aspects of adolescent nutrition and bone density.

BULIMIA NERVOSA

Bulimia nervosa is a disorder of over-eating rather than under-eating. The sufferer experiences a lack of control of appetite and will consume large quantities of food over short periods of time (bingeing). She (patients with bulimia nervosa are almost exclusively female) will then purge, usually with self-induced vomiting, in order to counteract the fattening effects of the binge. This behaviour is associated with cycles of uncontrollable tension followed by relief, followed by guilt. Depression is common.

Bulimia nervosa tends to onset slightly later in adolescence or early adulthood than anorexia nervosa and is less likely to come to medical attention; sufferers are normal weight and are usually ashamed of their eating difficulties. The prevalence is therefore probably underestimated, at around 2–3% of young women. Bulimia nervosa was first described in 1979 [19] as 'an ominous variant of anorexia nervosa'. Since 1979 there has been an exponential rise in numbers of cases presenting for treatment [20]. Russell saw the development of self-induced vomiting on weight recovery from anorexia nervosa as a poor prognostic sign, because of the association between purging and other types of self-harm. Certainly the severity of purging behaviour can be extreme, with serious medical complications. In addition the patient with bulimia nervosa is more likely to be overtly depressed than the anorexia nervosa sufferer. Overall though, now that more is known about bulimia nervosa and its treatment, it would generally be considered a less severe illness than anorexia nervosa in terms of morbidity and mortality. It is also more accessible to treatment, and management approaches are more clear-cut and validated.

Recognising bulimia nervosa

Bulimia nervosa is less obvious to recognise than anorexia nervosa, and may only come to light through suspicion of a family member or friend. If the sufferer herself seeks help it may be for a different problem, and hints about food and dieting may be the only clues. Irregular periods, callouses on the knuckles of forefingers due to abrasions from teeth during self-induced vomiting (Russell's sign) or erosion of dental enamel from stomach acid may be picked up. Adolescents living at home may find it harder to hide purging behaviour than adults living independently. There are no investigations that will confirm the diagnosis, only good interviewing skills.

Once recognised and acknowledged, the sufferer may be able to use one of the well-validated self-help manuals: *Overcoming binge eating* [21] or *Getting Better Bit(e) by Bit(e): A survival kit for sufferers of bulimia nervosa and binge eating disorders* [22]. Based on cognitive behavioural techniques these are as effective as therapist-led treatment in over half of cases, and are a useful adjunct to treatment in the remainder. Antidepressant medication also has a role in bulimia nervosa, regardless of whether the sufferer is also clinically depressed. Information about nutrition and control of appetite and the establishment of regular mealtimes are important educational components. The key to treatment lies in the recognition of triggers for binges and the establishment of alternative responses to those triggers.

OTHER EATING DIFFICULTIES ASSOCIATED WITH WEIGHT LOSS

The term 'food avoidance emotional disorder' (FAED) was coined by Higgs and Goodyer [23] to describe those children who avoid food sufficient to result in weight loss, for reasons other than fear of weight gain. Children with FAED can find it as difficult to eat as those with anorexia nervosa, although they often wish they could eat more. Depression may be present, but often the food avoidance exists as an isolated symptom.

Eating difficulties can be part of other disorders such as depression, obsessive compulsive disorder and pervasive developmental disorders. In addition, physical illness may often be associated with manifest loss of appetite, to which psychological factors can significantly contribute. We have come to use the term FAED when food avoidance is marked and merits treatment intervention in its own right. When comorbid disorders exist, either physical or psychological, they need to be addressed in addition to the eating difficulty.

In physical terms, the main differences between patients with FAED and those with early onset anorexia nervosa are in age at presentation (mean 11.8 versus 13.5 years) and in the gender ratio (approximately 2:1 girls to boys for FAED compared with 9:1 in anorexia nervosa) [24]. Psychologically the differences are more marked. Unlike anorexia nervosa patients, children with FAED know that they are underweight, would like to be heavier, and may not know why they find this difficult to achieve. They are more likely to have other medically unexplained symptoms, and their parents may attribute weight loss to an undiagnosed physical disorder. Addressing these concerns with a comprehensive physical assessment and an open mind is essential for successful treatment. FAED sufferers are also more likely than anorexia nervosa sufferers to show anxiety in other areas, unrelated to food. It is likely that children with FAED are a heterogeneous group of children, a minority of whom will later develop anorexia nervosa.

Clinical Paediatric Dietetics

Functional dysphagia is a term used for difficulty in swallowing associated with a fear of choking. The symptom can be found clinically in patients with FAED, selective eating and sometimes anorexia nervosa, or it may be a new symptom of acute onset, often following trauma. Failure to thrive should be considered when long term growth failure is seen in association with low weight, extending back to early childhood.

Recognising these more diffuse forms of food-related anxiety can be harder than recognising anorexia nervosa and bulimia nervosa. Often the presentation will be 'unexplained' weight loss. Clearly the priority is to exclude organic disorder, but the risk is that the child loses further weight during the course of investigations, or is traumatised by them (as can occur, for example, with endoscopy for the investigation of functional dysphagia). Equally distressing can be the 'there's nothing wrong with you – go and see the psychiatrists' response. The most direct route to opening discussion about causes is to ask parents what they think is wrong with their child. If they have no opinion, it may be helpful to ask specifically whether they think it is a gut-related problem, a cancer or other 'worst fear', or whether worry or an eating disorder may play some part. Psychological assessment can then be suggested as one of the possible investigations.

For all of these disorders, careful individualised assessment of the child and family is necessary in order to understand the origin and meaning of the symptom for the child in their particular context. A clear formulation of the problem is needed as a guide to treatment. Similarly, nutritional support may need to be carefully considered, taking into account the child's specific anxiety, and finding creative ways to encourage food intake while the child retains as much control as possible. In extreme cases nasogastric or other feeding can help take the pressure off while the child learns to overcome at his/her own pace his/her fear of eating.

EATING DIFFICULTIES WITH NORMAL WEIGHT

'Faddy eating' occurs in over 20% of toddlers [25], and can be considered normal at a particular developmental stage. In a small number, particularly boys, the behaviour persists into middle childhood and adolescence. This has been termed 'selective eating' [26].

In addition to the narrow range of foods, the consistent psychological characteristic is an extreme resistance or unwillingness to try new foods. Often selective eating exists as an isolated symptom. However, selective eating is found in a high number of children with neurodevelopmental difficulties such as autism. It is not unusual to find a mild degree of dyspraxia, language difficulty or social skills difficulty in a referred child with selective eating [27]. In addition, some show phobic anxiety about new things other than food.

The highly limited range of foods (generally 10 foods or less) seems to have no impact on growth and development, or on bone density (Nicholls *et al.*, unpublished data). Reassurance that the child is not doing him/herself any damage may be all that is required. However, particularly with approaching adolescence, the young person may be socially disadvantaged by eating, unable to go away on school trips or stay over at friends' houses. Alternatively, a parent may seek treatment anticipating social difficulties, while the child remains unconcerned.

For those children who are ready to change, a cognitive behavioural model of treatment, led by the child, can be rapidly effective. Over the years the child may have developed anticipatory nausea (with sight or smell triggers), fear of vomiting (textures), or a fear of choking at the sight of new foods. If the child is not committed to change, trying new foods during treatment will re-evoke anxiety and may result in even greater food avoidance. Suggesting they return at a later date may be appropriate if the child is not yet ready for treatment.

Hyperphagic short stature (HSS) [28] is a distinctive disorder in which children will eat voraciously, often scavenging for food, gorging and vomiting. Body mass index is in the normal range. The characteristic associated feature is growth failure (height below 3rd centile). Growth hormone secretion is suppressed but returns to normal on removal from or reduction of stress [29]. HSS is not usually considered with the eating disorders, but there are continuities with failure to thrive during infancy as well as with rumination disorders and pica.

THE ROLE OF THE DIETITIAN

Little has been said so far about specific nutritional aspects in the management of eating disorders. In part this comes from a belief that it is more important to empower the parents or adolescent to determine and decide their own food intake than for them to follow a prescribed regimen – treatment for many eating disorders involves abandoning dietary rules, rather than adopting them. In addition, wide cultural variations in eating habits as well as food content make it hard to contemplate a diet that would suit all.

That said, nutritional counselling is an important component of the comprehensive care of young people with eating disorders. While the sufferer from anorexia nervosa or bulimia nervosa may know a great deal about the nutritional content of food, they will have a very distorted view of their own dietary requirements, and unrealistic weight goals. One of the aims of treatment is for an adolescent to take more responsibility for his/her own nutritional intake. This means having factual information about daily nutritional requirements and some idea about energy balance, particularly if excessive exercising is one of the problem behaviours. In younger children, it may be the parents rather than the young person who need the ongoing support and advice.

Although iron, zinc and calcium deficiency have been reported in anorexia nervosa, these all normalise with refeeding and it is not part of standard treatment in the UK to add vitamin supplements. Calcium supplements are sometimes added when the disorder becomes chronic, because of the risk of falling bone density. As yet there is no empirical research to support this as part of treatment.

Many patients with anorexia nervosa are, or have become, vegetarian. Different treatment centres treat this issue in different ways. However, it is possible that the risks of hypo-oestrogenism (and therefore low bone density) are increased in vegetarians compared to non-vegetarians who are not menstruating due to low weight (H. Jacobs, pers. comm.).

Specific dietary expertise is needed when nasogastric or other feeding is necessary. This will usually be in an inpatient setting where monitoring for refeeding syndromes is possible. Following nutritional assessment, it is usual to increase feeding gradually over a few days, aiming at a weight gain of $^1/_2$–1 kg weight gain per week.

CONCLUSION

Eating disorders are psychiatric disorders that manifest through disturbances in eating. Early recognition can prevent serious physical complications, and also improves the outcome. Eating difficulties resulting in significant weight loss present the greatest risk. Nutritional counselling is one component of clinical management, and clear communication between members of the treating team can prevent professional isolation and collusion with the patient's anxiety. In early onset disorders nutritional counselling and education may be more appropriately offered to the parents than to the sufferer themself. The thrust of treatment for all eating disorders is to normalise eating as much as possible while providing a context in which the underlying emotional issues can be addressed. Collaborative work involving parents and the child/adolescent as much as possible produces the best results.

REFERENCES

1 American Psychiatric Association *Diagnostic and Statistical Manual of Mental Disorders – DSMIV*. Washington DC: American Psychiatric Association, 1994.

2 WHO. *ICD-10 Classification of Mental and Behavioural Disorders*. London: Churchill Livingstone, 1991.

3 Watkins E, Bryant Waugh R, Cooper P, Lask B *The Nosology of Childhood Onset Eating Disorders*. 2000 unpubl.

4 Lucas AR, Beard CM, O'Fallon WM, Kurland LT Fifty year trends in the incidence of anorexia nervosa in Rochester, Minnesota: a population-based study. *Am J Psychiatry*, 1991, **148** 917–22.

5 Fombonne E Anorexia nervosa. No evidence of an increase. *Br J Psych*, 1995, **166** 462–7.

6 Moller-Madsen S, Nystrup J, Nielsen S Mortality of anorexia nervosa in Denmark during the period 1970–1987. *Acta Psychiatr Scand*, 1996, **94** 454–9.

7 Nicholls D, de Bruyn R, Gordon I Physical assessment and complications. In: Lask B, Bryant-Waugh R (eds) *Anorexia Nervosa and Related Eating Disorders in Childhood and Adolescence*. Hove: Psychology Press, 2000.

8 Fosson A, Knibbs J, Bryant-Waugh R, Lask B Early onset anorexia nervosa. *Arch Dis Childh*, 1987, **62** 114–18.

9 Bryant-Waugh R, Lask B, Shafran R, Fosson A Do doctors recognise eating disorders in children? *Arch Dis Childh*, 1992, **67** 103–105.

10 Jacobs BW, Isaacs S Pre-pubertal anorexia nervosa: a retrospective controlled study. *J Child Psychol Psychiatry*, 1986, **27** 237–50.

11 Cole TJ, Freeman JV, Preece MA Body mass index reference curves for the UK, 1990. *Arch Dis Childh*, 1995, **73** 25–9.

12 Cole TJ, Donnet ML, Stanfield JP Weight-for-height indices to assess nutritional status – a new index on a slide-rule. *Am J Clin Nutr*, 1981, **34** 1935–43.

13 Treasure J *Anorexia Nervosa: A Survival Guide for Families, Friends and Sufferers*. Hove: Psychology Press, 1987.

14 Bryant-Waugh R, Lask B *Eating Disorders; A Parents' Guide*. London: Penguin, 1999.

15 Russell GF, Szmukler GI, Dare C, Eisler I An evaluation of family therapy in anorexia nervosa and bulimia nervosa. *Arch Gen Psychiatry*, 1987, **44** 1047–56.

16 Eisler I, Dare C, Russell GF, Szmukler G, le Grange D, Dodge E Family and individual therapy in anorexia nervosa. A 5-year follow-up. *Arch Gen Psychiatry*, 1997, **54** 1025–30.

17 Klibanski A, Biller BM, Schoenfeld DA, Herzog DB, Saxe VC The effects of estrogen administration on trabecular bone loss in young women with anorexia nervosa. *J Clin Endocrinol Metab*, 1995, **80** 898–904.

18 Weaver CM, Peacock M, Johnston CC Adolescent nutrition in the prevention of post-menopausal osteoporosis. *J Clin Endocrinol Metab*, 1999, **84** 1839–43.

19 Russell GFM Bulimia nervosa: an ominous variant of anorexia nervosa. *Psychol Med*, 1979, **9** 429–48.

20 Kendler KS, McLean C, Neale M *et al.* The genetic epidemiology of bulimia nervosa. *Am J Psych*, 1991, **148** 1627–37.

21 Fairburn C *Overcoming Binge Eating*. New York: Guilford Press, 1995.

22 Schmidt U, Treasure J *Getting Better Bit(e) by Bit(e)*. Hove: Psychology Press, 1994.

23 Higgs JF, Goodyer IM, Birch J Anorexia nervosa and food avoidance emotional disorder. *Arch Dis Childh*, 1989, **64** 346–51.

24 Nicholls D, Casey C, Stanhope R, Lask B Atypical childhood onset anorexia nervosa or food avoidance emotional disorder: physical and psychological characteristics. *R Coll Psych*, 1998, (Abstract).

25 Richman N, Lansdown R *Problems of Preschool Children*. Chichester: John Wiley and Sons, 1988, p. 243.

26 Bryant-Waugh R Overview of the eating disorders. In: Lask B, Bryant-Waugh R (eds) *Anorexia Nervosa and Related Eating Disorders in Childhood and Adolescence*. Hove: Psychology Press, 1999, pp. 27–41.

27 Nicholls D, Christie D, Lask B Selective eating: symptom, disorder or normal variant? *R Coll Psych Conf*, 1998, (Abstract).

28 Skuse D, Albanese A, Stanhope R, Gilmour J, Voss L A new stress-related syndrome of growth failure and hyperphagia in children, associated with reversibility of growth-hormone deficiency. *Lancet*, 1996, **348** 353–8.

29 Albanese A, Hamill G, Jones J, Skuse D, Matthews DR, Stanhope R Reversibility of physiological growth hormone secretion in children with psychosocial dwarfism. *Clin Endocrinol*, 1994, **40** 687–92.

USEFUL ADDRESSES

Child Growth Foundation
2 Mayfield Avenue, Chiswick, London W4 1PW. Tel. 020 8995 0257 8994 7625

Eating Disorders Association,
First Floor, Wensum House, 103 Prince of Wales Road, Norwich, NR1 1DW. Tel. (Helplines) 01603 621 414. Website: www.edauk.com

ACKNOWLEDGEMENT

The Child Growth Foundation, UK, supports the work of Dasha Nicholls.

CHAPTER 23

Obesity

SIMPLE OBESITY

Obesity is a relatively common problem in childhood and adolescence, which presents a difficult task and challenge for the clinician and dietitian to manage.

The definition of childhood and adolescent obesity remains unclear. This needs to be resolved so that the prevalence of childhood obesity can be examined [1]. Taitz has in the past defined obesity as 'an excess of adipose tissue, considered to be undesirable, or reach levels above those set arbitrarily, and based on a suitable anthropometric measurement' [2].

The prevalence of obesity, however, appears to be increasing in most parts of the world [3–6]. Between 1980 and 1996 the prevalence of obesity has more than doubled in the UK, increasing from 6 to 16% in men and from 8 to 18% in women [7]. There have been very few surveys of obesity among children from which secular trends could be ascertained. Studies in Tayside suggest that the prevalence of obesity is increasing in Scotland and may affect 20% of children and adolescents [8]. Furthermore, Hughes *et al.* have demonstrated that while English and Scottish children are getting taller for a given age, there is also a trend towards an increase in fatness [9]. However, in a more recent study of children aged 3–5 years, Reilly *et al.* found that the prevalence of overweight and obesity was significantly higher than expected with 15.8%, 20.3% and 18.7% of children overweight and 6%, 7.6% and 7.2% obese at 2, 4 and 5 years respectively [10]. The author also examined data in a study of 2630 English children, which showed that the frequency of being overweight was 22 and 31% for children aged 6 years and 15 years respectively and that of obesity ranged from 10% at age 6 years to 17% at 15 years of age. He also suggested that these figures will be an underestimate for various reasons [11].

Aetiology

The aetiology of obesity is complex and multifactorial. Organic causes of obesity, e.g. Cushing's syndrome and hypothyroidism, are rare. Prader-Willi syndrome is often associated with obesity and this condition is dealt with separately.

The understanding of the biological basis of obesity has grown rapidly in the last few years, especially with the identification of the genes associated with obesity and the hormone leptin [12]. The adipose cells primarily produce leptin and its importance appears to be in appetite regulation. There are some rare conditions where leptin may play a part in morbid obesity. Auwerx and Staels have summarised the advance in leptin research [13].

Both genetic and environmental factors contribute to the development of obesity. Many studies support the theory that obesity tends to run in families [14–19]. Children of non-obese parents have less than 10% chance of being obese, whereas this probability increases to 40% and 80% respectively when one or both parents are obese. Heredity and the degree of obesity in childhood and adolescence were found to have major influences on prognosis [20]. Being excessively overweight during puberty was associated with higher than expected morbidity and mortality in later life [21, 22]. Adults who were obese as children have increased mortality independent of adult weight [5]. A recent review article found the risk of adult obesity was at least twice as high for obese children as it was for non-obese children across all ages [23].

Lifestyle in the past few decades has changed considerably and this is reflected in eating habits, which tend to include more high energy 'fast foods' [24, 25]. The increase in television viewing, computer game use and other sedentary activities along with the decrease in priority given to physical education in schools means that many children are less physically active than in previous years [3, 26]. The government is currently investing more money in a variety of initiatives to develop youth and school sport and encourage increased participation in such activities. Children who take up sport in childhood may continue to pursue these activities into teenage years and adulthood [27]. Obese children are less active than their leaner peers [28, 26]; they are less fit and may feel embarrassed and uncomfortable when taking part in sporting activities.

Assessment

At the first clinic visit, baseline anthropometry should be obtained; weight and height measurements plotted on weight and height centile charts (e.g. Child Growth Foundation 1994, 1995, Tanner and Whitehouse revised 1995) and body mass index (BMI) charts (e.g. Child Growth Foundation 1997). Skinfold measurements, preferably taken by the same individual, using calipers will give a more accurate estimate of fatness and can be compared with centile charts [29]. In practice, the triceps skinfold is probably the most convenient measure of fatness in children and adolescents [30]. Generally a weight of more than two centiles higher than the height, or a weight for height index greater than 120% is considered to constitute obesity. In recent years there has been a great deal of discussion concerning the usefulness of BMI as a measure of overweight and obesity in children and adolescents [31]. The use of BMI with appropriate centile charts is now recommended by several groups – the International Obesity Task Force [32], the SIGN guidelines [33] and a recent European project that has been initiated to produce European standards [34].

Currently the cut-off points used to define overweight and obesity vary considerably and are still controversial; an international consensus is necessary to improve this predicament [35]. Charts have been developed with centile curves for BMI in British children from birth to 23 years; these are based on recently collated and nationally representative data. These suggest that for both boys and girls a BMI above the 98th centile constitutes obesity and a BMI

above the 91st centile indicates overweight [31]. However, different cut-offs are used in different countries to define overweight (e.g. 85th and 90th) and obesity (e.g. 95th and 97th) [3]. BMI charts are currently in use in some paediatric centres and are widely recommended for use in identifying the obese child.

At this first visit it is most important to get a detailed dietary history from both the child and the carer. Other details such as age of onset of obesity, eating pattern and family dynamics are also helpful. A recall diet history is most frequently used to determine current intake. It is advisable to ask specifically about take-away meals, snack foods and drinks consumed between meals since these are often overlooked. In addition, friends may share their food outside the home.

It is also advisable to ascertain the levels of activity that are normally undertaken. Advice can then be given regarding the levels required to assist in weight management. Simple achievable suggestions given to the family are helpful. Time spent playing computer games and watching television or video should also be estimated.

Management

To be successful, the school age child must want to lose weight, but this requires support and co-operation from the parents, grandparents, siblings and all who come into contact with the child. It is necessary to educate the child and the family so that they understand the aim of management – which is the need to change to a healthier lifestyle. This involves changing their eating habits, changing/reducing the types of food consumed as appropriate and increasing their activity level. The language and manner used to present these suggested changes is extremely important if we are to succeed. Emphasis should be on changing behaviour patterns and not on weight reduction alone. In addition, if children feel they have some control over choices this may improve the outcome. The use of weight loss versus weight maintenance will depend on the child's age, weight/height, BMI centile and the presence of medical complications [36].

Suggestions for specific dietary goals and activities for a particular family are often helpful. Children, if old enough, can be given one or two small suggestions for changes to their eating/activity pattern. These could be considered as targets to be met before their next appointment. Once these changes are established further goals can be given. Written information on a healthy dietary intake should be given, taking into account the child's current intake, age, social circumstances and family income.

A target weight can be agreed on if appropriate (although many centres are moving away from this approach) and a timescale can be planned for achieving this. In the overweight child the aim should be for the weight to remain static while BMI decreases so that the child will 'grow into' his weight. In the obese child the aim is to restrict the dietary intake so that weight loss is achieved without causing impairment of normal growth. Initially the emphasis should be on an energy deficit rather than a prescriptive regimen.

Frequent reinforcement is necessary in order to maintain interest and motivation. Ideally this should be carried out weekly or fortnightly and may be done by the school nurse, practice nurse or dietitian. In practice, however, this is not always achieved. One role of the dietitian is to ensure that a message of healthy eating and healthy lifestyle is conveyed to the child from parents, other family members, teachers and other carers. It is important that this is done in a positive, enthusiastic, non-judgemental and sensitive manner. If the child is the only family member who changes his eating habits or increases activity, he may feel deprived or resentful and, therefore, a relapse is more likely [36].

Attempts have been made to run group sessions for overweight and obese children, but on the whole these have not been successful, with a high drop-out rate.

'New generation' drugs for the treatment of obesity are being used in adults but these have not been licensed for use in children or adolescents in the UK.

Overweight and obese children are best managed on a long-term basis and with parental involvement rather than independently. This family-based therapy involves behaviour changes encompassing both the child's and family's lifestyle, which may result in benefits that last for 10 years or more [37, 38]. It is also important to consider psychosocial outcomes such as quality of life, as well as physiological outcomes. The effect of obesity during childhood and adolescence may have a lasting effect on self-esteem and body image [39].

Dietary treatment

Infants

It is difficult to overfeed a breast-fed infant, but bottle-fed infants can be persuaded to consume a greater volume than they require; in addition feeds can be made more concentrated than recommended or items such as cereal can be added to the bottle [40]. An infant is meant to be plump and naturally has more body fat than at other times in the lifespan; body fat content begins to decline after the first year of life. There is usually no need to restrict an infant's diet but advice may be needed if feeding practices are inappropriate or a slowing of weight gain is thought to be necessary.

The following advice may be helpful:

(1) Make sure that parents react appropriately to the infant's crying: often crying is perceived as indicating hunger, when in fact the baby may be bored, tired or uncomfortable.

(2) Avoid any additions to the infant's bottle (e.g. sugar or cereal).

(3) Make certain that the feed dilution is correct and that volume is appropriate for age.

(4) Solids should not be introduced before the age of 4 months.

(5) Weaning solids should have a low energy density (e.g. vegetables and unsweetened fruit).

(6) Reduced fat products can be used in the weaning diet, e.g. low fat yoghurts, reduced fat cheese.

(7) When a greater variety of foods is being consumed (e.g. lean meat, white fish and wholegrain cereals), the quantity of milk should be decreased.

(8) Infants should be introduced to a cup or teacher beaker from about 7–8 months and bottles omitted by one year of age. More milk is generally consumed when feeding from a bottle.

(9) Whole cow's milk can be used as the main milk drink from one year of age. Generally, skimmed and semi-skimmed milk should not be used before the ages of 5 and 2 years respectively. However, these lower fat milks are a useful way of decreasing energy intake in the overweight toddler. It is important that a supplement of vitamins A and D are given with these milks.

(10) Drinks of water should be offered with and in between meals. If the child is reluctant to drink

Table 23.1 General guidelines for reducing energy intake

1 Avoid fried foods (including chips and crisps), and added fat during cooking
2 Remove visible fat from meat and choose low fat product (e.g. low fat mince, sausages)
3 Use butter and margarine sparingly on bread and crispbread. A low fat spread is preferable. Do not add butter or alternatives to foods (e.g. cooked vegetables)
4 Avoid adding sugar to foods and drinks. An energy-free artificial sweetener (e.g. aspartame) may be used if required
5 Exclude as far as practical chocolate, sweets, cakes and biscuits
6 Give vegetables or salad at each meal
7 Use fruit (fresh, frozen, tinned in natural juice), low-calorie yoghurt and sugar-free jelly in place of desserts
8 Use low energy drinks and squash
9 Use semi-skimmed or skimmed milk (with care in children under 5 years). Do not exceed 600 ml daily
10 Use low fat cheese in place of full fat; use low fat fromage frais in place of cream
11 Avoid using diabetic foods except fruit squash

Table 23.2 Healthy intake for young children (1–5 years)

Milk – aim to give 300 ml daily, with a maximum of 600 ml. Semi-skimmed or skimmed can be used, provided that a supplement of vitamins A and D are given. Low fat yoghurts, milk puddings, white sauces, low fat hard cheese will all provide calcium if milk is disliked as a drink
Meat, fish, poultry, egg, cheese, beans and lentils – 1 to 2 portions should be given from this group daily. Low fat meats should be used, and meat should be grilled or baked, not fried
Cereal foods – breakfast cereal, wholemeal bread, brown rice, wholegrain pasta and crackers – at least one portion should be included at each meal. Avoid adding extra fat and sugar
Vegetables and fruit – at least four portions daily, raw or cooked

Sample menu

Breakfast	Wholegrain unsweetened cereal, porridge or muesli with milk (no sugar)
	Bread or toast with small amount of spread
	Milk or unsweetened fruit juice
Snack	Plain cracker or piece of fruit
	Water or low calorie squash
Lunch	Roll or bread, filled with tuna, meat, egg, low fat cheese or peanut butter/baked beans on toast
	Chopped salad or cooked vegetables
	Low calorie yoghurt or fruit
Snack	Fruit, raisins or small sandwich
	Water or low calorie squash
Evening meal	Meat, fish, cheese or pulse dish
	Vegetables or salad
	Potatoes, rice or pasta
	Fruit or low energy dessert
Bedtime	Milky drink (unsweetened)

water, pure unsweetened fruit juice, well diluted, can be given once or twice daily, with meals, although if the vitamin C content of the diet is adequate there is no nutritional need for this.

The pre-school child

In the under-fives a strict 'calorie counted' regimen is rarely appropriate. Written advice should be given to the parents on the avoidance of high-energy foods (Table 23.1) or on a balanced 'healthy' diet as outlined in Table 23.2. It is important that the whole family changes its eating habits and hopefully prevents the pattern of obesity continuing into later life.

Too much emphasis on diet in front of the child can lead to a feeling of victimisation and resentment and he may become very self-conscious about his size. It may be wise to send the child to play during part of the dietetic consultation.

Physical activity should be increased among the less active families/children: on occasions parents may be seen who still use a pushchair for an overweight child of 3–4 years because he walks too slowly! Other advice that may be offered includes the following:

- Crisps, sweets, chocolate and added sugar should be avoided
- Do not give food or sweets to a child as a reward or to console him.

Children over five years

The main aim of the diet must be to re-educate the child/family regarding their eating habits. The regimen prescribed is based on the current intake, and for a child whose consumption of chocolate, sweets, biscuits, crisps and chips is high then general guidelines (Table 23.1) are often initially all that is required. The establishment of a sensible eating pattern and regular physical activity should be the goal. Television viewing and computer game playing should be limited to 1 or 2 hours per day [41].

In moderate to severe obesity, a more formal approach is sometimes necessary. The reducing diet advised varies and those most frequently used are 1000–1500 kcal (4.2–6.3 MJ) daily. Diets of less than 1000 kcal are not usually advised. Most school-age children will lose weight on 1000 kcal (4.2 MJ) [42]. The diet suggested should be flexible, realistic and provide variety and sufficient food to stop the child pilfering or cheating. If the regimen is too strict the treatment will fail. Parents should be advised that weight loss is greatest in the first few weeks on the diet and thereafter the rate of weight loss declines. A realistic and achievable target weight should be set at each visit, if appropriate, usually 0.5–1 kg per month if the child is obese, less for the moderately obese or younger child.

High-energy foods as outlined in Table 23.1 should be avoided. Foods such as fruit, vegetables and whole grain cereals and bread should be encouraged. Many children unfortunately refuse to eat vegetables and fruit and parents may need advice on different forms of presentation. Home-made vegetable soup or vegetables incorporated into pasta sauce or casserole dishes may be more acceptable then plain vegetables; often one or two vegetables such as peas, sweetcorn kernels or tinned tomatoes will be eaten, and maximum use should be made of these. There are also a wide range of sugar-free and low energy products such as low calorie yoghurts, sugar-free jellies and low calorie soups that provide variety in the diet.

It is important to ensure that normal growth occurs when dietary intake is restricted. Adequate quantities of protein, vitamins and minerals should be taken; some children who dislike certain foods and do not consume a nutritionally adequate diet may need a supplement of vitamins or minerals (particularly iron and calcium). A reducing diet should provide at least 60% of the Estimated Average Requirement (EAR) for the child's age [43]. Written information in the form of a diet sheet, a list of unrestricted foods and a list of foods allowed may be given to the parents and child (Tables 23.3 and 23.4).

The question of school dinners should be addressed. Many overweight children regularly consume chips and pastry items/puddings for lunch at school. Fruit and low calorie yoghurt can replace dessert and the child should be advised to avoid

Table 23.3 Reducing diets

Meals should be chosen from the following foods

Lean meat	Vegetables	Fruit
Poultry	All varieties of	All varieties, fresh, frozen,
Fish	vegetables and salads	stewed without sugar,
Eggs		tinned in natural juice
Cheese		
Pulses		

Drinks
Low calorie squash and carbonated drinks
Mineral and soda water
Coffee, tea without sugar

Daily allowances
300–600 ml milk
30 g margarine or butter
. . . slices of bread or equivalent exchanges depending on energy content of diet

Exchanges for 1 slice of bread: 70 kcal (290 kJ) approximately
1 potato – baked, boiled or mashed
or 1 tablespoon boiled rice/spaghetti
or 3 tablespoons unsweetened breakfast cereal
or 1 Weetabix
or 2 crispbreads
or 2 crackers/large water biscuits
or 1 Digestive biscuit/2 Rich Tea

second helpings. However, the use of a 'treat' on a weekly or daily basis, if necessary, can help the child psychologically and provide motivation. It is easier to provide suitable food in the form of a packed lunch, although a certain amount of swapping of items often takes place.

The suggestion that money previously spent on sweets, chocolate etc. can be used for other items of the child's choice (e.g. games, books, clothing) is sometimes useful, particularly for indulgent grandparents.

Social eating

Eating out is usually a pleasurable activity and with a little planning and forethought, this is still possible on a healthy eating regimen. An invitation to tea with friends should not be turned down because of the 'diet', since a suitable choice of foods can usually be arranged.

Table 23.4 Low energy foods allowed freely

Vegetables

All green varieties and salads	Courgettes	Peas
Brussels sprouts	Celery	Peppers
French beans	Fennel	Swede
Runner beans	Leeks	Turnip
Cauliflower	Mushrooms	Tomato
	Onions	

Fruit

Bilberries	Gooseberries	Raspberries
Blackberries	Grapefruit	Redcurrants
Blackcurrants	Lemon	Rhubarb
Cranberries	Loganberries	Strawberries

Miscellaneous

Artificial sweeteners e.g. saccharin, Nutrasweet	Mineral and soda water
Coffee	Sugar-free drinks
Tea	Sugar-free jelly and chewing gum
Herbs	Stock cubes
Spices	
Seasonings	
Vinegar	

For birthday parties pastries, crisps and chocolate can be replaced with sandwiches, vegetable and fruit cocktail sticks, sugar-free jellies and unsweetened fruit. Low calorie drinks can be used for everyone. Prizes for games can be toys, notebooks, pencils, crayons and novelties in place of sweets.

Adolescents

Adolescents present the dietitian with the greatest challenge. Dietary prescription will depend on age and sex, with teenage boys requiring more energy generally than girls. Peer group pressure for consumption of snack foods is high and suggestions for alternative lower energy items is necessary. Adolescent girls may be at risk of developing anorexia nervosa or bulimia and an awareness of this is vital [44].

In general, slimming foods and drinks as a replacement for a meal are not appropriate, as they generally contain insufficient protein, minerals and micronutrients to meet the high requirements for this age group. Very low calorie diets (around 400–600 kcal) are specifically contraindicated.

Increasing energy expenditure

Increased physical activity on a regular basis should be encouraged in conjunction with a healthy dietary intake. Studies have shown that subjects treated with diet and exercise programmes continued to lose weight for longer than children treated by diet alone in the follow-up period [45, 46].

Physical exercise usually promotes a feeling of wellbeing and, in addition, it will keep the child/teenager occupied, avoiding boredom. Walking, jogging and swimming are useful activities for those who dislike team games.

Successful treatment of obesity demands a sustained commitment and effort from the whole family and the dietitian must endeavour to maintain a positive attitude and motivation towards weight control.

Preventative measures

There is evidence to suggest that we need to re-examine the ways in which obesity is managed and treated. Little work has been done on the prevention of obesity in childhood and adolescence. The available evidence to date suggests that the trends in obesity rates are related more to a reduction in energy expenditure than to an increase in energy intake [3]. There is a need to devise a scheme so that those children gaining excessive weight are identified at an early stage, particularly in overweight families. Public awareness schemes to increase physical activity and dietary change may be helpful in prevention [33]. Promotion of a healthy lifestyle must start in childhood if we are to reverse the current trend.

PRADER-WILLI SYNDROME

Prader-Willi syndrome (PWS) is a rare congenital disorder, the main characteristics of which are hypotonia, short stature, hypogonadism, a degree of mental retardation and an insatiable appetite leading to gross obesity if not controlled. Behavioural problems are encountered most often during adolescence [47–49] which add to the difficulties of treatment. The prevalence has been estimated at 1 in 25 000 births [50] making PWS the most common syndromal cause of obesity.

At birth infants present with hypotonia and feeding difficulties and subsequently fail to thrive (Fig. 23.1).

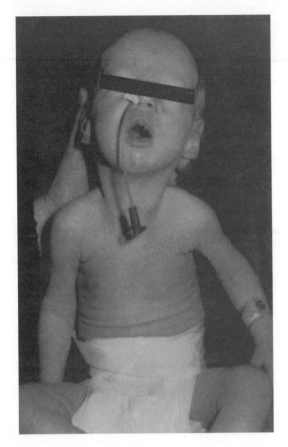

Fig. 23.1 Infant with Prader-Willi syndrome

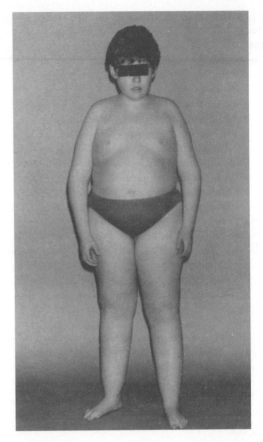

Fig. 23.2 Adolescent with Prader-Willi syndrome (same boy as in Fig. 23.1). With kind permission of Dr JK Brown

Tube feeding may be required during this period. Parents should be made aware of the two phases which are characteristic of the syndrome: from birth to approximately 2 years of age when weight gain is poor, and from 2–3 years onwards when weight is likely to escalate [51]. It is important that dietary intervention and advice is given at the onset of weight gain in order that excessive weight gain is curtailed. Consistent dietary advice from all professionals must be given to parents and carers and the need to adhere to this explained. This can prove very difficult because of the hyperphagia. Gross obesity often occurs during adolescence (Fig. 23.2) but can be controlled with comprehensive management. In addition, growth hormone treatment has been shown to be beneficial in reducing BMI significantly in PWS children [52]. Interestingly Crnic *et al.* believe that mainte-

nance of a lower body weight will improve intellectual performance [53].

Dietary treatment

The child with PWS requires a considerably lower energy intake than his or her normal peers. In order to achieve weight loss, energy intake must be 50% or less than expected for age (Table 1.8). Attempts should be made to check any potential sources of food (e.g. from neighbours or friends).

Much encouragement is required, but weight loss can be achieved with great vigilance. Weight should be monitored at monthly or three-monthly intervals. The diet presents great difficulty for the child, family, carers and school, due to the insatiable appetite; food is uppermost in the thoughts of most people with PWS. Bray *et al.* found that, when food was unrestricted, six of their adolescent patients consumed a daily average of 5167 ± 503 kcal (21.7 ± 2.1 MJ). Similar results were found in a more recent study [54]. Foraging for food is common and parents should be advised to lock the kitchen, cupboards and refrigerator. Many children get up during the night to eat and inappropriate foods such as bread for the birds or dog and cat food are commonly eaten. Interestingly, however unsuitable the foods that may be eaten, stomach upsets are rare.

Dietitians must be aware that medical and other health workers may not have encountered PWS previously and may lack the understanding necessary to give proper support to the family. Communication with other health professionals is essential to avoid misunderstanding.

Some activities are physically difficult for the PWS child due to poor muscle strength; however, walking and swimming can be accomplished by most and should be encouraged to increase energy expenditure. Contrary to some views it has been shown that during exercise, individuals with PWS require as much energy as others with simple obesity for the same level of work [55].

Multidisciplinary management, which includes dietary advice, behaviour modification and family support are advocated as an effective form of treatment [56].

A parents' self-help group exists, which parents may find helpful and supportive.

REFERENCES

1 Guillaume M Defining obesity in childhood: current practice. *Am J Clin Nutr*, 1999, **70** (Suppl) 126S–30S.

2 Taitz LS *Textbook of Paediatric Nutrition*, 3e. Edinburgh: Churchill Livingstone, 1991, p. 485.

3 Seidell JC Obesity: a growing problem. *Acta Paediatr*, 1999, **428** (Suppl) 46–50.

4 Prentice AM, Jebb SA Obesity in Britain: gluttony or sloth? *Brit Med J*, 1995, **311** 437–9.

5 Schonfeld-Warden N, Warden CH Pediatric obesity. An overview of etiology and treatment. *Pediatr Clin North Am*, 1997, **44** 339–61.

6 WHO Consultation on obesity. Global prevalence and secular trends in obesity. World Health Organisation. *Obesity preventing and managing the global epidemic.* Geneva: WHO, 1998, pp. 17–40.

7 *Obesity.* Report of the British Nutrition Foundation Task Force. A. Fehily (ed) Blackwell Science, 1999, p. 35.

8 White EM, Wilson AC, Greene SA *et al.* Body mass index centile charts to assess fatness of British children. *Arch Dis Childh*, 1995, **72** 38–41.

9 Hughes JM, Li L, Chinn S, Rona RJ Trends in growth in England and Scotland, 1972 to 1994. *Arch Dis Childh*, 1997, **76** (3) 182–9.

10 Reilly JJ, Dorosty AR, Emmett PM Prevalence of overweight and obesity in British children: cohort study. *Brit Med J*, 1999, **319** 1039.

11 Reilly JJ, Dorosty AR Epidemic of obesity in UK children. *Lancet*, 1999, **354** 1874–5.

12 Epstein LH Commentary: Future research directions in pediatric obesity research. *J Pediatr Psychol*, 1999, **24** 251–2.

13 Auwerx J, Staels B Leptin. *Lancet*, 1998, **351** 737–42.

14 Borjeson M The aetiology of obesity in children: a study of 101 twin pairs. *Acta Paediatr Scand*, 1976, **65** 279–87.

15 Stunkard AJ *et al.* An adoption study of human obesity. *New Eng J Med*, 1986, **314** 193–8.

16 O'Callaghan MJ, Williams GM, Anderson MJ, Bor W, Najman JM Prediction of obesity in children at 5 years: a cohort study. *J Paediatr, Child Health*, 1997, **33** 311–16.

17 Parsons TJ, Power C, Logan S, Summerbell CD Childhood predictors of adult obesity: a systematic review. *Int J Obes*, 1999, **23** (Suppl 8) S1–S107.

18 Whitaker RC, Wright JA, Pepe MS, Seidel KD, Dietz WH Predicting obesity in young adulthood from childhood and parental obesity. *N Engl J Med*, 1997, **337** 869–73.

19 Lake JK, Power C, Cole TJ Child to adult body mass index in 1958 British birth cohort: associations with parental obesity. *Arch Dis Childh*, 1997, **77** 376–81.

20 Garn SM, Clark DC Trends in fatness and the origins of obesity. *Paediatr*, 1976, **57** 443–56.

21 Mossberg HO 40-year follow-up of overweight children. *Lancet*, 1989, **ii** 491–3.

22 Must A, Jacques PF, Dallal GE, Bajema CJ, Dietz WH Long-term morbidity and mortality of overweight adolescents. A follow-up of the Harvard growth study of 1922 to 1935. *New Eng J Med*, 1992, **327** 1350–55.

23 Serdula M, Ivery D, Coates R, Freedman D, Williamson D, Byers T Do obese children become obese adults? A review of the literature. *Prev Med*, 1993, **22** 167–77.

24 Olsen L *Food Fight; A Report on Teenage Eating Habits and Nutritional Status.* San Francisco: Citizens Policy Centre, 1982, p. 124.

25 Young EA *et al.* Fast foods update: nutrient analysis. *Ross Laboratories Dietetic Currents*, 1986, **13** (6).

26 Bellisle F, Rolland-Cachera M-F *et al.* Three consecutive (1993, 1995, 1997) surveys of food intake,

nutritional attitudes and knowledge, and lifestyle in 1000 French children, aged 9–11 years. *J Hum Nutr Dietet*, 2000, **13** 101–111.

27 Strauss R Childhood obesity. *Curr Probl Pediatr*, 1999, **29** 1–29.

28 Durnin JV Physical activity by adolescents. *Acta Paediatr Scand*, 1971, **217** (Suppl) 133–5.

29 Tanner JM, Whitehouse RH Revised standards for triceps and subscapular skinfolds in British children. *Arch Dis Childh*, 1975, **50** 142–5.

30 *Obesity*. The Report of the British Nutrition Foundation Task Force. J Garrow (ed) Blackwell Science, 1999 3.

31 Cole TJ, Freeman JV, Preece MA Body mass index reference curves for the UK. *Arch Dis Childh*, 1995, **73** 25–9.

32 Dietz WH, Bellizzi MC The use of body mass index to assess obesity in children. *Am J Clin Nutr*, 1999, **70** (Suppl) 123S–5S.

33 Scottish Intercollegiate Guidelines Network (SIGN) *Obesity in Scotland: integrating prevention with weight management*. Edinburgh: Royal College of Physicians, 1996.

34 Lehingue Y The European Childhood Obesity Group Project: the European collaborative study on the prevalence of obesity in children. *Am J Clin Nutr*, 1999, **70** 166S–168S.

35 Dietz WH, Robinson TN Use of the body mass index as a measure of overweight in children and adolescents. *J Pediatr*, 1998, **132** 191–3.

36 Barlow SE, Dietz WH Obesity evaluation and treatment: expert committee recommendations (Electronic article). *Pediatr*, 1998, **102** (3) 29.

37 Epstein LH, Valoski A, Wing RR, McCulley J Ten-year outcomes of behavioural family-based treatment for childhood obesity. *Health Psychol*, 1994, **13** 373–83.

38 Epstein LH Family-based behavioural intervention for obese children. *Int J Obes Relat Metab Disord*, 1996, (Suppl) **1** S14–21.

39 Must A, Strauss RS Risks and consequences of childhood and adolescent obesity. *Int J Obes Relat Metab Disord*, 1999, **2** (Suppl) S2–11.

40 Taitz LS *The Obese Child*. Oxford: Blackwell Science, 1983.

41 American Academy of Pediatrics, Committee on communications: *Children, Adolescents and Television*, 1995, **96** 786–7.

42 Brooke OG, Abernethy E Obesity in children. *Hum Nutr: Appl Nutr*, 1985, **39a** (4) 304–14.

43 Bentley D, Lawson M *Clinical Nutrition in Paediatric Disorders*. London: Bailliere Tindall, 1988, p. 191.

44 Israel AC Commentary: Empirically supported treatments for pediatric obesity: goals, outcome criteria and the societal context. *J Pediatr Psychol*, 1999, **24** 249–50.

45 Epstein LH *et al*. Effect of diet and controlled exercise on weight loss in obese children. *J Paediatr*, 1985, **107** 358–61.

46 Reybrouck T *et al*. Exercise therapy and hypocaloric diet in the treatment of obese children and adolescents. *Acta Paediatr Scand*, 1990, **79** 84–8.

47 Whitman By, Accardo P Emotional symptoms in Prader-Willi syndrome adolescents. *Am J Med Genetics*, 1987, **28** 897–905.

48 Dykens EM, Kasari C Maladaptive behavior in children with Prader-Willi syndrome, Down's syndrome, and non-specific mental retardation. *Am J Men Retard*, 1997, **102** 228–37.

49 State MW, Dykens EM, Rosner B, Martin A, King BH Obsessive-compulsive symptoms in 'Prader-Willi and Prader-Willi-like' patients. *J Am Acad Ch Adol Psychiatry*, 1999, **38** 329–34.

50 Bray GA *et al*. The Prader-Willi syndrome: a study of 40 patients and a review of the literature. *Medicine*, 1983, **62** 69–80.

51 Wollmann HA, Shultz U, Grauer ML, Ranke MB Reference values for height and weight in Prader-Willi syndrome based on 315 patients. *Eur J Pediatr*, 1998, **157** 634–42.

52 Lindgren AC, Hagenas L, Muller J, Blichfeldt S, Rosenborg M, Brismar T, Ritzen EM Growth hormone treatment of children with Prader-Willi syndrome affects linear growth and body composition favourably. *Acta Paediatr*, 1998, **87** 28–31.

53 Crnic KA *et al*. Preventing mental retardation associated with gross obesity in the Prader-Willi syndrome. *Paediatr*, 1980, **66** 787–9.

54 Holland AJ, Treasure J, Coskeran P, Dallow J Characteristics of the eating disorder in Prader-Willi syndrome: implications for treatment. *J Intellect Disabil Res*, 1995, **39** 73–81.

55 Holm VA, Pipes PL Food and children with Prader-Willi syndrome. *Am J Dis Childh*, 1976, **130** 1063–7.

56 Wodarski LA, Bundschuh E, Forbus WR Interdisciplinary case management: a model for intervention. *J Am Diet Assoc*, 1988, **88** 332–5.

USEFUL ADDRESS

Prader-Willi Syndrome Association (UK)
2 Wheatsheaf Close, Horsell, Woking, Surrey GU21 4BP. Tel. 01483 724784.

Other Conditions Requiring Nutritional Support and Advice

CHAPTER 24

Epidermolysis Bullosa

INTRODUCTION

Epidermolysis bullosa (EB) comprises a rare group of genetically determined skin blistering disorders characterised by extreme fragility of the skin and mucous membranes, with recurrent blister formation. EB is broadly classified into three main types:

- Junctional (JEB) – lethal (Herlitz) and non-lethal (non-Herlitz)
- Dystrophic (DEB) – dominant (DDEB) and recessive (RDEB)
- Simplex (EBS) – Dowling-Meara and Weber-Cockayne subtypes.

At least 20 subtypes of EB have also been identified [1]. Each type of EB results from structural defects in the skin which allow separation between different layers, causing blistering and ulceration. Individually, they vary greatly in their impact from relatively minor handicap (e.g. limited ability to walk due to painful foot blisters) to death in infancy. Mild cases often remain undiagnosed, while the severely affected may die before a diagnosis is confirmed. Hence, it is difficult to assess the prevalence of EB. It affects the sexes equally and occurs in all races; mental development is normal. Blisters or lesions may be present at birth or develop soon afterwards; these occur both spontaneously and as a result of mechanical trauma. In the neonatal period, the appearance of the skin is a highly unreliable indicator of disease type, severity or prognosis. Blisters are not self-limiting and will extend indefinitely if they are not lanced as soon as they are detected. To minimise the area of the resultant raw lesion, carers are taught to pierce blisters, leaving the roof intact to protect the underlying wound. Dress-ings are applied both to damaged areas of skin and to parts vulnerable to injury.

A claim that EB can be cured by an exclusion diet combined with topical and systemic treatments was disproved in an open evaluation of the regimen [2]. Nevertheless, it is clear that early and proactive nutritional support can lead to significant improvements in growth, wound healing, resistance to infection, quality of life, morbidity and mortality. Much research is currently being undertaken to establish the molecular pathology of EB. Progress is good and researchers are cautiously optimistic that, within the lifetime of today's EB children, gene therapy will significantly improve their lives.

Optimising the nutrition of EB children now not only enhances their short term quality of life, but also increases the chances of their maximising the potential benefits of scientific advances. However, the dietitian cannot operate in isolation. Factors outside dietetic control, such as inadequate skin care, dental caries and periodontal disease, gastro-oesophageal reflux (GOR), faecal loading and overflow incontinence, psychological and psychosocial issues will sabotage the potential beneficial effects of nutritional intervention if left unaddressed. The collective expertise of a multidisciplinary team is crucial to achieve a holistic approach to optimal management of EB [3]. Even in spite of rigorous attention to the foregoing, the aetiology of EB is such that complications are inevitable to some extent. Some forms remain the most physically disabling and disfiguring of all diseases. Indeed, EB has been described as 'recalcitrant nutritional deprivation unparalleled in all of clinical medicine' (4). Although the dietitian may be shocked by the appearance of a severely affected patient, it is important not to relay this to the child or carers. Table 24.1 summarises the problems seen in the main types of EB and the nutritional interventions likely to be required.

Table 24.1 Main complications and nutritional interventions in different types of epidermolysis bullosa (EB)

EB Type	Complications	Nutritional intervention
Dominant dystrophic EB	Usually mild lesions with minimal scarring	Intervention is generally not indicated
Recessive dystrophic EB	Recurrent moderate to severe lesions heal with generalised scarring and contractures. Digits fuse. Internal contractures cause microstomia, dysphagia and oesophageal strictures. Anal erosions/fissures cause painful defecation and constipation	Aim for up to 115–150% EAR for energy and up to 115–200% RNI for protein when catabolic. Supplement iron, zinc, vitamins and fibre. Gastrostomy feeding often indicated – apply DRV for age and sex in stable patients
Non-lethal junctional EB	Recurrent mild to severe lesions heal without scarring and contractures, but often very slowly. May be genito-urinary involvement	As for recessive dystrophic EB. Gastrostomy placement may result in poor healing around entry site
Lethal junctional EB	Recurrent moderate to severe lesions heal without scarring and contractures. Laryngeal involvement, hoarse cry. Pain relief often exacerbates constipation. Failure to thrive frequently follows initial good weight gain	Intervention is of limited benefit. Maintain hydration, feed to appetite, correct deficiencies
Dowling-Meara subtype of EB simplex	Mild to severe lesions heal without scarring and contractures. Feeding problems mainly resolve after infancy. Lesions tend later to become confined to hands and feet. Anal erosions/fissures lead to painful defecation and constipation	Aim for up to 100–150% EAR for energy and up to 115–150% RNI for protein initially. Fibre, iron, zinc and vitamin supplementation may also be indicated. Beware of excess weight gain in later infancy/childhood
Weber-Cockayne subtype of EB simplex	Lesions usually confined to hands and feet, but may be severe, especially in hot weather	Supplementation is generally not indicated, but sufferers may require advice on weight reduction

FACTORS INFLUENCING NUTRITIONAL STATUS

Nutritional problems occur mainly in recessive dystrophic EB (RDEB), JEB and the Dowling-Meara subtype of EBS. There is controversy regarding the involvement of the internal mucosae. Whereas it has been suggested by some that the columnar epithelium of the gastrointestinal tract is affected [5], others consider the epithelial abnormality to be confined to stratified squamous epithelium, i.e. skin, mucous membranes, oesophagus, bronchus and anus [6]. Denudation of the intestinal epithelium has been said to lead to impaired absorption of amino acids and other nutrients [7]. However, malabsorption is very unlikely to be responsible for growth failure in RDEB at least, since many such children fed via gastrostomy can thrive on energy intakes comparable to their unaffected peers (see section on gastrostomy feeding later in this chapter). Strictures in the upper third of the oesophagus, where the diameter is narrowest, may result from the trauma of ingested food. Strictures in the distal oesophagus may reflect damage from reflux of gastric acid [8]. Although some adult RDEB patients report an improvement in dysphagia, many children and adults can tolerate only puréed food and liquids. Several studies have demonstrated inadequate dietary intakes with abnormal haematological and biochemical findings [9–12].

Two main factors potentially compromise nutritional status in EB:

- The hypercatabolic state in which open skin lesions with consequent losses of blood and serous fluid, increased protein turnover, heat loss and infection all contribute to increased requirements. As in the patient with thermal burns, nutrient needs reflect the severity of lesions [13].
- The degree to which oral, oropharyngeal, oesophageal and gastrointestinal complications (ulceration with or without stricture) limit intake. Faecal loading, chronic constipation and painful defaecation are extremely common and frequently cause apathy and secondary anorexia [10].

The interactions between causes and effects of nutritional problems in RDEB are shown in Fig. 24.1.

To form a feasible management plan, the dietitian must be aware of the patient's precise diagnosis and prognosis. This not only promotes proactive recommendations, but also avoids the setting of unrealistic targets. Indications for nutritional intervention are often governed as much by the clinical state and age of the patient as by the exact diagnosis. Thus, the information contained in this chapter is generally arranged in categories such as age, complications and requirements. Where the features of a specific EB type influence the course of dietetic management (e.g. in lethal JEB and RDEB) these are discussed in separate sections.

GENERAL AIMS OF NUTRITIONAL SUPPORT (MODIFY FOR LETHAL JEB, SEE BELOW)

- To promote wound healing
- To promote normal growth rates for age and sex
- To promote catch-up growth in those demonstrating growth failure
- To alleviate the stress associated with feeding difficulties
- To correct macro- and micronutrient deficiencies, e.g. hypoproteinaemia, zinc and selenium deficiency

- To alleviate constipation and promote normal bowel function.

When widespread lesions are present, particularly in association with sepsis, nutritional requirements are likely to be raised [9] and roles for an ever-increasing number of nutrients are being implicated in satisfactory wound healing [14]. Birge [12] has estimated energy requirement using a calculation based on weight-for-height age and taking into account the degrees of blistering, sepsis and requirement for catch-up growth. Although this method provides a working figure, the scoring of skin involvement is subjective and the formula is complex. Using dietary reference values [15], consistent increases in weight and height can be achieved by supplying 100–150% estimated average requirement (EAR) for energy and 115–200% reference nutrient intake (RNI) for protein.

Measurements of weight and height velocity is the most practical means of assessing growth, and these should be plotted regularly. Children should be weighed and measured three to sixth monthly, preferably on the same scales each time. Ideally, nutritional management should be undertaken by one dietitian so that a rapport can be established between dietitian and family. EB children and their parents need to be confident that their problems (those which impinge both directly and indirectly on nutrition) are understood by those offering dietetic advice. The aim is for the child to grow according to his genetic (and ethnic) potential. Predicted adult height can be calculated

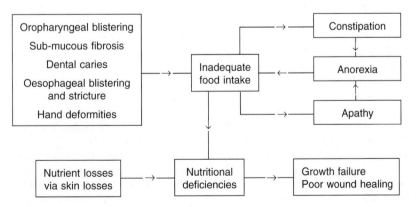

Fig. 24.1 Interactions between causes and effects of nutritional problems in severe epidermolysis bullosa. After Allman 1990 (see Nutritional information booklets at end of chapter)

from parental heights, using the formula described on current growth charts [16]. Pain and contractures around joints may lead to underestimated height measurements and EB children are more accurately measured using a supine stadiometer. The traditional 'rule-of-thumb' that disparity between weight and height should not be greater than two major centiles is generally applicable.

The importance of early nutritional support (modify for lethal JEB, see below)

The importance of providing optimal nutrition, starting as early as possible after birth, cannot be over-emphasised [3, 10]. Unfortunately, this area of management is often neglected, with priority given to other critical issues such as skin care and control of infection. The flawed assumption that either growth failure is an inevitable consequence of EB, or the baby will catch up later, means that valuable time is often lost before a dietetic referral is made.

Energy requirements usually range from 130 to 180 kcal (643–572 KJ)/kg actual body weight/24 hours (115–150% EAR), but can be as high as 225 kcal (940 KJ)/kg if the skin is septic or growth failure is profound. Protein requirements tend to be between 2.5 and 4 g/kg, (115–200% RNI), and fluid from 150 to 200 ml/kg. Babies with extensive blistering lose significant amounts of fluid from these open areas and may require correspondingly larger volumes of feeds. Breast feeding an EB baby is possible, and if it permits normal weight gain should be encouraged for the many benefits it confers [17]. However, rooting may cause, or exacerbate, facial lesions and blistering of the fragile mucous membranes of the mouth, tongue and gums. Babies should be allowed to suckle on demand and applying white soft paraffin or Vaseline to the lips and to the nipple reduces friction. For all but mild cases of EB, however, breast milk alone often fails to satisfy increased requirements, demonstrated by failure to gain weight.

As soon as possible, measures should be taken to provide a more nutrient-dense feed (see also section on lethal JEB). There are several ways in which this can be done (see Table 1.12 in Chapter 1). If facilities permit, the mother's own expressed breast milk (EBM) can be fortified with a proprietary whey-based powdered infant formula (e.g. Premium) at a concentration of 5 g/100 ml. A glucose polymer such as Caloreen can also be added (2–5 g per 100 ml) to increase further the energy content, giving a total carbohydrate content of 10–12 g/100 ml feed. Because of the small quantities of additions involved, fortifying EBM in this way may be practical only if a reasonable volume of milk can be treated each time. A low birthweight formula babymilk, e.g. SMA Low Birthweight Formula, can be used in hospital to supplement or replace breast milk. This can be fortified with glucose polymer to a maximum carbohydrate content of 12 g per 100 ml. Any feed modifications must be explained to parents and community medical and nursing personnel to avoid misunderstandings and conflicting advice. Alternatively, nutrient-dense ready-to-feed formulations such as Infatrini, Nutrini, Nutrini Extra or SMA High Energy Formula can be used, depending on the requirements of the individual baby. Regular review of weight and feed adequacy are essential.

Weights should be recorded on alternate days while a feeding routine is established in hospital. Although nude weight is ideal, the skin damage incurred during handling usually precludes this. If such precision is required, the baby can be weighed before a dressing change, and afterwards, the weight of the soiled dressings subtracted from this first weight. Weighings can be reduced to once weekly and then less frequently once the baby is discharged from hospital. Values should be plotted on a growth chart so that any 'fall-off' can be detected early and appropriate measures taken to modify the feeds.

Feeding teats should be moistened with cooled, boiled water or Vaseline before feeding to avoid the teat sticking to the lips and causing damage when it is removed. A Haberman Feeder® (Athrodax Healthcare International, Ross-on-Wye, UK) is extremely useful if the mouth is painful. The shape of this teat minimises trauma to the gum margin and the internal valve allows the carer to control the flow of feed, so that even a weak suck will deliver a satisfactory milk flow. Alternatively, the hole in a conventional teat can be enlarged using a sterile needle. Babies who cannot suck from a teat may need to be fed from a spoon or dropper or be fed by nasogastric tube (see later). In babies with extensive lesions and significant blood losses, iron and zinc status should be assessed and supplemented as required (see later sections on Iron and anaemia and Zinc).

Weaning (see also section on RDEB)

Weaning foods should be offered at the same time as for unaffected babies, i.e. around 4 months. However, babies whose mouths are very fragile, or who have experienced GOR or aspiration of feed, may be very reluctant to accept changes in texture or viscosity of foods. Carers should be reassured that this is not unusual, and advised that there is nothing to be gained, and much to be lost, by force-feeding. Community personnel may be overzealous in striving for 'normal' feeding milestones, and the practice of reducing the volume or the nutrient density of the feed to make the baby more hungry for solids should be strongly discouraged. Weaning foods of a suitable texture for unaffected babies are usually appropriate. However, hard or sharp foods such as baked rusks or crisp crusts are not suitable as these damage the mouth and gums. If growth is poor, carers should be advised regarding ways to increase the protein and energy content of the diet, without increasing its bulk. There is no evidence to suggest that long-term adherence to a liquid or puréed diet necessarily influences the course of dysphagia and oesophageal stricture. Babies who demonstrate swallowing problems from early on may be best to remain indefinitely on very soft or puréed foods.

Lethal junctional EB (LJEB) or Herlitz EB

The prognosis for LJEB is extremely poor, death usually occurring within the first year of life and often within weeks of birth. Paradoxically, skin lesions may initially be minimal, and weight gain deceptively good, on breast milk or normally reconstituted feeds. Almost invariably, however, this gives way to growth failure as new areas of skin become denuded, infection sets in and respiratory problems increase [18]. The dietitian must be aware of the prognosis, to try to minimise the disappointment parents will feel when feed modifications have little or no impact on growth or healing. Nutritional intervention (as for RDEB, see later) should be offered as a means of enhancing the quality, rather than the quantity, of life.

Mothers who have established breast feeding and wish to continue should not be discouraged from doing so even if weight gain is poor, as this is one of the few positive things they can do for a terminally ill baby. In terms of nutritional management, parents and medical and nursing staff should be discouraged from weighing the baby, as the disappointing result only adds to an already very distressing situation. However, pain relief is an important aspect of terminal care, and the baby may need to be weighed before the best regimen can be agreed.

Non-lethal junctional EB (JEB) or non-Herlitz EB

Some non-lethal JEB patients are mildly affected and survive into adulthood with relatively little handicap. Others, however, experience extreme nutritional compromise due to extensive and chronic ulceration, both externally and internally. Associated pyloric atresia and genito-urinary disease have been reported [19]. Nutritional support is the same as that recommended for RDEB (see later).

Recessive dystrophic EB (RDEB)

The complications of RDEB begin in infancy and, except in mild cases, progressively increase. In the more severe cases, prolonged and recurrent blisters with subsequent scarring gradually lead to tautness of the healed skin known as contractures. Contractures around joints progress to cause major walking difficulties and disability. Contractures in the mouth greatly limit opening and immobilise the tongue. Oesophageal scarring causes strictures – some sufferers experience periods when they are unable to swallow even their own saliva and require hospitalisation for rehydration. Anal scarring leads to fissures, extremely painful defecation and consequent fecal loading as defecation is postponed for lengthy periods [20, 21]. Self-feeding is greatly limited when fingers become fused and contracted. Specialised surgery is available to separate the fingers although the benefits are temporary. In many cases, without gastrostomy placement, the resulting nutritional compromise leads to profound malnutrition and growth failure [4, 12].

Patients with RDEB are at significantly increased risk of developing squamous cell (malignant) carcinoma. Despite the surgical removal of affected areas, the tumours metastasise rapidly, and without early identification the prognosis is generally extremely poor. It has been proposed that chronic malnutrition indirectly contributes not only to the metastasis of cancer cells, but also to the development of primary skin malignacies [7].

In the older child, a dietary assessment should be comprehensive and sensitively probing in order to elicit an authentic picture [3]. Judicious questioning regarding aspects such as the length of time taken to finish meals, whether the amount offered is actually all consumed and a demonstration of the child's maximum mouth opening capability and tongue thrust, all help to provide a complete picture. GOR and hiatus hernia are often neglected causes of dysphagia, the most serious complication of which is aspiration pneumonia [8, 21]. A history suggestive of these must be fully explored and medically treated. Fecal loading (with or without constipation) is invariably present to a greater or lesser extent, often from infancy. This frequently exerts a disastrous effect on appetite and tolerance of feeds and supplements, especially iron. Parents regularly omit to report symptoms of these, probably because they do not appreciate their detrimental impact on nutritional intake.

The dietitian should not assume that the child's medical/surgical carers have investigated these issues. Other professionals often fail to ask about such problems and parents do not mention them because they assume that they are inextricably linked to EB and therefore not treatable. What is frequently misinterpreted as non-compliance, manipulative behaviour or psychological disturbance is often explained by complications such as GOR or faecal loading.

The form shown in Fig. 24.2 summarises the points to address when carrying out a dietary assessment. The RDEB child with significant oral and oesophageal complications seldom achieves even the EAR for most nutrients using normal foods. Liquidised foods tend to be low in all nutrients, unless large volumes are consumed. Advice, in the first instance, should aim to improve the nutritional value of the child's normal food intake (see *Diet for Epidermolysis Bullosa – for Children over 1 Year*, DEBRA publication). As skin care and dressing changes can take up to 4 hours each day, dietary modifications must be practical and not overly time-consuming. The emphasis should be on increased protein and energy intakes, with improvements in vitamin and mineral intakes as indicated by dietary assessment

and laboratory results. In practice, milk often figures prominently in the diets of EB children, so protein and calcium intakes are generally satisfactory. Conversely, the intakes of those who dislike milk and who have difficulties chewing and swallowing meat invariably fall below the RNI, and will require supplementation.

Realistically, most severely affected RDEB children cannot consume adequate quantities of normal foods and must rely heavily on multinutrient supplements such as Build-up, Fresubin and Fortisip to make up the deficit. In the UK, the Advisory Committee on Borderline Substances (ACBS) authorises the prescription of many of these products for cases of dysphagia and disease-related malnutrition. Glucose polymers, e.g. Polycal, and fat emulsions, e.g. Calogen, are useful for the child who requires an increase in energy intake only. Strictly speaking, these are not prescribable for EB but most GPs are willing to do so. Children who consume multinutrient supplements on a regular basis will generally receive extra vitamins from these. This should be taken into consideration before a further vitamin supplement is prescribed. Those with anything more than the mildest EB should receive extra vitamins [10, 11] to achieve 150–200% of the RNI for age (see section on Vitamins later in this chapter).

Children who can maintain an adequate oral nutrition frequently do so only by the superhuman efforts of their parents. These efforts invariably demand disproportionate amounts of time and are often detrimental to family life. While it is important to impress on parents the key role played by nutrition in overall management, it is also vital not to set unrealistic targets and so engender guilt when these are unattainable due to the complications of the condition rather than to lack of parental diligence. The effect of any intervention should be monitored and an agreed time limit (e.g. 2 to 3 months) placed on assessing its efficacy. If significant improvement in nutritional intake is not achieved with oral supplementation, alternative intervention, e.g. gastrostomy placement (see section on Gastrostomy feeding later in this chapter) should be recommended [22]. Percutaneous endoscopic gastrostomies (PEGs) are not suitable because of the shearing damage to the oesophagus caused at their placement. Button devices inserted as a primary procedure are generally well tolerated, but should be placed via a laparotomy rather than endoscopically.

Date:

NAME: **dob:**   **HOSPITAL NUMBER:**

WEIGHT: kg   centile   **HEIGHT:**   cm   centile

PREFERRED CONSISTENCY OF FOOD: Normal   Soft   Liquidised   Fluid

REASON(S)   Oral blistering Yes/No   Microstomia Yes/No   Fixed tongue Yes/No

                       Dysphagia Yes/No   Oesophageal stricture Yes/No   Other

GASTROSTOMY *in situ*   Yes/No

TYPICAL   Breakfast:

                     Snack:

MEAL   Lunch:

                     Snack:

PATTERN   Evening:

                     Bedtime:

TIME TAKEN OVER AN AVERAGE MEAL   **FINISHES AMOUNT OFFERED?**   Yes/No

NUTRIENT-DENSE/ENERGY-DENSE SUPPLEMENT(S):   Preparation(s), dose, frequency

OTHER SUPPLEMENT(S):   Preparation(s), dose, frequency

          Iron   Zinc   Vitamins

          Carnitine   Selenium   Other

APPROXIMATE DAILY   Energy   kcal   Normal DRV* =   kcal
INTAKE: Protein   g   Normal DRV* =   g

EXCESS MUCUS PRODUCTION   Yes/No   **REGURGITATION**   Yes/No   **G-O REFLUX**   Yes/No

FAECAL LOADING   Yes/No   Frequency of BO   Pain   Yes/No

                          Bleeding p.r. Yes/No   Stool consistency
LAXATIVE(S)   Preparation(s), dose, frequency

FURTHER COMMENTS/ACTION:

* DRV = Dietary reference value

Fig. 24.2 Nutrition summary for epidermolysis bullosa

Dowling-Meara subtype of EB simplex

There is a wide range of severity in this type of EB. Death in the neonatal period is not uncommon, due to widespread blistering and feeding problems in which oropharyngeal blistering significantly compromises nutritional status. Nutritional support as outlined for RDEB earlier should be provided at this time. Aspiration of feeds, believed to be due to uncoordinated swallowing, is common, and GOR may be significant [23]; fortunately, these complications and the tendency to blister generally lessen with time. Even infants whose survival was seriously jeopardised in the neonatal period can proceed to thrive well. There may, however, be some degree of lifelong disability due to persistent and extremely painful blistering of the hands and feet. It is, therefore, important to guard against excessive weight gain in later infancy.

Vitamins

Infants who thrive on breast milk or normally reconstituted formula feeds tend to be those with minimal skin lesions, and their requirements for vitamins are unlikely to be greater than those of normal babies. However, if a satisfactory intake is in doubt, 5 drops daily of Mothers' and Children's Vitamin Drops A, D and C can be given [17], provided that total intake (particularly of vitamin A) does not exceed recommended safe upper limits [15]. Although requirements have not been determined, it may be assumed that more severely affected EB infants require increased amounts of all vitamins [11, 12], especially vitamin C, whose role in enhancing iron absorption [24, 25] and in collagen synthesis [26] is recognised. The provision of 150–200% of the RNI ensures that intakes are still within recommended safe limits.

Babies requiring feeds of increased concentration will automatically receive correspondingly increased amounts of all vitamins, possibly nearing 150% RNI if large volumes are consumed. Again, if a satisfactory intake is in doubt, and skin lesions are significant, a comprehensive preparation such as Ketovite liquid and tablets should be prescribed. Ketovite tablets can be crushed, mixed with a small amount of feed or water and given from a syringe or spoon. If this is not tolerated, a liquid preparation such as Abidec drops can be used, although this will not provide a complete range of vitamins. These preparations should be given at the normal recommended dose for age unless intake from other sources is substantial. When considering vitamin D intake, even fortified feeds may barely meet the normal RNI and it should be remembered that the skin of these babies may be largely covered with dressings and therefore receive minimal exposure to sunlight.

Older children who consume significant volumes of multinutrient supplements (e.g. Ensure Plus or Resource Shakes) on a regular basis will receive correspondingly significant amounts of vitamins from these. In cases where vitamin intake falls below the RNI, a supplement should be prescribed. Although the protective role of antioxidant vitamins in the development of malignancy in EB is unproven, it seems prudent to recommend an enhanced intake of these, while keeping within the currently accepted safe upper limits [15].

Iron and anaemia

As with many other features of EB, the severity of anaemia depends on EB type. RDEB and JEB sufferers experience continual losses from skin lesions and from the upper gastrointestinal tract. In the Dowling-Meara subtype of EB simplex, lesions in infancy can be extensive and blood loss significant. The resulting anaemia is usually microcytic and hypochromic, and is believed to be related to the 'anaemia of chronic disease' [24, 27]. This may not occur under 6 months of age in babies who were full term, presumably because of good iron stores at birth and an adequate iron intake from fortified baby milk and weaning foods. It is important that iron related parameters (see Table 24.2) are checked before this time, to establish baseline values, and iron should be supplemented if deficiency is indicated by reduced haemoglobin with low mean corpuscular volume (MCV), ferritin and high total iron binding capacity (TIBC). Care is required in the interpretation of laboratory results since factors such as infection can produce spuriously raised ferritin. If extra iron is indicated, a liquid form is preferable (e.g. Sytron® Link, Horsham, UK).

Opinion is divided as to the merits of daily [28] versus weekly iron administration [29]. The latter view relies on the hypothesis that a mucosal 'block' occurs in intestinal cells which then cannot absorb therapeutic daily doses of iron until they are renewed by cell turnover at roughly 3 day intervals. Since, in

Table 24.2 Biochemical and haematological investigations in children with epidermolysis bullosa (EB)

Investigation	Suggested frequency of sampling in stable patients
Urea and electrolytes	6–12 monthly
Creatinine	6–12 monthly
Calcium, phosphate	6–12 monthly
Total protein, albumin	6–12 monthly
Alkaline phosphatase, amino acids	6–12 monthly
Zinc, selenium	6–12 monthly
Vitamin B_1, carnitine	Yearly
Vitamin E	1–2 yearly
Serum iron, ferritin, full blood count	6–12 monthly
Hypochromic red blood cell	6–12 monthly
Transferrin receptors	6–12 monthly
Mean corpuscular volume (MCV)	6–12 monthly
Reticulocytes, red cell folate	6–12 monthly
Erythrocyte sedimentation rate (ESR)	6–12 monthly
Free erythrocyte protoporphyrin (FEP)	6–12 monthly
Vitamin B_{12}, folate	Yearly

practice, medications given on a less than daily basis are more likely to be forgotten, it is safer to prescribe on a daily basis so that administration is a part of the regular routine. Compliance is often poor due to the association between iron and constipation and gastric irritation. Dividing a daily dose into two may ease undesirable side effects. Constipation can be significantly reduced by an increase in fibre intake and correct prescription of laxatives and/or stool softeners [20]. To improve iron absorption, children whose oral mucosa is not irritated by a source of vitamin C can be advised to take this with the iron supplement.

Zinc

Zinc is an essential co-factor for over 200 enzymes and plays vital roles in growth, wound healing, immune function and membrane stability where its antioxidant properties are crucial [14, 30, 31]. These processes are especially important in EB, and zinc should be supplemented when skin lesions are severe. Biochemical estimation should be undertaken to provide a baseline, although the interpretation of plasma zinc concentration is notoriously difficult. For example, a low albumin level will cause an associated low zinc result. In such a situation, energy and protein intake should also be increased and a zinc sup-

plement concurrently prescribed. For ease of administration, a liquid supplement is preferable, such as 5–10 ml zinc sulphate solution (30 mg zinc in 5 ml) or a proprietary preparation such as $^1/_2$–1 effervescent tablet of Solvazinc® (Cortecs, Wrexham, UK) (45 mg zinc per tablet). To optimise absorption and minimise side effects of nausea, the daily dose should ideally be split into two. Some patients experience reduced feelings of nausea by sucking flavoured zinc lozenges, e.g. Holland & Barratt (Nuneaton, UK) (23 mg zinc per lozenge), which dissolve slowly in the mouth. The debate continues surrounding the merits of administering zinc supplements separately from iron supplements [32], with no clear consensus. Whichever regimen is adopted, it is important to establish that there is good compliance. Then, if the scheme proves impractical or the physiological response is poor, the regimen can be modified.

Selenium and carnitine

A small number of severely affected RDEB children have developed a fatal dilated cardiomyopathy, thought to be associated with deficiencies of selenium and carnitine [33]. These children had been suffering from generalised malnutrition, so the cause of their cardiomyopathy may have been multifactorial. More recent work [34] supported the hypothesis that selenium and carnitine are implicated in the development of dilated cardiomyopathy, although evidence remains inconclusive. Monitoring of selenium and carnitine status is advisable in all EB children whose nutrition is compromised and/or who rely on nutritional support (e.g. gastrostomy feeding). Where there is biochemical evidence of deficiency, supplementation should be provided. Selenium should be given as pure selenium (50 µg tablet daily). Preparations which also contain vitamin A should be given only if intake of vitamin A from other sources is not significant. 50–100 mg/kg daily of carnitine should be given as Carnitor Paediatric® solution (Shire, Andover, UK).

Biochemical and haematological estimations

Interpretation of blood tests in EB patients is rarely straightforward, due mainly to the inflammatory nature of the condition. Nevertheless, it is important to monitor certain parameters regularly. Table 24.2 lists the investigations which should be routinely carried out, with suggested sampling intervals. Frequency of sampling will vary depending on the disease severity of the individual case and the need to evaluate intervention such as selenium supplementation or gastrostomy placement with enhanced enteral nutrition. Care should be taken to ensure that results are compared with paediatric reference ranges.

Gastro-oesophageal reflux (GOR)

GOR is common in all types of EB and the corrosive action of gastric acid on the delicate oesophageal and oropharyngeal mucosae can cause severe, extensive and permanent scarring. Barium studies, milk scans and pH studies are difficult to perform in EB and, if GOR is suspected, anti-reflux medication should be prescribed even in the absence of positive results from such tests [23]. For infants, it may also be beneficial to provide thickened feeds in addition to medication (see p. 91).

Nasogastric (NG) feeding

Except as a short-term measure, NG feeding should not be undertaken routinely in EB since external as well as internal damage can occur in the securing and passing of the tube. If a long-term feeding problem seems likely, insertion of a gastrostomy should be considered (see Gastrostomy feeding in the next section of this chapter). Temporary NG feeding is indicated for babies who do not take satisfactory volumes of oral feeds and those whose mouths become excessively traumatised by suckling. It is also useful as an interim measure in the older RDEB or non-lethal JEB child who it is believed would benefit from gastrostomy placement, but who needs, or whose carers need, evidence of the effects of improved nutrition before agreeing to surgery. A 6–8 week period of NG feeding should be sufficient to demonstrate benefit.

A further example is in RDEB, where dental procedures frequently cause significant oral and pharyngeal blistering. Post-operatively, such trauma often precludes a satisfactory oral intake for several days. Since these procedures are undertaken under general anaesthetic, an NG tube can be passed in the operating theatre and the child fed by this route until an adequate oral intake is resumed. Whatever the age of the patient, the tube used should be as soft and of as narrow a gauge as possible, and it should not be

resited at every feed, but left in situ. Tubes should never be fixed to the skin with adhesive tape, since skin will be removed with the tape. Tubes can be secured with non-adhesive dressings such as Tubifast® (Seton Scholl, Oldham, UK), the tube being secured by winding a length of Tubifast around it where it enters the nostril. The edge of the nostril can be protected from trauma by applying Vaseline. The ends of the dressing are then tied together behind the head.

Gastrostomy feeding

For a review of gastrostomy feeding see Haynes [3, 22]. For many EB children, particularly those with RDEB, oral feeding is stressful, tedious and often painful, with none of the pleasurable associations enjoyed by non-sufferers. Enormous pressures are experienced by carers who spend protracted and frustrating periods encouraging feeding. Although some parents do succeed in nourishing their child well enough to maintain satisfactory short-term growth, this cannot be maintained indefinitely and is often detrimental to their quality of family life. Ideally, the decision to proceed with surgery should be taken before the child's growth deteriorates. Although many children with growth failure can achieve significant catch-up, they are often reluctant to persevere with oral nutrition, preferring to rely heavily on gastrostomy feeds. This probably reflects a long-term aversion to eating, an activity which they are relieved finally to stop. It should be possible, by sensitive questioning during dietary assessment, to determine which children would benefit from gastrostomy placement.

Many parents initially view the recommendation of a gastrostomy as a sign of their failure to nourish their child adequately and request continued information regarding alternative oral supplements. In fact, delaying placement only adds to their stress and frustration, engendering increased feelings of failure. With early intervention, the child is much more likely to continue with oral nutrition, albeit in small and varying quantities. This is important, not only for social reasons but also in anticipation of a time, after the pubertal growth spurt, when they may be able to take sufficient nutrition orally and the gastrostomy can be reversed. A nutrient-dense feed containing a mixed fibre source (e.g. Nutrini Fibre or Jevity Plus) should be chosen for gastrostomy feeds, and for children over the age of about 3 years, these are usually delivered overnight via a pump. Some children may require a combination of pumped overnight feeds and daytime bolus feeds. Using dietary reference values [15], consistent increases in weight and height can be achieved by supplying 100–150% estimated average requirement (EAR) for energy and 115–200% reference nutrient intake (RNI) for protein.

Constipation

There are a number of references which deal with the subject of constipation in EB: [3, 8, 20, 21] and see also section on RDEB earlier in this chapter. Chronic constipation (often more accurately termed fecal loading) with painful defecation is one of the most frequent, yet underestimated, complications of all types of EB. Even a moderately bulky stool can tear the delicate anal skin causing fissuring and extreme pain with subsequent bowel movements. Fear of defecation leads to infrequent and incomplete bowel emptying and the gradual accumulation of hard feces. It should be treated without delay if the vicious cycle of pain, conscious ignoring of the gastrocolonic reflex and secondary anorexia (Fig. 24.1) is to be avoided. In babies, extra fluid should be offered in the form of water, or if this is refused, one teaspoon of fresh fruit juice diluted in 100 ml water or ready-to-feed baby juice diluted with an equal volume of water. Alternatively, one teaspoon of sugar (anecdotal evidence suggests that brown is more effective than white) can be added to each feed. Lactulose should be prescribed, starting with 2.5 ml od to 2.5 ml bd. A pure fibre source, e.g. Resource Benefiber® (Novartis Medical Nutrition, UK) or a fibre-containing feed such as Paediasure with Fibre or Nutrini Fibre should be introduced at 6–8 months. Whether the infant is constipated or not, it is prudent to introduce a fibre source at 9–12 months of age, since constipation is such a likely complication of all types of EB, plus a stool softener such as lactulose. If the child then progresses onto a diet sufficiently high in fibre to promote comfortable defecation, the fibre source can be phased out.

Many older EB sufferers mistake overflow incontinence for diarrhoea, and reduce their prescribed laxative therapy, inadvertently exacerbating the situation. Oral lesions, dysphagia and requirement for a low bulk, nutrient-dense intake preclude their consuming a conventional high fibre diet. An increase in fibre intake is important, however, and a fibre containing feed (preferably one based on a mixed fibre source) should be introduced, orally or by gastrostomy, but only after the extent of fecal loading has been investigated and addressed. In addition to the feeds mentioned above, such products include Fortisip MultiFibre, Jevity, Jevity Plus, Enrich and Entera Fibre Plus.

The incorporation into feeds or foods of a fibre source, is extremely successful in normalising stool consistency and frequency of defecation. If an increase in both energy and fibre is indicated, this can be supplied by a product such as VibreCal. In the absence of UK recommended intakes of fibre for children and adolescents, the US formula of age (yrs) + 5–10 g daily [35] is a useful guideline. For example, a 3 year old child will require 8–13 g fibre per day. It is important to note that, if such preparations are introduced while the child remains fecally loaded, problems such as abdominal pain, GOR and vomiting will invariably ensue and compliance will be jeopardised. Therefore, firstly, intestinal transit time should be assessed. This can be done by giving a carmine dye marker and noting the time taken for it to appear in the stools [36]. Then, depending on the degree of fecal loading, this can be addressed by giving either a bowel-prep solution such as Klean-Prep® (Norgine, Harefield, UK) as a hospital inpatient, or a strong laxative such as Picolax® (Nordic Ferring, Langley, UK). Thereafter, some permutation of stool softener/laxative is generally necessary in the long term.

Dental aspects

The oral complications of JEB and RDEB often make it impossible to cleanse the teeth satisfactorily. Defective enamel seems to occur more frequently in these two groups than in DDEB and the simplex forms, although it is unclear whether this is due to structural defects or systemic conditions, e.g. anaemia, infection or abnormal nutrition [37]. The oral mucosa of many patients is generally too delicate to allow the use of a normal brush. Plaque collects around the teeth, leading to chronic marginal gingivitis. The removal of badly decayed teeth from a mouth with very poor opening may be extremely difficult even under general anaesthesia and often results in increased oral ulceration and scarring.

Unless a gastrostomy has been placed, a diet sufficiently high in energy to permit normal growth in EB generally means the consumption of considerable quantities of fermentable carbohydrate, especially sucrose, at regular intervals throughout the day. The frequency of such foods, especially coupled with the complications noted above, is highly conducive to the development of dental caries. This apparent conflict of interests between dietitian and dentist can lead to contradictory advice to the child and the carers. However, compromise is possible, and families must be taught from early on the importance of good oral hygiene. The advice of an experienced dentist should be followed regarding a fluoride supplement, fluoride toothpaste and a plaque-inhibiting mouthwash. Sweets and chocolate biscuits should ideally be restricted to the end of mealtimes and continuous sipping of sugary drinks outside mealtimes discouraged. However, in a severely affected child who relies on oral nutrition, this may be impossible as eating and drinking are extremely slow and one mealtime unavoidably merges into the next.

Oesophageal dilatation and colonic interposition

For many RDEB sufferers, dysphagia and oesophageal strictures are the main reasons for their failure to consume sufficient nutrition. In theory, dilatation of the strictures should relieve much of the problem. However, the pharyngeal and oesophageal mucosae are extremely fragile and may rupture; even in experienced hands, fatalities have occurred [38]. There is preliminary evidence that patients with high oesophageal strictures can benefit from serial balloon dilatations. However, any gains must be weighed against the risks. Colonic interposition and oesophagocolonoplasty have been undertaken with success [39]. Considering the technical complexity of the procedure and the significant mortality risk, this currently remains a last resort for those whose nutritional support cannot be maintained by any other means [40].

REFERENCES

1 Dunnill MGS, Eady RAJ The management of dystrophic epidermolysis bullosa. *Clin Exp Dermatol*, 1995, **20** 179–88.

2 Haber RM, Ramsay CA, Boxall LBH Epidermolysis bullosa. Assessment of a treatment regimen. *Int J Dermatol*, 1985, **24** 324–8.

3 Haynes L Nutritional support for children with epidermolysis bullosa. *J Hum Nutr Diet*, 1998, **11** 163–73.

4 Tesi D, Lin AN Nutritional management of the epidermolysis bullosa patient. In: Lin AN, Carter DM (eds) *Epidermolysis Bullosa: Basic and Clinical Aspects*. New York: Springer-Verlag, 1992, pp. 261–6.

5 Sehgal VN *et al.* Dystrophic epidermolysis bullosa. Interesting gastrointestinal manifestations. *Brit J Dermatol*, 1977, **96** 389–91.

6 Orlando RC *et al.* Epidermolysis bullosa: gastrointestinal manifestations. *Ann Int Med*, 1974, **81** 203–206.

7 Fine J-D, McGuire J Altered nutrition and inherited epidermolysis bullosa. In: Fine J-D, Bauer EA, McGuire J, Moshell A (eds) *Epidermolysis Bullosa. Clinical, Epidemiologic and Laboratory Advances and the Findings of the National Epidermolysis Bullosa Registry*. Baltimore: The Johns Hopkins University Press, 1999, pp. 225–35.

8 Ergun G, Schaefer RA Gastrointestinal aspects of epidermolysis bullosa. In: Lin AN, Carter DM (eds) *Epidermolysis Bullosa: Basic and Clinical Aspects*. New York: Springer-Verlag, 1992, pp. 169–84.

9 Lechner-Gruskay D *et al.* Nutritional and metabolic profile of children with epidermolysis bullosa. *Pediatr Dermatol*, 1988, **5** 22–7.

10 Allman SM *et al.* Nutrition in dystrophic epidermolysis bullosa. *Pediatr Dermatol*, 1992, **9** 231–8.

11 Fine J-D, Tamura T, Johnson L Blood vitamin and trace metal levels in epidermolysis bullosa. *Arch Dermatol*, 1989, **125** 374–9.

12 Birge K Nutrition management of patients with epidermolysis bullosa. *J Amer Diet Assoc*, 1995, **95** 575–9.

13 Gamelli RL Nutritional problems of the acute and chronic burn patient; relevance to epidermolysis bullosa. *Arch Dermatol*, 1988, **124** 756–9.

14 McLaren SMG Nutrition and wound healing. *J Wound Care*, 1992, **1** 45–55.

15 Department of Health Report on Health and Social Subjects No 41. *Dietary Reference Values for Food Energy and Nutrients for the United Kingdom*. London: The Stationery Office, 1991.

16 Freeman JV *et al.* Cross sectional stature and weight reference curves for the UK. *Arch Dis Childh*, 1995, **73** 17–24.

17 Department of Health and Social Security Report on Health and Social Subjects No. 32. *Present Day Practice in Infant Feeding*. London: The Stationery Office, 1988.

18 Lin AN, Carter DM Junctional epidermolysis bullosa: a clinical overview. In: Lin AN, Carter DM (eds) *Epidermolysis Bullosa: Basic and Clinical Aspects*. New York: Springer-Verlag, 1992, pp. 118–34.

19 Berger TG *et al.* Junctional epidermolysis bullosa, pyloric atresia and genitourinary disease. *Pediatr Dermatol*, 1986, **3** 130–34.

20 Haynes L, Atherton DJ, Clayden G Constipation in epidermolysis bullosa: successful treatment with a

liquid fiber-containing formula. *Pediatr Dermatol*, 1997, **14** (5) 393–6.

21 Clayden GS Dysphagia and constipation in epidermolysis bullosa. In: Priestley GC *et al.* (eds) *Epidermolysis Bullosa: A comprehensive review of classification, management and laboratory studies.* Berkshire: Dystrophic Epidermolysis Bullosa Research Association (DEBRA), 1990, pp. 67–71.

22 Haynes L *et al.* Gastrostomy and growth in dystrophic epidermolysis bullosa. *Br J Dermatol*, 1996, **134** 872–9.

23 Atherton DJ, Denyer J *Epidermolysis Bullosa. An Outline for Professionals.* Berkshire: Dystrophic Epidermolysis Bullosa Research Association (DEBRA), 1997.

24 Bothwell TH *et al. Iron Metabolism in Man.* Oxford: Blackwell Science, 1979, p. 431.

25 Seshadri A, Shah A, Bhade S Haematological response of anaemic pre-school children to ascorbic acid supplementation. *Hum Nutr: Appl Nutr*, 1985, **39A** 151–4.

26 Levene CI, Bates CJ Ascorbic acid and collagen synthesis in cultured fibroblasts. *Ann NY Acad Sci*, 1975, **258** 288–305.

27 Giardina PJ, Lin AN Hematologic problems in epidermolysis bullosa. In: Lin AN, Carter DM (eds) *Epidermolysis Bullosa: Basic and Clinical Aspects.* New York: Springer-Verlag, 1992, pp. 191–7.

28 Hallberg L Combating iron deficiency: daily administration of iron is far superior to weekly administration. *Amer J Clin Nutr*, 1998, **68** 213–17.

29 Beard JL Weekly iron intervention: the case for intermittent iron supplementation. *Amer J Clin Nutr*, 1998, **68** 209–212.

30 Halstead JA Zinc deficiency in man, the Shiraz experiment. *Amer J Med*, 1972, **53** 277–84.

31 Shankar AH, Prasad AS Zinc and immune function: the biological basis of altered resistance to infection. *Amer J Clin Nutr*, 1998, **68** (Suppl) 447S–63S.

32 Whittaker P Iron and zinc interactions in humans. *Amer J Clin Nutr*, 1998, **68** (Suppl) 442S–6S.

33 Melville C *et al.* Fatal cardiomyopathy in dystrophic epidermolysis bullosa. *Brit J Dermatol*, 1996, **135** 603–606.

34 Sidwell RU, Yates R, Atherton DJ Dystrophic epidermolysis and dilated cardiomyopathy. *Arch Dis Childh*, 2000, **83** 59–63.

35 Williams CL, Bollella M, Wynder EL A new recommendation for dietary fiber in childhood. *Pediatr*, 1995, **96** 985–8.

36 Denyer J *Care and Management of Children with Dystrophic Epidermolysis Bullosa.* Berkshire: Dystrophic Epidermolysis Bullosa Research Association (DEBRA), 1999.

37 Wright JT Oral manifestations of epidermolysis bullosa. In: Fine J-D, Bauer EA, McGuire J, Moshell A (eds) *Epidermolysis Bullosa. Clinical, Epidemiologic and Laboratory Advances and the Findings of the National Epidermolysis Bullosa Registry.* Baltimore: The Johns Hopkins University Press, 1999, pp. 236–56.

38 Griffin R, Mayou B The anaesthetic management of patients with dystrophic epidermolysis bullosa. A review of 44 patients over a ten year period. *Anaesthesia*, 1993, **48** 810–15.

39 Gryboski JD, Touloukian R, Campanella RA Gastrointestinal manifestations of epidermolysis bullosa in children. *Arch Dermatol*, 1988, **124** 746–52.

40 Fine J-D, Bauer EA, McGuire J The treatment of inherited epidermolysis bullosa. Nonmolecular approaches. In: Fine J-D, Bauer EA, McGuire J, Moshell A (eds) *Epidermolysis Bullosa. Clinical, Epidemiologic and Laboratory Advances and the Findings of the National Epidermolysis Bullosa Registry.* Baltimore: The Johns Hopkins University Press, 1999, pp. 374–406.

USEFUL ADDRESSES

The Dystrophic Epidermolysis Bullosa Research Association (DEBRA) is a charity which exists to help sufferers with all types of EB. DEBRA funds research into the molecular basis of EB, with the aim of finding a cure, and also dedicated nursing and dietetic support.

Dystrophic Epidermolysis Bullosa Research Association

DEBRA House, 13 Wellington Business Park, Dukes Ride, Crowthorne, Berkshire RG45 6LS. Tel. 01344 771961, Fax 01344 762661, E-mail debra.uk@btinternet.com, Website www.debra.org.uk

Nutritional information booklets published by DEBRA:

Allman, S (1990) *Diet for Epidermolysis Bullosa, For Children Over 1 Year.*

Haynes, L (1993) *Nutrition for babies with dystrophic epidermolysis bullosa.* (This information may be suitable for babies with EBS Dowling-Meara and JEB, but not LJEB.)

ACKNOWLEDGEMENTS

I would like to thank Dr David Atherton, Consultant Paediatric Dermatologist, and Jacqueline Denyer, Clinical Nurse Specialist in EB, for their support. I would also like to thank DEBRA who fund my post.

CHAPTER 25

Burns

The incidence of burns in children in the UK is not known. A recent American study suggests that some 70% of superficial burns occur in children under 5 years of age, with a peak incidence at 1–2 years [1]. These figures are likely to be comparable to what is seen in the UK.

ASSESSMENT OF INJURY

Burns are assessed from an accurate history of the incident. This should include the type of burn and whether there has been any smoke inhalation. The main causes and types of burn injury in children and adolescents are listed in Table 25.1.

Burns are classified as

- Partial thickness (superficial, deep dermal)
- Full thickness.

The total body surface area (TBSA) is determined using Lund and Browder charts [2]. In children a major burn is defined as being greater than 10% of body surface area, or if there is smoke inhalation.

METABOLIC RESPONSE TO BURN INJURY

Current thinking has moved away from the 'ebb and flow' response to injury. Historically it is likely that thermal injury resulted in greatly elevated energy requirements. Formulae for calculating requirements aimed to provide very high energy intakes [3, 4, 5]. Modern medical and nursing management, such as early excision and grafting, temporary wound cover, regular analgesia and control of ambient temperature, has had beneficial effects on the metabolic response to the burn injury. This has led researchers to

re-evaluate the nutritional requirements of this patient group.

AIMS OF NUTRITIONAL SUPPORT

The aim of nutritional support is to provide appropriate intervention to promote optimal wound healing and to maintain normal growth. It is well documented that improved nutritional status in the critically ill patient reduces the likelihood of complications (e.g. infection, poor wound healing), and length of stay in hospital [6, 7, 8, 9].

ASSESSMENT OF NUTRITIONAL REQUIREMENTS

Some of the factors influencing the nutritional requirements of a child with a thermal injury are listed in Table 25.2. A full assessment of nutritional requirements should be made taking these and any additional factors into consideration.

Energy requirements

Several researchers have investigated energy requirements in children with thermal injuries. Although the ideal way of calculating energy requirements would be to measure them on a daily basis, using indirect calorimetry and adjusting all nutritional support to meet these figures, the practicalities of this are prohibitive.

The Hildreth formula (Table 25.3), which takes account of age, weight, height and percentage burn surface area can be calculated at the bedside [10, 11]. It uses a nomogram to calculate body surface area (Fig. 25.1) [12]. A recent paper has suggested that

Table 25.1 Causes and types of burn injury

Type of burn	Cause of burn
Water	Kettle, teapot, cup, mug, bath, saucepan
Contact	Radiator, iron, oven, hot-water bottle
Flame	House fire, chip pan, electric/coal fire, barbecue
Fat	Chip pan, oven trays
Chemical	Cement, hair dye, cleansing agents, cytotoxic drugs
Electrical	Electrical appliances, overhead and underground cables
Other	Over-exposure to radiotherapy, frostbite, animal manure

Table 25.2 Factors influencing nutritional requirements

Age
Sex
Weight
Height/length
General nutritional status
Percentage burn surface area
Thickness of burn

Table 25.3 Hildreth formula for energy requirements

Infants <1 year	2100 kcal (8.8 MJ)/m² (SA) + 1000 kcal (4.2 MJ)/m² (BSA)
Children <12 years	1800 kcal (7.5 MJ)/m² (SA) + 1300 kcal (5.4 MJ)/m² (BSA)
Children >12 years	1500 kcal (6.3 MJ)/m² (SA) + 1500 kcal (6.3 MJ)/m² (BSA)

SA = surface area
BSA = burn surface area

energy requirements in children with burns rarely rise above the estimated average requirements (EAR) in the first 24 hours post-burn injury [13, 14]. An alternative may therefore be to aim for the EAR in injuries of a small surface area. All formulae are only guidelines and a point from which to start. Frequent reassessment and adjustment are required for an uneventful course and successful outcome.

Protein requirements

Investigators have documented the need for increased protein provision in thermal injury. Losses of lean muscle mass and negative nitrogen balance have both been recognised in studies investigating the nutritional needs of this patient group. It has been shown in several studies that appropriate wound healing is achievable in children receiving 2–3 g protein/kg/day [15, 16]. It has also been suggested that higher protein intakes of 23–26% of energy intake may contribute to an improved immune response in thermally injured children [17].

Moderate hypoalbuminaemia is common in children with thermal injuries and the literature suggests that this can be well tolerated. Increases in protein provision may be required to correct this; however, if the calculated protein requirement is being met then alternative medical management (e.g. albumin infusions) should be considered if levels are falling too low [18].

Vitamin and mineral requirements

This area is still very much in debate as there are few studies that specifically look at the requirements for vitamins and minerals in children with burns. It can be assumed, however, that requirements are increased for certain vitamins and minerals due to their role in the metabolic pathways of the body.

When assessing the requirements in burns patients the following should be considered:

- Vitamin A may have a role in the prevention of stress ulcers [19]
- Vitamin C is vital to collagen synthesis [19]
- B group vitamins are required proportional to energy intake
- Low levels of serum iron in most cases are not dietary related and may have a protective effect against infection [20]
- Both zinc and copper play a role in the wound healing process; however, the methods and benefits of supplementation require further investigation [21].

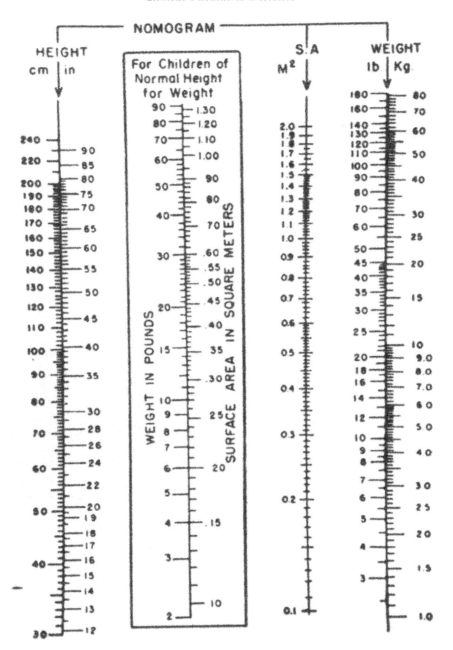

Fig. 25.1 Surface area nomogram, modified from data of E. Boyd by C. D. West; reproduced from *Nelson Textbook of Paediatrics*, 12e, London, W. B. Saunders Co., 1983

Before a vitamin and mineral supplement is considered it is important to check the nutritional composition and bioavailability of enteral and/or parenteral intervention, in conjunction with the appropriate biochemical parameters. Excessive supplementation may result in a nutritional imbalance, which could potentially result in toxicity of certain nutrients or interfere with the utilisation of other nutrients.

Novel substrates

Evidence of the benefits of these components of nutritional products is limited; however, the few published clinical trials are encouraging and offer therapeutic potential for the future. Optimal dosage, composition, timing and duration of these pharmacological nutrients require further research before comprehensive recommendations can be made [22, 23, 24, 25].

- *Glutamine* This is the most prevalent free amino acid in the human body and has a variety of functions. The reduction of the muscle free glutamine pool appears to be a common response to injury. Supplementation appears to have a protective effect on protein synthesis and tissue repair. It is also the main fuel source for gut enterocytes preserving the mucosal integrity and reducing bacterial translocation [26, 27].
- *Arginine* This amino acid has been shown to have an immune enhancing role in stressed patients [28].
- *Other substrates* These include nucleotides and omega-3 fatty acids. They are commonly referred to as immune-enhancing nutrients and have proven anti-inflammatory actions.

MEETING NUTRITIONAL GOALS

Several factors need to be considered before deciding the most appropriate method of achieving nutritional requirements. These are listed in Table 25.4.

Minor burns (<10%)

Children with minor burns should be encouraged to start eating and drinking as early as possible. Nutri-

Table 25.4 Factors influencing the achievement of nutritional requirements

Percentage burn surface area
Site of injury
Pre-existing clinical conditions
Previous nutritional status
Special dietary needs
Gastrointestinal function
Pain management and sedation
Pyrexia
Psychological distress

tious fluids such as milk, milk shakes and proprietary dietary supplements should be offered as opposed to juice or fizzy drinks. Every effort should be made to provide familiar foods in order to promote the child's appetite.

Daily food and fluid intake charts should be recorded by nursing staff. If these highlight difficulties in meeting the dietary targets alternative nutritional intervention may be necessary.

Major burns (>10%)

In major burns a nasogastric or nasojejunal feeding tube should be passed within the first few hours of treatment when other invasive procedures are taking place. Enteral feeds should then be commenced as early as possible and balanced against oral intake. It has been well documented that early enteral feeding of burns patients (within the first 6 hours) reduces the incidence of paralytic ileus. The many other benefits of early enteral feeding include maintenance of the integrity of the gastrointestinal tract thus reducing bacterial translocation, as well as improvements in immune status and wound healing [29, 30, 31, 32].

Nutritional management should consider treatment procedures, which may result in a decrease in nutritional intake. These can include surgical intervention, dressing changes, physiotherapy and medications.

Parenteral nutrition should be considered when enteral feeding is compromised. However, where possible minimal enteral feeds (as little as 2 ml/hour in children) should continue to be infused at a very low rate to maintain the brush border integrity of the gastrointestinal tract [33, 34]. The complications of total parenteral nutrition (TPN) are well recognised. Infection risks are already high in burns patients so special care must be taken when considering TPN. Other issues around TPN in children, such as electrolyte imbalances and hyperglycaemia, also require particularly close monitoring. Further guidance on enteral and parenteral nutrition support in children may be found Chapters 3 and 4.

Choice of oral and enteral feeds

The choice of feed will vary depending on the age of the child, the calculated requirements, any unrelated medical condition and the clinical course during admission. Some of the products available for use in the nutritional management of paediatric burns patients are outlined in Table 25.5.

MONITORING

All patients receiving nutritional support require regular monitoring to ensure optimal nutritional intake. It is important to note that a number of nutritional indicators are needed to give an overall view of nutritional status.

- This patient group has regularly changing nutritional needs related to the healing of their wounds. As the percentage burn surface area changes so the requirements should be reassessed.
- Regular weights (without dressings) and lengths should be recorded and plotted on appropriate centile charts. These should be compared with pre-admission measurements where available. Oedema may mask true weight early in the clinical course.
- Routine biochemistry should be monitored. Frequency will vary depending on the child's clinical course. Vitamin, mineral and trace element status should also be monitored. The recommendation for adult burn patients by the Burns Interest Group of the British Dietetic Association should be used as a guide at this time [19].

- C-reactive protein has recently been shown to predict sepsis in children with burn injuries [35]. This would suggest that it be included in routine monitoring in major burns where there is an increased risk of infection.
- Bowel motions should be recorded accurately indicating frequency and consistency. Adjustments to feeding regimens may be beneficial in normalising bowel habit.
- Monitoring of nutritional intake and overall nutritional status should continue post-discharge. Changes to the medical management of burns patients now results in early discharge home, even for quite major injuries. These children are still at risk of inadequate nutritional intake and therefore growth failure once at home [36].

Much work is still needed in the area of nutritional requirements of thermally injured children, particularly with respect to vitamin and mineral requirements. The Burns Interest Group of the British Dietetic Association is currently developing guidelines for the nutritional management of these patients. However, medical and nursing management is constantly advancing and therefore the effects on nutrition will continue to change.

CASE STUDY

An 18 month old toddler has sustained a 15% partial thickness scald as a result of pulling a jug of freshly boiled water over himself. His weight and length on admission are on the 25th centile for age.

A dietary history indicates that he takes approximately 500–600 ml of a follow-on milk, recommended as the family follows a lacto-vegetarian diet. There is no history of iron deficiency anaemia. He eats three meals plus supper daily and has no noted dislikes or food intolerance.

Calculating requirements

Energy: 1800 kcal (7.5 MJ)/m^2 (SA) + 1300 kcal (5.4 MJ)/m^2 (burn SA)
= (1800 × 0.48) + (1300 × 0.072)
= 958 kcal

Protein: 2–3 g protein/kg
= 24–36 g protein

SA = surface area

Table 25.5 Suitable feeds for paediatric patients

0–1 years	Low birth weight formula; infant formula; follow-on milk; high energy infant formula; protein hydrolysate formula
1–6 years	Paediatric enteral feeds; high energy paediatric enteral feeds; paediatric fibre feeds; age appropriate sip feeds
7–adult	As for 1–6 years; adult enteral feeds; high energy adult enteral feeds; adult fibre feeds; critical care enteral feeds; oral sip feeds
Others	Glucose polymers; fat emulsions; protein supplements; novel substrates

Achieving requirements

The following need to be considered:

- Site of injury – facial injury, therefore oral feeding may be compromised; a feeding tube should be passed on admission prior to facial swelling
- Percentage burn area – this is >10% and is therefore a major burn
- There is no medical history of note
- Previous nutritional status – good
- Special dietary needs – lacto-vegetarian
- No gastrointestinal problems
- Pain management – as a result of the injury the child is in a high degree of pain and has commenced opiate-based pain relief
- Pyrexia – none noted yet
- The child is scared and unsure of what is happening to him.

Method of feeding

An enteral feeding tube should be passed during the resuscitation period. Enteral feeds should commence within 6 hours of admission via this route, until such a time as the child is able to feed orally. Enteral feeds should gradually be replaced by oral intake to meet full nutritional requirements. Good oral hygiene should be maintained throughout.

Choice of feed

- A normal follow-on milk supplemented with glucose polymer and fat emulsions. The advantage of this option is familiarity and ease of regrading onto oral feeds. The disadvantage is the increased infection risk due to feed modification.
- A standard 1 kcal (4 kJ)/ml paediatric enteral feed. The advantage of this option is a nutritionally complete feed that will meet all nutritional requirements without modification. The disadvantage is the unfamiliarity of the product.

The final feeding regimen should be planned in conjunction with medical and nursing management.

Monitoring

- Dressings are changed twice weekly. The child should be weighed and the degree of healing

assessed. Nutritional support should be reassessed according to these criteria.
- Nutritional biochemical markers should be requested and monitored as necessary to 'fine tune' dietetic intervention and promote a positive outcome.
- A possible side effect of analgesia is constipation; bowel habits should be monitored closely.

REFERENCES

1 Dyer C, Roberts O Thermal trauma. *Nurs Clin Nth Am*, 1990, **25** 85–117.
2 Lund CL, Browder ND The estimation of areas of burns. *Surg Gynecol Obstet*, 1944, **78** 352.
3 Sutherland AB, Batchelor ADC Nitrogen balance in burned children. *Ann N Y Acad Sciences*, 1968, **150** 700.
4 Soloman JR Nutrition in the severely burnt child. *Progr Pediatr Surg*, 1981, **14** 653–79.
5 Grotte G *et al.* Parenteral nutrition. In: McClaren DS, Burman D (eds) *Textbook of Paediatric Nutrition*, 2e. Edinburgh: Churchill Livingstone, 1982.
6 Bagley SM Nutritional needs of the acutely ill with acute wounds. *Cri Care Nurs Clin North Am*, 1996, **22** 159–67.
7 Kiyama T *et al.* The route of nutrition support affects the early phase of wound healing. *J Parent Ent Nutr*, 1998, **22** 276–9.
8 Wallace E Feeding the wound: nutrition and wound care. *Br J Nurs*, 1994, **3** 662.
9 Kings Fund Centre *A Positive Approach to Nutrition as a Treatment*. London: Kings Fund, 1992.
10 Hildreth M *et al.* Calorie requirement of patients with burns under one year of age. *J Burn Care Rehabil*, 1993, **14** 108–112.
11 Hildreth M *et al.* Current treatment reduces calories required to maintain weight in paediatric patients with burns. *J Burn Care Rehabil*, 1990, **11** 405–409.
12 Behrman RE, Kliegman RM (eds) *Nelson Essential Paediatrics*, 3e. London: WB Saunders Co, 1990, pp. 805.
13 Childs C Studies in children provide a model to re-examine the metabolic response to burn injuries in patients treated by contemporary burn protocol. *Burns*, 1994, **20** 291–300.
14 Dept of Health Report on Health and Social Subjects No. 41. *Dietary Reference Values for food energy and nutrients for the UK*. London: The Stationery Office: 1991.
15 Cunningham JJ *et al.* Calorie and protein provision for recovery from severe burns in infants and young children. *Am J Clin Nutr*, 1990, **51** 553–7.
16 Prelack K *et al.* Energy and protein provisions for thermally injured children revisited: an outcome-

based approach for determining requirements. *J Burn Care Rehabil*, 1997, **18** 177–81.

17 Alexandra JW *et al*. Beneficial effects of aggressive protein feeding in severely burned children. *Ann Surg*, 1980, **192** 505–517.

18 Sheridan RL Physiologic hypoalbuminaemia is well tolerated by severely burned children. *J Trauma*, 1997, **43** 448–52.

19 British Dietetic Association Burns Interest Group *UK National Feeding Guidelines for Burns Patients*. Birmingham: BDA, 1992.

20 Ward CG *et al*. Iron and infection: new developments and their implications. *J Trauma*, 1996, **41** 356–64.

21 Cunningham JJ *et al*. Low ceruloplasmin levels during recovery from major burn injury: influence of open wound size and copper supplementation. *Nutrition*, 1996, **12** 83–8.

22 Saffle JR *et al*. Randomized trial of immune enhancing enteral nutrition in burns patients. *J Trauma*, 1997, **42** 793–800.

23 Weiman A, Baskan L Influence of arginine, omega 3 fatty acids and nucleotide-supplemented enteral support on systemic inflammatory response syndrome and multiple organ failure in patients after severe trauma. *Nutrition*, 1998, **14** 165–72.

24 Georgieff M, Tugtekin IF Positive role of immune nutrition on metabolism in sepsis and multiorgan failure. *Kidney Int Suppl*, 1998, **64** 580–83.

25 Fürst P New parenteral substrates in clinical nutrition. Introduction 1. New substrates in protein nutrition. *Eur J Clin Nutr*, 1994, **48** 607–616.

26 Houdijk AP *et al*. Randomised trial of glutamine enriched enteral nutrition on infectious morbidity in patients with multiple trauma. *Lancet*, 1998, **353** 772–6.

27 Souba WW Glutamine: a key substrate for the splanchnic bed. *Annu Rev Nutr*, 1991, **11** 285–308.

28 Barbul A The use of arginine in clinical practice. In: Cynober L (ed.) *Amino Acid Metabolism and Therapy in Health and Nutritional Disease*. Boca Raton, FL: CRC Press, 1995, pp. 361–72.

29 Chiarelli A *et al*. Very early nutrition supplementation in burned patients. *Am J Clin Nutr*, 1990, **51** 1035–9.

30 McDonald WS *et al*. Immediate enteral feeding in burn patients is safe and effective. *J Parent Ent Nutr*, 1991, **15** 578–9.

31 Hansbrough JF Enteral nutritional support in burn patients. *Gastrointest Endosc Clin N Am*, 1998, **42** 645–67.

32 Hunt D, Orr J Early nutritional intervention in a failure to thrive ex-premature infant with 15% full thickness radiator burns – a case in review. *ETRS Abstracts*, 1998, **14** 81.

33 Lucas A *et al*. Gut hormones and minimal enteral feedings. *Acta Paediatr Scand*, 1986, **75** 719–23.

34 Troche B, Harvey-Wilkes K Early minimal feedings promote growth in critically ill premature infants. *Biol Neonate*, 1995, **67** 1272–81.

35 Neely AN *et al*. Efficiency of a rise in C-reactive protein serum levels as an early indicator of sepsis in burned children. *J Burn Care Rehabil*, 1998, **19** 102–105.

36 Mittendorfer B *et al*. The 1995 clinical research award. Younger paediatric patients with burns are at risk for continuing post discharge weight loss. *J Burn Care Rehabil*, 1995, **16** 589–95.

ACKNOWLEDGEMENT

Thanks to Dr Peter King of the Burns Interest Group of the British Dietetic Association, for his comments.

CHAPTER 26

Nutrition for Children with Feeding Difficulties

Infants, children and adolescents with neurological, physical or sensory impairments are likely to experience difficulties in eating and/or drinking. Their ability to achieve their individual potential in growth and development will depend on the skills and intervention provided in the early years [1]. However, multidisciplinary teams have not focused on this particular problem, resulting in identification of nutritional problems at a later rather than an earlier stage of life. Webb [2] summarises:

'Nutrition for handicapped children is not a subject which generates much discussion probably because it is a difficult problem on which to speak in generalities. Classifications of handicaps usually consider only the major handicap, and thus labelling a child as having a particular disability gives little information on the food and nutrition problems which may be present.'

Impairments that result in limited oral motor or self-feeding skills will cause feeding difficulties. Social and physical issues affect the lives of these children and the services they may receive and provide a picture from which nutrition goals can be planned to help them achieve their potential. In this chapter the term carer describes parent, guardian, or staff in residential or educational locations.

Children with feeding difficulties require a multidisciplinary approach if the problems are to be assessed and managed successfully. The development of eating and drinking skills is important for several reasons, only one of which is nutrition.

- Efficient eating is necessary if the child is to consume adequate nutrition orally.
- Oral control, the patterns of movement of lips, tongue, jaw and breathing, are practised while

eating. This strongly influences the development of precise movements necessary for speech and control of saliva.
- Mealtimes provide opportunities for the development of posture, head control and eye/hand co-ordination.
- Mealtimes provide an ideal opportunity for language to be learned.
- Mealtimes provide ideal settings for social interaction where rules and social behaviour are learned and rehearsed.
- Social integration into mealtimes and eating out is easier as a child's competence improves.
- Independence can be gained through providing choice and control at mealtimes, allowing the child to develop self-esteem, independence and his or her own identity.

MAJOR NUTRITIONAL PROBLEMS

The major nutritional problems seen in these children are:

- Failure to thrive
- Low body weight for height
- Constipation
- Vitamin and mineral deficiencies
- Dental caries

Failure to thrive or low body weight has been well documented for children with developmental delay, neurological dysfunctioning and in particular for children with cerebral palsy [3–6]. Studies have been published showing the positive impact of nutrition intervention for children with cerebral palsy [7–10]. Sanders' prospective study demonstrated the importance of early intervention during the first year of

central nervous system (CNS) damage in order
to prevent or reverse growth deficits comparing
against older children [7]. Some studies have proposed that growth failure in children with cerebral
palsy is independent of nutrition [11, 12]. In addition,
beliefs that it is 'normal' for children with severe disabilities, particularly children with cerebral palsy, to
have poor stature and low weights has often been
'ascribed to their underlying cerebral deficit or
physical inactivity than to chronic malnutrition' [1].
Bax, in an editorial addressing this issue, was
'shocked' by the number of young disabled people
(40%) who had feeding problems [13]. Other studies
have shown that minimal oral-motor dysfunction
should be considered in non-organic failure to thrive
[14]. Stallings, in her summary of nutritional
assessment [15], states:

> 'Nutrition and growth status in children and adults
> with CP and other severe types of developmental
> disabilities is an essential component of care. While
> data are not available to provide precise definitions
> of the levels of severity of malnutrition and growth
> failure and their effect on long-term outcome, it is
> clear that many patients with moderate and severe
> CP and other disabilities have malnutrition and
> growth failure as the result of inadequate caloric
> intake.'

Special charts have been developed for children with
Down's syndrome [16] and Krick has proposed charts
for children with cerebral palsy [12]. Paediatric BMI
charts may be useful for showing the degree of underweight; however, a height measurement is essential.
Accurate height/length is often difficult to obtain due
to the child's impairments (e.g. spastic or dystonic
cerebral palsy). Alternative measurements such as
upper arm and lower leg lengths and knee heights can
be used to estimate height [15]. However, there is
no general consensus on best clinical practice. Height
can be measured by the physiotherapist when
monitoring use of a standing frame or lying board.
Other measurements such as mid arm circumference
and skinfold thickness may provide more accurate
assessment and monitoring of nutritional status.

Constipation is a common problem for children
with feeding difficulties. It may be as a result of inadequate fluid intake, excessive fluid loss via spillage,
poor lip closure, poor head control or dribbling,
immobility, poor gut motility, side effects of medication, or occasionally lack of dietary fibre. As a

consequence constipation will have a negative
effect on appetite, behaviour and general wellbeing;
anecdotally it has been reported to trigger seizures.
Vigorous assessment and treatment is necessary in
order to avoid further nutritional compromise [17].

Studies on vitamin and mineral intakes and deficiencies in children with feeding problems are not
well documented. However, nutritional assessment
based on a good diet history will highlight inadequate
intake due to poor variety, small quantities of food
eaten and potential vitamin losses through liquidising
foods or long cooking methods.

Dental caries can be a problem for a number of
reasons – poor dental hygiene due to hypersensitivity
to teeth cleaning, medications, inability to clear the
mouth of food after eating, reduced saliva production
and frequent consumption of foods containing sugar
may all contribute. A dilemma exists in the management of children with feeding difficulties because
small, energy-dense meals and drinks given regularly
throughout the day are often contrary to the advice
given to prevent dental caries. A compromise may be
necessary and discussion with the child's dentist will
not only help to prevent contradictory messages being
given, but may offer alternative preventative dental
treatment. Dental treatment can be dangerous, time
consuming and very frightening for some children
with disabilities and therefore prevention should
always be considered. In addition, a child with dental
caries who cannot communicate his pain will more
than likely exhibit negative behaviours around food
and drink thus increasing his feeding difficulties.

CAUSES OF FEEDING DIFFICULTIES

The main causes of feeding difficulties can be broadly
divided into four groups:

- Oral dysfunction resulting from either structural
  abnormalities such as cleft palate, high roof of the
  mouth, enlarged tongue or neurological disturbances such as those seen in cerebral palsy
- Physical disabilities such as cerebral palsy
  where the child finds it difficult to co-ordinate
  the passage of food and fluids to and in the
  mouth
- Sensory impairment where one or more of the
  senses are affected
- Learning disabilities or developmental delay,
  where some children may take longer than their

chronological peers to learn the skills necessary for eating and normal masticatory patterns.

As a guide, the more severe the disability and the presence of multiple disabilities, i.e. two or more of the above, the greater the likelihood of feeding difficulties.

OTHER FACTORS

Medication

Some children may be on medication with side effects which directly or indirectly have a negative effect on their nutrition. Some forms of anti-convulsant therapy affect appetite, induce nausea and gastro-intestinal irritation, cause drowsiness and affect utilisation of vitamin D. In addition, changes in medication may negatively or positively impact on oral skills, e.g. the introduction of a muscle relaxant may alter the position of the child during feeding/drinking.

Ill health

Repeated periods of ill health may be common for some children, e.g. recurrent chest infections, GOR, constipation, seizures. This not only affects the appetite but also decreases the opportunities for learning or practising eating skills and possibly increases nutritional requirements.

Social issues

The social issues which can affect a child's nutrition are obviously the same as for any other child, but disability heightens the effect. Financial commitments are greater in a family where a person has a disability. Eating socially, eating out in popular peer group venues, picnics, school meals and cookery classes are all limited for a child with feeding difficulties, thus reducing the opportunities to learn and eat the variety of foods and drinks available to other children.

Pressures on the carer

Pressures on the carer responsible for providing and delivering food and drink are enormous. Not only are they expected to provide an adequate, varied diet of the correct consistency and texture, but also to know how to help the child develop the necessary oral and motor skills. Time is a major consideration; it takes longer to feed a child with feeding difficulties. Some children may take up to an hour to eat a meal, leaving all concerned tired and bored with the event. Gisel [18] found that in a study group of children with cerebral palsy and oral motor dysfunction, some required up to 18 times longer to eat a normal mouthful of food. Learning to eat and drink independently with a degree of dexterity occurs within the first 3 years but for some children with developmental delay this period is extended and may even be doubled or trebled; some may never achieve the goal. It is potentially an anxious, frustrating and messy business for both child and carer.

The time factor has to be weighed against all the other activities that carers are required to perform for their child. The more severe the disability, particularly for those with multiple disabilities, the greater is the time and energy invested in the caring and educational role. Appointments with the multitude of professionals, specialists and researchers from all statutory and voluntary agencies can make the daily timetable very difficult to adhere to. Privacy can be a rare commodity in families where the child has input from a large number of people.

Communication

Requesting and signalling needs and desires for food provide cues for the carer. An infant who is unable to cry for food, a child who is unable to demand food, is obviously at risk of inadequate feeding. In addition, children with feeding difficulties may be incorrectly interpreted at meal times, e.g. it is accepted that an infant of 4–6 months (without feeding difficulties) may initially reject lumpy food because he cannot yet manage the consistency; however an older infant, toddler or child (with unrecognised feeding difficulties) doing the same may be misinterpreted as disliking the food, being fussy, stubborn, awkward or lazy. Carers may not report that the child has a feeding problem, but describe him as fussy or naughty at mealtimes. Thus it might appear that among the other problems that occur, carers just accept the feeding difficulties and do not ask for help. Without thorough investigation of exactly what the carer means by 'fussy' or 'naughty' the severity of the problem may be overlooked or even accepted as normal for that particular medical diagnosis.

STAGES OF EATING AND DRINKING

Four stages are necessary in order to achieve the safe and efficient passage of fluid or solids to the stomach:

- *Preparatory stage* This involves the activities before feeding takes place, which include understanding that feeding will happen, the ability to self-feed, and an attitude to meals and feeding. Children may have difficulty at this stage due to past unpleasant experiences associated with feeding, poor sensory development, learning difficulties, inability to self-feed, stressful and difficult mealtimes, and poor ability to communicate. Problems at this stage include fear, food refusal and lack of interest.
- *Oral stage* This consists of controlled head and jaw movements, good lip closure, complex tongue movements, the ability to separate liquids from solid, and the ability to collect food together and pass it to the third stage. Problems include excessive food and fluid loss, involuntary biting of utensils, slow movement of food to the swallowing position, and food and fluid passing uncontrolled into the pharynx.
- *Pharyngeal stage* This involves an appropriate swallowing reflex for liquids and solids, and the ability to propel the bolus safely into the oesophagus and to laryngeal closure. Problems at this stage include coughing, choking, gagging and aspiration.
- *Oesophageal stage* This depends on the appropriate opening and closing of the cardiac sphincter. Problems at this stage include loss of tone in the cardiac sphincter and gastro–oesophageal reflux (GOR).

NUTRITION AND FEEDING ASSESSMENT

Nutrition and feeding problems are identified by measuring, observing and questioning. A nutritional problem is the failure to obtain and utilise sufficient nutrients to maintain adequate growth and health. A feeding problem is having difficulty with food and fluid textures and amounts. A multidisciplinary feeding assessment draws together the skills and expertise from carer, speech and language therapist, occupational therapist, physiotherapist, dietitian and psychologist.

Observation

A whole meal should be observed to assess what is being offered, how it is presented, how much is eaten, how the child copes with the meal and child/carer interaction.

There are various models that can be used, all involving observing the child eat and drink. Individual people may assess independently and make recommendations or one or two key people observe the child eating and drinking or the whole team observes the child eating/drinking. A video assessment can be useful and less invasive to the child. It provides a visual record that can be analysed and discussed by the group and carer without the child being present or distracted by people watching him eat. A video also provides an objective record for reviewing whether goals have been achieved; the carer can keep the video as a reminder of progress and to retain some confidentiality.

The venue and timing of the observation and the health of the child need to be considered carefully if a true picture of the child's capabilities is to be extracted. Sometimes videos of the child eating in two familiar places, such as home and school, can elicit useful information.

Observation of meal – observing the child

- Interest in own and others' food
- Reaction to the presentation of food
- Desire to self-feed/drink
- Quantity, texture and range of food eaten and lost
- Ability to concentrate and persevere
- Ability to communicate needs
- Control and autonomy issues
- Reaction to parents' behaviour
- Time taken to eat.

Observation of meal – observing the carer

- Control over child's table behaviour
- Management style – distraction, encouragement, force, passivity
- Emotional state – anxiety, anger, frustration, detachment, patience, warmth

- Awareness of child's needs and demands
- Quantity, texture and range of food/fluid offered
- Ability to tolerate mess.

Beliefs and expectations

- Others' estimations of food eaten/drunk in comparison with observation
- Expectations of ability to develop skills, change or grow.

Nutrition assessment

Height and weight should be measured and plotted to assess the growth trajectory using height, weight, BMI (for children over 1 year old) or growth velocity charts. Biochemical and haematological measurements such as full blood count, vitamin D, ferritin, folate and vitamin C may be indicated. Activity level should be assessed to predict energy needs. A medical history and clinical assessments are made by a paediatrician. Clinical investigation – dentition, barium swallow, chest X-ray, 24 hour pH monitoring, videofluoroscopy, endoscopic assessment – are carried out as clinically indicated.

Assessment of feeding problems – the biological context

Carers should be questioned about intake over the last 24 hours (including overnight) to gain appreciation of the amount, range and textures of food and fluid consumed:

- Food diaries and 24 hour recall of food and drink intake, i.e. the child's appetite, fluid intake, amount, range and textures of foods eaten, and food preferences.
- Salivation – does the child lose fluids through excessive salivation, inability to swallow saliva, or poor lip closure and head control? Or does the child have a dry mouth?
- Medication – some medication may cause drowsiness, nausea and vomiting, or gastric symptoms.
- Seating and feeding position assessed by an occupational therapist/physiotherapist preferably at a seating clinic.
- Oral skills and motor skills assessed by a speech and language therapist.

- Feeding history, child's early feeding experiences – problems with swallowing, choking, gagging, co-ordination of sucking and breathing; problems with chewing, oral motor skills in co-ordination; repeated vomiting, retching, nausea; lack of appetite; GOR, pain; bloating; constipation, diarrhoea; allergic reaction.
- Hand to mouth co-ordination assessed by an occupational therapist.
- Age of onset of feeding problems.
- Developmental patterns of feeding.
- Patterns of tube feeding, i.e. quantity and timings.

Assessment of feeding problems – the social context

The multidisciplinary team should ideally have access to a clinical psychologist for the maximum benefit to be derived from this assessment:

- Where does the child usually eat? Are there distractions?
- Parents' eating history and attitude to food
- Early attachment difficulties, especially with an ill child
- Marital/family stress, life events, social support, family networks
- General child management and skills of parents
- Parent-child relationship and interaction
- Advice and attitude of health professionals
- Past and present parental mental health
- Parental level of anxiety and obsessions
- Ethnic and cultural beliefs and values
- Finance.

Documentation

A clear picture of the child's feeding capabilities should be documented. Assessment tools [19, 20] based on normal development provide an excellent aid to identifying the movement and sensory patterns that create limitations. With this information precise short and long term goals can be set.

NUTRITIONAL REQUIREMENTS

Nutritional requirements for macronutrients are based on height age, current weight and mobility/activity. Generally, chronological age is used to estimate micronutrient requirements. Height age is a crude estimation of bone age. Bone age is used as the basis for calculating nutritional requirements.

Use the following three steps to estimate a child's height age:

- Measure height
- Using a decimal age growth chart, read off the decimal age when the height meets the 50th centile age; this represents the child's height age.
- Note whether the child is weighed wearing spinal jackets, splints, calipers, second skins.

Energy

Children with physical impairments

Using the child's height age and current weight, calculate the child's energy requirements (kcal/day) using one the formulae below. These have been adapted from Krick's proposed formula [21] and dietary reference values [22]:

Birth to 10 years old
*EAR × LPAR × BTR × GRR

11–17 years old
*BMR × PAR × BTR × GRR

* see Table 26.1

Children with Down's syndrome

It is suggested that energy requirements are calculated on kcal/cm. Culley has advocated 16.1 kcal (67kJ) /cm/day for boys and 14.3 kcal (60 kJ)/cm/day for girls [23]. Pattison and Walberg Ekvall endorse this figure in their nutrition assessment of children with Down's syndrome [24].

Protein

Requirements may be calculated by using:

Current weight (kg) x protein requirement for height age per kg body weight.

Refer to Tables 26.2a and 26.2b for quick reference. For catch-up growth, protein should supply at least 9–15% of total energy intake.

Table 26.1 Calculating energy requirements of children with physical impairments

EAR	Estimated average requirements for energy. This is used instead of basal metabolic rate as there are no values for children under 10 years of age	See Tables 26.2a and 26.2b for quick reference	
LPAR	Low physical activity ratio is used if the child is immobile. If the child is mobile do not include LPAR in calculation	Birth–8 months	0.90
		9 mnths–12 mnths	0.85
		1yr–3yrs	0.77
		4yr–5yrs	0.71
		6yr–10yrs	0.74
BTR	Body tone ratio is used for children with muscular-neurological features where most limbs are hypertonic, normal or hypotonic	Hypertonic	1.10
		Normal	1.0
		Hypotonic	0.9
GRR	Growth rate ratio is used if there is a need for weight management for overweight, or to promote normal or catch-up growth and weight	Overweight	0.8
		Normal	1.0
		Catch-up	1.2–1.5
BMR	Basal metabolic rates are available for children 11 years and over	Males	17.7 wt + 657 kcal/d
		Females	13.4 wt + 692 kcal/d
PAR	Physical activity ratio is used in conjuction with the BMR for children 11 years and over	Children who are:	
		not able to sit, crawl or walk	1.15
		not able to crawl or walk	1.20
		not able to walk	1.25
		able to walk	1.30

Table 26.2a Energy and protein requirements for boys

Age (years)	Average weight for age (kg)	Energy (kcal/kg/day) EAR for energy by age and current body weight	Energy (kcal/day) EAR for energy by age	Adjustment for low PAL*	Protein g/kg/day
1 month	4.2	115	480	0.90	2.1
3 months	6.1	100	610	0.90	2.1
6 months	8.0	95	760	0.90	1.6
9 months	9.3	95	880	0.85	1.5
12 months	10.1	95	960	0.85	1.5
18 months	11.4	95	1080	0.77	1.1
24 months	12.5	95	1190	0.77	1.1
30 months	13.5	95	1280	0.77	1.1
36 months	14.5	95	1380	0.77	1.1
4 years	16.2	94	1520	0.71	1.1
5 years	19.5	88	1720	0.71	1.1
6 years	21.5	84	1810	0.74	1.1
7 years	22.3	84	1890	0.74	1.0
8 years	25.0	79	1970	0.74	1.0
9–10 years	29.0	70	2040	0.74	1.0
11–14 years	43.1	51	2220	0.74	1.0
15–18 years	64.5	43	2775	0.74	0.85

Adapted from *Nutritional Requirements for Children in Health and Disease 2000*. London: Great Ormond Street Hospital for Children NHS Trust.
* PAL physical activity level

Table 26.2b Energy and protein requirements for girls

Age (years)	Average weight for age (kg)	Energy a (kcal/kg/day) EAR for energy by age and current body weight	Energy d (kcal/day) EAR for energy by age	Adjustment for low PAL	Protein g/kg/day
1 month	4.0	115	460	0.90	2.8
3 months	5.7	100	570	0.90	2.8
6 months	7.5	95	710	0.90	1.8
9 months	8.6	95	820	0.85	1.5
12 months	9.6	95	910	0.85	1.5
18 months	10.7	95	1020	0.77	1.1
24 months	11.9	95	1130	0.77	1.1
30 months	12.9	95	1230	0.77	1.1
36 months	13.9	95	1320	0.77	1.1
4 years	16.8	87	1460	0.71	1.1
5 years	18.9	82	1550	0.71	1.1
6 years	21.3	76	1620	0.74	1.1
7 years	22.8	75	1680	0.74	1.0
8 years	25.0	70	1740	0.74	1.0
9–10 years	29.0	62	1790	0.74	1.0
11–14 years	44.0	42	1845	0.74	1.0
15–18 years	55.5	38	2110	0.74	0.82

Adapted from *Nutritional Requirements for Children in Health and Disease 2000*. London: Great Ormond Street Hospital for Children NHS Trust.

Fluid

The current weight is used to calculate fluid requirement:

Children under 10 kg
150 ml/kg for first 5 kg + 50 ml/kg thereafter

Children over 10 kg
100 ml/kg for first 10 kg + 50 ml for second 10 kg + 20 ml/kg thereafter

Fibre

In the absence of contradictory clinical evidence use the normal guidelines for calculating fibre requirements for children (g/day):

$$\frac{\text{Daily Energy (kcal) required to maintain current weight} \times 18}{2000}$$

where 18 (g/day) is the suggested fibre intake for adults (g/day) and 2000 represents the average adult energy requirement.

Vitamins and minerals

Use the reference nutrient intakes for chronological age and sex.

MEDICAL CONDITIONS CAUSING FEEDING PROBLEMS

Cerebral palsy

Cerebral palsy is non-progressive brain damage in the cerebral cortex that occurs before birth or within 5 years of birth. Cerebral palsy lesions cause neuromuscular problems producing abnormal muscle movement or tone (Table 26.3). Additionally, children with cerebral palsy are likely to have multiple impairments; sensory impairments (vision, hearing,

Table 26.3 Classification of cerebral palsy

Classification by muscle tone	Description
Hypertonic or spastic	Increased muscle tone with increased resistance to stretch
Hypotonic or atonic	Decreased muscle tone causing 'floppiness'
Rigid	Stiff and inflexible muscle tone
Dystonic	Problems with muscle tone that cause excessive increase in tone when the muscle is being used and hypotonia when it is at rest. This usually causes abnormal posture

Classification by movement	Description
Athetoid	Uncontrolled and continuous involuntary movements
Choreiform	Rapid, jerky movements
Ataxic	Poorly co-ordinated, but voluntary movements

Classification by area affected	Description
Monoparesis	One limb affected
Hemiparesis	Involves one side, but the arm is more affected
Diparesis	Involves one side, but the leg is more affected
Quadriparesis	Affects all four limbs

Adapted from Erenberg G Cerebral palsy: current understanding of complex problem. *Postgraduate Medicine*, 1984, **75** 87–93.

touch); perceptual difficulties resulting in impaired sensory interpretation; learning disabilities; limited communication; and medical conditions such as respiratory difficulties, epilepsy and gastro-oesophageal reflux. The incidence of cerebral palsy is 3 in every 1000 live births and the likelihood of feeding problems is very high. A small but detailed study showed that of 49 children living in the community, 45 had clinically significant oral motor dysfunction. The more severe the cerebral palsy the higher the incidence of oral motor dysfunction [25].

Children with cerebral palsy often display both retained and abnormal patterns of movement, which are sometimes excessively strong or brisk. These reflexes prevent children developing more mature and controlled patterns of movement and will affect their feeding capabilities. Examples of these reflexes are extensor thrust, gag and bite reflex. A child with extensor thrust will throw their head back, spine arched, legs straight and arms tight. The result is that it is hard to position the child for feeding; assisted or self-feeding is more difficult in this stiff position; chin thrust prevents efficient swallowing and may cause choking; jaw thrust prevents mouth closure and interferes with normal sucking or chewing movements. The gag and cough reflex is a protective mechanism; however, a hypersensitivity to food may cause frequent coughing and will override all other eating patterns. A brisk gag reflex at the front of the mouth reduces the tolerance to food. The bite reflex is typified by sudden jaw closure in response to front gums or teeth being touched. This results in an inability to open the mouth and co-ordinate jaw movement while introducing food into the mouth. Table 26.4 summarises the types of feeding problems a child with cerebral palsy may experience.

Down's syndrome

A number of studies have been carried out to ascertain the frequency of feeding problems in children with Down's syndrome. Van Dyke *et al.* [26] review the American based studies and suggest that eating problems are common but usually are minor in nature. Subsequently Spender [27] has found significant impairments in oral motor function among children with Down's syndrome. Surveys of parents [26] suggest that 60% are totally independent in feeding by early childhood and the most common problems

are slight oral hypotonia, tongue thrust, difficulties in chewing, poor lip seal, and choking and gagging on food. However, it is noted that this feeding success may be partly as a direct result of feeding programmes and not simply a natural developmental step, thus reinforcing the need for assessment and management programmes.

Subsequently Hopman [28] has noted that solids were introduced at a later stage compared with controls, possibly due to low parental expectations of developmental ability. Foods requiring less chewing were given, thus further inhibiting oral motor development. Bolders-Frazier [29] found that children with Down's syndrome have increased oral sensitivity, interfering with the acceptance of new foods and a high incidence of aspiration which is possibly related to the high incidence of respiratory disease. Other authors [30] suggest that normal motor development follows a systematic timetable.

Severe feeding difficulties secondary to hypotonia, placidity, weak suckling and rooting reflex may occur at birth. The main reasons why children with Down's syndrome may experience feeding difficulties are due to multiple cranial skeletal differences. The palate is often short and narrow, and this underdevelopment of the maxilla may alter the position of the muscles used for chewing. The tongue may be large or appear large due to a small oral cavity secondary to midfacial hypoplasia. Many children with Down's syndrome are mouth breathers, due to a small oral cavity, enlargement of the tonsils and/or decreased nasal passages. This will have an effect on the development of efficient oral skills. Generalised facial/oral hypotonia also contributes to poor lip closure, poor suck, poor tongue control, and difficulties with jaw stability.

In addition, infants with Down's syndrome with congenital heart defects may have the combined problems experienced by infants with heart abnormalities (p. 183) and poor oral skills stated above. Other medical problems that may be present and have a direct effect on nutrition assessment are compromised immune systems and hypothyroidism. In addition Down's syndrome has been associated with immune-related disorders such as a high incidence of coeliac disease [31, 32].

Anthropometric assessment of children with Down's syndrome is complicated because the disorder is associated with a number of abnormalities related to growth, e.g. short stature, decreased head circumference, and altered growth patterns. Cronk

Table 26.4 Type of feeding difficulty and the nutritional consequence

Causes	Symptoms	Consequences
Communications difficulties		
Inability to request food or drink	Food refusal	Prolonged mealtimes
Distorted requests	Distress	Inadequate nutritional intake
Inability to express preferences	Fear	Specific nutrient deficiencies
	Irritability	Failure to thrive
	Lack of interest	Dental caries
		Pulmonary disease
		Increased risk of infection
		Upper respiratory tract infection
		Urinary tract infections
Gross motor impairment		
Cannot seek out food	Dependency	
Inability to self-feed	Difficulty in feeding position	
Poor head/trunk control		
Oral motor dysfunction		
Difficulty in sucking, munching, chewing and swallowing	Excessively long mealtimes	
Poor bolus formation and manipulation	Excessive food loss and drooling	
Poor oral hygiene	Spitting	
	Dental pain and caries	
Pharyngeal dysfunction		
Aspiration of food and liquid	Coughing	
Slow pharyngeal transit time	Choking	
Reduced peristalsis	Gagging	
Delayed or absent swallow reflex	Noisy respiratory patterns	
Reduced laryngeal closure	Altered phonation	
Incomplete clearance of residue	Upper respiratory tract infection	
Oesophageal dysfunction		
Gastro-oesophageal reflux	Regurgitation	
Delayed gastric emptying	Vomiting	
Oesophagitis	Constipation	
Aspiration of GOR	Dehydration	

Taken from Reilly S Feeding problems in children with cerebral palsy. *Curr Paediatr*, 1996, **3** 209–13.

[33, 34] suggests that while height in people with Down's syndrome is significantly lower than the norm, the period in which most significant growth failure occurs is during the first five years of life. Longitudinal studies [35] corroborate this but show that growth velocity of children aged 7–18 years was not significantly different to the norm. Cronk [33] has produced growth charts for children with Down's syndrome based on these studies and Taylor-Baer [36] has reviewed studies around these problems.

A 10–15% lower resting metabolic rate but equivalent expenditure above resting has been found in prepubescent children with Down's syndrome [37]. The same group had lower energy and micronutrient intakes and lower energy expenditure when compared with the control group; 20% were considered to be at risk of vitamin A and C deficiency and 50% for vitamin E deficiency. Obesity is a common concern; Cronk [33] found nearly 30% of young children showed weight greater than one standard deviation above length by 36 months. Crino [38] reports 66% of pubertal children were obese. Medlin's papers [39, 40] expand on weight management and food related behaviours.

Low levels of calcium have been reported in Down's syndrome [41] which may be related to poor vitamin D absorption. A study using analysis of trace metal levels in hair reported lower levels of calcium, copper and manganese [42]. There is no consistent evidence of vitamin deficiencies but the reported deficiencies of certain vitamins and minerals in some of the literature has been proposed to be due to malabsorbtion of nutrients rather than dietary insufficiency. There is little clinical evidence to suggest that megadoses of vitamin supplementation have significant beneficial effects on health outcome or intellectual functioning [43, 44]. At the time of writing interest is in targeted nutritional intervention to improve intellectual functioning. The treatment is based on a biochemical hypothesis, which is not supported by clinical trials, that people with Down's syndrome have excess activity of superoxide dismutase which leads to an overproduction of hydrogen peroxide. It is suggested that this oxidative stress causes brain cell death and increases susceptibility to infection. Large amounts of antioxidants are proposed to slow down the process. The commercial preparations available and marketed towards people with Down's syndrome also contain amino acids and digestive enzymes. There are currently no known clinical trials on such preparations.

Cleft palate

Clefting is one of the most common birth defects, and the most common affecting the face and oromotor mechanism. A cleft is a separation of parts of the mouth usually joined together during the early weeks of fetal development. A cleft lip is separation of one or both sides of the upper lip, and often the upper dental ridge. The cleft can be incomplete, affecting primarily the lip and not extending into the nasal cavity. A complete cleft includes separation of the dental ridge and the lip and extends through the nasal cavity. A bilateral cleft occurs on both sides of the nose.

Clefts of the palate may occur in the bony hard palate or in the soft palate at the back of the mouth. It may occur with or without a cleft lip. It can occur as a unilateral complete cleft through both soft and hard palate on one side or bilaterally. A submucous cleft occurs when the tissue connecting the two sides of the hard or soft palate is incomplete even though the surface tissue is intact. The latter is invisible to the eye.

Clefts are repaired by surgery, and the timing is dependent on the severity of the cleft, child's condition and surgeon's preference.

Feeding is the most immediate issue facing carers: some infants have few feeding problems but others will experience great difficulty. The majority of infants will be fed orally; however the carer will require help to obtain adapted drinking utensils and the optimum position to prevent choking. Bottle feeding is generally preferred to spoon feeding in the early months. Breast milk can be given as expressed milk and some mothers have managed to establish breast feeding.

The main problem experienced by the child is difficulty with sucking and maintaining an adequate suction. In addition, because the nose and mouth cavities are not fully separated by the palate, food may back up and run out of the child's nose causing coughing, choking, spitting or vomiting.

Weaning would normally occur in the same sequence as for other children; however, as these transitions may occur before surgical closure of the cleft the infant will need to learn how to control lumps as they arrive at the palate opening. Infants with clefts will normally learn to eat proficiently with modifications for positioning, equipment and speed of presentation of food, as they will compensate for difficulties of the cleft. Children who do not may have other developmental problems.

Rett syndrome

Rett syndrome is a neurological disorder that only affects girls and is caused by a genetic mutation on the X chromosome. The prevalence is estimated at 1 in 10 000–15 000 female births and Rett syndrome is thought to account for 10% of all profound disability in females. The prevalence is approximately the same in all ethnic groups. Diagnosis is purely on clinical symptoms and features of the condition are listed in Table 26.5 [46]. Infants are normal at birth and for about the first 6 months of life. Regression occurs by the end of the first year and feeding skills as well as other abilities are lost. There is a large variability in motor disability with about 80% of adult women unable to walk. Appetite is generally good and children (and adults) with Rett

Table 26.5 Diagnostic criteria for Rett syndrome

Essential criteria for diagnosis
Normal development up until approximately 6 months of age
Deceleration of head growth between 5 months and 4 years
Progressive loss of acquired hand skills between 6 and 30 months of age
Development of severe psychomotor retardation
Stereotypic hand movements such as hand-wringing, clapping, tapping etc.
Gait and truncal apraxia

Other features
Breathing dysfunction – intermittent hyperventilation/breath-holding
Air swallowing, leading to 'air bloat'
Oromotor dysfunction
Epilepsy
Scoliosis
Growth retardation
Spasticity, muscle wasting and dystonia
Hypotrophic small feet

syndrome usually derive great pleasure from food. Self-feeding skills may be regained after an initial period of regression.

A number of feeding difficulties and nutritional problems have been noted, including chewing and swallowing difficulties [47], constipation, gastro-oesophageal reflux and inability to co-ordinate breathing and feeding [48]. Although appetite is usually good, factors such as air bloat caused by air swallowing and drugs used to treat seizures may depress the desire to eat. A typical pattern of growth occurs in Rett syndrome, with normal growth initially. After symptoms of the condition begin to appear, weight gain slows and weight loss may occur, particularly during illness, and many young girls are underweight. After puberty weight may increase to normal or, in physically inactive women, to obese levels.

Nutritional requirements are generally normal, although girls with high activity or continued repetitive movements may have a higher energy requirement than normal for their size. A ketogenic diet has been tried with some success to control seizures in Rett syndrome [49]. Management of nutritional problems is according to symptoms. Some girls who are prone to frequent infections and weight loss have a gastrostomy but most can be managed using energy supplements and thickened drinks.

NUTRITIONAL MANAGEMENT OF FEEDING DIFFICULTIES

Increasing energy

This should be based on the same dietetic principles as for other children who are failing to thrive or are underweight. However, caution should be taken where failure to thrive occurs when epilepsy is evident or is associated with a particular syndrome, as undocumented clinical experience suggests that some children with severe feeding difficulties and poor energy intakes may be ketotic. Thus suddenly increasing energy intake may increase the risk of seizures (p. 231). Energy dense foods of the correct consistency should be offered regularly throughout the day. Carers familiar with current healthy eating messages are often concerned about the use of high fat milks, the addition of margarine to foods or the frequent use of energy rich desserts, e.g. chocolate mousses. Supplementation with a glucose polymer can often be the most practical method to increase energy intake. For some children the use of proprietary high energy drinks/sip feeds may be appropriate. However, the frequent use of sugar has to be balanced against the risk of dental caries.

Fluids

Inadequate consumption or excessive loss of fluids is a feature common to many children with feeding difficulties. Advice should be based on careful assessment of why the child is not consuming adequate fluids. Sometimes the carer will offer the child the same number and quantity of drinks as other children forgetting that a large percentage of the fluid offered is being lost. By simply reminding carers to offer a second cup, or more frequent drinks, this problem may be overcome. However, this does add to the time taken to drink. The long term goal would be to help the child develop better oral skills, e.g. improve lip closure in order to reduce saliva and fluid loss and improve the movement of fluids to the back of the mouth.

For some children thickening drinks to the consistency of a 'thick shake' or thick sauce can enable them to be successful. Thin fluids are the most difficult consistency to manipulate in the mouth. The child with a poor swallow is more likely to aspirate thin fluids than thick ones. Numerous thickened milk shake type drinks are now commercially available; they are not only useful but are also acceptable to peers. Other fluids can be thickened using a range of familiar products such as thick yoghurts, ice cream, instant powdered desserts, instant sauce granules, smooth puréed fruit and jars of puréed baby food fruit desserts. Cornflour, blancmanges and custard powder can be used, but are time consuming to prepare. A range of proprietary thickening agents are now available on prescription such as Instant Carobel, Nestargel, Thixo D, Vitaquick, Thick and Easy, Nutralis and Resource, although they may not be prescribable or appropriate for use in infants or small children. Many carers do have fears about offering thick drinks as they perceive this as 'not quenching his thirst'; their use should be fully discussed.

For children who manage food better than fluids, a method of increasing their fluid intake is to offer foods with a high water content between meals, e.g. fruit-based baby foods, puréed fruit, thick yoghurts, fromage frais, ice cream and ice lollies. Jelly can be useful; however, it does dissolve immediately on entering the mouth resulting in the same problems as thin fluids.

Indications that the fluid intake has increased will be incidentally reported by carers as: more wet nappies, less urinary tract infections, and softer or more regular bowel movements. Some children are unable to tolerate large volumes of fluid and require small volumes frequently. Increasing the fluid intake via gastrostomy can sometimes be considered. Despite all efforts some children still find it extremely difficult to achieve an acceptable fluid intake.

Increasing cereal fibre

The use of cereal fibre to help with constipation should only be considered if the child is consuming adequate fluids. Breakfast cereals, e.g. Weetabix, softened with hot milk or incorporated into desserts, or soft wholemeal breadcrumbs added to main courses, smooth savoury egg custards and sauces can be eaten by some children. The use of natural bran or high bran foods should be avoided and should only be considered in the most extreme cases with an older child who is known to be drinking more than adequate fluids and when all other sources of dietary fibre have been considered. Prescribable sources of fibre may also be considered.

Anecdotally the use of proprietory probiotics has relieved the problem of chronic constipation in some children with feeding difficulties.

Challenging foods and drinks

If a child is to develop oral skills, sensory tolerance or self-feeding, foods that are liked but present a challenge to the child need to be incorporated into the meal. For some children the emphasis may be on ensuring a safe texture to reduce the risk of aspiration. One approach identifies three methods of introducing challenging foods [50]:

- Start with challenging food while appetite is strong and modify the food to easy at a later stage in the meal
- Start with easy (to allay strong eating patterns and appetite) and then introduce challenging food
- Alternate easy and challenging food throughout the meal.

It is important to remember when using this approach that the helper must persevere and keep offering the challenge when unsuccessful in the initial periods. Whenever possible foods should be chosen which make challenges fun, for example soft chocolate bars and jelly based sweets. Move a child through challenges gradually, always including easy foods so that not all meals are hard work.

Texture

The food texture required by the child should be assessed by a speech and language therapist. One useful system for classifying food textures is shown in Table 26.6. In the absence of a nationally agreed classification of textures, refer to the local speech and language terminology. The carer should be provided with numerous ideas on the foods within that group to help provide variety in the diet. Specific brands of commercial products may be advised for their particular useful texture. Where the child requires thick, smooth, paste-type consistency to ensure safe swallowing, the thickness required can be demonstrated by using easily available foods such as instant mashed potato or powdered baby foods.

Table 26.6 Food textures

Challenging foods			Easier foods	
Thickness	Thin fluids	e.g. water, juice	Thick fluids	e.g. drinking yoghurt, milkshake, thin custard
	Thin and watery	e.g. thin yoghurt, thin gravy	Thick and creamy	e.g. creamed potatoes, semolina, ground rice, creamed pulses, thick sauces, thick gravy, thick custard, fromage frais, thick creamy yoghurt
	Swimming foods	e.g. sponge cake swimming in custard, carrots and meat in gravy. Overcooked lumpy scrambled egg		
	Thin and lumpy	Dilute Stage 2 baby food, thin rice pudding	Thick and lumpy	e.g. meat/fish and veg in thick sauces, macaroni cheese, sieved meals
Texture			Single texture	e.g. Stage 1 baby food, mashed vegetables, mashed bananas
	Crunch and crumble/ splinter	e.g. crisp raw apple, raw carrot, crisps, cream crackers, nuts, digestive biscuits	Crunch and dissolve	e.g. cheese puffs, Sugar Puffs, wafers, sponge fingers
	Bite and stick	e.g. white bread	Bite and dissolve	e.g. sponge cake, chocolate buttons
	Hard chew	e.g. tough meat, dry fish, toffee, chewing gum	Soft chew	e.g. soft raw apple, boiled potato, boiled carrot, processed meat (e.g. corned beef), brown bread and spread
	Stringy and husky	e.g. spinach, runner beans, shredded meat, chicken, celery		
	Bite and slip	e.g. tinned peaches, oranges, jelly	Soft slip and swallow	e.g. tinned spaghetti, ice cream, mousse, Angel Delight
Temperature	Very hot/very cold		Warm	
Taste	Acid Bitter Savoury meat		Bland Mild Sweet	

Presentation

The way food is presented to the child is important to success. Food should be given slowly and rhythmically allowing time to finish each mouthful and anticipate the next one. Small mouthfuls are more likely to be successful; however, for some children the spoon needs to be heaped towards the tip of the spoon to provide sensory cues for the lips. The spoon should normally be presented horizontally from the front and, depending on the techniques being practised at the time, it could be centrally or towards the side of the mouth when encouraging chewing. Scraping food off the spoon with the top teeth should be avoided. The speech and language therapist or occupational therapist can suggest other methods to help the child to learn to take food from the bowl of the spoon.

EQUIPMENT

The choice of equipment will have an enormous effect on whether or not the child is successful in feeding. Occupational therapists normally have the expertise to assess the child's needs and they have numerous catalogues from which to choose the appropriate pieces for each individual. For some children standard equipment with slight adaptations will meet their needs, while for others a wide range of specialised equipment is available.

Spoons that are soft, strong and shatter-proof, made of plastic or polycarbonate, are preferred. A flat or shallow-bowled spoon facilitates removal of food with the lips and a small-sized spoon helps direct the food to the side of the mouth. Hard metal, brittle or poorly shaped spoons can stimulate a bite reflex or cause discomfort. For some children it may be more appropriate to use a fork, spatula or fingers rather than a spoon as it is easier to direct food to the side of the mouth than with a broad or deep-bowled spoon.

Angled spoons help some children with limited hand or arm movement to achieve independent or assisted feeding. Children with a poor grasp can be assisted to develop independent self-feeding skills by using cutlery with built-up or shaped handles to suit the child's hand; sometimes a strap may be used to maintain grasp. Training knives and forks with an indent for the index finger can be used to encourage correct holding of cutlery.

Plates to assist independent self-feeding include high-sided plates or plate guards, and sloping plates with a curved edge such as the Mannoy plate. Divided and heated plates encourage better visual presentation and temperature of food. Divided plates also discourage the helper from mixing all flavours and textures together. Non-slip mats provide more stability for a child who finds the plate runs away when eating.

The choice of drinking utensils is crucial to successful fluid intake. Experimentation with teats is necessary to find one that provides adequate stimulation. Bulbous cherry-topped teats can stimulate swallowing but for some children they may produce a gag reflex. Extended use of bottles, however, can prevent the development of oral skills as it promotes an imma-

ture sucking action. Teats for children with cleft palates include long soft teats with enlarged holes, allowing the milk to trickle into the mouth. The Rosti bottle, a soft plastic bottle with a teat shaped like a spoon or scoop, may be preferable for infants who have difficulty in sucking (Fig. 7.2).

A wide variety of commercially available training beakers is available. The correct balance has to be found between those that offer independent drinking, e.g. a cup with a wide flat training nozzle and a lid, and those that develop immature drinking patterns, e.g. beakers with drinking spouts. Soft plastic cups are more comfortable, particularly if the child has sensitive teeth. Slanted cups can facilitate good lower lip seal and control of unwanted tongue movements. Straws are sometimes the preferred choice and special straws may help the child who has difficulty in maintaining lip seal.

Positioning

The child's position at mealtimes is vital to success. He needs to be secure and symmetrical to obtain optimum trunk, limb, head and oral control. The position should be assessed by the physiotherapist or occupational therapist and may be either on the carer's lap (infants and small children) or in adapted seating. For some children a personalised seating system is necessary.

The helper needs to adopt a position that is comfortable, and safe for his back, particularly if the meal takes a long time, and that facilitates the techniques necessary to help the child. Sometimes this will require the helper to experiment with different positions until they have the best arrangement for them both.

Prompts

The use of prompts at mealtimes prepares a child for eating or drinking. It helps him to understand what is expected of him and he is therefore more likely to be successful. Prompts can be given visually, e.g. an environment with other people eating, mirrors, and seeing the food being prepared or arriving at the table. Physical prompts such as the smell of food, stroking the lower lip with the spoon or giving very small amounts allowing time for the child to experience the taste, texture and temperature of the food, can all be used. Verbal prompts promote the awareness of the concepts of eating, telling the child what he is doing as it occurs. Repetitive phrases throughout the meal help the child know what he is doing e.g. 'bite', 'chew' and 'swallow.' Object recognition, e.g. a spoon is placed in the child's hand prior to each meal in order to help the child to understand and anticipate that a food is on its way. Assessment will suggest which combination will be preferred by the child; however, consistency by all helpers is important.

Eating with other people

Eating with other people is important for children with feeding difficulties; however, limitations may prevent this from happening, for instance the special chair will not fit under the family table. The problems should be identified in the assessment and the physiotherapist or occupational therapist alerted to this problem. In some cases the carer finds it easier to give the child his meal before everyone else. Practical ways in which the child can join in on some family meals need to be identified. The time or stress involved with meal preparation can be reduced (by using convenience foods) and this time spent with the child at the table; other members of the family can be asked to help feed the child. If it is the child's behaviour that is identified as the problem then a psychologist/behavioural nurse's expertise would be indicated. Eating out may be a problem; however, familiarisation with popular commercial menus will provide ideas for the carer. For example, many venues serve thick shakes which, if transferred to the appropriate cup, can provide a perfect consistency for some children requiring thickened drinks.

Helpers

All people who could possibly be involved with feeding the child should be identified. Total reliance on one main carer should be discouraged as this can be so frustrating. Other members of the family – grandparents, friends, respite care, social service family support, students, volunteers – can all give support at mealtimes. The carer should be encouraged to let another person help with at least one meal a week. Liaison with the health visitor or social worker and statutory agencies, such as a meal at a family centre once a week, gives this needed respite. Training and support should be offered to the helpers and they should be involved in the assessment

and review process. Clear details of the current programme must be given to all involved with feeding.

Small goals

Skills should be broken down into small, short term goals as these are more likely to enable the child to succeed, e.g. 'encourage him to chew by placing toys and hard foods such as sticks of carrot between the gums, in the side of the mouth once a day' could be a goal to help him develop chewing skills. Regular review of the child's progress will provide the baseline for building on these skills. Ideally, more small goals will be added according to the child's needs, speed of learning, and opportunity to practise. When a child has been unable to achieve a goal it needs to be assessed whether he has been given long enough to practise, whether the task has been impractical for the carer to carry out and why, and whether the carer has understood the purpose of carrying out the task. The goal may need to be redesigned after checking that the carer feels able to carry it out. Possibly other carers, in school for example, can practise the skill with the child.

Demonstrating technique

A model of how the task is best carried out provides the carer with a clear picture of what is expected. Also, this can increase the empathy of the demonstrator by briefly experiencing the difficulties experienced by the feeder at every meal.

Support literature

Pre-printed diet sheets rarely accommodate the needs of children with feeding difficulties. Individualised lists of foods of the correct consistency, including suggestions and/or recipes for meals and snacks, are the most useful to a carer. This is particularly important if a child cannot eat commonly used foods such as bread. Foods which can quickly be added to instant mash – for example grated cheese, cream cheese, mashed tinned fish, corned beef, paté, avocado pear, frozen chopped spinach – all provide variety without too much preparation time. As many convenience foods as possible should be included when compiling food and drinks lists in order to help reduce the time involved with the preparation of foods and to help reduce the guilt that some carers may feel when relying heavily on convenience foods. Carers should be helped to select value-for-money convenience foods that can be easily modified to the correct texture for the child.

ENTERAL TUBE FEEDING

Tube feeding may be indicated for some children as a result of an inability to consume adequate nutrition and/or fluid and/or aspiration of food/fluid or stomach contents. It can provide either partial or total fluid or nutrition depending on oral nutritional intake and risks of aspiration.

Short or long term feeding should be considered for children who are failing to thrive with severe feeding difficulties. This must be weighed against the evidence that tube feeding has severe impacts upon the child [19, 50]. The Norah Fry Research Centre study documents the problems encountered by disabled children, their families and those providing health, social care and education services, suggesting 'serious and unintended social deprivations resulting from the need to be tube fed' [51]. Their national survey shows a lack of both co-ordination of services and health/social policy resulting in the provision of ineffective support to the child and families. The recommendations from this study to improve the services to children who are tube fed should be encompassed by all statutory agencies nationally.

The choice of nasogastric versus gastrostomy feeding has to be carefully assessed for the child with feeding difficulties. The first is highly likely to interfere with the child's already compromised oromotor skills and respiratory patterns, such as increasing sensitivity and gagging. A gastrostomy can increase the opportunities to improve oral and enteral intake but has surgical and site risks. For some the surgical risks are deemed too high, or parents feel that they cannot consent to such invasive procedures. Given the right information and support [51] children with feeding difficulties and their families can find that tube feeding enhances health and quality of life [52].

When total tube feeding is chosen as a result of medical confirmation of aspiration of food/fluids, it must be remembered that this will not prevent aspiration of oral secretions or gastric contents. In fact in some children the placement of a tube will result in a reduction in the lower oesophageal sphincter pressure and subsequent development or increase of GOR. Thorough assessment of the presence or potential development of GOR [19, 50] prior to tube feeding should be carried out.

Management

Bolus versus continuous feeding needs to be carefully planned, balancing the child's tolerance of larger volumes and the impact of feeding in the social context. A combination of both bolus and continuous overnight feeding may suit some children. However, one of the common problems is the inability to tolerate adequate volumes of feed. These children normally do best with very slow rate continuous feeds, gradually increasing the rate/volume according to tolerance.

Initially calculating the proposed nutritional content and volume of the feed may cause some concern, particularly for a child with severe failure to thrive and low tolerance to food/fluids. Both the nutritional requirements and the actual intake are assessed using previously described methods. If intolerance to an increased intake is anticipated, feeding should be commenced with a product that is isocaloric and the same volume as the oral intake. Both energy and volume are gradually increased towards the child's estimated requirement. Vitamin and mineral intake supplied by the feed is calculated and supplemented as necessary to meet the RNI for chronological age.

Conservative measures to treat GOR [53] using positioning during and after food/fluid, thickening feeds/food, small frequent volumes, and medication including those to speed up stomach emptying, can be effective. However, for some children conservative approaches will not be effective, and surgical procedures to tighten the semi-valve formed by the oesophagus and the fundus of the stomach, e.g. fundoplication, may be considered. This type of surgery will resolve the problems of aspiration of stomach contents but not of oral or upper respiratory secretions. In addition, it does not resolve slow gastric emptying and may frequently be associated with bloating. Behavioural programmes may be necessary for some children who may use GOR as an aid in communication [19].

Exclusive use of tube feeding without concurrent efforts to provide oromotor simulation will result in regression of oral motor patterns and management of oral secretions and increased oral hypersensitivity [51]. Programmes that address the oral and social requirements will help counteract these disadvantages [19, 54, 55]. Where tube feeding is used as an aid to improve nutrition/fluids while a child improves their oral motor skills the use of continuous overnight feeding may be indicated. Evans Morris provides a 13 point holistic oral motor treatment programme for tube fed children [19].

MONITORING

Systematic monitoring by a multidisciplinary team is crucial. This may be achieved through correspondence, hand-held records or a multidisciplinary feeding review. The latter, although seemingly time consuming, can work effectively if a systematic evaluation of specific goals is taken on a regular basis. This works particularly well in venues such as schools.

REFERENCES

1 Rosenbloom L, Sullivan P The nutritional and neuro-developmental consequences of feeding difficulties in disabled children. In: *Feeding the Disabled Child.* Clinics in Developmental Medicine no 140, Sullivan P, Rosenbloom L, 1996, Mackeith Press, pp. 33–9.

2 Webb Y Feeding and nutrition problems of physically and mentally handicapped children in Britain: a report. *J Hum Nutr*, 1980, **34** 241–85.

3 Karle IP *et al*. Nutritional status of cerebral palsied children. *J Amer Diet Assoc*, 1961, **38** 22–6.

4 Krick J, Van Duyne M The relationship between oral-motor involvement and growth: a pilot study in paediatric population with cerebral palsy. *J Amer Diet Assoc*, 1984, **84** 555–9.

5 Tobis J *et al*. A study of growth patterns in cerebral palsy. *Arch Phys Med*, 1961, **42** 475–81.

6 Thommessen M *et al*. Feeding problems, height and weight in different groups of disabled children. *Acta Paediatr Scand*, 1991, **80** 527–33.

7 Sanders KD *et al*. Growth response to enteral feeding by children with cerebral palsy. *J Parent Enter Nutr*, 1990, **14** 23–6.

8 Thommenssen M *et al*. The impact of feeding problems on growth and energy intake in children with cerebral palsy. *Europ J Clin Nutr*, 1991, **45** 470–87.

9 Corwin DS *et al*. Weight and length increase in children after gastrostomy placement. *J Am Diet Assoc*, 1996, **96** 874–9.

10 Samson-Fang, Stevenson R Linear growth velocity in children with cerebral palsy. *Dev Med Child Neurol*, 1998, **40** 874–9.

11 Stevenson RD *et al*. Clinical correlates of linear growth in children with cerebral palsy. *Dev Med Child Neurol*, 1994, **36** 135–42.

12 Krick J *et al*. Pattern of growth in children with cerebral palsy. *J Am Diet Assoc*, 1996, **96** 680–85.

13 Bax M Editorial: Eating is important. *Dev Med Child Neurol*, 1989, **31** 285–6.

14 Matisen B *et al*. Oral-motor dysfunction and failure to thrive among inner city infants. *Dev Med Child Neurol*, 1989, **31** 293–302.

15 Stallings V Nutritional assessment of the disabled child. In: *Feeding the Disabled Child.* Clinics in Developmental Medicine no 140, Sullivan P, Rosenbloom L, 1996, Mackeith Press, pp. 62–76.

16 Cronk CE *et al*. Growth charts for children with Down syndrome: 1 month to 18 years of age. *Pediatr*, 1988, **81** 102.

17 Clayden G Constipation in disabled children. In: *Feeding the Disabled Child.* Clinics in Developmental Medicine no 140, Sullivan P, Rosenbloom L, 1996, Mackeith Press, pp. 106–16.

18 Gisel E, Patrick J Identification of children unable to maintain a normal nutritional state. *Lancet*, 1988, **1** 283–6.

19 Evans Morris S *Pre-feeding Skills: A Comprehensive Resource for Feeding Development.* (Therapy Skill Builders). Buckinghamshire: Winslow Press, 1987.

20 Harvey Smith M Nutrition care in developmental disorders: nutritional assessment. *Topics Clin Nutr*, 1993, **8** 7–33.

21 Krick J *et al*. Proposed formula for calculating energy needs of children with cerebral palsy. *Dev Med Child Neurol*, 1996, **43** 481–7.

22 *Nutritional Requirements for Children in Health and Disease 2000*. London: Great Ormond Street Hospital for Children NHS Trust.

23 Culley W *et al*. Caloric intake of children with Down's syndrome (mongolism). *J Pediatr*, 1965, **66** 722.

24 Patterson B, Walberg Ekvall S Down syndrome. In: *Pediatric Nutrition in Chronic Diseases and Developmental Disorders: Prevention, Assessment and Treatment*. New York: Oxford University Press, 1993.

25 Reilly S *et al*. Prevalence of feeding problems and oral motor dysfunction in children with cerebral palsy: a community survey. *J Pediatr*, 1996, **129** 877–82.

26 Van Dyke D *et al*. Problems in feeding. In: Van Dyke DC *et al*. (eds) *Clinical Perspectives in the Man-*

agement of Down Syndrome. New York: Springer-Verlag, 1990.

27 Spender Q *et al*. An exploration of feeding difficulties in children with Down syndrome. *Dev Med Child Neurol*, 1996, **38** 681–94.

28 Hopman E *et al*. Eating habits of young children with Down syndrome in the Netherlands: adequate nutrient intakes but delayed introduction of solid food. *J Am Diet Assoc*, 1998, **98** 790–94.

29 Bolders Frazier J *et al*. Swallow function in children with Down syndrome: a retrospective study. *Dev Med Child Neurol*, **38** 695–703.

30 Alexander R *Early Feeding, Sound Production and Pelinguistic Cognitive Development in their Relationship with Gross Motor Development*. Madison, WI: Curative Rehabilitation Center, 1980.

31 Janasson U *et al*. Down's syndrome and coeliac disease. *J Paediatr Gastroenterol Nutr*, 1995, **21** 443–5.

32 Gale L *et al*. Down's syndrome is strongly associated with coeliac disease. *Gut*, 1997, **40** 492–6.

33 Cronk CE *et al*. Growth charts for children with Down syndrome 1 month to 18 years of age. *Pediatr*, 1988, **81** 102.

34 Cronk CE Growth of children with Down syndrome: birth to age 3 years. *Pediatr*, 1978, **61** 564.

35 Rarick GL, Seefeldt V Observations from longitudinal data on growth in stature and sitting height of children with Downs syndrome. *J Mental Defic Res*, 1974, **18** 63.

36 Taylor Baer M *et al*. Nutrition assessment of the child with Down syndrome. In: Van Dyke DC *et al*. (eds) *Clinical Perspectives in the Management of Down Syndrome*. New York: Springer-Verlag, 1990.

37 Luke A *et al*. Nutrient intake and obesity in prepubescent children with Down syndrome. *J Am Diet Assoc*, 1996, **96** 1262–7.

38 Crino A *et al*. Growth pattern and pubertal development in Down syndrome: a longitudinal and cross sectional study. *Dev Brain Dysfunction*, **9** 72–9.

39 Medlin J Weight management in Down syndrome – the early childhood years. *Down Syndrome News and Update*, 1999, **1** 181–4.

40 Medlin J Weight management in Down syndrome – the school age and adolescent years. *Down Syndrome News and Update*, 1999, **1** 185–8.

41 Cabana M *et al*. Nutritional rickets in a child with Down syndrome. *Clin Pediatr*, 1997, 235–7.

42 Barlow P *et al*. Hair trace metal levels in Down's syndrome patients. *J Ment Defic Res*, 1981, **25** 161.

43 Smith G *et al*. Use of megadoses of vitamins in Down syndrome. *J Pediatr*, 1984, **105** 228–34.

44 Weathers V Effects of nutritional supplementation on IQ and certain other variables associated with Down syndrome. *Am J Ment Defic*, 1983, **88** 214–17.

45 Bennet F Vitamin and mineral supplementation in Down's syndrome. *Pediatr*, 1983, **72** 707–713.

46 Hagberg B Rett syndrome: clinical peculiarities and biological mysteries. *Acta Paediatr*, 1995, **84** 971–6.

47 Morton RE, Bonas R, Minford J, Kerr A, Ellis RE Feeding ability in Rett syndrome. *Dev Med Child Neurol*, 1997, **39** 331–5.

48 Budden SS Rett syndrome: habilitation and management reviewed. *Europ Child Adoles Psychiat*, 1997, Suppl 1 103–107.

49 Rice MA, Haas RH The nutritional aspects of Rett syndrome. *J Child Neurol*, 1998, **3** Suppl S35–S42.

50 Winstock A *The Practical Management of Eating and Drinking Difficulties in Children*. Buckinghamshire: Winslow Press, 1994.

51 Townsley R, Robinson C *Food for Thought? Effective support for families caring for a child who is tube fed* – Summary and Recommendations, 1999. Birstol: Norah Fry Research Centre (full report in press).

52 McCurtin A *The Manual of Paediatric Feeding Practic*. Bicester, Oxon: Winslow Press, 1997.

53 Monohan P *et al*. Effect of tube feeding on oral function. *Dev Med Child Neurol Supp*, 1988, **57** 7.

54 Luiselli J A behaviour analysis approach toward chronic food refusal in children with gastrostomy – tube dependency. *Topics Early Childh Spec Educ*, 1995, **15** 1–18.

55 Nardella M *Practical Tips on Tube Feeding for Children*. Nutrition Focus for children with special health care needs. Washington: Child Development and Mental Retardation Center, University of Washington, 1995, **10** 1–8.

USEFUL ADDRESSES

Scope for People with Cerebral Palsy
6 Market Road, London N7 9PW. Tel. 020 7619 7100, Web: www.scope.org.uk

The Bobath Centre for Children with Cerebral Palsy
Bradbury House, 250 East End Road, London N2 8AU. Tel. 020 8444 3355.

Crisp
NICOD, Malcolm Sinclair House, 31 Ulsterville Avenue, Belfast BT9 7AS. Tel. 01232 666188.

National Institute of Conductive Education
Cannon Hill House, Russell Road, Moseley, Birmingham B13 8RD. Tel. 0121 449 1569. Web: www.conductive-education.org.uk

Advisor Service Capability Scotland (ASCS)
111 Ellersly Road, Edinburgh EH12 6HY. Tel. 0131 346 7864.

The Scottish Centre for Children with Motor Impairments
Craighalbert Centre, 1 Craighalbert Way, Cumbernauld G68 0LS. Tel. 01236 456 100.

Norah Fry Research Centre
3 Priory Road, Bristol BS8 ITX. Tel. 0117 923 8137. Web: www.bris.ac.uk/Depts/NorahFry/

Rett Syndrome Association UK
113 Friern Barnet Road, London N11 3EU. Tel. 020 8361 5161. Web: www.rettsyndrome.org.uk

CHAPTER 27

Failure to Thrive

The term 'failure to thrive' (FTT) is applied to infants and young children who do not achieve a normal or expected rate of growth. Early this century, the miserable state of many deprived infants and young children in institutions was observed. During the 1940s, Spitz termed this disorder 'hospitalism' [1], suggesting emotional deprivation and retarded growth leading to irreversible developmental delays.

Classically FTT has been subdivided into two groups: 'organic' and 'non-organic' failure to thrive. This dichotomy is no longer thought to be appropriate as undernutrition is the primary cause of failure to grow appropriately in all cases of non-organic failure to thrive and in the majority of organic cases [2]. In medical conditions such as gastrointestinal disease, neurological disorders and congenital heart disease, growth failure is due to an inadequate nutritional intake compared with requirements but only 5% of children who are failing to thrive have an organic condition. FTT in the absence of physical disease is the result of a combination of environmental factors which may include neglect and abuse. Growth failure in these children is still due to a low energy intake and inadequate nurturing, not emotional deprivation [3]. A number of children have minor conditions such as asthma or recurrent otitis media, but the majority of them with poor growth have major social problems [4]. Thus no clear distinction can be drawn between organic and non-organic FTT, as both physical and psychosocial factors can co-exist.

WHEN DOES GROWTH RETARDATION BECOME A CAUSE FOR CONCERN?

Normal growth is usually defined in relative terms. Centile charts allow a child's growth to be viewed in relation to the growth of a normal population. When plotting growth, corrections for prematurity should always be made. It has been suggested by Edwards *et al.* that the child's maximum weight centile achieved between 4 and 8 weeks is a better predictor of the centile at 12 months than is the birth centile [5]. Birthweight centile is largely determined by maternal influences such as age, parity, nutrition, smoking and alcohol habits during pregnancy. The child's own genotype may exert a greater influence by 4–8 weeks of age.

Abnormal growth patterns in FTT

Traditionally, concern has been shown for children below the third centile but a fall across centiles, plateauing or fluctuating weight should also raise concern. Batchelor and Kerslake [6] have described several patterns of growth in children who are failing to thrive.

Falling centiles   A classic feature of FTT is a downward deviation in weight across one or more major centile lines.

Poor parallel centiles   In many children who fail to thrive, their centile position initially falls and growth for both height and weight follows a lower parallel centile line having adapted to poor nutrition.

Height and weight centiles markedly discrepant   Where there is a marked discrepancy between height and weight centiles and between the individual child and other family members, FTT should be suspected.

Discrepant family patterns   Children who fail to thrive frequently show marked discrepancies from the parents' attained height centiles. Parental height is influenced by a number of factors including whether the parents failed to thrive as children.

Retrospective rise   Improvement in the child's centile position may occur if nutrition is improved after severe illness or malnutrition, demonstrating catch-up growth.

Saw-tooth pattern   This is also referred to as 'dipping'. A child's weight fluctuates, crossing and recrossing centile positions. Dips in weight may be related to periods of intercurrent illness but commonly reflect other problems.

RECOGNITION OF FTT

To assess changes in weight, regular and accurate measurements should be monitored and plotted on centile charts. A child's length/height is not measured routinely in clinics but the recent working party on Child Health Surveillance [7] recommended a single height measurement at age 3 years or sooner if the opportunity occurs. However, if there is concern about a child's weight, measurement of length/height and head circumference is essential both at assessment and for serial growth monitoring. Mid upper-arm circumference (MUAC), which indirectly assesses nutritional status by estimating body fat and muscle bulk, is also a useful measurement (Table 27.1).

Batchelor and Kerslake [6] showed that one in three children whose weight had fallen below the third centile were not recognised by health professionals as children who had FTT. The reason for non-recognition included:

- A general lack of awareness of the problem
- Social class – a child from an owner-occupying two parent family was more likely to be considered small

Table 27.1 Mid upper-arm circumference of 1–5 year olds [8]

<14.0 cm	Very likely to be a significantly malnourished child
14.0–15.0 cm	May be malnourished (likelihood greater if age nearer 5 than 1 year)
>15.0 cm	Nutrition likely to be reasonable

- A well-cared for child – showing no signs of physical neglect
- No reported feeding difficulties
- Under-use of growth charts
- Lack of treatment facilities.

Early recognition of FTT is the goal of all health professionals involved. The routine use of growth charts, proactive health visiting and acknowledgement of abnormal growth patterns will help more children before poor patterns of nutrition and growth become firmly entrenched.

CONSEQUENCES OF FTT

Nutrition in the early years of life is a major determinant of growth and development and it influences future adult health [9]. In FTT, not only growth is compromised but deficits may be seen in the child's emotional and intellectual development. A child's growth including brain growth is rapid in the first 2 years of life. Studies have shown that severe growth retardation in the first year influences later mental development. The longer the duration of growth retardation, the greater the effect on mental development [10].

PREVALENCE OF FTT

The incidence of FTT in the population depends very much on how FTT is defined. It is suggested that it affects 5% of infants in deprived inner city areas but occurs across a wide social range [11].

CONTRIBUTING FACTORS

FTT is caused by inadequate energy intake which can arise when food is not available or alternatively from insufficient food intake resulting from feeding and behavioural difficulties. The aetiology of FTT is complex and many factors contribute to the problem. In some children, medical conditions are clearly the principal reason for undernutrition (Table 27.2).

Despite an often seemingly adequate intake, gastrointestinal disorders may lead to failure to thrive due to malabsorption, e.g. coeliac disease. Children with congenital cardiac or respiratory defects may show FTT due to decreased nutritional intake

Table 27.2 Organic factors in FTT

- Inability to digest or absorb nutrients
  - coeliac disease
  - cystic fibrosis
- Excessive loss of nutrients
  - vomiting
  - chronic diarrhoea
  - protein-losing enteropathy
- Increased nutrient requirements due to underlying disease
  - chronic cardiac or respiratory failure
  - chronic infection
- Inability to fully utilise nutrients
  - metabolic disease
- Reduced intake of nutrients
  - functional problems
  - suck/swallow inco-ordination
  - oral hypersensitivity

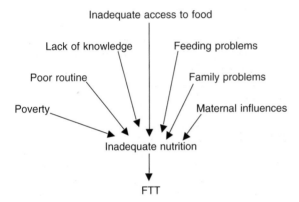

Fig. 27.1 Factors contributing to failure to thrive

because of anorexia, breathing problems or increased energy requirements caused by their disease. Children with neurological dysfunction may have problems with oromotor development which can affect the ability to suck and swallow. They may also suffer from oral hypersensitivity and therefore refuse to feed. Children with metabolic disorders can present with FTT as a result of poor feeding or inability to utilise energy correctly.

Energy needs in the earliest months of life are great with a high proportion required for growth. A combination of many factors that limit or affect intake can contribute to FTT (Fig. 27.1).

Weaning

Parents may lack knowledge about food, cooking and children's dietary needs. A child can fail to thrive at any age but for many the problem starts around the time of weaning. Between 4 and 6 months, a young infant's oromotor skills develop allowing the acceptance of new tastes and textures. If this opportunity is missed, the progression through weaning towards the acceptance of more solid textures can be difficult leading to an overdependence on milk. Intake is then restricted, inappropriate for age and with insufficient energy for normal growth.

Feeding problems

Many parents of children who fail to thrive report feeding difficulties in their children such as holding food in the mouth, spitting food out or vomiting [12]. The child may show no signs of being hungry, nor is there apparent eagerness to feed when food is offered [13]. Excessive consumption of fluids whether milk or juice can also exacerbate the problem [14, 15]. There are many reasons for food refusal including excessive temperatures of food, inappropriately sized pieces, insensitive feeding or reluctance of parents to allow the child to feed itself and make the inevitable 'mess'.

Behaviour problems in some children frustrate parents who will differ in their ways of dealing with these feeding difficulties. The nature of the interaction between the child and parent can affect the child's behaviour at mealtimes and consequently the child's intake.

Family problems

Many studies have focused on psychosocial characteristics of the family and the environment of the child failing to thrive. Parents of children with FTT have been described as having disorganised, disrupted or chaotic lifestyles. Family conflict before the age of seven has been shown to have a strong and significant association with slow growth [16].

Maternal influence

Characteristics of the mother include depression, anxiety, social isolation, low intelligence level, eating disorders and a family cycle in which the mother received inadequate nurturing during her own childhood. Maternal attitudes towards food and feeding also have an influence on the eating habits of children. McCann *et al.* reported that mothers of children who fail to thrive showed greater dietary restraint both concerning what they ate themselves and what they were prepared to offer their children [17].

Poverty

The link between deprivation and failure to thrive is well documented [18] but it has been shown that children from severely deprived backgrounds, devoid of almost all stimulation, recovered weight rapidly when energy intake was 50% greater than normal requirements [19].

MANAGEMENT OF FAILURE TO THRIVE

Overall assessment

FTT is a multifactorial disorder, so there is much to recommend a multidisciplinary team approach to its management [20, 21, 22] with a clear focus on feeding. This will allow for assessment of medical and nutritional status, feeding history, dietary intake, oral function, and psychosocial and developmental aspects. Potential members of a multidisciplinary feeding team are given in Table 27.3. Joint working is ideal enabling discussion of individual cases, and close co-operation between professionals is also very important.

It is important to construct a complete picture of all aspects of and influences on the child's feeding. Dietary assessment will include feeding history,

dietary recall of present intake and completion of a food diary. Food diaries are a powerful tool in nutritional assessments, revealing invaluable quantitative information as well as helping to establish the nature of dietary inadequacies [23] (Table 27.4).

Food diaries can reveal important information regarding the quantities and quality of foods consumed, number of meals and the time intervals in between, frequency and amounts of fluids, routines and daily variation. Health conscious parents may report a high fibre, low fat diet which is unsuitable for these young children [24]. Some parents report what they would like their children to eat and record excessively large quantities at any one meal. These are termed 'food lies' and can be recorded for many reasons which need to be investigated.

Behavioural assessment

In many cases of FTT, the lack of adequate nutritional intake is compounded by behavioural problems. Assessment by the clinical psychologist will provide insights into the child's behavioural feeding problems. Observation of the child being fed by the parent or carer in the normal feeding environment will provide crucial information about how the child feeds, parent-child interaction and the emotions surrounding feeding (Table 27.5). Behaviour problems, including food refusal, can be caused by a number of factors [25], as follows.

Learned food aversion

The child may have had an experience of vomiting which is associated with ingestion of a particular food, even though the vomiting may not have been caused by the food.

Table 27.3 Multidisciplinary feeding team

Paediatrician
General practitioner
Community medical officer
Dietitian
Clinical psychologist
Speech and language therapist
Nurse
Social worker
Health visitor
Others e.g. nursery key worker
               family aide worker

Table 27.4 Food diary information

Food frequency
Quality of food
Food quantity
Fluids – type and frequency
Feeding routine – variation between days
Food refusal
'Food lies' – overreported quantities

Table 27.5 Mealtime observation

Observation of child	Observation of parents
Interest in own and others' food	Awareness of child's needs and demands
Desire to feed or drink by themselves	Ability to tolerate mess
Quantity, texture and type of food eaten	Quantity, texture and type of food offered
Ability to concentrate and persevere	Management style e.g. force, encouragement
Ability to communicate needs	Emotional state e.g. frustration, anxiety
Reaction to parent's behaviour	Control over child's behaviour

Lack of positive learning experiences with certain foods

If a child has not been exposed to a wide range of tastes in the earliest weaning months when taste preference is acquired through dietary experience, refusal to eat a wide variety of foods may occur.

Developmental stage

A child, particularly over 12 months, may be showing independence wanting to self-feed and refusing both to be fed or to accept new foods.

Poor parent-child interaction

The child needs to control their own behaviour, e.g. needs to signal satiety. If the parent does not respond to these satiety signals the child may then increase abnormal behaviour, e.g. screaming, turning away, spitting, throwing food. Once a child is showing signs of satiety, i.e. refusing any more food, further attempts to get the child to eat more are unlikely to succeed.

Assessment of oromotor function

It is important for a speech and language therapist to assess oromotor function in children with FTT, exhibiting food refusal and neurodevelopmental problems. Such assessments, often in conjunction with video-fluoroscopy, will identify children who are unable to co-ordinate the suck/swallow reflex. These children are likely to aspirate feeds and will require non-oral feeding. They will also detect oral hyper-sensitivity and be able to help with desensitisation programmes.

NUTRITIONAL MANAGEMENT

Assessment of requirements

Following assessment of anthropometry and nutritional intake, a strategy for catch-up growth has to be planned. Diets which only cover age-specific requirements for energy and protein [26] will not provide for catch-up growth. Diets based on normal requirements will usually allow for maintenance of growth along the centile to which the child has fallen. Additional protein and energy will be required for catch-up growth. A formula for predicting energy requirements for catch-up growth in infants and young children has been suggested [27]:

$$\text{kcal(kJ)/kg} = \frac{120 \times \text{ideal weight for height (kg)}}{\text{actual weight (kg)}}$$

This may mean an intake of 1.5 to 2 times the normal recommended energy requirements for age.

Additional protein above the reference nutrient intake (RNI) for age will be needed for periods of increased growth velocity. A minimum of 9% energy from protein has been shown to be necessary in order to achieve maximum nitrogen retention in malnourished children [28], although care must be taken when advising high protein intakes if there is any risk of renal insufficiency.

Vitamins, minerals and trace element requirements are increased during periods of rapid growth and a suitable supplement should be included if the child's intake is thought to be inadequate. No guidelines exist, but intakes should be at least appropriate for the proposed energy intake. Anaemia is common in children who are failing to thrive and in one study in Leeds, one third of the sample had iron deficiency anaemia [29].

Achieving nutritional requirements

Information from the dietary assessment will allow discussion with the parents or carers on appropriate intervention. The most suitable method of achieving an adequate nutritional intake will depend on the individual needs of the child.

In a young breast fed infant who is failing to thrive, the maternal diet needs to be assessed and its quantity and quality improved. Supplementation of breast feeds may be necessary but this should be done under dietary supervision and with caution as it may suppress production of breast milk. For formula fed infants, options include increasing the volume of feed, adding energy supplements to infant feeds or the use of a high energy formula.

Children with FTT as a result of organic disease or functional problems often respond quickly to adequate refeeding once the underlying problem is diagnosed and appropriate nutritional treatment given, both in terms of nutrients required and route of administration, e.g. infants with oromotor dysfunction may require nasogastric or gastrostomy feeding.

In general, young children have a high energy requirement relative to their size. In cases of FTT, when catch-up growth is the aim, requirements are 'supernormal'. This is difficult to achieve as many children have small appetites, consuming small food portions at any one time. The following ways of increasing energy intake must be considered:

- Regular meals
- Frequent snacks
- Use of energy dense foods
- Fortification of foods.

Provision of regular feeding

Meals alone will not enable catch-up growth. Regular snacks as well as meals will help these children to increase their interest in food, improve appetite and therefore energy intake. Excess juice consumption encountered in many young children should be discouraged with solids being offered first.

Energy dense foods

Children still need to consume as wide a variety of foods as possible from the five food groups (bread, other cereals and potatoes; meat, fish and alternatives; milk and dairy foods; fruit and vegetables; fatty and sugary foods) with a greater emphasis on the energy dense foods. Foods high in fibre are bulky and may contain high phytate levels compromising both energy intake and the bioavailability of micronutrients.

Fortification of foods

Extra energy, e.g. butter, margarine or cheese, can be added to popular foods. Dried full fat milk powder can be used to fortify puddings, soups and milk. Iron status of young children can be improved through dietary modification by using iron fortified foods and if necessary by giving supplementary iron.

Supplements

The use of dietary supplements is not recommended for children with non-organic FTT. The use of these products can medicalise the problem and give the impression to parents or carers that they do not have a role in helping their child to improve nutritional intake.

In children where growth retardation is due to organic disease, dietary supplements may be necessary and can be prescribed. Supplements of carbohydrate, fat or protein can be used to enrich foods or for some children prepackaged nutrient and energy-dense drinks may be appropriate food. The principle of frequent feeding, regular meals and snacks, use of energy dense foods and fortification of solids with extra energy still applies.

For all children who are failing to thrive, advice tailored to individual needs is important, starting with foods the child is happy to eat. Initially weight gain may be rapid, followed by a gradual deceleration until the child's normal centile is reached. Caution needs to be exercised during the period of catch-up growth in stunted children against carers not limiting intake, because of fears that the child will become obese. Usually, weight is regained before an increase in linear growth occurs [3].

Use of enteral feeding

If the child has severe FTT and it is not possible to achieve a reasonable intake orally, enteral feeding (nasogastric or gastrostomy) will be required initially. The use of overnight feeds is preferred as this leaves the daytime for establishing oral feeding. If tube feeding is initiated to supplement a child's nutritional status, then psychological management is crucial so that tube feeding is recognised as maintaining nutrition while oral feeding is established and improved.

Behavioural management

FTT in a number of children is compounded by behavioural problems. Any attempts to improve nutritional intake to achieve catch-up growth in these children should be improved by a behavioural modification programme. The helping of parents must be done in a sensitive way, offering support and constructive advice, with no blame attached and no criticism of their parenting. The therapy programme includes:

- No force feeding
- Relaxed mealtimes
- Positive reinforcement of good feeding behaviour; aberrant behaviour should be ignored, e.g. by turning the face away from the child
- A time limit for mealtimes
- Closely spaced mealtimes are a possibility, to maximise the opportunity for feeding practice and to reduce the pressure to eat at any one meal.

Failure to thrive is a failure to grow physically, intellectually, emotionally and socially. To thrive, children need adequate nutrition and appropriate nurturing. Abnormal growth patterns must be recognised in child health surveillance.

Many factors contribute to a child's poor growth and intervention benefits from a multidisciplinary team approach encompassing any diagnosis of underlying organic cause and assessment of nutritional intake, oromotor function and feeding and behavioural difficulties. Early intervention is crucial, with a clear focus on improving the child's nutrition to enable catch-up growth.

REFERENCES

1 Spitz RA Hospitalism. *Psychoanalytic Study of the Child*, 1945, **1** 53–7.
2 Skuse D Failure to thrive: current perspectives. *Current Paediatr*, 1992, **2** 105–10.
3 Frank DA, Zeisal SH Failure to thrive. *Pediatr Clin N Am*, 1988, **34** 1187–206.
4 Wright CM, Talbot E Screening for failure to thrive – what are we looking for? *Child: Care and Development*, 1996, **22** 223–34.
5 Edwards AGK *et al.* Recognising failure to thrive in early childhood. *Arch Dis Childh*, 1990, **65** 1263–5.
6 Batchelor JA, Kerslake A *Failure to Find Failure to Thrive*. London: Whiting & Birch, 1990.
7 Hall DMB *Health for all Children.* A programme for child health surveillance. Oxford: Oxford University Press, 1989.
8 Hobbs CJ *et al. Child Abuse and Neglect – A Clinician's Handbook*. Edinburgh: Churchill Livingstone, 1999.
9 Barker DJP The fetal and infant origins of adult disease. *Brit Med J*, 1990, **301** 1111.
10 Illingworth RS *The Development of the Infant and Young Child*, 8th edn. Edinburgh: Churchill Livingstone, 1983.
11 Wright CM *et al.* Effect of deprivation on weight gain in infancy. *Acta Pediatr*, 1994, **83** 357–9.
12 Iwaniec D *et al.* Social work with failure to thrive children and their families. Part 1: Psychological factors. *Brit J Social Work*, 1985, **15** 243–59.
13 Skuse D *et al.* Psychological adversity and growth during infancy. *Eur J Clin Nutr*, 1994, **48** (Suppl 1) S113–30.
14 Smith MM, Lifshitz F Excess fruit consumption as a contributing factor in non-organic failure to thrive. *Paediatr*, 1994, **93** 438–43.
15 Hourihane JO'B, Rolles CJ Morbidity from excess intake of high energy fluids: the 'squash drinking syndrome'. *Arch Dis Childh*, 1995, **72** 141–3.
16 Montgomery SM *et al.* Family conflict and slow growth. *Arch Dis Childh*, 1997, **77** 326–30.
17 McCann JB *et al.* Eating habits and attitudes of mothers of children with non-organic failure to thrive. *Arch Dis Childh*, 1994, **70** 234–6.
18 Frank FA, Drotar D Failure to thrive. In: Reece RM (ed.) *Child Abuse: Medical Diagnosis and Management*. Philadelphia: Lea & Febiger, 1994.
19 Whitten C *et al.* Evidence that growth failure from maternal deprivation is secondary to undereating. *J Amer Med Assoc* 1969, **209** 1675–82.
20 Hobbs C, Hanks HGI A multidisciplinary approach for the treatment of children with failure to thrive. *Child: Care and Development*, 1996, **22**: 273–84.
21 Peterson KE *et al.* Team management of failure to thrive. *J Am Dietetic Assoc*, 1984, **84** 810–15.
22 Blithoney WG *et al.* The effect of a multidisciplinary team approach on weight gain in non-organic failure to thrive children. *Dev Behav Pediatr*, 1991, **12** 254–8.
23 Moores J Non-organic failure to thrive – dietetic practice in a community setting. *Child: Care and Development*, 1996, **22** 251–9.
24 Department of Health *Weaning and the weaning diet*. RHSS 45. London: The Stationery Office, 1994.
25 Harris G, Booth IW The nature and management of eating disorders in pre-school children. In: Cooper P, Stein A (eds) *Monographs in Clinical Paediatrics; Feeding Problems and Eating Disorders*. Switzerland: Harwood Academic Publishers, 1991.

26 Department of Health *Dietary Reference Values for Food and Nutrients for the UK*. RHSS 41. London: The Stationery Office, 1991.

27 Maclean WC *et al*. Nutritional management of chronic diarrhoea and malnutrition: primary reliance on oral feeding. *J Paediatr*, 1990, **97** 316–23.

28 Jackson AA Protein requirements for catch-up growth. *Proc Nutr Soc*, 1990, **49** 507–16.

29 Raynor P, Rudolf MCJ What do we know about children who fail to thrive? *Child: Care and Development*, 1996, **22** 241–50.

FURTHER READING

Batchelor JA *Failure to Thrive in Young Children: Research and Practice Evaluated*. The Children's Society, 1999.

CHAPTER 28

Children from Ethnic Minorities and those following Cultural Diets

The UK is the home to a multicultural and multiethnic society. Immigration occurred mainly during the late 1950s and early 1960s in response to labour shortages. Therefore, the main ethnic minority communities are situated near large industrialised cities. The immigrants introduced a wide variety of cultures, including dietary beliefs and practice that had to fit into their new lifestyles. Nutritionally adequate diets can be hard to achieve when people suddenly find themselves in an environment very different from their homeland.

Infants and children of any age have special dietary requirements. It is therefore essential that religious and cultural attitudes towards diet are known in order to achieve optimal growth and development among these populations. Assessment of intake must be accurate and advice must be relevant to dietary custom so that it is both realistic and achievable.

Children are subject to many outside influences and often start to develop westernised dietary ideas. With time these ideas are taken home and adopted by other members of the family. The extent of adoption of dietary practices differing from traditional customs is variable; therefore, all diets must be individually assessed.

VEGETARIAN AND VEGAN DIETS

Vegetarianism and veganism are common dietary practices among many religious and ethnic groups. In addition, increasing numbers of the indigenous population are also restricting their intake of meat and animal products for either humanitarian, ethical or health reasons. Table 28.1 gives a classification of vegetarian and vegan diets. Providing careful attention is given to ensuring nutritional adequacy, these diets will support normal growth and development [1, 2,

3]. In general, the greater the degree of dietary restriction the greater the risk of nutritional deficiency [4].

Infant feeding

Breast feeding is commonly practised amongst the indigenous vegetarian and vegan population. Providing the maternal diet is adequate, breast milk will be nutritionally complete for the first 4–6 months of the infant's life. Specific attention must be paid to the mother's vitamin D, calcium and iron intakes. Vegan mothers may require additional supplementation with vitamin B_{12} [5]. Neurological damage in infancy has been associated with severe vitamin B_{12} deficiency [6]. If breast feeding is not the chosen method of feeding a suitable infant formula must be given (Table 28.2). Infants should not be given home-made or unmodified soya milks, as these are often deficient in energy, protein, vitamins and minerals [5]. Goat's and ewe's milk are also contraindicated due to their nutritional inadequacy, high renal solute load and doubtful microbiological safety [5, 7].

Weaning

Breast milk or infant formula will provide sufficient nutrition until the infant is 4–6 months of age [7]. After this period, solids should be gradually introduced, increasing flavours and textures with time (Table 28.3). Fruit, vegetables and pulses should be cooked with the skin on to preserve nutrients. This should then be removed to avoid an excessive fibre intake, which adds too much bulk to the diet and may also bind certain nutrients, inhibiting their absorption [8]. Pulses should be thoroughly cooked to destroy toxins such as trypsin inhibitors and haemaglutinins

Table 28.1 Classification of vegetarianism and veganism

	Foods excluded	Protein source		Nutrient at risk of deficiency
Partial vegetarian	Red meat Offal	Poultry Fish Milk Cheese Yoghurt	Eggs Beans Lentils Nuts	Iron
Lacto-ovo vegetarian	Red meat Offal Fish Poultry	Milk Cheese Yoghurt Eggs	Beans Lentils Nuts	Iron
Lacto vegetarian	Red meat Offal Poultry Fish Eggs	Milk Cheese Yoghurt	Beans Lentils Nuts	Iron Vitamin D
Vegan	Red meat Offal Fish Poultry Eggs Milk Cheese Yoghurt	Beans Lentils Nuts		Protein Energy Iron Fat-soluble vitamins Vitamin B_2 Vitamin B_{12} Calcium Zinc

Table 28.2 Infant formulas suitable for vegetarian and vegan children

Milk based	Soya based
Cow & Gate Premium	InfaSoy*
Cow & Gate Plus	Wysoy*
SMA Gold	Prosobee*
SMA White	Farley's
Farley's First Milk	Soya formula isomil
Farley's Second Milk	
Aptamil First	
Aptamil Extra	
Milumil	
Enfamil	
Enfamil AR	
SMA High Energy	
Infatrini	

Protein hydrolysates (for therapeutic use only)
Alfare
Nutramigen
Pregestimil
Pepti-Junior
Neocate*

* Suitable for vegans

Table 28.3 Suitable vegetarian and vegan weaning foods [5, 15]

3–4 months	Baby rice** Fruit and vegetable purées (cooked)
4–7 months	Rusk** Weetabix Pulse and lentil purées (well cooked) Pulse and vegetable purées Pulse and cereal purées Fruit purées Milk puddings or custards (cow's* or soya milk based)
7–9 months	Introduce lumps to the above foods Wholegrains Bread (white and wholemeal) Pasta and rice Finely ground nuts Dried fruits Cheese e.g. cheese sauces* Eggs e.g. savoury egg custards* Tofu and Quorn*

* Suitable for vegetarians only
** Milk-free varieties for vegans

that may cause diarrhoea and vomiting [5]. As the child gets older he should be encouraged to take at least 500 ml of full fat cow's or approved soya milk daily or the equivalent in cheese or yoghurt [5].

Children

Milk gradually provides less of the total nutrient intake and, therefore, extra care is needed to ensure nutritional adequacy. There have been many conflicting studies examining the dietary intake and growth of vegan children [9, 10]. Therefore, regular assessment of growth and development is of paramount importance.

To provide optimal nutrition a vegetarian and vegan diet should be well balanced, containing two or three protein foods and cereals, vegetables, fruits and fats daily (Table 28.4). Vegetable and pulse proteins have a lower concentration and range of essential amino acids than protein from animal or fish sources. Therefore, careful planning of menus with pulse and cereal combinations is necessary to provide sufficient protein of high biological values [5, 9]. The intake of energy dense foods may also be low in the vegan diet, which can lead to failure to thrive [11]. Regular

Table 28.4 Sample vegetarian or vegan menu plan

Breakfast	Cereal + milk or milk substitute
	Wholemeal OR white bread + margarine + peanut butter OR yeast extract
	Egg*
	Diluted fresh orange juice
Dinner	Bean OR nut based dish OR cheese* based dish
	Vegetables OR salad
	Bread, potato, pasta OR rice
	Fruit OR fruit crumble/pie/sponge* + custard (cow's* or soya milk) OR milk pudding (cow's milk* or soya based)
Tea	Lentil or bean burgers OR bean soup OR baked beans OR egg*
	Bread + margarine
	Fruit OR yoghurt OR fromage frais (cow's milk* or soya based)
Snacks	Nuts, toast, biscuits, crisps, fruit, cake

* Suitable for vegetarians only

Table 28.5 Sources of nutrients at risk of deficiency in a vegan diet [11, 15, 25]

Nutrient	Vegan sources	
Riboflavin	Wheat germ	Avocados
	Almonds**	Soya beans
	Green leafy vegetables	Fortified soya milk
	Yeast extract* e.g. Marmite Tastex	
Vitamin B$_{12}$	Fortified cereals	Yeast extracts*
	Fortified soya milk	Tofu
	Soya meat analogues	
Vitamin D	Fortified margarine	Fortified cereals
	Fortified soya milk	Sunlight
Calcium	Fortified soya milk	Hard water
	Green leafy vegetables	Sunflower seeds**
	Legumes	Sesame seeds
	White bread	Almonds**
	Cashew nuts**	
Iron	Fortified cereals	Nuts**
	Wholegrain cereals	Dried fruit
	Wholegrain bread	Molasses
	Green leafy vegetables	Cocoa
	Pulses	Curry powder
	Legumes	Quorn
	Tofu	
Essential fatty acids	Oils	Nuts**
	Wholegrains	Seeds

* Should be used with care in children under the age of 2 years due to high salt content
** Should not be given to children under the age of 2 years unless finely ground

assessment of growth and development is therefore of paramount importance. The protein and energy content of the diet can be increased with the use of nuts, beans and oils. Nut butters can be used to increase the energy content of finger foods; however, the nuts should be finely ground to avoid the danger of inhalation [5].

The main micronutrients at risk of deficiency in the vegan diet are shown in Table 28.5. A daily vitamin supplement such as Abidec is beneficial for both vegetarian and vegan children and should be given from the age of 6 months to 5 years [7]. In addition, vegan children may require a daily supplement of 1–2 µg vitamin B$_{12}$ [5, 9].

There may also be poor bioavailability of zinc [12] and iron from vegetarian and vegan dietary sources, therefore a higher intake than is usually advised may be required. It is also important to ensure that a food rich in vitamin C is given alongside the iron containing food to increase its bioavailability.

When considering the NACNE [13] and COMA [14] recommendations for dietary fat intake, a vegan diet is often regarded as 'healthy'. The resultant diet may, however, as well as being low in total fat, also contain a very poor quality of fat. Docosahexaenoic acid (22:6n-3), which is believed to play an important role in the health of the retina and central nervous system, has been found to be absent from vegan diets. For this reason, it has been suggested that vegans should use oils with a low linoleic:alpha-linolenic acid ratio such as rapeseed oil [10].

Zen macrobiotic diets

The Zen macrobiotic principle originates from Japan and is based on the correct balance between Yin (positive) and Yang (negative) foods. This balance is believed to keep spiritual, mental and physical wellbeing. The individual works through ten levels of dietary elimination. Animal products, fruits and vegetables are gradually removed from the diet until the ultimate goal is achieved of consuming only brown rice. Fluids are also severely restricted [15].

This type of diet is nutritionally inadequate for a child of any age, being severely deficient in energy and most other nutrients. Marked growth retardation, associated with muscle wasting and a delay in gross motor and language development, have been documented in infants fed macrobiotic weaning diets [16, 17]. Growth failure [18] and reduced bone mass [19] have also been documented in older children. Deficiencies of vitamins B_{12}, D and thiamin and of the minerals calcium and iron have also been observed [20, 21, 22, 23]. Improved growth has been reported in children previously following macrobiotic diets, following the consumption of fatty fish, dairy products or both [24]. This finding suggests that linear growth retardation in children on macrobiotic diets is caused solely by nutritional deficiencies.

Fruitarian diets

Fruitarian diets are based on fruit and uncooked fermented cereals and seeds. These diets are nutritionally inadequate for children of any age and can lead to severe protein energy malnutrition, anaemia and multiple vitamin and mineral deficiencies [9].

ASIAN DIETS

The Asian community represent the largest ethnic minority group in the UK. The communities consist of people who migrated directly from India, Pakistan and Bangladesh and those who came via East Africa [26]. Immigration is now strictly limited by legislation. The population, however, continues to expand because of families being born in the UK. Dietary customs are largely based on the religious and cultural beliefs of the three main religious groups (Moslems, Hindus and Sikhs). Great dietary variance is also observed within these groups, as income and geographical area [26, 27, 28] affect the diet in the homeland.

Hindus

Approximately 30% of the Asian population in the UK are Hindu. The majority came from the Gujarat region of India, although some are from the Indian Punjab and East Africa [26, 29, 30]. Hindus believe that the soul is eternal and, therefore, believe in reincarnation.

Dietary customs

The caste system dictates who can prepare and serve food [26]. A restriction on eating beef was introduced in 800 BC because Hindus regard the cow as sacred. It is also unusual for pork to be eaten as the pig is thought to be unclean, though other meats are acceptable (Table 28.6). Devout Hindus believe in the doctrine of Ahisma (not killing) and are, therefore, vegetarian. Some will eat dairy products and eggs, while others refuse eggs on the grounds that they are potential sources of life. A minority of Hindus practice veganism.

Wheat is the main staple food eaten by Hindus in the UK. It is used to make chapattis, puris and parathas. Ghee (clarified butter) and oil are used extensively in cooking [26].

Most Hindus fast on 3 days a year to celebrate the birthdays of the Lords Shiva (March), Rama (April) and Krishna (August). In addition to these days, orthodox Hindus may also fast once or twice every week (often on Tuesdays and Fridays). Fasting lasts from dawn to dusk and varies from avoiding all foods except those considered pure (e.g. rice, fruit and yoghurt) to total food exclusion [26, 29].

Table 28.6 Asian religious groups [26, 27, 28]

Group	Religion	Language	Staple	Dietary customs
Hindus	Hinduism	Hindi Gujarati	Millet Wheat Rice	No beef Often no pork No alcohol Often vegetarian or vegan
Moslems	Islam	Urdu Bengali Gujarati Punjabi	Rice Millet Wheat	No pork Halal meat No alcohol No fish without scales
Sikhs	Sikhism	Punjabi Hindi	Wheat	No beef Often no pork No Halal meat

Moslems

Moslems comprise approximately 30% of the Asian population in the UK, the majority originating from Pakistan and Bangladesh [26, 30]. Moslems practice the Islamic religion; Allah is their god and the prophet Mohammed his final messenger.

Dietary customs

The Koran provides Moslems with their food laws. The consumption of pork, alcohol, carnivorous animals, fish without scales and some birds is forbidden [26]. These foods which are strictly avoided are called Haraam. All meat and poultry must be ritually slaughtered (bled to death and then blessed) to render it Halal and, therefore, legitimate to eat [26, 30]. Wheat, usually in the form of chapattis, is the staple cereal eaten by Moslems from Pakistan, whereas those from Bangladesh eat more rice [26, 28]. Cooking oil is used in preference to ghee.

During the lunar month of Ramadan, Moslems fast between sunrise and sunset. Children under the age of 12 and the elderly are exempt from fasting. People who are ill, pregnant, menstruating or on a long journey are also excused, but are however expected to fast at a later date. Unfortunately, many pregnant women will fast with the rest of the family during Ramadan as they find it more convenient [26, 29]. The Koran also dictates that children should be breast fed up to the age of two years [26].

Sikhs

The remaining 40% of the Asian population in the UK are Sikh. Sikhism is a relatively new religion, originating as a reformist movement of Hinduism, in the Indian Punjab in the sixteenth century. Sikhs believe in reincarnation and in one personal god who is eternal, the creator of the universe and the source of all being [26, 29]. Devout Sikhs undergo Amarit, a special kind of confirmation where certain practices must be followed. Prayers must be said every day and Sikhs must not drink alcohol, smoke or eat Halal meat. They must also adhere to a strict ethical code and wear the five signs of Sikhism: Kesh (uncut hair), Kara (steel or silver bangle), Kanga (comb), Kirpa (small symbolic dagger) and Kaccha (special undergarments).

Dietary customs

Most Sikhs will not eat pork or beef but some will eat lamb, poultry, fish, eggs and dairy produce. Vegetarianism is common, with eggs and dairy produce usually being eaten [26, 29].

Wheat and, to a lesser extent, rice are the main staples eaten, and ghee and oil are used in cooking [26]. Devout Sikhs will fast once to twice weekly and most will fast on the first day of the Punjab month or when there is a full moon. This again varies from total food exclusion to eating only pure foods [29].

Common Asian dietary customs

Many of the Asian people in the UK share dietary customs, despite their varying religious and geographical background (Table 28.7). Many older members of the Asian community, especially those originating from Pakistan and Bangladesh, have retained traditional dietary customs. There is, however, an increasing consumption of westernised foods, especially convenience foods. The extent of adoption of these foods is variable, tending to be greater in the younger generations and in those who have lived in the UK for some time [26].

At breakfast time chapatti, paratha, bread and occasionally hard boiled or fried eggs are traditionally eaten. The two main meals, usually eaten at lunchtime and in the evening, are based around the staple, usually served with a curry [27, 28, 29]. Most curries are based on vegetables, pulses, nuts and seeds. Even if allowed, very little meat, fish or poultry is used. Most foods, including spices, are usually fried before adding to the curry, which is then served with home-made chutneys, side salads of tomatoes and onions and yoghurt [29, 30]. Very little hard cheese is eaten; paneer, an Indian soft curd cheese, is preferred [29]. Meals are usually served with tea, which is made with hot milk and sugar, although English tea is becoming popular [29]. Traditionally Asians rarely eat snacks, although western snack foods are increasing in popularity. Traditional Asian savoury snacks (usually reserved for celebrations only) are high in fat and the sweets are often very high in refined sugar.

Many Asians believe that foods have heating and cooling effects on the body. These hot and cold foods should be eaten in the correct balance to achieve a healthy state. Certain hot foods can cause symptoms

Table 28.7 Foods commonly eaten by the Asian population in the UK [31, 32, 33]

Food	Nutrients	Method of cooking		Food	Nutrients	Method of cooking
Cereals				*Fruits*		
Wheat	Energy	Chapatti	Samosa	Guava, lychee, mango	Vitamin A	Raw
	B vitamins	Paratha	Pakora	Paw paw/papaya	Vitamin C	Curries
		Popadom	Poori	Indian gooseberries	Fibre	Chutneys
		Bhagi		Dried fruits		
Rice		Boiled	Fried	*Meat and fish*		
Semolina		Porridges		Many types	Protein	Curries
Ground rice		Sweetmeats		(see Table 28.6)	Fat-soluble	Roast
					vitamins	
Tubers					Iron	
Arvi/colocasia root	Energy	Boiled				
Cassava		Fried		*Dairy products*		
Taro tuber		Curries		Milk	Energy	Drinks
Yam				Yoghurt	Protein	Raw
				Cheese/paneer	Vitamin A	Boiled
Vegetables				Eggs	Riboflavin	Fried
Ackee Okra	Vitamin A	Boiled			Nicotinic acid	
Bringal Pepper	Riboflavin	Fried			Vitamin D	
Cho cho/chayote	Folic acid	Curries			Iron	
Fenugreek leaves	Vitamin C	Chutneys			Calcium	
Bitter gourd/darela	Iron	Pickles				
Kantola	Calcium			*Fats and oils*		
Patra leaves	Fibre			Ghee/clarified butter	Energy	Frying
Spinach				Vegetable oil	Essential fatty	Spreading
				Margarine	acids	
Peas, beans and nuts						
Balor/valor beans	Energy	Curries				
Blackgram/urad gram	Protein	Dahls				
Chickpeas/bengal gram	B vitamins					
Cluster beans/guar	Iron					
Coconut	Calcium					
Red lentils/masur dahl	Fibre					
Mung/moong beans						
Papri beans						
Pigeon peas/red gram						
Lima beans						

such as constipation, sweating and body fatigue, while certain cold foods can lead to strength and happiness. Foods may also be used to treat a condition, for example hot foods should be avoided during pregnancy and cold ones avoided when breast feeding [27, 29].

Infant feeding

Early studies consistently reported a lower breast feeding rate among Asians in the UK when compared with the Caucasian population [34, 35, 36, 37] and Asians in the Indian subcontinent [38, 39]. However, high incidences of breast feeding among Bangladeshi, Indian and Pakistani mothers compared with white mothers have more recently been reported [40]. In this large survey, which sampled 95% of the Asian population in the UK, Bangladeshi and Pakistani mothers were, however, less likely to continue breast feeding their babies beyond 8 weeks of life when compared with Caucasian mothers. Interestingly, of mothers who were born outside the UK, 30–40% who either bottle fed initially or who stopped breast feeding to bottle feed reported that they would have fed their babies differently had they not been born in the UK. Unfortunately, for some bottle feeding is perceived as the western ideal and therefore better for the baby. There is also often a lack of education promoting breast feeding in the Asian community [26, 34, 36]. This problem is compounded by communication difficulties and overcrowded housing [5], making it difficult for a mother to breast feed in privacy.

Higher hospital admission rates for bottle fed Asian babies have been reported. This may be due to difficulties in understanding the instructions on infant formula tins that can lead to poor hygiene and incorrect dilution of feeds [41].

Weaning

Social disadvantage, the varying quality, expense and availability of familiar Asian weaning foods and the pressures of westernisation may compromise good weaning practice. Late weaning and prolonged breast feeding are commonly practised in infants who are born on the Indian subcontinent and those who have only been in the UK for a short time [35, 36, 37, 38, 41, 42]. On the Indian subcontinent it is considered safer to leave the infant on breast milk and wean straight onto adult foods. In the UK late weaning may be partly due to the poor availability of suitable foods and the lack of adequate and appropriate advice [40, 43]. Some Asian infants born in the UK are weaned earlier [36, 37, 38, 39], but are commonly given sweet proprietary weaning foods that are low in protein and iron [35, 36, 42]. This mainly occurs because many mothers do not know the composition of savoury weaning products and often will not use these foods unless they are vegetarian [26]. Because of these problems, mothers should be encouraged to cook savoury weaning foods at home. Suitable home-made Asian weaning foods are given in Table 28.8. The practice of sweetening milk and adding foods such as rusk, honey, Weetabix and baby rice to bottles is also common [26, 36, 40] and should be discouraged.

Many Asian infants are given cow's milk from the age of 5 months [26, 40]. This practice can lead to a higher saturated fat and salt intake and a reduced vitamin D and iron intake than if breast milk or infant formula were continued [7]. Feeding development is often delayed because of late conversion from bottle to cup and very late progression onto family foods [26, 36, 42]. Although fewer Asian than white

Table 28.8 Suitable Asian weaning foods

4–6 months	
Puréed	Cauliflower and potato*
	Cauliflower and pea*
	Pea and potato*
	Aubergine and potato*
	Green vegetable and potato*
	Vegetable and cheese*
	Lentil and rice*
	Chickpea and marrow*
	Porridge
	Fruit purée
6–12 months	
	Introduce small lumps to the above foods
	Mild spices, e.g. cumin and coriander may be used
	Introduce finger foods, e.g. small pieces of chapatti

* A small amount of meat, poultry or fish may be added if eaten

mothers have been reported to experience feeding problems when the infant was approximately 9 weeks old, more reported problems when the child was between 5 and 15 months old [40]. It is not unusual for a two year old to derive the majority of his nutrition from bottles of cow's milk and sweetened fruit drinks.

Very few differences have been reported between the diets of first and second generation Asians [44]. It has been suggested that this may be due to the cohesive nature of the community and because all young children are subject to similar dietary and cultural expectations and pressures. Therefore, infant feeding practices among the Asian population can still be improved:

- The teaching curriculum of all catering and health-related training should include ethnic cultures, food and diet, so that effective education on all aspects of infant feeding can be given [42]. This training should be updated regularly [36].
- Communication barriers must be overcome. Practical demonstrations, the use of bilingual interpreters and written advice in the Asian languages should be available [26, 36, 42].
- Education promoting breast feeding should reach the parents before pregnancy, and support should be given while breast feeding [36].
- Breast or formula milk should be given up to 1 year of age [36].

- Sugary drinks should be avoided [36].
- Infants should be weaned at 4–6 months of age [7].
- Weaning advice should include the use of appropriate family foods in addition to commercial baby foods [26, 36].
- Salt, sugar, honey or hot spices should not be added to bottles or weaning foods [27].
- Advice should be given on foods rich in vitamin C, vitamin D and iron, as these nutrients may be at risk of deficiency [36].
- The cup should be introduced between 6 months and 1 year of age [36].
- Vitamin drops should be given from the age of 6 months up to 2 years and preferably up to 5 years [7].

Further research is required to study nutrient intake and the nutritional status of Asian infants, children and adolescents as the population changes. Regular studies, such as that by Thomas and Avery [40], concerning lifestyle and health perceptions are required to ensure that nutritional advice is culturally acceptable.

Nutritional problems commonly found in Asian children

Failure to thrive

Dietary intake is the major influence on growth. However, to a lesser extent family income, housing standards, maternal education, psychological distress and morbidity are also influences [26, 35]. Low birth weight has been reported in the Asian population, both in this country and in the country of origin [38, 43, 45, 46]. Genetic factors and maternal undernutrition may be to blame [26, 45]. Birth weight has, however, increased over the last 15 years, suggesting that genetic factors do not have a major influence. Longer birth intervals, fewer teenage pregnancies and improved nutrition are thought to be contributing factors [26].

Despite lower birth weights, some studies show that Asian babies and children grow as well as the indigenous population [26, 38, 40, 45, 47]. In one study Sikh children were found to be taller than children from other Asian subgroups and Caucasians [48]. In contrast, others suggest that growth failure is common [41, 49, 50]. Because of these conflicting observations it is important that growth and the need

for nutritional supplementation are assessed for the individual.

Iron deficiency anaemia

Iron deficiency anaemia has been described in Asian infants [41, 51, 52, 53]. Inadequate dietary intake of iron is commonly related to the early introduction and excessive use of unfortified cow's milk in children who already have low iron stores [26]. Prolonged use of a baby bottle and the mother being born outside the UK has also been shown to have a negative influence on the iron status of Asian children [53]. There is, however, conflicting evidence regarding the adequacy of dietary iron intakes [35]. It is therefore essential that the diets of Asian children are assessed individually. Advice should include information on the use of foods rich in iron and also vitamin C, as the diets of Asian children are unlikely to regularly contain fresh vegetables [40].

Megaloblastic anaemia

Megaloblastic anaemia due to vitamin B_{12} deficiency has been observed in some strict vegetarian and vegan Asians [30, 54]. Education regarding vitamin B_{12} sources in the vegetarian diet is required and supplementation may be needed in the vegan diet.

Rickets

The steady decline in rickets in the UK was halted in the late 1960s and early 1970s when a number of cases appeared in immigrant families, mainly of Asian origin [41, 42, 55, 56, 57]. There is now evidence that the incidence is in decline following large scale vitamin D supplementation [26]. However, low plasma vitamin D levels are still observed in some members of the Asian population, especially those of Pakistani origin, those who also have low haemoglobin levels and those who do not take routine vitamin supplements [58, 59, 60]. There have been conflicting results from studies comparing the dietary vitamin D intake of Asian and Caucasian children [9, 26, 35].

In addition to dietary intake of vitamin D, other factors such as low sunlight exposure, skin pigmentation, late weaning, high fibre and high phytate intakes may also contribute to the development of rickets in Asian children [9, 26, 41]. Until we have more information on the causes of rickets, vitamin supplementation is advisable for both infants and deficient pregnant women to prevent neonatal hypocalcaemia and rickets [5, 26]. The need for supplementation in young children has been emphasised in the COMA report on bone health [61]. The weaning diets of infants should include foods rich in vitamin D such as milk, eggs, oily fish, liver, fortified cereals and margarine [5, 25, 30, 62]. Children should also be encouraged to play outside [62].

Dental caries

Traditionally, sugary foods are reserved for celebrations and, therefore, do not play a major role in Asian diets. However, with increasing westernisation, over-consumption of refined sugar has become a problem. Indeed, a high incidence of dental caries has been observed in Asian pre-school children [63]. Asian mothers often add sugar to babies' bottles and give sweetened drinks via the bottle for prolonged periods. These drinks, as well as being full of sugar, are acidic which can easily lead to tooth decay [36]. Education regarding infant feeding with the restriction of quantity and frequency of sugar intake, the use of fluoride-containing drops and toothpaste and frequent dental visits will help to reduce the incidence of dental caries.

Obesity

With the increasing consumption of high sugar and fat foods the prevalence of obesity is increasing. In addition to restricting these foods, advice on acceptable Asian food alternatives and appropriate cooking techniques must be given. Dietary fat intake can be reduced by avoiding deep fried foods, reducing the amount of oil or ghee used in cooking and restricting or not adding fat to chapattis. Avoiding the popular sweet sugary tea and Asian sweetmeats will reduce dietary sugar.

AFRO-CARIBBEAN DIETS

The Afro-Caribbean community is the second largest ethnic minority group in the UK [26, 64].

Dietary patterns

The two main meals are taken at breakfast time and in the evening [65, 66]. Traditional breakfasts include fried plantain, cornmeal dumplings and fried dumplings. However, many dietary practices have now been adopted from British culture and toast and cereals have largely replaced these foods. The evening meal is more likely to contain traditional foods, especially with the younger generation who seem keen to retain their identification and culture. Cereals and tubers such as rice, green banana, yam and sweet potato form the main part of the diet [64]. These starchy foods are served with small amounts of meat or fish [65]. Traditionally, preserved meat, fish and milk are eaten, as the tropical climate in the homeland makes it difficult to keep these foods fresh [64]. Peas, beans, nuts and green leafy vegetables are widely used, often being made into home-made soups and stews which are well seasoned with herbs and spices [26]. Boiling, baking, frying, stewing, steaming and roasting are all commonly used cooking methods for meat, fish and vegetables [64] (Table 28.9).

Rastafarians

A minority of the Afro-Caribbean population within the UK are Rastafarians. Dietary beliefs are based on laws laid down by Moses in Genesis that state that certain types of meat should be avoided. However, many Rastafarians avoid meat completely to obey the commandment 'thou shalt not kill'. Vinegar, raisins, grapes and wine are also avoided by some Rastafarians as the Nazarite law states that fruits of the vine should not be eaten. Dietary restrictions are followed with varying degrees of strictness. The most orthodox follow a vegan diet and will only eat 'Ital' (natural) foods; chemicals and additives are thought to pollute the body and soul [64]. In addition, salt is also prohibited. Many Rastafarians are socially deprived and often unemployed and are, therefore, unable to provide adequate nutrition for their children within the dietary code [26]. Less orthodox Rastafarians, although accepting the central tenets of 'Ital', will eat dairy products, small amounts of fish with scales, sea salt and other seasonings. The nutritional adequacy of these diets is much easier to achieve.

Infant feeding

Information on infant feeding in Afro-Caribbean communities in the UK is scanty; feeding is mainly influenced by the place of birth, knowledge of

Table 28.9 Foods commonly eaten by the Afro-Caribbean population in the UK [64, 67]

Food	Nutrients	Method of cooking	Food	Nutrients	Method of cooking
Cereals			*Fruit*		
Wheat	Energy	Boiled	Avocado	Vitamin C	Fresh
Oats	B vitamins	Dumplings	Cashewfruit		Stewed
Maize		Porridges	Guava		
Rice		Bread	Oranges		
			Paw-paw		
			Sapodilla		
Tubers			Mango		
Green banana	Energy	Mashed	Cane sugar		
Sweet potato	B vitamins	Fried	Grapefruit		
Bread fruit	Vitamin C	Roasted	Oteheite apple		
Yams		Stewed	Passion fruit		
Cassava			Pineapple		
Plantain			Soursop		
			Coolie		
Peas, beans and nuts			*Meat and fish*		
Red peas	Protein	Stews		Protein	Fry
Pigeon peas	B vitamins	Boiled		Fat-soluble	Steam
Coconut	Calcium		Mainly chicken	vitamins	Roast
Almonds	Iron		Many types of fish	Iron	Boil
Sesame seeds	Fibre				Stewed
Black eyed peas					Bake
Broad beans					
Channa			*Eggs*		
Cashews				Protein	Scrambled
Pumpkin seeds				Vitamin A	Cake
				Vitamin D	Fritters
				Iron	Puddings
Dark green leafy vegetables					
Cabbage	Vitamin A	Stews	*Fats and oils*		
Carrot	Vitamin C	Stir fry	Coconut oil	Essential	Frying
Egg plant	Calcium		Olive oil	fatty acids	Spreading
Okra	Iron		Margarine		Baking
Callaloo			Lard		
Dasheen leaves			Vegetable oil		
Karela			Butter		
Pumpkin			Suet		

traditional practices and advice from relatives. In the homeland over 90% of women breast feed their babies initially. However, even in Africa, this is often short-lived and exclusive breast feeding is rare [64]. The large scale marketing of infant formulas and the early return of women to work are implicated. Many Afro-Caribbean mothers avoid giving their infants colostrum and in its place give water, which is thought to cleanse the body before the breast milk is given. This practice may reduce breast milk production and,

therefore, also contribute to the low exclusive breast feeding rate both in this country and in Africa.

Weaning

Infants are traditionally weaned as early as 1 month of age and 45% are reported to be receiving food by 3 months [64, 65, 66]. In contrast, late weaning is commonly observed within the orthodox Rastafarian

Table 28.10 Suitable Afro-Caribbean weaning foods

4–6 months	Rice or oat porridge
	Puréed fruit
	Puréed vegetables, e.g. yam, peas, okra
	Puréed vegetables and meat or fish
	Puréed rice and vegetable
	Egg custard
7–12 months	Introduce:
	Small lumps to the above foods
	Mashed family foods avoiding highly seasoned foods
	Finger foods, e.g. toast, biscuits, fruit

population [5]. Common weaning solids include high starch foods with a low nutrient density such as corn-meal, oats or rice porridge. This practice may lead to energy, protein, vitamin and mineral deficiencies if continued for a long time [5, 29, 68, 69]. More suitable weaning foods are shown in Table 28.10. There are also many suitable commercial baby foods that are now being used [64]. The common practice of adding thin porridge to bottles should be discouraged as it can lead to a delay in the weaning process. It is also common for infants to be given bush teas (infusions of herbs and leaves) as a cure for minor ailments [65]. Care should be taken to ensure that these are not given instead of milk.

By the age of 9 months most infants are eating family foods with the diet having both traditional and western influences [65].

Nutritional problems found in Afro-Caribbean children

Obesity

With the adoption of British dietary customs there has been an increase in the consumption of high sugar and fat convenience foods and drinks. This has led to an increased prevalence of obesity in Afro-Caribbean children. Advice given should take into consideration both traditional and westernised dietary practice.

Iron deficiency anaemia

Iron deficiency anaemia has been observed in Afro-Caribbean children living in the UK. The main causes are thought to be prolonged bottle feeding, late weaning onto foods with a low iron content and the early introduction and excessive use of cow's milk [26].

Megaloblastic anaemia

There have been reports of megaloblastic anaemia in Rastafarian children living in Jamaica [70, 71]. Vegan children may require vitamin B_{12} supplementation.

Rickets

Rickets has been seen in Afro-Caribbean children [26, 69]. Advice on dietary sources of vitamin D and calcium and vitamin D supplementation is beneficial.

Lactose intolerance

There is a high incidence of lactose intolerance because of hypolactasia among the Afro-Caribbean population. A reduction in, and occasionally the avoidance of, the consumption of milk and other foods containing lactose will usually reduce symptoms (p. 81).

CHINESE DIETS

Chinese people represent the third largest ethnic minority group in the UK [72]. Over 25% are British born; the rest originate from the Caribbean, Hong Kong, Taiwan, China, Malaysia and Singapore [72]. Dietary habits vary according to the country and region of origin. Very few foods are avoided, with the exception of pork which is not eaten by the Chinese Moslem population. Northern China has a cool climate favouring the growth of wheat, maize, sorghum and millet. These staples are often made into steamed bread, dumplings, pancakes or noodles [29, 72]. Meals are often based on root vegetables such as sweet potato and turnip, with very little meat being eaten. In contrast, because of its high rainfall, rice is the staple in southern China. Fresh vegetables and fruit are also found in abundance [72]. In the east, because of the long coastline, fish and shellfish are plentiful. In the west, livestock is reared and, therefore, the consumption of meat, milk and cheese is much higher [72].

Dietary patterns

Traditional breakfasts include rice porridge (congee), served either plain or with liver, meat, salted fish, salted eggs or Chinese cheese and a soup made from rice and meat [29, 72]. These traditional foods are, however, slowly being replaced by western alternatives. The midday and evening meals consist of boiled rice or noodles and a variety of highly seasoned dishes such as fried or steamed meat and fish and stir-fried vegetables. Raw food is rarely eaten, as fertiliser in China commonly contains human manure. Meals are usually served with either China tea or a thin soup and then followed with fruit. Sweet foods are usually reserved for special occasions [29, 72].

The main health concerns are the high salt intake associated with many of the preserved foods and seasonings used and the high fat and refined sugar intake associated with the increasing consumption of western foods, especially by the younger generation [72]. A high incidence of lactose intolerance, due to hypolactasia, is also becoming apparent with the increasing consumption of milk and other dairy products [72].

Yin and Yang foods

To Chinese people health is perceived as the maintenance of a sound body and mental state, rather than absence of disease. Traditional Chinese medicine states that good health relies on the body's balance of two opposite elements, Yin (cold), which represents female energy, and Yang (hot), which represents male energy [29, 72]. In illness the balance becomes disturbed and the body becomes either too hot or too cold. Tolerance of Yin and Yang increases with age; thus an adult can eat a much wider variety of foods than can a child. The classification of foods varies: in general meat, duck, goose, oily fish, potatoes, coffee, nuts, herbs, spices, alcohol and fats are regarded as hot foods; fish, rice and some vegetables are neutral foods; chicken, certain fruits and vegetables and barley water are cold foods. Stewing, deep fat frying, grilling and roasting makes foods hotter, steaming neutralises and boiling and stir-frying have a cooling effect [29, 72].

During pregnancy and after childbirth the woman's body is thought to become cool and therefore cold foods are avoided. Alcohol, ice cream, mutton, beef and fizzy drinks are also avoided. In addition, if the woman is breast feeding, green vegetables and fruit are avoided because of concern that they may give the baby diarrhoea. As a consequence breast feeding mothers often have a high protein intake [72].

Infant feeding

In the UK, Chinese women often return to work soon after childbirth, which has led to a decrease in the rate and duration of breast feeding. Low breast feeding rates in the Chinese population living in other countries have also been observed [73, 74]. Soya bean oil, which is a poor source of essential fatty acids, is a major source of fat in the Chinese diet. Because of this, breast milk has been found to have a low concentration of docosahexaenoic acid (DHA) and arachidonic acid (AA) [75]. It has, therefore, been suggested that mothers who are breast feeding their infants should supplement their diet with a good source of DHA and AA such as fish oil.

Because infant formula is regarded as hot, bottle fed babies are often given frequent cooling drinks such as water and barley water. Most infants are weaned at 3 months of age and traditionally rice-based porridges are introduced but more recently commercial baby foods are being used [72]. In general, infants are thought to have a hot equilibrium and, therefore, neutralising or cooling foods are considered best for them. It is common practice for children to be given afternoon tea consisting of cooling foods such as bread, biscuits, cake, barley water and herb teas to counteract the heating effect of school meals [72].

VIETNAMESE DIETS

Some 75% of Vietnamese settlers in the UK are ethnic Chinese and, therefore, share many of the Chinese traditions [72].

Food habits

There are no forbidden foods; however, certain unfamiliar foods such as lamb, ox liver, tinned or cooked fruit and some root vegetables may be avoided [29]. Rice is the main staple food and is served either boiled or fried with small amounts of meat or fish. Like

Chinese food, main dishes are often heavily seasoned and vegetables are lightly steamed or stir-fried in oil or lard. Very little fresh milk, butter, margarine and cheese are used, due to both their lack of availability in Vietnam and the high incidence of lactose intolerance. Snacks of roasted nuts, sweet potatoes, rice or noodle soup, spring rolls and fresh fruit are frequently eaten. Common beverages include tea, coffee and fruit juice and alcohol is taken on special occasions [29]. Generally, the Vietnamese diet is low in fat and high in unrefined carbohydrate [76]. However, with increasing westernisation, the intake of high sugar and fat snack foods is increasing, especially in the younger generation. This has led to an increase in dental caries in the Vietnamese population, both in the UK [77] and other countries [78].

The Vietnamese people observe hot and cold food principles, similar to the Chinese. In contrast to the Chinese, however, pregnancy is regarded as a hot condition and therefore women eat less red meat and fish. A traditional stew called Keung Chow, made from pigs' trotters, boiled eggs, vinegar and ginger, is given to women after childbirth to help recovery and to celebrate the birth of the child. After childbirth, women are encouraged to eat hot foods to regain their strength [29].

Infant feeding

Since their arrival in westernised countries, including the UK, Vietnamese mothers have abandoned traditional infant feeding practices in favour of more modern bottle feeding methods [78, 79, 80]. Hence the incidence of breast feeding is low and there is a need for culturally sensitive health education programmes to support breast feeding in this group.

Nutrients at risk of deficiency

Calcium

Children are at risk of calcium deficiency, especially if minimal milk and associated products are eaten [29]. The rice traditionally grown in Vietnam is a good source of calcium, but is unavailable in Britain. Traditional Vietnamese fruit and vegetables also contain more calcium than British varieties [29].

Vitamin D

Deficiency of vitamin D has been noted in Vietnamese children. For this reason children may need vitamin D supplementation [29].

REFERENCES

1 Hebbelinck M, Clarys P, De Malsche A Growth, development, and physical fitness of Flemish vegetarian children, adolescents, and young adolescents. *Am J Clin Nutr*, 1999, **70** 579S–85S.
2 Sanders TA Vegetarian diets and children. *Pediatr Clin North Am*, 1995, **42** 955–65.
3 O'Connell JM *et al.* Growth of vegetarian children: the farm study. *Pediatr*, 1989, **84** 475–81.
4 Hackett A, Nathan I, Burgess L Is a vegetarian diet adequate for children? *Nutr Health*, 1998, **12** 189–95.
5 Taitz LS, Wardley BL Dietary variants. In: *Handbook of Child Nutrition*, 2nd edn. Oxford: Oxford University Press, 1990, pp. 47–56.
6 Von Schenck U, Bender-Gotze C, Koletzko B Persistence of neurological damage induced by dietary vitamin B_{12} deficiency in infancy. *Arch Dis Childh*, 1997, **77** (2) 137–9.
7 Committee on Medical Aspects of Food Policy *Present day practice in infant feeding*. Report of a Working Party of the Panel on Child Nutrition. London: The Stationery Office, 1988.
8 British Dietetic Association. *Children's Diet and Change*. Birmingham: BDA, 1987, pp. 29–32.
9 Francis D *Nutrition for Children*. Oxford: Blackwell Science, 1986, pp. 49–54.
10 Sanders TAB, Manning J The growth and development of vegan children. *J Hum Nutr Diet*, 1992, **5** 11–21.
11 Sanders TA Growth and development of British vegan children. *Am J Clin Nutr*, 1988, **48** 822–5.
12 Gibson RS Content and bioavailability of trace elements in vegetarian diets. *Am J Clin Nutr*, 1994, **59** 1223–32.
13 National Advisory Committee on Nutrition Education. *Proposals for Nutritional Guidelines for Health Education in Britain*. London: Health Education Council, 1983.
14 Committee on Medical Aspects of Food Policy. *Diet and Cardiovascular Disease*. DHSS Report on Health and Social Subjects. London: The Stationery Office, 1984.
15 Thomas B (ed.) In: Vegetarianism and veganism. *Manual of Dietetic Practice*. Oxford: Blackwell Science, 1988, pp. 303–306.
16 Dagnelie PC *et al.* Nutritional status of infants aged 4–18 months on macrobiotic diets and matched omnivorous control infants: a population based mixed longitudinal study. II: Growth and psychomotor development. *Eur J Clin Nutr*, 1989, **43** 325–38.

17 Dagnelie PC *et al*. Do children on macrobiotic diets show catch up growth? A population based cross sectional study in children aged 0–8 years. *Eur J Clin Nutr*, 1988, **42** 1007–1016.

18 Van Dusseldorp *et al*. Catch-up growth in children fed a macrobiotic diet in early childhood. *J Nutr*, 1996, **126** 2977–83.

19 Parsons TJ *et al*. Reduced bone mass in Dutch adolescents fed a macrobiotic diet in early life. *J Bone Miner Res*, 1997, **12** 1486–94.

20 Herens MC *et al*. Nutrition and mental development of 4–5 year old children on macrobiotic diets. *J Hum Nutr Diet*, 1992, **5** 1–9.

21 Dagnelie PC *et al*. Nutritional status of infants aged 4–18 months on macrobiotic diets and matched omnivorous control infants: a population based mixed longitudinal study. I: Weaning patterns, energy and nutrient intake. *Eur J Clin Nutr*, 1989, **43** 311–23.

22 Dagnelie PC *et al*. Increased risk of vitamin B$_{12}$ and iron deficiency in infants on macrobiotic diets. *Am J Clin Nutr*, 1989, **50** 818–24.

23 Dagnelie PC *et al*. High prevalence of rickets in infants on macrobiotic diets. *Am J Clin Nutr*, 1990, **51** 202–208.

24 Dagnelie PC *et al*. Effects of macrobiotic diets on linear growth in infants and children until 10 years of age. *Eur J Clin Nutr*, 1994, **48** S103–11.

25 Paul AA, Southgate DAT *McCance and Widdowson's The Composition of Foods*, 4th edn. London: The Stationery Office, 1978.

26 Health Education Authority *Nutrition in Minority Ethnic Groups: Asians and Afro-Caribbeans in the United Kingdom*. London: HEA, 1991.

27 *Weaning*: an information pack for those working with Asian communities. Bolton, Lancs: Bolton Health Authority Health Promotion Service, 1989.

28 Price SR Observations on dietary practices in India. *Hum Nutr: Appl Nutr*, 1984, **38A**, 383–9.

29 Thomas B (ed.) In: Cultural minorities. *Manual of Dietetic Practice*. Oxford: Blackwell Science, 1988, pp. 307–12.

30 Hunt S Traditional Asian food customs. *J Hum Nutr*, 1977, **31** 245–8.

31 Holland B *et al*. *McCance and Widdowson's The Composition of Foods*, 5th edn. London: Royal Society of Chemistry/MAFF, 1991.

32 Tan SP, Wenlock RW, Buss DH *Immigrant Foods*. The Second Supplement to *McCance and Widdowson's The Composition of Foods*. London: The Stationery Office, 1985.

33 Jaffrey M *Indian Cookery*. London: BBC Books, 1988.

34 Treuherz J, Cullinan TR, Saunders DI Determinants of infant feeding practice in East London. *Hum Nutr: Appl Nutr*, 1982, **36A** 281–6.

35 Warrington S, Storey DM Comparative studies on Asian and Caucasian children. 2: Nutrition, feeding practices and health. *Eur J Clin Nutr*, 1988, **42** 69–80.

36 Sahota P *Feeding Baby: Inner City Practice*. Bradford: Horton Publishing, 1991.

37 Goel KM, House F, Shanks RA Infant feeding practices among immigrants in Glasgow. *Brit Med J*, 1978, **2** 1181–3.

38 McNeill G Birth weight, feeding practice and weight/age of Punjabi children in the UK and in the rural Punjab. *Hum Nutr: Clin Nutr*, 1985, **39C** 69–72.

39 Evans N *et al*. Lack of breast feeding and early weaning in infants of Asian immigrants to Wolverhampton. *Arch Dis Childh*, 1978, **51** 608–12.

40 Thomas M, Avery V *Infant Feeding in Asian Families*. Office for National Statistics. London: The Stationery Office, 1997.

41 Jivani SKM The practice of infant feeding amongst Asian immigrants. *Arch Dis Childh*, 1978, **53** 66–73.

42 Jones VM Current weaning practices within the Bangladeshi community in the London Borough of Tower Hamlets. *Hum Nutr: Appl Nutr*, 1987, **41A** 349–52.

43 Alvear J, Brooke OG Foetal growth in different racial groups. *Arch Dis Childh*, 1978, **53** 27–32.

44 Parsons S *et al*. Are there intergenerational differences in the diets of young children born to first- and second-generation Pakistani Muslims in Bradford, West Yorkshire? *J Hum Nutr Diet*, 1999, **12** 113–22.

45 Warrington S, Storey DM Comparative studies on Asian and Caucasian children. 1: Growth. *Eur J Clin Nutr*, 1988, **42** 61–7.

46 Chetcuti P, Sinha SH, Levine MI Birth size in Indian subgroups born in Britain. *Arch Dis Childh*, 1985, **60** 868–70.

47 Duggan MB, Harbottle L The growth and nutritional status of healthy Asian children aged 4–40 months living in Sheffield. *Br J Nutr*, 1996, **76** 183–97.

48 Gatrad AR, Birch N, Hughes M Preschool weights and heights of Europeans and five subgroups of Asians in Britain. *Arch Dis Childh*, 1994, **71** 207–10.

49 Harris RJ *et al*. Nutritional survey of Bangladeshi children aged under 5 years in the London Borough of Tower Hamlets. *Arch Dis Childh*, 1983, **58** 428–32.

50 Rona R, Chinn S National study of health and growth: social and biological factors associated with height of children from ethnic groups living in England. *Ann Hum Biol*, 1986, **13** 453–71.

51 Ehrhardt P Iron deficiency anaemia in young Bradford children from different ethnic groups. *Brit Med J*, 1986, **292** 90–93.

52 Hunt S *The Habits of Asian Immigrants*. Burgess Hill, West Sussex: Van der Berghs and Jurgens, 1975, pp. 40–41.

53 Lawson MS, Thomas M, Hardiman A Iron status of Asian children aged 2 years living in England. *Arch Dis Childh*, 1998, **78** 420–26.

54 Chanarin I *et al*. Megaloblastic anaemia in a vegetarian Hindu community. *Lancet*, 1985, **2** (8465) 1168–72.

55 Hunt SP *et al*. Vitamin D status in different subgroups of British Asians. *Brit Med J*, 1976, **2** 1351–4.

56 Goel KM *et al*. Reduced prevalence of rickets in Asian children in Glasgow. *Lancet*, 1985, **ii** 405–407.

57 Dunnigan MG *et al*. Prevention of rickets in Asian children: assessment of the Glasgow campaign. *Brit Med J*, 1985, **291** 239–42.

58 Lawson MS, Thomas M, Hardiman A Dietary and lifestyle factors affecting plasma vitamin D levels in Asian children living in England. *Eur J Clin Nutr*, 1999, **53** (4) 268–72.

59 Lawson M, Thomas M Vitamin D concentrations in Asian children aged 2 years living in England: population survey. *Brit Med J*, 1999, **318** 28.

60 Iqbal SJ *et al*. Continuing clinically severe vitamin D deficiency in Asians in the UK (Leicester). *Postgrad Med J*, 1994, **70** (828) 708–14.

61 Department of Health. *Nutrition and Bone Health: With particular reference to calcium and vitamin D*. Report on Health and Social Subjects 49. London: The Stationery Office, 1998.

62 Wharton BA Low plasma vitamin D in Asian toddlers in Britain. *Brit Med J*, 1999, **318** 2–3.

63 Holt RD *et al*. Caries in pre-school children in Camden 1993/94. *Br Dent J*, 1996, **181** 405–10.

64 Douglas J *Caribbean Food and Diet*. Cambridge: National Extension College for Training in Health and Race, 1987.

65 Kemm J, Douglas J, Sylvester V Afro-Caribbean diet survey interim report to the Birmingham inner city partnership programme. *Proc Nutr Soc*, 1986, **45** (3) 87A.

66 Kemm J, Douglas J, Sylvester V A survey of infant feeding practice by Afro-Caribbean mothers in Birmingham. *Proc Nutr Soc*, 1986, **45** 87A.

67 Holland B, Unwin ID, Buss DH *Vegetables, herbs and spices*. The fifth supplement to *McCance & Widdowson's The Composition of Foods*, 4th edn. London: Royal Society of Chemistry/MAFF, 1991.

68 Springer L, Thomas J Rastafarians in Britain: a preliminary study of their food habits and beliefs. *Hum Nutr: Appl Nutr*, 1983, **37A** 120–27.

69 James JA, Clark C, Ward PS Screening Rastafarian children for nutritional rickets. *Brit Med J*, 1985, **290** 899–900.

70 Campbell M, Lofters WS, Gibbs WN Rastafarianism and the vegan syndrome. *Brit Med J*, 1982, **285** 1617–18.

71 Close GC Rastafarians and the vegan syndrome. *Brit Med J*, 1983, **286** 473.

72 Goodburn PC, Falshaw M, Hughes H *Chinese Food and Diet*. Cambridge: National Extension College for Training in Health and Race, 1987.

73 Fok D Breast feeding in Singapore. *Breast Feeding Rev*, 1977, **5** 25–8.

74 Leung S, Davies DP Infant feeding and growth of Chinese infants: birth to 2 years. *Paediatr Perinat Epidemiol*, 1994, **8** 301–13.

75 Xiang M, Lei S, Li T, Zetterstrom R Composition of long chain polyunsaturated fatty acids in human milk and growth of young infants in rural areas of northern China. *Acta Paediatr*, 1999, **88** (2) 126–31.

76 Carlson E, Kipps M, Thomson J An evaluation of a traditional Vietnamese diet in the UK. *Hum Nutr: Appl Nutr*, 1982, **36** 107–15.

77 Todd R, Gelbier S Dental caries prevalence in Vietnamese children and teenagers in three London Boroughs. *Br Dent J*, 1990, **168** 24–6.

78 Harrison R *et al*. Feeding practices and dental caries in an urban Canadian population of Vietnamese preschool children. *ASDC J Dent Child*, 1997, **64** 112–17.

79 Rossiter JC Promoting breast feeding: the perceptions of Vietnamese mothers in Sydney, Australia. *J Adv Nurs*, 1998, **28** 598–605.

80 Sharma A, Lynch MA, Irvine ML The availability of advice regarding infant feeding to immigrants of Vietnamese origin: a survey of families and health visitors. *Child Care Health Dev*, 1994, **20** 349–54.

Appendices

Manufacturers of Dietetic Products

A full list of drugs and their manufacturers appears in the *British National Formulary* (BNF), a joint publication of the British Medical Association and the Royal Pharmaceutical Society of Great Britain.

Abbott Laboratories Ltd
Abbott House, Norden Road, Maidenhead, Berkshire SL6 4XE

Baxter Healthcare Ltd
Caxton Way, Thetford, Norfolk IP24 3SE

Bio Diagnostics Ltd
Upton Industrial Estate, Rectory Road, Upton-under-Severn, Worcestershire WR8 0XL

The Boots Company PLC
1 Thane Road, Nottingham NG2 3AA

B Braun (Medical) Ltd
Brookdale Road, Thorncliffe Park Estate, Sheffield S35 2PW

Cadbury Ltd
PO Box 12, Bournville Lane, Bournville, Birmingham B30 2LU

Cow & Gate Nutricia Ltd
White Horse Business Park, Trowbridge, Wiltshire BA14 0XQ

Eastern Pharmaceuticals Ltd
Coomb House, 7 St Johns Road, Isleworth, Middlesex TW7 6NA

Farley
(See Heinz)

Fresenius Ltd
Melbury Park, Birchwood, Warrington WA3 6FF

Fresenius Kabi Ltd
Parenteral Nutrition Division, Davy Avenue, Knowlhill, Milton Keynes MK5 8PH

General Dietary Ltd
PO Box 28, Kingston upon Thames, Surrey KT2 7YP

Gluten Free Foods Ltd
Unit 10 Honeypot Business Park, Parr Road, Stanmore, Middlesex HA7 1NL

Heinz H J Co Ltd
Hayes Park, Hayes, Middlesex UB4 8AL

Mead Johnson Nutritionals
Division of Bristol-Myers Squibb Pharmaceuticals Ltd, 141–149 Staines Road, Hounslow, Middlesex TW3 3JA

Milupa Ltd
White Horse Business Park, Trowbridge, Wilts BA14 0XQ

Nestle Clinical Nutrition
St George's House, Croydon, Surrey CR9 1NR

Novartis Consumer Health
Wimblehurst Road, Horsham, West Sussex RH12 5AB

Nutricia Clinical Care
Nutricia Ltd, White Horse Business Park, Trowbridge, Wiltshire BA14 0XQ

Paines & Byrne Ltd
Yamanouchi House, Pyrford Road, West Byfleet, Surrey KT14 6RA

Rhone-Poulenc-Rorer Ltd
RPR House, 50 Kings Hill Avenue, Kings Hill, West Malling, Kent ME19 4AH

Searle
PO Box 53, Lane End Road, High Wycome, Bucks HP12 4HL

SHS International Ltd
100 Wavertree Boulevard, Wavertree Technology Park, Liverpool L7 9PT

SMA Nutrition
Huntercombe Lane South, Taplow, Maidenhead, Berks SL6 0PH

SmithKline Beecham Healthcare
SB House, Brentford, Middlesex TW8 9BD

Sutherland Health Ltd
Unit 1 Rivermead, Pipers Way, Thatcham, Berkshire RG19 4EP

UCB Pharma Ltd
Star House, 69 Clarendon Road, Watford, Herts WD1 1DJ

Ultrapharm Ltd
PO Box 18, Henley-on-Thames, Oxon RG9 2AW

Unigreg Ltd
Enterprise House, 181–189 Garth Road, Morden, Surrey SM4 4LL

Vitacare Ltd
Freepost 121, Enfield, Middlesex EN1 3BR

Vitaflo Ltd
11 Century Building, Brunswick Business Park, Liverpool L3 4BL

Warner Lambert Consumer Healthcare
Lambert Court, Chestnut Avenue, Eastleigh, Hants SO5 3ZQ

APPENDIX II

Dietetic Products

Abidec	Warner Lambert	Enfamil	Mead Johnson
Al 110	Nestle	Enfamil AR	Mead Johnson
Alfare	Nestle	Enfamil Lactofree	Mead Johnson
Aminex	Gluten Free Foods	Enfamilk breast milk fortifier	Mead Johnson
Aminogran Food Supplement	UCB Pharma	Enlive	Abbott
Aminogran Mineral Mixture	UCB Pharma	Enrich	Abbott
Analog LCP	SHS	Ensure Plus	Abbott
Aproten	Ultrapharm	Entera Fibre Plus	Fresenius
Aptamil Extra	Milupa	Eoprotin	Milupa
Aptamil First	Milupa	Essential Amino Acid Mix	SHS
Bi-Aglut	Novartis	Farley's First Milk	Farley/Heinz
Build-up	Nestle	Farley's Follow-on Milk	Farley/Heinz
Calogen	SHS	Farley's Second Milk	Farley/Heinz
Caloreen	Nestle	Farley's Soya Formula	Farley/Heinz
Calsip	Fresenius	Forceval	Unigreg
Caprilon	SHS	Formance	Abbott
Casilan 90	Heinz	Fortijuce	Nutricia
Clinutren 1.5	Nestle	Fortimel	Nutricia
Clinutren ISO	Nestle	Fortisip	Nutricia
Coffee-mate	Nestle	Fortisip Multifibre	Nutricia
Comminuted Chicken Meat	SHS	Forward Follow-on	Milupa
Complan	Heinz	Frebini	Fresenius
Complete Amino Acid Mix		Fresubin	Fresenius
(Code 124)	SHS	Fresubin Isofibre	Fresenius
Dalivit	Eastern	Fructose Formula	SHS
Dialamine	SHS	Galactomin 19	
Diocalm Junior	SmithKline	Galactomin 17	SHS
	Beecham	Generaid Plus	SHS
Dioralyte	Rhone-Poulenc-	Glycerol Trioleate Oil	SHS
	Rorer	Hypostop	Bio-Diagnostics
Duobar	SHS	Impact	Novartis
Duocal	SHS	InfaSoy	Cow & Gate
Electrolade	Eastern	Infatrini	Nutricia
Elemental 028	SHS	Instant Carobel	Cow & Gate
Elemental 028 Extra	SHS	Intralipid	Fresenius Kabi
Emsogen	SHS	Isomil	Abbott
Ener-G	General Dietary	Isosource Energy	Novartis
Energivit	SHS	Isosource Fibre	Novartis

Isosource Junior	Novartis	Nutrison Pepti	Nutricia
Isosource Standard	Novartis	Nutrison Standard	Nutricia
Jevity	Abbott	Omneo Comfort	Cow & Gate
Jevity Plus	Abbott	Oral Impact	Novartis
Juvela	SHS	Osmolite	Abbott
Kabimix II	Fresenius Kabi	Osterprem	Farley/Heinz
Ketovite	Paines & Byrne	Paediasure	Abbott
Kindergen PROD	SHS	Paediasure with Fibre	Abbott
Lipfundin	Braun	Paediatric Seravit	SHS
Liquigen	SHS	Paediatric Seravit (flavoured)	SHS
Locasol	SHS	Pepdite	SHS
Lofenalac	Mead Johnson	Pepdite 1$^+$	SHS
Loprofin	SHS	Peptide Module 767	SHS
Lorenzo's Oil	SHS	Pepti-Junior	Cow & Gate
Lucozade	SmithKline Beecham	Phlexy-10	SHS
Maxijul	SHS	PK Aid 4	SHS
Maxijul LE	SHS	PKU 2	Milupa
Maxijul Liquid	SHS	PKU 3	Milupa
Maxipro HBV	SHS	Plus	Cow & Gate
MCT Duocal	SHS	Polycal	Nutricia
MCT Pepdite 0–2	SHS	Polycal Liquid	Nutricia
MCT Pepdite 2+	SHS	Polycose	Abbott
Metabolic Mineral Mixture	SHS	Pregestimil	Mead Johnson
Milumil	Milupa	Prejomin	Milupa
Modulen IBD	Nestle	Prematil	Milupa
Monogen	SHS	Premcare	Farley/Heinz
MSUD Aid III	SHS	Premium	Cow & Gate
MSUD Analog	SHS	Primene	Nestle
MSUD Maxamaid	SHS	Progress	SMA Nutrition
MSUD Maxamum	SHS	ProMod	Abbott
Nanny	Vitacare	ProSobee	Mead Johnson
Neocate	SHS	Protein Forte	Fresenius
Neocate Advance	SHS	Protein-free diet powder	Mead Johnson
Nepro	Abbott	(80056)	
Nesquik	Nestle	Protifar	Nutricia
Nestargel	Nestle	Provide Xtra	Fresenius
Novasource Forte	Novartis	Pulmocare	Abbott
Novasource GI Control	Novartis	Rehidrat	Searle
Novasource Junior	Novartis	Resource	Novartis
Novasource Peptide	Novartis	Resource Benefiber	Novartis
Novasource Start	Novartis	Resource Dessert Energy	Novartis
Nutralis	Nutricia	Resource Fibre	Novartis
Nutramigen	Mead Johnson	Resource Junior	Novartis
Nutrini	Nutricia	Resource Protein Extra	Novartis
Nutrini Extra	Nutricia	Resource Shake	Novartis
Nutrini Fibre	Nutricia	Resource Thickened Drink	Novartis
Nutriprem	Cow & Gate	Resource Thickened Squash	Novartis
Nutriprem breast milk	Cow & Gate	Resource Thicken Up	Novartis
fortifier		Rite-Diet	Nutricia
Nutrison Energy Plus	Nutricia	Scandishake	SHS
Nutrison MCT	Nutricia	Seravit	SHS

SMA breast milk fortifier	SMA Nutrition	XMet Analog	SHS
SMA Gold	SMA Nutrition	XMet Maxamaid	SHS
SMA High Energy	SMA Nutrition	XMet Maxamum	SHS
SMA Lactofree	SMA Nutrition	XMTVI Amino Acid Mix	SHS
SMA Low Birthweight	SMA Nutrition	XMTVI Analog	SHS
SMA White	SMA Nutrition	XMTVI Maxamaid	SHS
Sno Pro	SHS	XMTVI Maxamum	SHS
Step-Up	Cow & Gate	XP Analog	SHS
Suplena	Abbott	XP Maxamaid	SHS
Thick & Easy	Fresenius	XP Maxamaid Bar	SHS
Thixo-D	Sutherland	XP Maxamum	SHS
Ultra	Ultrapharm	XPhen, Tyr Analog	SHS
Valpiform	General Dietary	XPhen, Tyr, Met Analog	SHS
Vaminolact	Fresenius Kabi	XPhen, Tyr Maxamaid	SHS
VibreCal	Vitaflo	XPhen, Tyr Maxamum	SHS
Vitajoule	Vitaflo	XPhen, Tyr, Met Maxamaid	SHS
Vitapro	Vitaflo	XPhen, Tyr, Met Maxamum	SHS
Vitaquick	Vitaflo	XPT Tyrosidon	SHS
Wysoy	SMA Nutrition	XPTM Tyrosidon	SHS
XMet Amino Acid Mix	SHS		

Index